MAJOR'S

PHYSICAL DIAGNOSIS

Eighth Edition

Edited by

MAHLON H. DELP, M.D.

Peter T. Bohan Professor of Medicine, Emeritus
The University of Kansas School of Medicine,
Kansas City, Kansas

and

ROBERT T. MANNING, M.D.

Professor of Medicine and Associate Professor
of Biochemistry
Eastern Virginia Medical School
Norfolk, Virginia

W. B. SAUNDERS COMPANY

Philadelphia • London • Toronto

W. B. Saunders Company: West Washington Square
Philadelphia, Pa. 19105

1 St. Anne's Road
Eastbourne, East Sussex BN21 3UN, England

833 Oxford Street
Toronto, M8Z 5T9, Canada

Library of Congress Cataloging in Publication Data

Major, Ralph Hermon, 1884-
      Major's Physical diagnosis.

      Includes bibliographies and index.
   1. Physical diagnosis.   I. Delp, Mahlon, ed.   II. Manning, Robert T., ed.
[DNLM: 1. Diagnosis.   WB200 M234p]
RC76.M3   1975   616.07′54   74-9430
ISBN 0-7216-3012-X

Major's Physical Diagnosis   ISBN 0-7216-3012X

Last digit is the print number: 9   8   7   6   5   4

Contributors

ROBERT E. BOLINGER, M.D. Professor of Medicine; Director, Department of Endocrinology and Metabolism, University of Kansas School of Medicine, Kansas City, Kansas.
Examination of the Endocrine System

LARRY L. CALKINS, M.D. Former Clinical Professor of Ophthalmology, University of Kansas School of Medicine, Kansas City, Kansas.
Examination of the Eyes

MAHLON H. DELP, M.D. Emeritus Peter T. Bohan Professor of Medicine, University of Kansas School of Medicine, Kansas City, Kansas.
The Clinical Process

MARVIN I. DUNN, M.D. Professor of Medicine, University of Kansas School of Medicine, Kansas City, Kansas.
The Cardiovascular System

STANLEY R. FRIESEN, M.D., Ph.D. Professor of Surgery, University of Kansas School of Medicine, Kansas City, Kansas.
Consultant, Veterans Administration Hospital, Kansas City, Missouri.
Examination of the Abdomen

ROBERT P. HUDSON, M.D. Associate Professor and Chairman, Department of History and Philosophy of Medicine, University of Kansas School of Medicine, Kansas City, Kansas.
Perspectives

C. FREDERICK KITTLE, M.D. Professor of Surgery, Rush Medical College. Senior Staff, Rush–Presbyterian–St. Luke's Medical Center, Chicago, Illinois.
Examination of the Breast

KERMIT E. KRANTZ, M.D. Professor of Anatomy and Obstetrics and Gynecology, University of Kansas School of Medicine, Kansas City, Kansas.
Examination of the Female Genitalia

ROBERT T. MANNING, M.D. Professor of Medicine and Associate Professor of Biochemistry, Eastern Virginia Medical School, Norfolk, Virginia.
The Clinical Process

HERBERT C. MILLER, M.D. Professor of Pediatrics, University of Kansas School of Medicine, Kansas City, Kansas.
Pediatric Examination

LEONARD F. PELTIER, M.D., Ph.D. Professor of Surgery; Head, Section of Orthopedic Surgery, The University of Arizona College of Medicine, Tucson, Arizona.
Examination of the Back and Extremities

G. O'NEIL PROUD, M.D. Professor and Chairman, Department of Otorhinolaryngology, University of Kansas School of Medicine, Kansas City, Kansas.
General Principles of the Ear, Nose, and Throat Examination

DAVID W. ROBINSON, M.D. Distinguished Professor of Plastic Surgery, University of Kansas School of Medicine, Kansas City, Kansas.
Examination of the Head and Neck

WILLIAM E. RUTH, M.D. Professor of Medicine, University of Kansas School of Medicine. Vice-Chairman for Medicine and Director, Division for Pulmonary Disease, Kansas University Medical Center, Kansas City, Kansas.
Examination of the Chest, Lungs, and Pulmonary System

GORDON C. SAUER, M.D. Clinical Professor of Medicine (Dermatology), University of Kansas School of Medicine, Kansas City, Kansas. Attending Dermatologist, Kansas City General Hospital, St. Luke's Hospital, and Research Hospital, Kansas City, Missouri.
Examination of the Skin

WILLIAM L. VALK, M.D. Professor of Surgery Emeritus, University of Kansas School of Medicine, Kansas City, Kansas.
Examination of the Male Genitalia and Rectum

SLOAN J. WILSON, M.D. Professor of Medicine, University of Kansas School of Medicine, Kansas City, Kansas.
Examination of the Hemic and Lymphatic Systems

DEWEY K. ZIEGLER, M.D. Professor, Department of Neurology, University of Kansas School of Medicine, Kansas City, Kansas. Osawatomie State Hospital, Osawatomie, Kansas, Kansas City General Hospital and Veterans Administration Hospital, Kansas City, Missouri.
Examination of the Nervous System

Preface

Major's Physical Diagnosis continues its traditional function as a textbook of physical diagnosis. Modifications are in keeping with this comment Dr. Major made in the preface to the fourth edition: "While the fundamental facts of physical diagnosis are as true today as they were in the days of Auenbrugger, Laennec, and Skoda, new facts and new interpretations have made their importance obvious, as our understanding of physiology, both normal and abnormal, has deepened our knowledge of disease and of the changes it produces in the human body." This philosophy has resulted in perpetual, gradual change over the 37-year life of the book. Significant changes dealing with various body systems were made in the eighth edition. This revision gives early attention to aims and goals of the book. We believe students at any level learn more readily and more certainly if they are initially provided with objectives of the exercise. It is hoped this effort renders study of the text more meaningful.

With the death of Dr. Major a new contributor, Dr. Robert Hudson, has revised the chapter on the History of Physical Diagnosis. Dr. David Robinson, distinguished professor of plastic surgery, has revised the section on the Head and Neck. All chapters have been revised and a reordering of the chapter sequence has been accomplished. This rearrangement has been a deliberate attempt to introduce the student to the total patient as quickly as possible in his move from basic science to the clinical environment. Early requirements are for presentation of an overview of the patient and those procedures of physical examination required to complete the study of even the first patient encountered. Dr. Richard E. Davis has been instrumental in assisting the editors in weaving into the text an understanding and awareness of the human, personal aspects of history taking and physical examinations.

In this edition, the basic steps and logic utilized in data analysis and diagnostic synthesis are again analyzed. Here the process rather than the conclusion is accented. We believe that when teachers of clinical medicine ignore description and discussion of the intellectual processes involved in making a diagnosis they perpetuate the myth and mystique of clinical acumen and thus encourage careless skip-step practices. The completed diagnosis, often likened to a finished picture, reveals a complex structure of many essential details. The clinical syndrome may thus be viewed as a vignette, less detailed, less complex, but serving as an excellent instrument to illustrate the process of diagnosis. Each chapter dealing with the body systems is followed by a listing of related clinical syndromes.

Medical school curriculum changes involving abbreviated schedules, early patient contact, and emphasis upon illness and its social aspects, rather than exclusive preoccupation with disease alone, highlight the need for more appropriate student guidance. In parallel with the ferment in curriculum has come renewed interest in improved methods of collecting and recording information from the patient. In real sympathy with these ideas, the editors incorporate in this edition the concepts of the structured history and problem-oriented record.

Satisfactory medical communication requires a common vocabulary. A beginning in this area is made during basic science instruction, but clinical conversation does not mature until the student is introduced to clinical medicine in physical diagnosis and clerkships. In an effort to assist with this goal, each chapter dealing with the various systems is followed by a selected list of common clinical terms.

Finally, the change in the physical format of the book reflects our desire that the reader use it as a readily accessible reference as he sees patients—not only his first ones but also those who pose a diagnostic challenge as he gains more experience as a clinician. Two publications appearing in 1969, *The Clinical Approach to the Patient* by Morgan and Engel, and *Medical*

Records, Medical Education and Patient Care by Weed, should have tremendous impact upon clinical learning, understanding, and patient care. No text dealing with physical diagnosis can disregard these contributions. The editors have drawn upon these sources extensively, and other excellent texts, particularly those of McBryde and Blacklow, Harvey and Bordley, Judge and Zuidema, and DeGowin and DeGowin, have been very useful.

MAHLON H. DELP

ROBERT T. MANNING

Contents

1

PERSPECTIVES 1
Robert P. Hudson

2

THE CLINICAL PROCESS 20
Robert T. Manning and Mahlon H. Delp

Introduction to Clinical Medicine 20
    Approach to the Patient 24
    Study of the Patient 26
    Physical Examination 46
The Diagnostic Process 54
    Diagnosis by Method of Hypotheses 55
    A Formal Diagnostic Logic 57
    The Medical Record 72

3

EXAMINATION OF THE SKIN 88
Gordon C. Sauer

Examination of the Skin 92
Primary, Secondary, and Special Skin Lesions 95
    Primary Lesions 95

xi

Secondary Lesions 108
Special Lesions 112

4

EXAMINATION OF THE NERVOUS SYSTEM 118

Dewey K. Ziegler

Behavior and Consciousness 119
Higher Functions 123
    Spontaneous Speech 124
    Further Testing of the Patient for
        Aphasia and Apraxia 127
    Other Tests of Higher Functions...................... 129
    Judgment and Abstraction Ability 130
Motor Function 131
Reflex Examination 142
Sensory Examination 149
    Test Objects and Testing Techniques 150
    Discriminatory Sensation.............................. 152
    Patterns of Sensory Dysfunction 154
Cranial Nerves... 159
Ancillary Examinations of the Nervous System 170

5

EXAMINATION OF THE HEAD AND NECK 175

David W. Robinson

The Head 175
    Face.. 179
    Facial Bones... 189
    Hair 190
    Lips.. 191
    Teeth and Gums... 196
    Tongue 202

Breath 209
Buccal Cavity 210
The Neck 212

6

GENERAL PRINCIPLES OF THE EAR, NOSE,
AND THROAT EXAMINATION 230

G. O'Neil Proud

The Ear 230
The Nose 236
The Pharynx and Larynx 240

7

EXAMINATION OF THE EYES 242

Larry Calkins

Appraisal of the Visual Acuity 242
Examination of the Ocular Media 245
The Fundus Examination 252
The Pupillary Reflex 255
External Examination 257
Diseases of the Eye 270

8

EXAMINATION OF THE CHEST, LUNGS,
AND PULMONARY SYSTEM 301

William E. Ruth

Topographical Anatomy 301
History 304
General Evaluation 305
Examination of the Chest 311
Inspection 312

Palpation.. 320
Percussion of the Chest................................ 325
Auscultation 334

9

THE CARDIOVASCULAR SYSTEM 358

Marvin I. Dunn

The Heart.. 358
Inspection, Palpation, and Percussion
    of the Heart... 359
Blood Pressure and Pulse.................................... 384
    Blood Pressure 384
    The Pulse 390
Auscultation of the Heart 413
    Sound and Hearing 415
    Listening to the Heart.................................. 416
    The Heart Sounds.. 420
    Gallop Rhythms 432
    Friction Sounds.. 433
    Cardiac Murmurs 434
    Systolic Murmurs 439
    Diastolic Murmurs....................................... 444
    Functional Murmurs 456
    Auscultation of Blood Vessels......................... 459
Physical Findings in Cardiovascular Disease 460
    Pericarditis.. 460
    Arteriosclerotic Heart Disease 466
    Hypertensive Heart Disease........................... 470
    Cor Pulmonale 471
    Myocarditis and Myocardial Disease 473
    Heart Failure 474
    Chronic Valvular Heart Disease....................... 475
    Endocarditis 482

Congenital Heart Disease 484
The Electrocardiogram................................. 491
The X-Ray in the Diagnosis of
    Cardiac Disease....................................... 492
Peripheral Vascular Disease 493
    History 493
    Physical Examination..................................... 495
    Diseases of the Lymphatic System 498
    Diseases of the Veins.................................... 500
    Diseases of the Arteries................................ 502
    Aneurysm 506

10

EXAMINATION OF THE BREAST.............................. 517

C. Frederick Kittle

History of the Patient... 518
Examination of the Patient.................................... 519
Breast Cancer... 532
Intraductal Papilloma 535
Paget's Disease of the Breast 535
Fibroadenoma... 537
Cystic Disease of the Breast 538
Breast Hypertrophy 538
Breast Infections... 541
Traumatic Fat Necrosis.. 543

11

EXAMINATION OF THE ABDOMEN 548

Stanley R. Friesen

Inspection 550
Palpation.. 566
Percussion.. 582

Auscultation 584
Physical Findings and Diagnostic Probabilities....... 585

12

EXAMINATION OF THE MALE GENITALIA
AND RECTUM... 590
William L. Valk

Inguinal Area.. 590
Genitalia 591
Rectal Examination 601

13

EXAMINATION OF THE FEMALE GENITALIA 605
Kermit E. Krantz

Patient's History 605
Pelvic Examination 607
Speculum Examination.. 617
    The Vagina... 622
    The Cervix 623
Bimanual Examination 628
Preventive Medicine 635

14

EXAMINATION OF THE BACK AND
EXTREMITIES 637
Leonard F. Peltier

General Inspection... 638
Gait and Stance.. 639
Joint Motion 640
Examination of Muscles....................................... 645

Examination of the Cervical Spine 647
Examination of the Back 649
Examination of the Shoulder 657
Examination of the Elbow 662
Examination of the Wrist 664
Examination of the Hand 666
Examination of the Hip and Lower Extremities 673
    The Hip 673
    The Knee 681
    The Leg 687
    Ankle and Foot 689

15

EXAMINATION OF THE ENDOCRINE SYSTEM 700
    Robert E. Bolinger

    The Thyroid Gland 700
    The Parathyroid Glands 706
    The Adrenal Cortex 708
    The Adrenal Medulla 712
    The Pancreas 713
    The Gonads 715
    The Pituitary Gland 717
    Miscellaneous Syndromes 721

16

EXAMINATION OF THE HEMIC AND
LYMPHATIC SYSTEMS 724
    Sloan J. Wilson

    General Inspection 724
    The Skin 727
    The Mouth 732

The Eyes 733
The Chest.. 733
The Extremities 734
The Lymph Nodes... 734
The Abdomen, Liver, and Spleen............................ 737
Bones and Joints 737
Neurological Examination...................................... 739

17

PEDIATRIC EXAMINATION 742

Herbert C. Miller

Anthropometric Measurements............................. 745
The Newborn 745

INDEX... 761

1
PERSPECTIVES

For the beginning physician, physical diagnosis is the bridge between the study of disease and the management of illness. Making a distinction between disease and illness may strike some students as strange, and indeed the two words frequently appear as synonyms. But there are important reasons to conceive them differently.

In pathology you study disease; in clinical training you work with illness. In making this transition you will need to remind yourself that diseases, as defined in pathology, do not exist in reality; they are abstractions, albeit useful ones. Tuberculosis, for instance, is defined variously by basic scientists. The microbiologist emphasizes the staining qualities of the tubercle bacillus and its fastidious eating habits on culture media. The pathologist speaks of a tissue reaction featuring caseous necrosis and Langhans' giant cells. It is convenient and even necessary to begin the study of tuberculosis in these terms.

But tuberculosis—the illness—is more. It is the totality of signs (objective findings) and symptoms (subjective feelings) that together characterize a *single patient's* response to infection by the tubercle bacillus. Tuberculosis the illness is the *patient's* reaction, not merely his tissue reaction. Each such illness is a unique event in the history of man. It happens to a single individual over a restricted period of time and will never happen again in precisely the same way. Disease, then, is an abstraction; illness, a process.

Ideally, the physician will think in terms of both disease and illness, but our educational process makes such a proper balance difficult to come by. Medical teaching is compartmentalized in ways that have little to do with what the physician does in practice. Indeed, the educational separation of disease and illness creates obstacles in this regard which can be overcome only by conscious effort.

Students who never conceptualize the distinction between disease and illness will make one of two errors, neither of which has much to recommend it over the other. The first is to mistake the disease for reality, the second is not to see the illness at all. The first error leads to what might be termed cookbook medicine, a rigid pseudoscience which is usually more comforting to physicians than to patients. A blood pressure reading of 150/95 becomes a disease rather than a sign of possible illness. If no other cause can be found the patient is given a disease label, essential hypertension, and the recipe for this label calls for, among other things, a diet low in salt. Never mind that the patient is eighty-four years old and that his chief remaining joys in life are his daily trips to the festive board. The physician who has a balanced view of *disease and illness* will see the elevated blood pressure as only a sign of disease, not the thing itself. Whether he recommends salt restriction will depend on many factors peculiar to this particular patient, including, one hopes, the patient's own estimate of the value of a few more weeks of life achieved at the expense of tasteless food.

There are equal dangers in thinking only in terms of illness. There is indisputable merit in understanding the total social and psychological forces impinging on the patient, but this alone is not enough. It does no good to discover that a patient will have trouble affording his antihypertensive medication if the physician overlooked obvious physical findings indicating that the hypertension was secondary to a tumor of the adrenal gland. To put it another way, the patient may want a physician who is expert at managing a terminal illness, but not one whose ignorance of disease unduly hastens that end.

Both are needed, then—the science of understanding disease and the art of managing illness. The seasoned physician merges the two without thinking. But in the process of becoming a physician you will have to consciously identify the two and determine which is dominating your thinking at any given time. In making a diagnosis and assessing the objective findings as time passes you will call on your knowledge of disease. In deciding on management you will come to think largely in terms of illness, of the total impact the affliction is having on this particular human being and those close to him.

In a general way the history and the physical examination also share this disease-illness dichotomy. The patient's reaction to disease is mainly subjective and is reflected in the answers to the physician's questions, the history. He has little interest in such labels as tuberculosis. He wants only to be reassured that he will survive and that he has not infected his wife and child.

But disease leaves objective tracks as well. These may not be apparent to the patient, but it is the physician's job to seek them out. The method here is the physical examination and the tools are those of physical diagnosis. Traditionally, the process is divided into looking (inspection), feeling (palpation), tapping or thumping (percussion), and listening (auscultation). Our professional progenitors relied on smelling (the "mousy" odor of typhus fever) and tasting as well (the sweetness of diabetic urine), but these have diminished importance in modern Western medicine.

The potential of physical diagnosis did not begin to be realized until the early nineteenth century. This surprises many students, but then so does the fact that as recently as 100 years ago physicians did not know the cause of a single important human disease. There were complex reasons for this late appearance of understanding in medicine generally, but the principal reason related to the way physicians conceived of disease. During roughly the first half of written history, disease was viewed almost entirely as supernatural in origin. Disease was inflicted on man by the gods or through the medium of a shaman as punishment for sin or breaking a tribal taboo. In truth, this belief still dominates the thinking of much of the Earth's population today.

As long as man perceived disease as supernatural there was

by definition no need for anatomical or physiological understanding. It does not matter that pain is transmitted via the sciatic nerve if you believe that pain derives from a whimsical god and can be relieved only by divine intervention. Feeling no need to understand anatomy and pathology, early medicine men would perceive no need for physical diagnosis in our sense of the term. A radical change in thinking would have to precede any scientific approach to understanding disease.

"Always the Greeks," some scholar once muttered in a moment of understandable pique. And so it was with the first great conceptual leap in the history of medicine, the notion that disease was natural, not divine. By our standards the Greeks studied nature with both hands tied. They had but two tools, observation and rationalization. Their limited technology is exemplified by the clepsydra or water clock which could be used for counting the pulse. In their broad-ranging study of nature it is not surprising that the Greeks questioned why man sickened and died. It is nonetheless awesome that they concluded that disease was natural, because as the beginning medical student soon learns there is nothing at all obvious about the cause of disease. Consider epilepsy as one example. If any condition has the appearance of a blow from the gods it is the grand mal seizure of epilepsy. A vigorous chieftain, sitting at the fire glorying in the aftermath of a victorious battle, suddenly utters an eerie cry, drops to the ground in a frothing bone-jarring convulsion, loses control of bladder and bowels, and chews blood from his tongue. After a ten minute seizure he lapses into a deep sleep and awakens an hour later unable to recall the episode and suffering no apparent effects whatever. Who but the gods could produce such a mysterious and frightening display? Yet here is what a Greek writer had to say of epilepsy some four hundred years before Christ:

It is thus with regard to the disease called Sacred: It appears to me to be nowise more divine nor more sacred than other diseases, but has a natural cause from which it originates like other affections.

If disease was natural, reasoned the Greeks, it followed that it could be studied and its course predicted just as learned astronomers could forecast an eclipse. Their method of study was essentially the same as that used today in clinical medicine. The bedside study of disease is still sometimes called the Hippocratic method after the man we revere as the father of medicine. The Greeks' case descriptions were so accurate that with near certainty we can diagnose a number of them 2500 years later. The cases became part of the Hippocratic Corpus, a collection of some seventy surviving books. These volumes, along with others since lost, formed the nucleus of a library around which medicine became a profession in today's sense of the word.

Despite its greatness the Greek system contained a flaw that was bound to limit the development of physical diagnosis. In keeping with their holistic philosophy, the Greeks theorized that all disease had a single cause, an imbalance of the fluid portions of the body, more specifically the Four Humours: yellow bile, black bile, blood, and phlegm. At first glance the Doctrine of the Four Humours, or humoral pathology as it came to be called, would appear hostile to advances in physical diagnosis. Why search for or assign any importance to localized signs if disease derives from an imbalance in the body's fluids as a whole? As a matter of fact, there is nothing inherently contradictory in using localized changes to reveal the nature of the imbalance in the Four Humours. There is no reason why a disease might not originate generally and still have localized manifestations, just as we now agree that diseases arise locally, but may have generalized manifestations. Thus, paradoxically, while the Greeks did not think in terms of specific diseases, they observed and recorded physical findings so precisely that any senior medical student easily assigns them specific disease names.

Still the conception of disease as generalized discouraged the development of anatomy and pathology almost as surely as the idea that disease is supernatural. If disease resulted from an imbalance of the Four Humours and could be treated only by restoring the previous balance, there was no incentive to determine the relationship between, say, the kidney, the ureters, and the bladder. Accordingly, the Hippocratics developed little knowledge of anatomy and pathology, the two sciences that are the sine qua non of physical diagnosis.

The Doctrine of the Four Humours developed slowly over some eight centuries and was pulled together in so convincing a fashion by Galen (A.D. 130–188) that humoral pathology dominated medical thinking for some 1500 years. During this time the artful science of physical diagnosis could make little real progress. For physicians of the Middle Ages and Renaissance, diagnosis centered around astrology, a complicated and fanciful pulse lore, and uroscopy, in which disease was diagnosed by careful observation of a flask of urine, at times with the patient not even present.

To reiterate, medical men could not begin thinking in terms of localized disease until they had a sound knowledge of anatomy and were in the habit of thinking anatomically. Though he made many genuine contributions, the anatomy Galen passed to his successors was not based on human dissection. It was replete with such errors as the pores he had to postulate in the septum of the heart to make possible his erroneous notion of the movement of the blood.

During the Renaissance a number of factors conjoined to revive medical interest in anatomy and physiology. The spirit of the time—*Zeitgeist* the Germans call it—favored the launching of that epochal event we call the scientific revolution. The origins of this momentous movement cannot be reviewed here. For our purposes we need only note that the biological sciences were swept up in the scientific revolution, though they lagged behind accomplishments in physics, mathematics, and astronomy.

Human anatomy was brought to the level of a science at this time by the work of Andreas Vesalius (1514–1564), the first truly great medical scientist after Galen. Vesalius was German by blood, though Flemish born. He studied medicine first in Paris, and then, because of war, fled to Padua in Italy. There he completed his medical degree, and immediately was appointed to direct anatomy and surgery at the University of Padua. At the time he was only twenty-three and he soon put his youthful brashness to good purpose by writing an entirely new anatomy rather than simply issuing a new version of Galen as his publisher wished. *De Humani Corporis Fabrica Libri Septem,* or the *Fabrica* as it came to be called, appeared in 1543. In preparing his book, Vesalius departed a long medieval tradition and did his own dissecting. Prior to this the learned anatomy professors had limited themselves to sitting perched above the cadaver reading from Galen while an assistant did the dissecting and tried to square what he saw in the cadaver with what Galen said should be there. Though there were occasional lapses, the merit of looking for oneself—direct experimentation—was never lost on medical men after Vesalius.

Others had dissected before, but not with the genius of Vesalius. Garrison struck the mark when he said that Vesalius "alone made anatomy what it is today—a living, working science." William Osler called the *Fabrica* the "greatest book ever written, from which modern medicine dates." Strong words, but less so when one traces the effects of an accurate anatomy to what we now see as one of the most fruitful notions in the history of medicine, the *anatomical idea.*

The anatomical idea, of itself, has an almost naive ring to the modern medical ear. In essence it says nothing more than that the human body is composed of anatomical units. Defined in this way, today's student not only wonders why the idea was so long taking hold, but may even have trouble seeing what all the fuss is about. The fuss relates not so much to the idea itself, but to the almost inescapable extensions that derive from anatomical thinking. If the body is composed of definite structures having certain relationships to one another, it follows that understanding the functions of these structures may be enhanced by noting their anatomical relationships. Galen himself had taken this lead many times with brilliant success, for instance, when he tied off the ureters and proved that urine was formed in the kidneys rather than settling in the bladder by a sort of condensation. But the method died with Galen's overwhelming bequest of humoral pathology. Vesalius himself was quick to revive the idea that function is dependent on structure, devoting the last chapter of the *Fabrica* to physiological experimentation. But there was a difference with Vesalius; now the anatomy was accurate.

The spread of anatomical thinking did not stop at physiology. If normal structures related to normal function, was it not possible that altered structure could determine signs and symptoms of disease? If true, the anatomical idea could lead on to gross pathology and physical diagnosis. What was lacking at this point was autopsy experience. After Vesalius, dissection became increasingly commonplace, at first motivated by an irate desire on the part of ardent Galenists to prove Vesalius wrong. But a dissection is not always an anatomical investigation any more than it is necessarily an autopsy. The man with the scalpel takes away from dissection largely what he goes after, and in Renaissance dissection the goal was normal anatomy and its variations. Autopsy experience accumulated slowly and in the eighteenth century a man came on the scene who transcended previous "pathologists" as much as Vesalius had towered above his predecessors. He was Giovanni Battista Morgagni (1682–1771), who worked for 50 years before publishing his magnum opus, a studied caution that would not carry him very far up today's academic ladder. Morgagni's labor consisted of a systematic compilation of what we now term clinical-pathological correlations. The first step was a careful notation of the signs and symptoms his patients exhibited in life. The key second phase took place at the autopsy table where he related the pathological findings to his ante mortem observations.

From these efforts Morgagni reached a monumental conclusion. Disease was not generalized in origin as physicians had believed for more than 2000 years. Rather, it arose in the organs; it was localized in origin. Morgagni published his conclusions in 1761 in a book entitled *On the Seats and Causes of Disease.* In so doing he initiated perhaps the single most fruitful movement in man's understanding of disease, the process of localizing disease at ever finer levels. After Morgagni, the Frenchman Xavier Bichat (1800) fixed the origin of disease in the tissues. Rudolph Virchow (1858) extended the idea to the level of the cell. The process continues in present concepts of subcellular pathology and the end is not in sight.

What has all this to do with physical diagnosis? For the moment it is better to ask what good Morgagni's discovery was to practicing physicians. The answer is that it was all but valueless.

Humoral pathology remained firmly entrenched and, in any event, what difference did it make if disease was localized in an organ? The vital organs, those in which disease produced significant morbidity or mortality, were not accessible to the physician's senses. The brain, heart, lungs, liver, and spleen were encased in bony boxes generally beyond the reach of inspection or palpation. It is true that a careful follower of Morgagni's method might have been better able to interpret the patient's symptoms, what the disease did to him subjectively, but that was imperfect help. Tools were needed to provide objective evidence, methods that would bring the vital but inaccessible organs into contact with the physician's senses.

The first such tool came at the hands of Leopold Auenbrugger (1722–1809), the son of an Austrian innkeeper, an occupational fact that is not without significance to our story. In 1761 Auenbrugger published a tiny volume called *Inventum Novum.* His "new invention" was the diagnostic tool we call percussion.

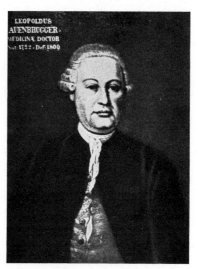

Figure 1–1. Leopold Auenbrugger.

Percussion depends on the physical fact that sounds produced by tapping over hollow structures differ from those over a solid. The sound that results from tapping over normal, air-filled lung is drumlike, and Auenbrugger used precisely this analogy in his book. Even to the uninitiated such a sound is distinctly different from the percussion note over a lung turned solid by pneumonia or one in which fluid is interposed between the percussing finger and underlying aerated lung tissue.

It is often said that Auenbrugger conceived percussion by recalling how his father slapped the sides of wine kegs to determine the level of that ancient ferment Galileo described as "Moisture held together by fire." This story gains credence from Auenbrugger's words in the third observation in *Inventum Novum*:

These variations depend on the cause which can diminish or increase the volume of air commonly in the thoracic cavity.

Such a cause whether it be in a solid or a liquid mass produces what we observe for example in casks, which, when they are empty, resound at all points; but, when filled, lose just so much of this resonance as the volume of air which they contain has been diminished.

To the novice, percussion seems a crude and awkward exercise, and he is likely to wonder if it can ever be more. At this point he is well advised to recall his first kiss with malice aforethought, and how rapidly he improved with practice. The method can be remarkably productive in seasoned hands. Lacking the eye of the x-ray, some nineteenth century physicians became incredibly expert at the art of percussion. Necessity is the mother of perfection as well as invention.

We have seen then that two great medical books appeared in the same year, 1761. They were, in the words of historian Henry Sigerist, " . . . expressions of an identical movement, expressions of the advancing anatomical idea. Morgagni laid the foundations of pathological anatomy, and Auenbrugger laid the foundations of anatomical diagnosis."

The two books shared another feature. As it had with Morgagni's before him, Auenbrugger's idea fell on barren ground. In the late eighteenth century Galen's humoral pathology, now dressed up a bit, continued to dominate men's thinking about disease. It was a chicken-and-egg situation. The idea of localized disease was not likely to catch on until its value to practicing physicians could be demonstrated by improved tools of physical diagnosis. Yet there could be no perceived need for new methods of physical diagnosis as long as disease was seen as a generalized imbalance of bile, phlegm, and blood. An impasse developed which lasted for more than a quarter of a century. It was not the first or only instance in medical history wherein time had to elapse before new truth could take hold.

By the turn of the nineteenth century the yeast of centuries finally stirred genuine ferment in medicine. The center of world medicine had shifted from Edinburgh to France, in part because French clinicians were the first to realize the potential in Morgagni's conception of localized disease and Auenbrugger's "new invention." What would come to fame as the "French clinical school" was based on an unprecedented marriage of physical diagnosis, the autopsy table, and the first sophisticated use of statistical methods. In the process of burying galenic pathology these brilliant French clinicians elevated physical diagnosis to the level of a science.

The key event in this climactic chapter took place around the turn of the century when a French physician, Jean Nicolas Corvisart (1755–1821), happened on a reference to Auenbrugger's still obscure *Inventum Novum.* Corvisart perceived the possible merit of percussion and set about testing it with the method that finally proved phenomenally fecund in the hands of French clinicians — percuss, record, test the conclusions at post mortem examination. After many painstaking exercises of this nature Corvisart was convinced. In 1808 he published the *Nouvelle Méthode pour reconnaître les Maladies internes.* In the preface Corvisart wrote,

I could have raised myself to the rank of author by revamping the work of Auenbrugger, and by publishing a work on percussion. But by that, I should sacrifice the name of Auenbrugger to my own vanity. I have not wished that; it is he, it is his beautiful and rightful discovery (inventum novum, as he says justly) which I have wished to make live again.

The book at once popularized percussion and assured Auenbrugger's immortality. Corvisart was barely in time, for Auenbrugger died the following year.

Corvisart's talent and fame attracted a number of gifted students. Chief among them was a slight young man who was born in Quimpier in 1781, René Théophile Hyacinthe Laennec. Under Corvisart's tutelage, Laennec was thoroughly indoctrinated in clinical-pathological correlation. In 1816 Laennec invented the stethoscope, the instrument that came to symbolize

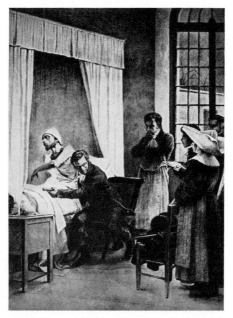

Figure 1-2. *Laennec examining a patient at the Necker Hospital.*

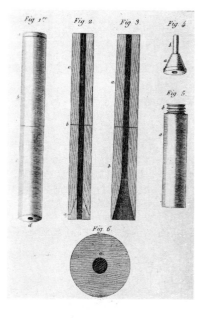

Figure 1–3. Laennec's stethoscope.

the bedside physician. As it had with Auenbrugger, chance and childhood played a role in Laennec's discovery. According to his friend Lejumeau de Kergaradec,

The author told me himself, the great discovery which has immortalized his name was due to chance . . . . One day walking in the court of the Louvre, he saw some children, who, with their ears glued to the two ends of some long pieces of wood which transmitted the sound of the little blows of the pins, struck at the opposite end. . . . He conceived instantly the thought of applying this to the study of diseases of the heart. On the morrow, at his clinic at the Necker Hospital, he took a sheet of paper, rolled it up, tied it with a string, making a central canal which he then placed on a diseased heart. This was the first stethoscope.

It should be noted that Laennec did not invent auscultation. The practice of listening to sounds in the patients by placing the ear directly on the chest, immediate auscultation, was known to ancient Greek physicians. Laennec himself called attention to relevant passages in the Hippocratic writings: "In hydrops of the lungs . . . if applying your ear against the chest, you listen for some time, *it boils within like vinegar*" (râles); and again, "when the lung falls against the ribs, the patient has a cough . . . he feels pain in his chest . . . a sound like that of leather is heard" (friction rub).

But immediate auscultation had serious limitations. The sounds were too soft and too diffuse, particularly in obese patients. After numerous experiments Laennec settled on wood as the best material for his stethoscope, usually ebony or cedar. For three feverish years (literally as well as figuratively, since he already exhibited signs of the tuberculosis that finally claimed him), Laennec tested his device in the crucible of clinical-pathological correlations. In 1819 he published his famous *De l'Auscultation Médiate.* Concerning this book, Major wrote:

> It was far more than a manual for the stethoscope. It was, also, a treatise on diseases of the lung and of the heart, a mine of information on the clinical aspects of pulmonary and cardiac disease, with an accurate description of the pathological anatomy of these conditions. Laennec heard with his stethoscope sounds never before heard or described and for which no terms existed in medical literature. He was the creator of a large number of words now currently employed in physical diagnosis, such as râles, bronchophony, pectoriloquy, and egophony. His book, unlike Auenbrugger's *Inventum Novum,* did not wait 47 years for recognition. It was immediately accepted as an epoch-making work, and auscultation was soon used in medical clinics throughout the world.

In full knowledge that his furious pace was shortening his life, Laennec produced a second edition of *De l'Auscultation Médiate* in 1826, then returned for the last time to his home in Brittany where he died on August 13 in the prime of middle age.

Even the most dedicated humoralists could not long hold out against the look-for-yourself evidence of Corvisart and Laennec. For the first time in living patients physicians could differentiate the dread tuberculosis from pneumonias, bronchiectasis, and other pulmonary afflictions. Laennec, as Brown

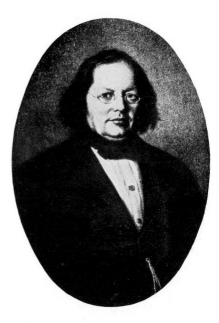

Figure 1-4. Josef Skoda.

said, "found phthisis pulmonalis a conglomeration of disease, pulmonary and general, and left it a clear-cut entity." In this way during the nineteenth century medical practice came to be dominated by the conception of localized disease made useful by new methods of physical diagnosis.

Thanks in part to another talented clinician, Josef Skoda, Vienna was destined to succeed Paris as the medical center of the world. Skoda consolidated the achievements of the French school and placed physical diagnosis on a firm scientific base, even to using the laws of physics to explain the findings of percussion and auscultation. He also possessed the quality that distinugishes the scientist from the zealot—he recognized the limitations of his methods. "Diseases which are entirely different," he said, "may show the same findings on percussion and auscultation and vice versa, the same disease may show a great variety of findings when we percuss or auscultate, because sound depends not upon the chemical but upon the anatomical state of the organs." It might be said that Laennec and Auenbrugger *cum* Corvisart established the methodology of physical diagnosis and Skoda perfected its philosophy. This he accomplished with the publication of *Abhandlung über Perkussion und Auskultation* in 1839, and with that book the essential history of physical diagnosis ends. The method had been proved and its limitations recognized. The basic goal remained unchanged — to make sensible the inaccessible. What was left was largely a matter of improving technology. To the stethoscope were added the laryngoscope, bronchoscope, ophthalmoscope, sigmoidoscope, and many others.

In the beginning the demand for improved tools of physical diagnosis was linked inseparably to extension of the notion that disease is localized. But as Skoda had recognized, there were limits to percussion and auscultation. As the seat of disease moved from organs to tissues and on to cells and subcellular structures, the limitations of physical diagnosis were not only apparent but intolerable. Physical diagnosis could help differentiate between tuberculosis and pneumonia, but not between uncomplicated infectious pneumonia and that caused by an early bronchial cancer. Further, certain important structures, such as the brain, pancreas, and kidneys, remained largely inaccessible to the most sophisticated application of physical diagnosis. Finally, it became clear that many serious human diseases produce changes in organs that cannot be felt, heard, or seen, e.g., diabetes mellitus and glomerulonephritis. Clearly something else was needed. That something was laboratory diagnosis, a story that can only be touched on here.

A convenient starting point is the period 1867 to 1869. During that time Adolph Kussmaul, who was professor of internal medicine at the University of Freiburg, inserted a stomach pump in treating acute gastric dilatation. Kussmaul quickly realized that the gastric contents so withdrawn might serve diagnostic as well as therapeutic purposes. Kussmaul's lead was taken up by Ottomar Rosenbach, who later substituted a flexible tube for the unwieldy stomach pump. Rosenbach's work led him to coin the term "ventricular insufficiency," by which he meant a disproportion between the muscular power of the stomach and the amount of work demanded of it. The term persists today principally with the heart, but Rosenbach's idea of studying the function of organs ushered in the whole study of the physical and chemical changes produced by disease — laboratory testing, which plays such a large part of diagnosis today.

In addition to chemical diagnosis the science of physics contributed such innovations as the x-ray, discovered by Wilhelm Röntgen in 1895, and the electrocardiogram, for which Willem Einthoven received the Nobel prize in 1924.

A few men had decried the mechanization they saw in interposing Laennec's stethoscope between the doctor and his patient. As chemistry and physics permitted increasingly earlier and more precise diagnoses in many diseases, some gloom-seers predicted the end altogether of traditional physical diagnosis. In truth, the phonocardiograph could time murmurs with a precision few clinicians could achieve, and the x-ray did outline the cardiac shadow better than percussion. But new technology is not a threat to existing diagnostic methods. The best tools will survive and the others should go. The historical problem more commonly has been one of overzealousness — of claiming more for a new method than the technique could deliver. Laennec's stethoscope is a case in point. Finding that certain heart murmurs correlated with autopsy findings of damaged heart valves, Laennec placed undue significance on the importance of blowing murmurs, many of which we now know are physiological rather than pathological. In his second edition Laennec corrected this error, in fact overcorrected it by concluding the *bruit de soufflet* (blowing murmur) had no significance whatever. Thus Laennec condemned himself, as Potain observed, to "a new error worse than the first." But Laennec's initial conclusion was widespread by this time, and an unknown but probably large number of cardiac neurotics were created because they had a harmless blowing murmur. Similar confusion took place in the early years of chest x-rays, as physicians pronounced dire diagnoses on the basis of normal hilar shadows produced by bronchi and blood vessels.

The most recent technological bugaboo is the suggestion that electronic computers will replace physicians in taking the patient's history. This is as unlikely as earlier fears proved to be. The reason is that computers necessarily deal in the cold literal aspect of words while physicians are trained to search for hidden meanings and to weigh the patient's responses in the total affective context. To the question, "Is your pain bothering you now?" the computer records "Yes" even when the patient is smiling broadly as he responds. The physician reads far more into such a "yes" than a simple affirmative response.

In many ways the computer is less efficient than an experienced physician. In localizing abdominal pain the computer may have to instruct the patient in the requisite anatomy, then ask a half-dozen questions. In two seconds the physician obtains more accurate information by having the patient put his finger on the origin of his pain. The computer's problem is even more unwieldy when the pain radiates through to the back as it can in pancreatic and gallbladder disease.

There is another and more important reason why the computer and other technology will not replace the physician in taking the history and performing the physical examination. It is erroneous to assume that the sole purpose of physical diagnosis is to gather facts. Obtaining data is an important part of this function, but by no means the only one. The history and physical examination frequently mark the first contact between patient and physician. It is the ideal time to initiate the friendly partnership which can decide whether the physician eventually will help his patient. Further, a significant amount of therapy takes place in this setting as well. The woman who finally finds someone who believes her story of backache and whose detailed questioning demonstrates that he truly cares for her and her problem is on the way to recovery long before the physician reaches for a prescription pad. Technology can never fill this function as well as a sympathetic and knowledgeable health professional.

This is not meant to deprecate the likes of computers. Computers have certain superior capacities and these should be utilized. They can screen piles of electrocardiograms without the mental fatigue man is heir to. Their superior memory can remind us of reasonable but obscure diagnostic possibilities, an important function as increasing world travel confronts the physician with disease entities which formerly were admired in pathology texts for their exotic names and then forgotten. There is no reason why computers should not be used for historical screening. But they can replace the physician only at the loss of something near the heart of whatever it is when human beings fall ill and turn to other human beings for help.

BIBLIOGRAPHY

Garrison, F. H.: History of Medicine. 4th ed. Philadelphia, W. B. Saunders Co., 1929.

Laennec, R. T. H.: De l'Auscultation Médiate. Paris, Brosson et Chaudé, 1819.

Laennec, R. T. H.: Traité de l'Auscultation Médiate. Paris, J. S. Chaudé, 1826.

Major, R. H.: Classic Descriptions of Disease. Springfield, Illinois, Charles C Thomas, 1932.

Skoda, J.: Abhandlung über Perkussion und Auskultation. Vienna, Mosle & Braumüller, 1839.

2
THE CLINICAL PROCESS

INTRODUCTION TO CLINICAL MEDICINE

The content of this section deals with matters belonging to "the art of medicine." As a logical first step in preparation for a career in health care, you study the biological science and then follow with the acquisition of new attitudes, skills, and knowledge that extend your capabilities beyond an understanding of biological systems and disease processes. Finally, you must develop your understanding and action capabilities relative to the emotional components of human illness and the attitudes and behavior that inevitably influence the patient-physician relationship.

Though learning experiences occur in the classroom, situations involving patients with whom you can develop a patient-physician relationship are essential to your professional maturation. A broad encounter with the manifestations of disease is important but relatively less so than experience in patient approach and methods of examination. These procedures of information gathering, recording, and analysis of data through which the mature physician synthesizes a problem solution require practice, discipline, repetition, and continual verification. The personal self-confidence generated by such a process is of great significance in creating in your patient a source of trust and a spirit of cooperation at a time when he or she is likely to be frightened, anxious, or otherwise in a fragile emotional state.

Although the primary purpose of this text is to share with you successful approaches to patient evaluation, there is a secondary, more general objective. It is to convey to you something of the emotional turmoil frequently generated in the patient by this information-gathering process. The majority of similar texts tend to ignore the human dimension engendered by verbal and physical probing of one human being by another. Yet physician-patient interaction is rarely more delicately experienced — at least by the patient — than during the health examination.

All that a physician need do to refresh the intense personal significance of such an experience is to submit to it by a fellow physician. However sophisticated and educated he or she may be, there is a feeling of humility, bordering on helplessness, as one submits to nakedness, cold instruments, and casual, if professional, disinterest in those exposures we have so preciously kept to our own discretion. A personal, thorough physical examination for the physician is an abrupt reminder of what every person experiences during such a professional encounter.

One physician described an enlightening experience this way: "I still recall a woman fearfully and angrily clasping her clothing to her bare front as I foolishly walked into the examining room without first knocking. 'Get out of here until I'm dressed!' she shouted. And I did. She later reminded me that although this may have been my tenth examination that day, it was her first in a year. I have never forgotten her reminder that each patient contact is unique to that patient and highly personal, particularly to the individual who is being examined."

The novice physician has such a huge task of learning that it is easy for the most sensitive and compassionate of us to become too accustomed to patient examination, to treat it as an academic fact-finding tour and forget fears hidden behind those frequent patient smiles. It is similarly easy for us to take for granted the rare privilege extended to us by society and the individual patient when they permit us, even encourage us, to examine and question in a manner which if employed by another unlicensed person would probably lead to arrest, jail, and conviction for assault and battery.

The privileges given to you as a physician by society are truly remarkable. Individuals who permit you to ask searching personal questions and to physically manipulate their bodies give you license given to few human beings. With the patient's sanction you are given the legal and moral right to exercise awesome freedoms; of jabbing sharp steel into their flesh; of slicing open the abdomen of another human being and removing vital organs. You will be allowed, and expected, to ask the most personal questions, questions that other people would be shunned for asking. You will have the privilege of handling the most private parts of another human's body and may well be part of a team that explores the very bowel, heart, and brain of the human you are examining and treating. You will share secrets that may not be shared within the most private counsels of the patient's family. In short, with proper credentials from society and the permission of an individual, you will be permitted action accorded no other category of man.

You are given permission to ask a relative stranger of either sex to disrobe, to assume the most awkward and humiliating of positions, to accept the introduction of foreign materials into their body, and often to tolerate discomfort or even pain, while expressing no resistance.

With these privileges go the responsibility to remain sensitive and considerate of your patients' feelings, both emotional and physical, and to adequately inform them of the reasons for such scrutiny. Of equal importance to such study is an understanding that however well motivated your actions are, they may at times be misunderstood by alarmed and dismayed patients.

This combination of unique privileges and responsibilities demands not only that one develop skill and consideration in examining a patient, but also that physicians develop stability and character to a point where all requests to the patient are clearly addressed to the patient's benefit, and are not disguised devices of rewarding the physician's need for approval or advantage.

A frequently ignored responsibility of medical education is to help the medical student (and practitioner) learn and understand how his or her own inner feelings and behavior can benefit—or damage—the physician-patient relationship. Knowing that anger, physical attraction, repulsion, overprotection, inconsiderateness, and so forth, are emotions or attitudes experienced by all humans during their daily interaction (and, contrary to some contemporary beliefs, "humans" include physicians) is particularly significant for the responsible physician.

After honest self-recognition of one's inner reaction to patient behavior, the physician can learn constructive and successful ways to cope with such inevitable responses. The skillful physician will discover ways to translate these potentially destructive feelings into positive measures for helping a patient who may be living a provocative life style. However, should the problem lie more in the physician's own misinterpretation and subsequent inappropriate reaction, rather than in the patient behavior and attitude, then this too needs recognition and change.

Accepting these hang-ups as occasional but inescapably painful facts of life, and knowing one's own inner feelings with reasonable accuracy, gives opportunity for planning for successfully coping with such behavior for the patient's benefits, rather than reacting with righteous rage and rejection. It is common knowledge that a large proportion of malpractice suits initiate from poorly handled physician-patient relationships, rather than from gross malpractice.

These are tremendous educational and personal responsibilities—to learn to know oneself well enough to fairly serve the sick. Even the mature physician continually reinforces his early indoctrination regarding such goals. Rights and obligation granted the physician may enhance his self-esteem, but should do so only as they enhance his humility, for this nearly sacred trust the public has placed in the physician is there for one purpose only, to assist a more helpless human, who is ill. However long one practices medicine, however routine the procedures and activities become over the years, the physician must retain a dominant sense of duty to the patient and the latter's benefit, while depreciating any drive toward personal promotion.

Dr. Karl Menninger in his book *A Psychiatric Case History*

summarized the physician's attitude well. "It might be summed up as one [attitude] of respect for the dignity of the individual human being and of reverence for the mystery of pain, of impaired life and growth. With this, too, goes the respect for the responsibility and authority of the role of the physician — a self-respect, and the respect for one's associates and their predecessors, for the accumulation of medical science, and for that quality and the nature of human beings that leads them to turn in trust to some of their equally fallible fellow creatures and place their fate in our hands. Such respect dictates a pervasive humility and an earnest dedication to a task approaching a function of divinity."

You are urged to keep the human dimension in mind while you acquire the necessary facts and skills to adequately perform in the physician's role. You will find occasional reference to such factors throughout this text, as a reminder that examination of the fifth left intercostal space with a stethoscope is important in terms of accurately interpreting the sounds, but it is equally important to the patient that the stethoscope first be warmed by the physician's hand so that there is not the unexpected shock of a cold piece of metal introduced against skin of the often uneasy patient. Such a dimension is compatible with the best in medical practice, where the art and the science of medicine are so entwined.

Approach To The Patient

Peculiar to the educational experience involving patients is the understanding that the relationship between patient and physician must promote a free disposition in the patient to share information. You must assume the role of a physician, grasp the inherent obligations and responsibilities, and proceed with your study of the patient, his illness and disease.

The clinical setting. The office, the clinic, the hospital ward are all clinical laboratories.

Each area is a social environment of varied physical characteristics populated by a team of health workers.

Student-patient relationship. In determining your approach to a patient, you must give consideration to the following factors which influence the student-patient relationship.

TYPES OF PATIENTS
1. Casual—insurance examination, school examination.
2. Acutely ill—e.g., pneumonia, myocardial infarction, injured.
3. Chronically ill—e.g., diabetic, arthritic, hypertensive for follow-up.
4. Periodic health examination.
   —the well and the worried well, e.g., preventive health care, prospective health care.
   —chronically ill with stable problem seen for annual reevaluation.

FACTORS INFLUENCING THE PATIENT'S BEHAVIOR
1. His need for help.
2. His previous experience as a patient.
3. His past experience in relating to other persons.
4. His fears concerning illness.
5. Social, cultural, educational, and economic determinants.

FACTORS INFLUENCING THE STUDENT-PHYSICIAN'S BEHAVIOR
1. His insecurity in the new role.
2. His youth and inexperience.
3. His personal attitudes and psychology and problems.

Obligations of the clinical clerk. The obligations of the clinical clerk include his duty (1) to the patient, (2) to the patient's family and visitors, and (3) to ward and clinic personnel.

Privileges of the clinical clerk. The privileges of the clinical clerk are to interview, to examine, to carry out minor procedures, to ask for help, to examine charts, to speak with other personnel, and to gain acceptance into patient care groups.

Characteristics of the complete physician. The ideal physician is humane, sympathetic, systematic, observant, and understanding of basic principles; he uses reason and logic, knows his limitations, respects information, and his approach is confident, gentle, and competent.

Study Of The Patient

Physician-patient relationships.   Patients present themselves to physicians because they have a problem and want help. Indispensable to a successful conclusion of this consultation is creation of a suitable patient-physician relationship. Such a relationship makes possible observation and study of disease and promotes the involvement of the patient in active efforts to manage his illness.

The reason for a patient's visit to a physician (the iatrogenic stimulus) is an essential element in knowing your patient. The visit may be casual, or urgent. The patient may be present because it is required of him, he may have been coerced by a family member, he may be worried because a friend has recently died, or he may be suffering pain, discomfort, or other symptoms.

Economic, cultural, educational, and social elements may influence a patient's behavior and must be expected, recognized, and accepted by the physician and other members of the health team. Easily understood is the patient's fear concerning his illness, but less often considered is the patient's possible unfavorable past experience as a patient. Puzzling indeed is the patient who is simply inept at relating to anyone, but the student or physician must adapt and resolve the circumstances. Life and death situations may not permit the understanding, sympathetic approach. Here the patient's emergent need solves many emotional barriers, but even then the patient expects and respects a confident, gentle approach.

If a patient's visit to a physician is not occasioned by some incidental problem, such as a periodic health examination, he comes voicing in words and phrases his description of some discomfort. His portrayal may be fragmentary and disconnected, but even so represents invaluable evidence frequently intimating underlying disturbances or disease. Clues contained in such words should be used as leads which can be followed to the actual seat of the illness.

With presentation of a patient at any point in the health care system, and usually before the physician sees him, certain pertinent personal data such as age, sex, race, height, weight, blood pressure, temperature, and pulse rate are collected and become the first step in the study of the patient and his health problem. Current trends suggest that more and more data will be assembled before contact with the physician in a dispersal of health care responsibilities to those capable of extending the arm of the physician. The second step in the study of the patient is the medical interview and development of the history. Usually conducted by the physician or student physician, this duty in many instances is even now delegated to other trained members of the health care team. This history, the second portion of the patient's record, is really a brief medical biography of his life, presented with special reference to his physical ailments, personal problems, hereditary characteristics, habits, and social environment. Information contained in the history is recorded and then supplemented by a physical examination and certain laboratory data. All are recorded, evaluated, analyzed, and interpreted. Hypotheses are raised and tested against the collected data in an intellectual exercise commonly known as differential diagnosis. A pretherapeutic diagnosis is finally made and subsequently used in making a prognosis and as a guide in making a plan for management. Continued observation and even therapeutic response may modify preliminary conclusions. All such observations, hypotheses, and conclusions are duly entered in the chart, which is little different than the bench scientist's notebook.

The following steps provide a systematic sequence for collection, analysis, synthesis, and recording of data derived from patient study.

OBJECTIVES FOR PERSONAL EVALUATION

Every participant in a learning venture is influenced and guided by criteria for assessment of progress. In clinical medicine these features may be obscure; however, it is possible to list them, although values vary from discipline to discipline.

1. Histories and physicals.
2. Initiative.
3. Interest.
4. Knowledge of subject.
5. Judgment.
6. Tact.
7. Teamwork.
8. Responses to criticism.
9. Willingness to seek help.
10. Sense of humor.
11. Attendance at teaching sessions.
12. Self-confidence.

Regrouping of these features, ranked in order:
1. Degree of involvement (attitudinal).
2. Medical knowledge and skills (cognitive, manipulative).
3. Human relations skills (attitudinal).
4. Student role (attitudinal).
5. Personal traits (attitudinal).

Structuring the Interview

Dispute concerning the order in which information should be elicited serves no useful purpose. A patient consults a physician because of pain, discomfort, or apprehension which is troubling him at that particular moment. It is the present and not the past upon which his attention is focused. He has little interest in the ailments he had while a child and none at all in diseases of his forefathers—although both may be important and aid the physician in his diagnosis. If the physician, on hearing that his chief problem is "shortness of breath," asks him next what caused his father's death, the patient is unable to see any logical connection between the two questions and may promptly lose interest in the entire procedure as well as confidence in the physician. In practically all instances, it is better to ask the patient for all the details regarding his discomfort such as: Where is it? What is it like? How extensive or severe? When did it begin and how has it progressed or diminished? Under what circumstances did it occur or recur? What alleviates or worsens the problem? Are there other associated or related symptoms? When this investigation has been completed, the examiner may, without any loss of interest on the part of the patient, proceed to other matters of the history such as: past history, family history, social and personal history, and the system review.

Following these comments is an item by item display of a sequentially outlined format arranged for narrative development as most histories are; however, in the authors' institution a structured history, the completion of which results in a standard and uniform data base, is used for all first visit patients. In its published form this instrument requires a minimum of narration and can be completed quite rapidly. This is greatly appreciated by the patient and also contributes to accuracy, since the interrogator has his attention fixed upon obtaining facts free of many of the worries of composition. More will be said of this history form in the section dealing with the record.

The interview is a deeply personal experience and will often result in a completely sterile, meaningless collection of details unless accomplished with a certain degree of sophistication. It has been said that any house-officer can do a physical examination and secure highly reliable and reproducible findings, but that similar skill in obtaining a history comes much later.

Conducting the Interview

Numerous items regarding the method of collecting data deserve comment. It is always desirable to conduct the interview in privacy, if possible. However, there are instances in which the history must be supplied by a relative or a friend, as with the comatose patient or a child. The attitude of the physician toward the patient, and the reverse, markedly colors the outcome. This is a situation which a skilled interviewer has largely under his control. Acceptance of the patient and genuine, sympathetic interest on the part of the physician or student is extremely desirable. Manifestation of unhurried understanding, warmth, and sympathy, with an attempt to demonstrate to the patient that his problem is now the most important one with which you are concerned, will do much toward making the interview successful.

Time devoted to the interview is important in several ways. Sufficient time must be given, but spending an hour in getting an elaborate history from a patient with obvious dermatitis due to poison ivy, or from a patient with an obvious fracture of the arm, is totally inappropriate.

Prepared questionnaires submitted to a patient before the interview may in time become a useful supplement to this form of data collection. It may save time and add to the objectivity and completeness of the history, but it must not replace the personal approach.

Thoughtful formulation of questions in a manner designed to convey exactly what information is wanted is quite necessary and may require rephrasing the question many times. Lack of sophistication and unfamiliarity with common medical terms may pose a real block to communication. For example, a patient exhibiting many signs of small bowel obstruction repeatedly gave a negative response to "Have you been vomiting?" but quickly responded with "Oh, I've been 'puking' all night" when he finally understood the physician's question. Making the patient understand your questions is no more important than knowing exactly what he means in his response. Reliability, uniformity, consistency, precision, and objectivity are absolutely necessary features in this two-way communication exercise.

Disease entities, when studied detached from the patient as a frame of reference, may seem to have remarkable uniformity; but each illness, in contradistinction to each disease, is unique. It is made so by the invariable dissimilarity in human beings. This requires a patient-oriented, rather than a disease-oriented, approach to every health problem. A holistic concept of illness with recognition of the influence of both the psyche and soma in any given departure from health is highly desirable.

In expressing time relationships, the onset of each symptom should be fixed by date, if possible. Leading questions should be avoided as far as possible in eliciting the history, since the desire to be cooperative often causes the patient to reply with answers that he believes the physician wants, thereby creating a misleading picture of his illness. Also, there is a common tendency for the patient to conceive of his illness as having started later than it actually did. Certain questions such as "When did you last feel perfectly well?" or "When did you have to quit work?" may help in defining the onset and speed of progression of the disease.

Telling his life story may be an intense personal experience for the patient. Therefore, the physician who will listen attentively and sympathetically, with few interruptions, will usually gain his confidence. It is necessary, however, for the physician to aid the patient in minimizing irrelevant discussion and in the elaboration and clarification of pertinent factors, such as complaints of "dizziness," "biliousness," "strain," "cold," and "stomach trouble." When the patient's description of symptoms and signs is clear and graphic, it is often advantageous to quote it. Particular symptoms and signs are defined by describing such features as onset, duration, recurrence, periodicity, character of sensation, site, radiation, factors producing exacerbation or relief, associated symptoms or activities, confinement to bed, and response to therapy. Pain, for example, is described by stating its location, radiation, character (sharp, colicky, burning, dull, gnawing), severity (requiring morphine, causing doubling-up or crying-out), duration (constant, intermittent, or periodic), and time of occurrence. Record the pain's relation to (relieved, aggravated, or produced by) meals, bodily functions, exertion and rest, heat and cold, anxiety, and medications; its association with other symptoms (e.g., nausea, vomiting, diarrhea, chills, fever, cough, sweating, prostration); and its interference with work, sleep, and meals.

Emotional and somatic aspects of illness coexist and may be interrelated. In the course of the examination, therefore, observe closely the behavior and appearance of the patient, noting his expressions, anxieties, perplexities, and general emotional reactions. It is important to anticipate the effect of a question on the patient and to phrase it in such a manner as not to frighten or otherwise disturb him.

It may be a serious error to rely on the history as obtained from the patient alone, since he may be unable to describe his illness and may falsify or omit important information. No history should be considered complete, therefore, until it has been verified by information obtained from the patient's relatives, physician, employer, or friends.

Chief complaint. This should be stated as briefly as possible and in the patient's own words. The complaint, however, and not the diagnosis should be recorded. The patient should be urged to tell what his symptoms are, why he seeks relief, and not what the diagnosis of another physician has been. The chief complaint should not be recorded as "diabetes" or "heart trouble," but as "excessive urination" or "shortness of breath."

The statement that the chief complaint should be recorded in the patient's "own words" assumes that these words contain a clear expression of thought, a concise statement of his symptoms, and not vague phrases such as "heart trouble," "lung trouble," or "kidney trouble."

Present illness. The method that should be followed in obtaining a history of the present illness varies with the patient and with the illness from which he is suffering. You should strive when possible to allow the patient to tell his story just as he wishes and to emphasize the features which he considers important. Some patients have the unfortunate tendency to ramble on and on and never give a clear or concise recital of their ailments. In such cases you must, by skillful questioning, direct the story along the proper lines. Take care, however, not to suppress the thoughts of the patient and not to substitute your own instead. We are all familiar with the physician who can make the patient give the desired history by laying undue emphasis on certain details and by suppressing others altogether. In percussing a patient's chest, as Friedrich Müller remarked, we should not percuss our ideas into it. Similarly, in taking a history we should not force our own thoughts into the patient's mind.

PAIN. The most common complaint that causes the patient to seek medical advice is pain or its closely related symptom, discomfort. We should distinguish carefully between the two. A sharp pain in the stomach after eating has an entirely different significance from a dull, heavy feeling in the abdomen. The other most common types of complaints are nervousness, loss of weight, and weakness. The history of the present illness must obviously vary with the complaint. The following queries, however, are usually valuable.

DURATION. First, we should ask how long the patient has been ill. In other words, is the trouble acute or chronic? Some diseases have a sudden onset with a rapid termination; others begin slowly and insidiously. In some diseases the patient can tell almost the exact minute he had his first symptoms; in others he cannot tell within a week or two when his symptoms first began.

If the patient has been ill for a month, he is not suffering from lobar pneumonia; if he was well yesterday, and quite ill today, his illness is not pernicious anemia.

LOCATION. The importance of the pain or discomfort is obvious. If the pain is in the head, neck, chest, abdomen, or extremities, the site directs our attention to a certain organ. Does the pain remain localized, or does it travel or radiate to some other region?

PROGRESS. The progress of the symptoms is closely related to their duration. Has the trouble developed rapidly or slowly? Have the symptoms become worse or better? Are they better at times and worse at other times?

CHARACTER. Note the character of the pain or discomfort of which the patient complains. Is the pain sharp, or dull? Is it really pain, or is it discomfort? Does it appear suddenly and disappear quickly, or does it gradually increase in intensity and slowly subside?

RELATION TO PHYSIOLOGICAL FUNCTION.   Ascertain the effects of certain normal activities upon the symptoms. What is the effect of posture? Are the symptoms worse when the patient is standing or sitting or lying down? What effect does exercise produce? Are the symptoms worse when the patient walks? The effect of posture or exercise upon symptoms due to disease of the circulatory or respiratory system is usually striking. Equally striking is the distress produced by exercise in patients with severe anemia.

If disease of the digestive system is suspected, the effects of eating should be noted. In some diseases, eating relieves the symptoms; in other diseases, it aggravates them.

The relationship of the symptoms to sleep is important. Some symptoms appear while the patient is asleep and wake him from a sound sleep. In other cases, sleep brings relief from distressing symptoms.

EFFECTS OF DISEASE.   The effects produced by a disease process vary greatly. Some diseases quickly produce prostration, loss of weight, failing appetite, and extreme nervousness, causing the patient to appear quite ill and wretched. Other diseases, even after days or weeks, produce little change in the patient's general condition or appearance. Some may produce little change for weeks or months and then quickly cause catastrophic symptoms and rapidly change the appearance of the patient.

After obtaining the history of the onset of the present illness, its duration, location, progress, and character, carefully inquire as to its effects generally and then about its effects upon the systems of the body. Has the patient become weak and lost weight? Does he have fever or chills or sweats? Has he headaches, shortness of breath, indigestion, loss of appetite, vomiting, distention of the abdomen, polyuria, painful urination, or constipation?

It is important to know whether the patient has been treated for his ailment and also what the treatment was. Often a patient with a relatively minor complaint has taken some powerful drug and is suffering from the effects of the treatment rather than from the initial complaint. Examples are overdosage with digitalis and susceptibility or sensitivity to drugs, antibiotics, or biological agents. The untoward effects of corticosteroid therapy may produce numerous bizarre physical manifestations.

Personal history. The personal history, as Herrmann has emphasized, "should reveal the individual as a whole, his personality, his mental make-up." It is not sufficient to record merely his physical complaints, the various diseases from which he has suffered. It is important to know whether the patient is habitually depressed or elated and to know his reactions to his environment, to his social contacts, to his work, and to his family and friends.

The patient's social, religious, and economic background, his education, his feeling of achievement or of frustration—all are important factors to evaluate. Patients who are emotionally unstable are particularly disposed to be on the alert for any symptoms that may, in their self-analysis, be the warning of an impending serious illness. We should never forget that many patients complaining of severe symptoms are anatomically and even physiologically sound. Their symptoms are not the result of organic disease, but belong entirely to the class of emotional disorders.

Since in today's complicated society a great many environmental factors influence a patient's health, some prefer to group these features under the heading of social history. General environmental factors such as education, occupation, income and its source, as well as the ethnic group to which the patient belongs, are of obvious importance. Such matters as the physical aspects of marriage, human relationships in the family, adjustment to the job, and indulgence in various habits are important features of the immediate environment. From this elicited information, estimate which factors really have a bearing on the health problem and whether they are supportive or stressful influences.

HABITS. The habits of the patient may give important

clues to diagnosis. There are certain diseases to which alcoholics are especially prone and certain diseases which primarily attack particular groups of workers. The excessive use of tobacco and alcohol may produce a train of symptoms whose significance is entirely missed unless the patient's habits of smoking and drinking are known. Such terms as "moderate smoker" or "moderate drinker" should be avoided because they are inexact and misleading. Moderation for one person may be excess for another. The patient's daily consumption of tobacco should be recorded in numbers of cigars, cigarettes, or pipes smoked, and his daily consumption of alcohol should be recorded in terms of pints or quarts of wine, beer, or whiskey.

Many patients develop the habit of taking drugs for minor complaints, a practice which should be carefully noted. Patients often take irritating cathartics for constipation and develop severe diarrhea followed by constipation, thus perpetuating the constipation and cathartic habit. Some tranquilizers produce severe moodiness and depression; withdrawal from others can result in convulsive seizures.

Family history. The family history is important in many diseases, particularly those of the nervous system. Some diseases are always hereditary. Diabetes shows a hereditary tendency; hemophilia is invariably passed on by an affected mother to her sons; migraine is usually transmitted by the mother to the children; allergic diseases are commonly hereditary; a cancer often stalks through generation after generation of the same family; neurasthenic parents beget neurasthenic children. Arterial hypertension shows a marked tendency to appear in certain families—there are few diseases outside of hereditary nervous affections that show a more striking hereditary factor. The classic answer to the question of preventing arterial disease is "to be born of the proper parents." Life insurance actuaries have long since given preferential treatment to policy holders who are children of long-lived parents. Physicians, as a class, need no indoctrination by the advocates of eugenics, although they may question seriously the practicability of the eugenicist's program.

In taking the family history, it is important to note whether the father and mother are living and well. The health of the brothers and sisters should be ascertained.

System review. The infectious diseases noted in the outline may all have a definite effect upon the patient's later health. The same holds true for operative procedures and hospitalizations.

HEAD AND EYES. If a patient is suffering from a headache, it is important to know where it is localized and to know of anything that increases its intensity or relieves it. The importance of inquiries regarding the eyes is obvious. The laity recognizes the association of eyestrain and headache.

EARS AND NOSE, THROAT, AND MOUTH. The patient's history of disease of the ears and throat is of particular importance in affections due to streptococci, since such may be the pathogenesis for rheumatic heart disease or nephritis.

RESPIRATORY AND CARDIOVASCULAR SYSTEMS. Inquiries regarding the history of the cardiorespiratory system are of great importance. A history of chronic cough with expectoration and hemoptysis is obviously suggestive of tuberculosis or carcinoma of the lungs, while shortness of breath and palpitation of the heart, especially upon exercise, suggest the presence of a heart affliction. If this history of dyspnea is associated with the history of a past attack of rheumatic fever, the suspicion of heart disease becomes almost a certainty.

GASTROINTESTINAL SYSTEM. In diseases of the gastrointestinal tract the diagnosis is usually made from the history and the x-ray findings. Physical examination and laboratory examinations usually play minor roles. For this reason the history must be taken with extreme care. The outline indicates the type of questions to be asked.

GENITOURINARY SYSTEM. Abnormalities of urination are first considered. It is important to know whether the patient gets up at night to urinate (one of the early signs of prostatism) and if so, how often. The past history of possible gonorrhea, and particularly of syphilis, should be gone into with great care. The diagnosis of gonorrhea is usually obvious from the patient's history. The diagnosis of syphilis may be difficult from his account.

The physician today appreciates, as never before, the role

played by environment in the production of disease. Environment was previously considered only in the form of the patient's occupation. Today we realize that its scope is far more extensive and includes every phase of the patient's life — including his success or failure in his work and his family life and marital relations. A more complete discussion of the neuropsychiatric interview will amplify these brief comments concerning emotional features of illness.

NEUROPSYCHIATRIC HISTORY. It has often been said that functional illnesses make up the majority of a physician's practice. Certainly they constitute an important field, and taking the history of a patient with a functional disorder requires accuracy, tact, industry, and boundless patience. If the physician finds no physical abnormality, he should not begin by telling the patient that there is nothing wrong with him and that all his trouble is in his head. Such remarks usually infuriate the patient and also are not true. Patients do not consult physicians unless there is something the matter with them. The trouble may not be organic, but that is for the physician to explore and decide.

A patient's general attitude comes under scrutiny immediately upon his arrival in the consultation room, and impressions are gained by his state of consciousness, lethargy, or alertness. Every physician should learn much from the facial expression. It often is the picture of pain, but may also be that of anxiety and depression. The flat, expressionless face of the severely depressed is almost as pathognomonic as that in myxedema. The state of dress, neat or slovenly, and the degree of motor activity, such as restlessness and agitation, may tell much. Constant drumming of the fingers may be very tangible evidence of underlying tension not otherwise obvious. Whether the patient is interested and attentive to the physician's inquiry concerning his illness is quite important.

Quite often the patient with an organic brain syndrome is seen by several persons in the large, crowded hospital wards before it is discovered he has no correct idea of his whereabouts. Orientation as to time and place may be established during the routine questioning, but not always, and its extreme value must not be slighted by careless oversight.

In the beginning the physician should play down as much as possible his role as an interrogator, an examiner, a prober, or an investigator and assume the attitude of a seeker — a fellow seeker who joins in the search for possible clues to unravel the patient's difficulty. The clarity of a patient's stream of thought is best established by attentive listening to the patient's story with minimal interruption or priming. A patient's distraction from the main theme of his story by minimal external stimuli and his failure to regain this with help from the interviewer suggest an organic brain syndrome, such as severe cerebrovascular disease. The manic stage of a manic-depressive psychosis may be suggested by the excessive speed of a veritable torrent of words.

The patient's family history and background, the emotional stability or instability of parents, brothers, and sisters, may be important. The patient's sense of security or insecurity, satisfaction with his efforts, plans and hopes for the future, satisfaction with domestic life, satisfaction or dissatisfaction with sexual relations, attraction to a member of the opposite sex, married or unmarried, are topics to be examined, albeit without haste and with the maximum of tact. These various topics could be fairly accurately grouped under the question, "Is the patient reasonably satisfied with life as it is?"

The waking mental state is constantly engaged in interpreting numerous external stimuli. Disturbances in the ability to correctly perceive result in illusions characterizing some mental illnesses. The patient falsely interpreting the backfire of an automobile as someone shooting at him is having an illusion. If, on the other hand, there is no outside object giving rise to this false perception, it is said he suffers from hallucinations. Most common is the hallucination of voices speaking to or about the patient in otherwise quiet surroundings. Other illusional fields of sensation may occasionally be encountered, and we speak of these as olfactory, gustatory, or tactile. Rarely is it wise to ask questions directly about these disturbances.

Irrelevant or inappropriate comments or phrases in the patient's responses may demonstrate an incoherence of thought suggestive of toxic brain states or schizophrenia. There is a normal and orderly fashion in which ideas follow one another in conversation. Deviation from this orderliness becomes significant if there is no cultural or educational barrier between the physician and the patient being interviewed.

An incorrect assumption or belief based upon a false premise held by an individual is traditionally known as a delusion. The uninitiated always feel that they can easily set the patient straight by explanation, but no amount of argument will dissuade the victim. Occasionally a delusion takes a more complex form in which the patient believes others are influencing him or his thinking through mysterious external means, such as the radio.

Reference has already been made to the importance of the patient's mood. Such elements of mood as euphoria, anxiety, apathy, and depression are all quite self-evident, since they are emotional sensations common alike to patient and physician, and hopefully they stand out in objective relief to the physician-interviewer.

An important group of emotional manifestations, very resistive to change but clear indicators of psychoneurosis, are the phobias, obsessions, and compulsions. The fear of being in a room with a closed door is a common phobia. Constant preoccupation with a thought, the absurdity of which even the patient recognizes, constitutes an obsession. The patient who for years was tortured with the thought of killing her husband with the heavy weights in the grandfather's clock illustrates this emotional aberration. A physician who throughout his life would not open a door unless with a gloved hand for fear of microbial contamination illustrates the term compulsive and the absurdity of its manifestations. It is not necessary that these manifestations of psychoneurosis be disabling or have more than a remote bearing upon the illness for which the patient presents himself; if tension and anxiety are evident, eventually these features will need uncovering.

A patient's ability to understand at least in part why he is ill and to recognize that help is needed is clinically called insight. While most frequently used in reference to purely emotional states, it has broad implications in each and every illness. The emotional implications of even a fractured leg may, under proper circumstances, be tremendous, and these must be recognized by both physician and patient.

It is an old adage that a single diagnosis in a patient is more likely to be correct than multiple diagnoses. This is a valuable adage but should not be followed slavishly. A patient with organic disease may suffer from functional disturbances brought on by fear or by pain. Also, a patient with a marked psychoneurosis may develop an organic disease which has little relationship to the psychoneurosis.

As the history and physical examination are completed, the collected data should be recorded in precise descriptive words and phrases free of diagnostic terminology and all other elements likely to involve bias. The whole must then be subjected to careful analysis during which the irrelevant is discarded and the relevant arranged and ordered so that an evaluation of the data may be carried out to achieve a diagnosis. This has greater likelihood of accomplishment if the information in its recorded form has objectivity, precision, consistency, uniformity, reliability, validity, reproducibility, and freedom from bias. If these characteristics hold, utilization of the rules of logic becomes useful and reasonable. Every student and physician should develop the sharpest of skill in the basic methods of observation, analysis, and interpretation of clinical data so that specific criteria and classifications of disease and illness may be extended and the great number of diseases now recognized with such uncertainty can be diminished.

The interview as an encounter may be described as a skillful art which approaches a science. The process requires motivation of the patient to talk, control of the situation, and evaluation of the information. Usually the patient sincerely desires help, so that his motivation is positive. Control of the situation is accomplished stepwise by "breaking the ice," taking the initiative through neutral and open-end questions and then proceeding to direct, loaded, or leading questions. Supplementary comments, remarks, or gestures may encourage spontaneous amplification. Responses must be evaluated by observing nonverbal clues.

The interview is the first step in the procedure of making a diagnosis: an objective upon which all definitive treatment and fruitful management depends.

Outline: The Medical History

The patient's name, age, sex, ethnic extraction, marital status, occupation, place of residence, and referring physician represent information usually recorded by clerical assistants prior to the time the patient reaches the consultation room. Record the time and place of the examination. If not the first visit, then the number and dates of other admissions should be recorded. Append a statement as to the apparent reliability of the patient or informant. Finally, the history and examination should carry the signature and status of the examiner.

Chief complaint. A very brief statement, in the patient's own words if possible, of what concerns the patient most and how long he has been ill. Avoid if possible words or phrases representing a diagnosis or of purely diagnostic implications. Attempt to secure in terminology of *symptoms* and *signs.*

Present illness. When, why, and how did the patient become ill? Detail in concise chronological order all information relevant to the onset and course of the illness. The patient's understanding of his illness and his expectations of the visit should be elicited if possible.

Family history

1. *Family background:* Ages of parents, state of health, past physical and emotional illnesses, and important events coupled with the patient's age at the time. Include queries concerning grandparents and other household members.

2. *Siblings:* Number of mother's pregnancies; number of brothers and sisters: sex, state of health, illnesses or other problems; patient's age position in group of brothers and sisters.

3. *Marital history:* A statement about the patient's spouse and children, including ages, state of health, illnesses or other problems, and emotional relationships.

4. *Familial history:* Incidence of arthritis, allergy, cancer, diabetes mellitus, bleeding disorders, hypertension, epilepsy, kidney disease, migraine, nervous or mental disorders, rheumatic fever, peptic ulcer, and other dominant patterns of illness.

Social and environmental history

1. Education, military service, and religious activity. Describe when pertinent.

2. Occupational history: Describe activities both inside and outside the home, including a typical day's routine.

3. Living arrangements: Describe the physical and social aspects of the home.

4. Features relating to this illness: Consider finances, changes in work and at home, sexual outlets, use of alcohol, drugs, and tobacco. Particularly evaluate emotional reaction to this illness.

Past medical history

1. Birth and early development: Summarize patient's knowledge about his birth, feeding, growth, behavior and environment, emphasizing interpersonal relationships and major events of early life.

2. Past illnesses, childhood and otherwise: Communicable diseases and sequelae; immunizations; allergic and hypersensitivity reactions; drug reactions.

3. Operations, injuries, accidents, hospital admissions: Give dates and circumstances. Elicit comments about anesthesia, drug reactions, and results of treatment.

4. Drugs, medications, habits: Inquire about tea, coffee, alcohol, tobacco, laxatives, or any drugs used regularly.

5. General health: Simply the patient's evaluation as good, average, or poor.

Review of systems.   Record all pertinent signs, symptoms, and values. Utilize the system review to gain information which might have been omitted by oversight.

1. *Skin, hair, nails:* Changes in character, consistency, or pigmentation; pruritus; eruptions, hives, sores.

2. *Head:* Characterize headaches, vertigo, syncope, trauma.
   a. Eyes—visual acuity, corrective lenses, photophobia, diplopia, inflammation.
   b. Ears—pain, discharge; deafness; tinnitus.
   c. Nose—epistaxis; discharge; obstruction; sense of smell; sinusitis.

   d. Mouth and throat—status of teeth, gums, dentures; leuko-
      plakia or sores; sore throats; hoarseness; tonsillectomy;
      adenoidectomy.
   3. *Respiratory:* Cough, sputum, hemoptysis—amount and character; use of tobacco, or other respiratory tract irritants; chest pain; dyspnea; cyanosis; tuberculosis; asthma; pneumonia; dates of chest x-ray
studies.
   4. *Circulatory:* Angina pectoris; congestive failure; dyspnea upon
exertion; orthopnea; edema; disturbance of cardiac rhythm; intermittent claudication; leg cramps; blood pressures changes.
   5. *Gastrointestinal:* Appetite, eating habits; dysphagia; nausea,
vomiting; jaundice; bowel habits, diarrhea, constipation, character of
stools, blood in stools, melena; abdominal pain.
   6. *Urinary:* Frequency, urgency, dysuria, hematuria, nocturia;
hesitancy; colic; dribbling; incontinence; calculi; enuresis.
   7. *Reproductive:* Female—menarche, menstrual history; pregnancies; abnormal pain, vaginal bleeding or discharge; breast; venereal
disease; frigidity or impotence. Date of last menses and previous menstrual period. Male—libido, potentia, fertility, venereal disease.
   8. *Musculoskeletal:* Deformities; arthritis; fractures; pain, limitation of motion, weakness, wasting, tremors.
   9. *Neurological:* Headaches; syncope; seizures; aphasia; loss of
sensation; pain; ataxia; weakness or paralysis.
   10. *Hematopoietic:* Anemia; transfusions; hematinics; abnormal
bruising or bleeding; lymphadenopathy.
   11. *Metabolic and Endocrine:* Growth and development; normal
weight, weight at 18 years of age; temperature intolerance, nervousness, sweating; glycosuria; polydipsia, polyuria; voice change,
change in hair distribution or amount.
   12. *Psychological:* Childhood behavioral problems; "nervous break-
downs"; anxiety; depression; irritability; insomnia; alcoholism; psychosexual adjustment and maturity.

Physical Examination

   The examination begins the instant the patient comes
under observation with the examiner's use of one of the basic
maneuvers of physical diagnosis, inspection, and continues

throughout the various stages of a systematic collection of basic data. Instead of becoming less valuable, in this age of technological advance, this part of the study has become even more fertile. The many precision instruments used to supplement the examination have served in a very effective manner to stimulate expertness and sophistication in examiners. This is so aptly demonstrated in a resurgence of interest and facility in cardiac auscultation prompted by the widespread use of phonocardiography.

Preservation of the patient rapport and relationship achieved during the medical interview is desirable and in fact may be extended by a complete, efficient, and professional utilization of the basic maneuvers of inspection, palpation, percussion, and auscultation as appropriate. Of first importance in this phase of study is sincere respect for the patient's body and person. Avoid unnecessary embarrassment or discomfort. Retain the dignity the circumstance demands.

Physical diagnosis may be defined as that exercise through which disease is identified by use of the traditional stratagems listed above, but since the days of Auenbrugger and Laennec, certain instruments have added refinement to the observations and the beginning student should provide himself with certain equipment. The needed list should include: stethoscope, sphygmomanometer, ophthalmoscope, otoscope, flashlight, percussion hammer, tuning fork (128 cycles per second), tape measure, pocket hand lens, tongue blade, and thermometer. In the physical examination that follows, the appropriate instrument is noted in the area most likely requiring its use. The same indications are made for the basic maneuvers of inspection, palpation, percussion, and auscultation.

With the patient prepared for the examination in a manner suitable to avoid needless exposure and embarrassment, initiate the procedure by feeling the pulse and checking the blood pressure. Then in a systematic manner conduct a complete regional survey beginning with the head and neck and including the chest, the heart, the abdomen, the extremities, and finally the pelvic and rectal area. Many details of the various system examinations are elaborated in subsequent sections of the text.

Outline: The Physical Examination

Preparing for examination.

EQUIPMENT. Stethoscope, sphygmomanometer, ophthalmoscope and otoscope, flashlight, percussion hammer, tuning fork (128 cps), tape measure, pocket hand lens, tongue blade, thermometer, (tonometer).

PREPARE THE PATIENT. Avoid embarrassing and needless exposure.

INITIATION OF EXAMINATION. Feel pulse, take blood pressure.

Basic maneuvers

INSPECTION. Each region of the body is inspected for:

1. Skin
   a. Color and pigmentation in general.
   b. Lesions.
   c. Superficial vascularity.
   d. Edema.
   e. Moistness, dryness, or oilyness.
   f. Characteristics of hair and nails.
2. Mucous membranes
   a. Color and pigmentation in general.
   b. Lesions.
   c. Superficial vascularity.
   d. Edema.
   e. Moistness and secretions.
3. Architecture
   a. Size and shape
   b. Symmetry or deformity, localized bulging or swelling.
   c. Muscular development.
4. Movement
   a. Muscles, bones, joints.
   b. Respiratory
   c. Vascular.
   d. Peristaltic.
   e. Other.
5. Position

PALPATION. Each region of the body is palpated for:

1. Confirmation and extension of observations made by inspection.

2. Data revealed primarily by palpation:
   a. Tenderness: superficial; deep; rebound; referred.
   b. Tones of muscles: increased resistance; spasm; rigidity.
   c. Tumor (mass): lymph nodes, or underlying organs that are usually felt but not seen. Evaluate each for:
      (1) Location and relationship to other structures.
      (2) Architecture: size, shape, symmetry, surgence, edge.
      (3) Consistency, fluctuation.
      (4) Tenderness, redness, heat.
      (5) Mobility and attachment.
      (6) Pulsation.

PERCUSSION. The technique of tapping an area of the body and noting the sounds produced and the resistance encountered.

1. Classification of percussion sounds:
   a. Resonance.
   b. Dullness.
   c. Flatness.
   d. Tympany.

AUSCULTATION. The technique of detecting sounds arising from various organs accomplished by listening to the surface of the body, either by direct application of the examiner's ear or with a stethoscope.

1. Classification of sounds heard over the chest:
   a. Breath sounds: vesicular; bronchovesicular; bronchial; cavernous or amphoric.
   b. Voice sounds:
      (1) Spoken: normal vocal resonance; bronchophony; egophony.
      (2) Whisper: normal whisper; whispered pectoriloquy.
   c. Adventitious sounds:
      (1) Interrupted discrete sounds: râles (fine, medium, coarse).
      (2) Continuous sounds: ronchi (low pitch); wheezes (high pitch).
      (3) Friction rubs: pleural (inspiratory; expiratory); pleuro-pericardial.
      (4) Succussion splash.

2. Classification of sounds heard over the heart:
   a. S_1: First heart sound, associated with closure of the mitral (M) and tricuspid (T). M normally precedes T.

b. S_2: Second heart sound, associated with closure of the aortic (A) and pulmonary (P) valves. A normally precedes P. A_2 and P_2 refer to the aortic and pulmonic components of S_2.

c. OS: Opening snap.

d. S_3: Physiological third heart sound.

e. S_3G: Third sound gallop.

f. S_4: Physiological fourth heart sound.

g. S_4G: Fourth sound gallop.

h. Systolic sounds: early, mid, late.

i. Murmurs:

(1) Systolic: early; mid; late; holosystolic.

(2) Diastolic: early; mid; late; holodiastolic.

j. Clicks.

Suggested order of procedure. In the routine data collection process the following order of observation is suitable; however, such a stepwise systematic approach could be grossly inappropriate in an emergency state.

VITAL SIGNS. Record the temperature, pulse rate, respiratory rate, blood pressure (indicate position and arm). Also record height and weight when possible.

APPEARANCE AND BEHAVIOR. This should be an accurate description of the patient as an individual, including the following information:

1. Mental state: State of consciousness, orientation, mood, attitude, attention, memory.

2. Language: Quality of speech, content, coherence.

3. Posture: Position in bed; dress and appearance.

4. Physique: Constitution; nutritional status; hydration; color; edema, if present.

5. Apparent severity and duration of illness.

6. Attitude and emotional state in relation to illness and to the examiner.

INTEGUMENT. Basic maneuvers—inspection, palpation.

1. Skin: Complexion, texture, turgor, pigmentation, eruptions, petechiae, tumors, or nodules.

2. Nails: Color, clubbing.

3. Hair: Color, texture, distribution.

LYMPH NODES. Basic maneuvers—inspection, palpation.

1. General: Local or generalized enlargement, discrete or matted; mobility, tenderness.

2. Location: Anterior and posterior cervical; pre- and postauricular; occipital; supraclavicular; axillary, epitrochlear; iliac, inguinal, femoral.

HEAD. Basic maneuvers—inspection, palpation, percussion, auscultation. Instruments—stethoscope.

1. Scalp: Tenderness, scars.
2. Skull: Configuration, depressions, or exostoses.

EYES. Basic maneuvers—inspection, palpation. Instruments—flashlight, ophthalmoscope, (tonometer).

1. General: Exophthalmos, ocular tension.
2. Lids: Ptosis, lid lag.
3. Sclerae: Jaundice, hemorrhages.
4. Conjunctivae: Pallor, injection, petechiae.
5. Cornea: Scars, ulcerations, arcus senilis.
6. Pupils: Size, shape, equality; reaction to light and accommodation; extraocular movements.
7. Vision: Acuity; visual fields by confrontation; color perception. If glasses are worn, note defect and type of correction.
8. Fundi: Optic discs, arteries, hemorrhages, exudates.

EARS. Basic maneuvers—inspection, palpation. Instruments—otoscope, tuning fork.

1. External: Tophi, discharge.
2. Internal: Canal walls, tympanic membranes; fluid behind drums.
3. Auditory acuity: Bone versus air conduction.

NOSE. Basic maneuvers—inspection, palpation. Instruments—flashlight, nasal speculum.

Shape, septum, congestion, discharge, polyps, patency of airways, sinus tenderness, transillumination.

MOUTH AND THROAT. Basic maneuvers—inspection, palpation. Instruments—flashlight, tongue blade, laryngeal mirror.

1. General: Breath, hygiene.
2. Lips: Color, cyanosis, cheilosis, cold sores.
3. Teeth: Number, caries, dentures.
4. Mucous membranes and gingivae: Pallor, ulceration, pigmentation, enanthem.
5. Tongue: Color, papillary atrophy, deviation, tremor, ulceration.
6. Pharynx: Tonsils, epiglottis, palatal movement.

NECK. Basic maneuvers—inspection, palpation, auscultation. Instruments—stethoscope.

1. General: Mobility, meningismus.
2. Blood vessels: Engorgement of veins; carotid pulsations, abnormal pulsations; scars.
3. Thyroid: Size, nodules, bruit.
4. Trachea: Position, tracheal tug.

BREASTS.   Basic maneuvers—inspection, palpation.

Symmetry, masses, scars, nipples, secretion, pigmentation, tenderness.

CHEST AND LUNGS.   Basic maneuvers—inspection, palpation, percussion, auscultation. Instruments—stethoscope, tape measure.

1. Inspection: Shape, symmetry, contour of rib cage, anterior-posterior diameter, expansion (note quality of expansion).
2. Palpation: Tactile fremitus, measured expansion.
3. Percussion: Resonance, descent of diaphragms, supraclavicular spaces.
4. Auscultation: Breath sounds, prolongation of expiration; râles, rhonchi, post-tussive râles; friction rub.

HEART.   Basic maneuvers—inspection, palpation, percussion, auscultation. Instruments—stethoscope, tape measure.

1. Inspection: Pulsations, peripheral jugular, carotid, apical impulse, precordial bulge.
2. Palpation: Radial pulse, carotid pulse; confirm position of apical impulses, thrills, precordial heave.
3. Percussion: Map out cardiac size—RCD (relative cardiac dullness), ACD (absolute cardiac dullness), and other areas of abnormal density. Percuss parallel to expected line of dullness.
4. Auscultation: Rate, rhythm, sounds; first sound, second sound, splitting, murmurs, friction rubs, clicks.

ABDOMEN.   Basic maneuvers—inspection, palpation, percussion, auscultation. Instruments—stethoscope, tape measure.

1. Inspection: Shape, scars, veins, peristalsis, distension.
2. Palpation: Liver, spleen, kidneys, colon, bladder, uterus; tenderness, rebound tenderness and referred rebound tenderness, costovertebral angle tenderness; tone (spasm, involuntary guarding, rigidity); masses, hernias.
3. Percussion: Liver, spleen, and bladder; shifting dullness, fluid wave; size and shape of masses.
4. Auscultation: Peristalsis; gastric succussion splash.
5. Other signs of peritoneal irritation; rebound tenderness.

6. Hernia: Psoas spasm, inguinal (direct, indirect), femoral, incisional.

GENITALIA. Basic maneuvers—inspection, palpation. Instruments—vaginal speculum.

1. Male: Distribution and amount of pubic hair; foreskin (circumcised?), adhesions; penile scars, inflammation, discharge; urethral stricture; testes and epididymes; size, masses, undescended testes; varicocele, hydrocele.

2. Female: Distribution and amount of pubic hair; external genitalia; size of clitoris; glands, urethra; introitus, pelvic relaxation; inflammation, discharge, vagina, cervix, uterus, adnexa.

ANUS AND RECTUM. Basic maneuvers—inspection, palpation. Instruments—rubber glove, light proctoscope.

Sphincter tone, hemorrhoids; prolapse, fissure, fistula; prostate, masses; presence or absence of blood on examining finger.

EXTREMITIES. Basic maneuvers—inspection, palpation, auscultation. Instruments—tape measure, stethoscope.

1. Upper: Color of palms, moisture; joint swelling, inflammation, deformity; fractures, irregularities, limitation of function; nodules.

2. Lower: Equality of leg lengths; mobility, swelling, inflammation, deformity of joints; fractures; measure circumference and length of extremities when indicated.

PERIPHERAL VESSELS. Basic maneuvers—inspection, palpation, auscultation. Instruments—stethoscope, tape measure, sphygmomanometer.

Palpate and describe major vessels and describe amplitude, character, and equality of pulsations (note particularly posterior tibial and dorsalis pedis arteries); color and temperature of feet; edema, varicose veins, venous engorgement, abnormal vascular patterns, thrills, bruit.

BACK AND SPINE. Basic maneuvers—inspection, palpation, percussion. Instruments—tape measure.

Posture; mobility curvature, tenderness, root pain, meningismus, pilonidal sinus.

NERVOUS SYSTEM. Basic maneuvers—inspection, palpation, percussion, auscultation. Instruments—percussion hammer, ophthalmoscope, tuning fork, tape measure, (taste and temperature tests).

1. Cranial nerves: Brief survey numerically unless performing a detailed, formal neurological examination.

2. Motor system: Muscle tone, strength, wasting, contracture, fasciculations, involuntary movements; power, spasticity; clonus.

3. Reflexes: Deep tendon reflexes; superficial and plantar reflexes; abnormal signs (Babinski, Hoffmann, Chvostek, Trousseau, and so forth).

4. Sensation: Touch, pain, vibration, joint position; Romberg's sign.

5. Coordination: Stance; ataxic, spastic, or festinant gait.

6. Autonomic nervous system: Sweating, flushing, blanching.

THE DIAGNOSTIC PROCESS

For traditional and present reasons, the *diagnosis* is of prime importance for the purpose of definition of the pathological processes in a detached or impersonal manner. Equally important is an evaluation of the physical and emotional reactions of the patient. The first identifies the *disease*, while the second gives recognition to the *illness* and usually embodies a concept known as the prognosis.

The diagnostic study of a patient is in reality a combination of intellectual and manipulative procedures through which *disease* is identified and *illness* evaluated. Procedures involved include history taking, physical examination, and various technical diagnostic observations. The accumulated information becomes the data base from which conclusions emerge.

The history yields information concerning the patient's subjective sensations (e.g., dyspnea, nausea, pain), his emotional sensations (e.g., fear, despair, or irritability), changes in his bodily appearance (e.g., yellow skin, edema, or tumor mass), and changes in bodily functions (e.g., paralysis, decreased urine output, or inability to carry out his daily routine).

Clinical manifestations of illness are known as *symptoms* and *signs*. *Symptoms* are those subjective sensations and alterations in functions reported by the patient, while *signs* are the abnormal findings detected by the physician in the physical examination.

The diagnostic process itself involves a systematic analysis of all information in the *data base*, utilizing age old methods of reasoning and logic. Study of the data includes: (1) identification of the abnormal findings; (2) localization of the abnormal findings in anatomical terms; (3) interpretation of those findings in structural and functional terms; (4) consideration of etiology; (5) subjection of data to method of hypotheses; (6) classification of the disease; and (7) formulation of a prognosis.

Diagnosis By Method of Hypotheses

Differential diagnosis, like scientific research, is based on the method of hypothesis first described by Plato, not Hippocrates. He is the father of the reasoning process we use today in scientific investigation and in diagnosis. This method provides for the logical selection of one or more hypotheses from a group of alternatives. Far more than a historic relic, it is the cornerstone of diagnostic reasoning.

Performed so often and apparently so effortlessly by physicians, the diagnostic process becomes spontaneous and nonconscious to the skilled clinician. Seemingly ordinary clinical illnesses are as easy to recognize as the faces of relatives. The facility with which these accomplishments occur is misleading to both the performer and the audience. It is not intuitive and neither is it occult; it is a combination of pattern recognition combined with polished deductive reasoning.

To use deductive reasoning with a minimum of error we must be aware of the logical traps into which the diagnostician may fall. Correct diagnoses are based on *correct information*, as well as valid reasoning.

Analysis of any case begins during the medical interview. It continues during the physical examination; it directs the choice of tests and special studies and continues during the course of the patient's illness. As data are accumulated their significance is weighed in terms of reliability, pertinence, and degree of abnormality. Analysis then selects signal items or constellations of features, such as jaundice or anemia. Years ago, Richard Cabot described this diagnostic analysis in these words: "When for example, a patient pronounces the word, headache, a group of causes should shoot into the field of attention like the figures on a cash register. . . . Each clue or combination of clues should come to possess it's own set of radiations or 'leadings.' " Dr. Cabot's clues led to possible causes, and thus a list of alternative diagnoses was devised. Today we are properly satisfied with clues leading us first to categories such as biochemical, physiological, or anatomical syndromes, rather than directly to diseases. Such identification may point more quickly to an acceptable plan of action, both diagnostic and therapeutic. Obviously, recognition of congestive failure and institution of management immediately is much more logical than risking life while obsessively searching for a cause. This method of *differential diagnosis* remains perfectly sound.

We are still faced with making a diagnostic choice between alternatives, dismissing the unlikely and trying to establish one (or more) to be certain. In the method under discussion one tries to solve a problem, whether it be that of scientific research, medical diagnosis, or even that of criminal detection. In each situation a list of alternatives is made. The clinician lists his possible diagnoses, the scientist his hypotheses, and the detective his suspects.

The clinician tests each hypothetical diagnosis in turn, trying to dismiss the unlikely and to verify the correct. He does this by asking two questions: Does the diagnosis explain all the findings? Are the expected findings present?

First we look at the illness to see if it fits a class (the disease or syndrome) proposed as the hypothetical diagnosis. Next we reverse our approach and we examine the class to see if the characteristics of the class (diagnostic criteria) are consistent with the illness which we are viewing. The patient and his illness are real and certainly do exist as our senses discern; the disease, as described in textbooks, is only a frequently observed and repeatedly described construction of logical dimensions. It does not exist in any other form. However, if this "logical construct" is to be useful, your observations of the illness must be accurate and complete.

A Formal Diagnostic Logic

The role of the physician in modern diagnosis.   What may be called scientific methods are used in many areas of modern day medicine to obtain information needed for diagnosis. The fundamental role of the physician remains, however, in the artful assembly and interpretation of these data to the ill person. We believe, therefore, that this role of the physician is not endangered and can only gain by application of the rules of logic, probability, and decision theory, and by the use of computers in the manipulation of data derived from clinical and laboratory study of patients.

Scientific medicine must be tempered by the art of medicine, as has been so well said by Chesterton:

A man can understand astronomy only by being an astronomer; he can understand entomology only by being an entomologist (or, perhaps, an insect); but he can understand a great deal of anthropology merely by being a man. He is himself the animal which he studies. Hence arises the fact which strikes the eye everywhere in the records of ethnology and folklore — the fact that the same frigid and detached spirit which leads to success in the study of astronomy or botany leads to disaster in the study of mythology or human origins. It is necessary to cease to be a man in order to do justice to a microbe; it is not necessary to cease to be a man in order to do justice to men. That same suppression of sympathies, that same waving away of intuitions or guesswork, which make a man preternaturally clever in dealing with the stomach of a spider, will make him preternaturally stupid in dealing with the heart of man.

The diagnostic process.   The word diagnosis (derived from the Greek *dia* = through or part of, and *gnoscien* = to know) is usually taken to mean to know apart, that is, to separate things or persons into groups for purposes of description, study, or action. In this manual, however, we emphasize the meaning of to know through. That is, to diagnose is to know patients through what they say about their illness (their symptoms), to know patients through the various manifestations that disease produces in their physical being (the physical signs of illness), and to know them through the skills of laboratory science and radiology.

The ultimate intellectual function of the physician is to combine the information obtained about a patient from all relevant sources into a diagnosis. This diagnosis should be simple enough to be understood, and complete and correct enough to form a logical basis for decisions regarding therapy, management, and prognosis. A fundamental problem of this diagnostic function is that the information available to the physician is frequently inadequate, irrelevant, and of varying accuracy and precision.

As your experience increases, you will recognize that each of a great many groups of findings has been labeled with a name called "the diagnosis." This diagnosis may imply some etiological factor, as in streptococcal pharyngitis or alcoholic cirrhosis; or it may imply some change observed in the tissues, such as arteritis. It may suggest a predominantly functional derangement, such as schizophrenia; it may simply recognize a peculiar manifestation, such as disseminated lupus erythematosus; or it may be an eponymic designation, such as Parkinson's disease. Once again, the purpose of stating any diagnosis is to identify the patient as belonging to a given disease category so that the physician may make significant statements regarding treatment, prognosis, or other factors of interest.

Diagnostic classifications, as do all classifications, proceed from the general to the singular, from the less certain to the more certain. As has been masterfully stated by R. L. Engle and R. J. Davis, diagnoses are of five orders of certainty, which we summarize as follows:

DIAGNOSIS OF FIRST ORDER OF CERTAINTY. Gross anatomical defects: trauma, such as leg fracture; harelip; genetic abnormalities, e.g., sickle cell anemia.

DIAGNOSIS OF SECOND ORDER OF CERTAINTY. Infection with microorganisms; malnutrition; chemical poisoning. Pictures may vary greatly, as with pneumonia.

DIAGNOSIS OF THIRD ORDER OF CERTAINTY. Largely descriptive, easily recognized, but little is known about etiology and pathogenesis, such as peptic ulcer, essential hypertension, cirrhosis.

DIAGNOSIS OF FOURTH ORDER OF CERTAINTY. While the

general type of reaction may be recognized, the specific cause is unknown, and individual as well as environment variations occur. Benign and malignant tumors fit into this category. Chiefly identified by microscopic cell changes, they offer even the pathologist much trouble.

DIAGNOSIS OF FIFTH ORDER OF CERTAINTY.   These are based on groups or collections of signs and symptoms which make up the disease picture, but the etiology remains obscure. Examples are infectious mononucleosis, sarcoidosis, and systemic lupus erythematosus.

It is the purpose of this book to recount in some detail those personal methods of obtaining diagnostic information. Contrasted with these methods are impersonal techniques, such as analysis of the urine or blood or inspection of an x-ray photographic image. Specifically, this section describes a logical process for evaluating items of diagnostic information.

The evaluation of observations.   Classically, the methods and techniques of clinical diagnosis are presented in descriptive form without much attempt at demonstration of the methods whereby these maneuvers are used in synthesizing a diagnosis. We would suggest that the following diagram illustrates the steps that a physician ordinarily passes through in reaching a "diagnosis" (Fig. 2–1).

It is important to note that when a physician reaches a diagnosis based on study of a patient, he believes that this diagnosis describes the actual state of that patient. It is the goal of clinical medicine to insure that the diagnosis made by the physician corresponds as often as possible to the actual disease that is producing the patient's illness.

The possible error inherent in every diagnosis arises from the fact that all knowledge of human origin is uncertain. The distinguishing characteristic of scientific knowledge is not that it is more certain than nonscientific knowledge, but that the degree of uncertainty can be rather well determined. Indeed, the most reliable of all knowledge is that which includes a realistic self-appraisal. Since observation, be it qualitative or quantitative, is the basis for all scientific truths or facts, the reliability of these

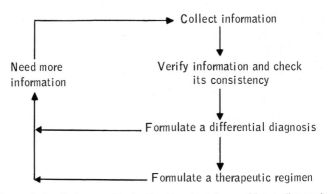

Figure 2–1. A diagram illustrating the steps in reaching a diagnosis.

observations determines the reliability of any resultant principles, classifications, or diagnoses.

Logical manipulation of information gained from examination of patients develops intuitively in the artful human physician. Perhaps in this regard it is true that good clinicians are born, not made. We can, however, demonstrate that the rules of reasoning that the physician uses are no different from the rules that the good investigator uses in the laboratory, that the astute businessman uses in his economic manipulations, or that any other person involved in making decisions uses in evaluating the information available to him.

In order to clearly and concisely describe the rules for evaluation of observations, it is necessary to introduce a few symbols.

First, let us agree that we will represent any diagnosis by the letter D and some subscript number or letter — D_1, D_2 ... D_i, D_k. For example, given a list of diagnostic possibilities

D_1	Appendicitis
D_2	Rheumatoid arthritis
D_3	Tonsillitis
D_4	Diabetes mellitus
D_5	Arteriosclerotic heart disease

we could refer to any specific diagnosis by writing D and the appropriate subscript; i.e., D_2 = rheumatoid arthritis. In general, we will say that our diagnostic list has k elements numbered 1 through k. In the example, $k = 5$. Therefore, if k is infinite we are concerned with all the diagnostic possibilities. Practically, we will restrict our considerations to a finite number of diagnoses, the differential diagnosis.

The credibility of diagnoses.   As you study medicine via lectures, textbooks, and patients, you will gradually develop your own list of diagnoses, which will relate to your locale and experience. Attached to each of the diagnoses in the list will be an appraisal of the frequency with which each might be encountered in any given patient. You might, for example, believe that it would be quite unusual to see a native Kansas patient with schistosomiasis or that it would be most odd to be confronted by an infant who had carcinoma of the lung. Ten years ago poliomyelitis was a common disease of children and young adults, but now it is a rarity because of immunization programs. It is, therefore, no longer in the forefront of diagnostic considerations for the young person with fever and a stiff neck. Thus, when you first observe any patient you begin your thinking with a group or set of possibilities within which you can reasonably expect your patient's disease process to fit. Those that are very unlikely are placed at the bottom of the list of diagnostic possibilities.

Specifically, a 70 year old man might credibly be expected to have cancer, heart disease, or cerebrovascular disease but not childhood infections, Wilms' tumor of the kidney, or glomerulonephritis. This diagnostic estimate is made before any examination of the patient and concerns your prior knowledge and experience with disease processes in this age group.

It is convenient for purposes of discussion if we design some means of representing the strength of our belief in any specific diagnosis for a given patient. Let us agree, therefore, that we will discuss the credibility of a diagnosis and, furthermore, that if a diagnosis is absolutely not credible we will say it has a credibility of zero (0) and if it is totally believable it has a credibility of one

(1). We could, therefore, rank according to the degree of credibility all the items of the diagnostic lists that we develop. It is essential to realize that these credibilities are developed prior to evaluation of any specific patient and arise from the body of experience that each physician gains about his medical environment. Moreover, one physician's estimates of credibilities may or may not coincide with another's estimates of the same diagnostic list. For example, the list of diagnoses conceived by a physician practicing in metropolitan New York would certainly differ from a list evaluated by a rural physician in Montana or a medical missionary in central Africa.

Finally, let us assume that each diagnostic consideration (D_1, D_2, D_3 . . . D_k) has an exclusive and independent credibility such that the sum of credibilities from any specific list is 1 and that only one diagnosis from such a list can be "true" at any given time. For example, suppose we believe that a patient has a sore throat due either to a streptococcal infection (D_1), which we rank on our credibility scale at 0.6, or to a viral infection (D_2), which we rank at 0.2. Now, how believable is it that he has either a streptococcal infection or an upper respiratory viral infection? By our rule it is equal to the sum of the individual credibilities or, in this case, $0.6 + 0.2$ or 0.8. Since we are not certain that he has one or the other of these, their sum is not 1; i.e., he might have something else. The likelihood that he has something besides these two is 0.2 since $1.0 - 0.8 = 0.2$. In dealing with credibilities we use the symbol $\cup$ to indicate either/or and $\cap$ to indicate and. Thus, symbolically:

$$C(D_1 \cup D_2) = C(D_1) + C(D_2) \text{ if and only if } C(D_1 \cap D_2) = 0$$

i.e., they are mutually exclusive.

In words, this equation states that the credibility that either diagnosis 1 or diagnosis 2 is correct is equal to the sum of their individual credibilities provided diagnosis 1 and diagnosis 2 cannot occur simultaneously, i.e., provided that they are independent and mutually exclusive.

Partition of the diagnostic possibilities. Let us now apply these rules to an example. Suppose that you are called to see a 42 year old man who has collapsed while at work. Using as a basis your past medical experience with regard to the causes of collapse in middle-aged men and any prior information that you may have about the work this man did, or his social, economic, and medical background, you would develop a list of diagnostic possibilities.

Consider the following:

Diagnostic List	Credibility of Diagnosis
D_1 Myocardial infarction	$C(D_1) = 0.5$
D_2 Cerebrovascular accident	$C(D_2) = 0.3$
D_3 Cardiac arrhythmia	$C(D_3) = 0.1$
D_4 "Something else"	$C(D_4) = 0.1$
$k = 4$	$\Sigma C(D_k) = 1$

You will note that the sum of these credibilities is equal to 1; the inclusion of the diagnostic consideration that he has "something else" makes the list all-inclusive. The arrangement of the diagnostic considerations in this fashion is called a partition of the possible diagnoses; that is, the patient must have one and only one of the disorders we have listed.[1] We have stipulated, in other words, that the patient cannot have both myocardial infarction and a cerebrovascular accident and that if we add together all the diagnostic possibilities he must have one of them. This may be written as $\Sigma C(D_k) = 1$. The Greek sigma (Σ) is the notation saying "add all of the terms from $C(D_1)$ to $C(D_k)$." In our instance k is equal to 4. In classic textbook descriptions, this list of credible diagnoses is called a differential diagnosis.

In Figure 2–2, this partition is illustrated by relating the credibility of the various diagnoses to the area representing each in the circle. Note that this partitions the circle and that no overlap occurs between any of the areas.

---

[1] As a commonplace example, the suits of a deck of cards form a partition of the deck. If we add all the spades, hearts, diamonds, and clubs together we have an entire deck of cards, and a card cannot be a spade and a diamond at the same time. The same is true for our set of diagnostic possibilities in this example.

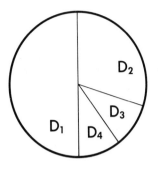

Figure 2–2. A diagrammatic representation of the partition of diagnostic possibilities.

Conditional probabilities. The next logical step is to obtain information about the patient by inquiry, physical diagnostic techniques, and laboratory tests. Now once again we must call on past experience, both personal and general, to evaluate the findings that would be uncovered if the patient actually had any of the given disorders. For example, if he had suffered a myocardial infarction, we would expect that he would complain of severe substernal pain, of being cold, pale, and perhaps sweaty, and quite likely he would show some arterial hypotension. We believe it possible, but less probable, to observe this particular group of signs and symptoms if he had suffered a stroke or if he had something else. For this diagnostic partition (the differential diagnosis), we establish a series of considerations or a series of statements regarding the probability of observing certain clinical manifestations. (See Table 2–1).

Tables like this appear in most textbooks of medicine and in medical literature and represent appraisals of the signs or symptoms experienced by patients who have specific diseases and resulting illnesses. Much of your study of medicine will be directed toward establishing for yourself a large series of such probability tables for the signs and symptoms of various diseases. These probabilities are manipulated by the same rules as credibilities of diagnosis; that is, if something is totally improbable ("never occurs"), we say that its probability is 0. If some event

TABLE 2–1. PROBABILITY STATEMENTS FOR THE SAMPLE DIAGNOSTIC PARTITION

Symptom	Myocardial Infarction	Cerebro-vascular Accident	Cardiac Arrhythmia	"Some-thing Else"
Severe chest pain	Very probable	Unlikely	Possible	Unlikely
Cold and sweaty	Probable	Probable	Probable	Possible
Hypotension	Probable	Improbable	Possible	Possible
Irregular pulse	Possible	Unlikely	Very probable	Unlikely
Weakness on one side of the body	Unlikely	Probable	No	Unlikely

always occurs, we say that it has a probability of 1; thus, all probabilities by definition lie between 0 and 1. We also will note that the probability of one or another finding's occurring is equal to the sum of their individual probabilities if the two events are mutually exclusive. These statements can be summarized as follows:

$$1 \geqslant P(S_1) \geqslant 0 \text{ (S stands for sign or symptom)}$$
$$P(S_1 \cup S_2) = P(S_1) + P(S_2) \text{ if and only if}$$
$$P(S_1 \cap S_2) = 0$$

These statements are identical to those made regarding credibilities.

Thus, study of patients with specific diseases leads to the observation that specific signs and symptoms occur in such patients, and we should be able to appraise the frequency of occurrence of each sign or symptom. Such statements about probabilities of findings, given a specific diagnosis, are called conditional probabilities. Thus, the presence of a specific disease may or may not alter the probability of observing a certain finding or group of findings. As in our table, if we know that a myocardial infarction has occurred, we feel it is very probable that we may elicit a history of severe chest pain, whereas if the patient has had a cerebrovascular accident, this is unlikely.

Thus, estimates of the probability of these various signs and symptoms are conditioned by our consideration of the disease that may be present. These conditional probabilities are written as: $P(Sign/D_k) = ?$

This asks the question, "What is the probability of observing some sign given the condition that a specific diagnosis (D_k) is present?"

Evaluation of the findings.   Let us now return to our example and consider that we have examined the patient as completely as possible and have obtained a group of findings. We evaluate the probability of observing this specific group of findings for each of the conditions under consideration; in other words, we evaluate the conditional probabilities for our set of examination results. We evaluate these as follows:

P(These exam findings/if he had infarction) $= 0.6 = P(Exam/D_1)$
P(Exam findings/cardiac arrhythmia) $= 0.4 = P(Exam/D_2)$
P(Exam findings/stroke) $= 0.2 = P(Exam/D_3)$
P(Exam findings/something else) $= 0.2 = P(Exam/D_4)$

These conditional probability statements are termed the posterior information, since the information is evaluated after the examination of the patient.

Note that we would like to find some sign or symptom or group of observations that has $P(Exam/D_k) = 1$. Or in other words, we would like to find a group of observations that is always evident if a certain disease is present. If an observation may only be made when a certain disease is present, the observation is called a "pathognomonic finding." Conversely, $P(Exam/D_k) = 0$ indicates that the set of findings never occurs if disease D_k is present.

Return now to the partition of the diagnosis list as illustrated in Figure 2–3. Superimposed on this figure is a hatched area representing the information obtained by examining the patient. Note that this area is made up of the intersection of each diagnosis of the partition and the examination information. This is another way of saying that the results of the examination

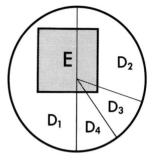

Figure 2-3. *The intersection of the diagnostic possibilities with the findings upon examination of the patient.*

are compatible with more than one diagnosis. Each intersection, represented graphically as a surface of intersection, is symbolically represented by P(Exam ∩ D_k). In other words, any given intersection represents the probability that this set of examination results and the corresponding diagnosis from our list will occur together.

Now, by inspection and intuitively, the conditional probability of obtaining these examination results if any specific diagnosis is present is equal to the probability that the examination results obtained and that particular diagnosis will occur together, divided by the credibility of that diagnosis, or

$$P(Exam/D_k) = \frac{P(Exam \cap D_k)}{C(D_k)}$$

Inspect Figure 2-3 to verify this. Note that if D_1 is known to be present, then the probability that the examination result will be observed is equivalent to the area of intersection divided by the area of D_1 (which represents the credibility of D_1).

Now, rearrangement gives $C(D_k)$ P(Exam/D_k) = P(Exam ∩ D_k). But, as noted, the area representing the probability of obtaining the examination is equal to the sum of the intersection of each diagnosis and the examination; thus, P(Exam) = P(Exam ∩

D_1) + P(Exam D_2) + P(Exam $\cap$ D_3) + P(Exam $\cap$ D_4) and, from the preceding equality, this is equal to adding the following:

$$C(D_1) \; P(Exam/D_1)$$
$$C(D_2) \; P(Exam/D_2)$$
$$C(D_3) \; P(Exam/D_3)$$
$$C(D_4) \; P(Exam/D_4)$$

or we may represent this sum as

$$\sum_{k=1}^{4} C(D_k) \; P(Exam/D_k).$$

This is evaluated numerically in the third column of Table 2–2. We wish now, at the culmination of the diagnostic process, to ask the question: If we obtain a given set of findings on examination, what is the credibility of each of the diagnoses from our list of possibilities; i.e., what is $C(D_k/Exam)$?

As has been demonstrated, the probability of obtaining this examination is equal to

$$C(D_k) \; P(Exam/D_k).$$

For each separate diagnosis, then,

$$C(D_j/Exam) = \frac{C(D_j)P(Exam/D_j)}{\sum\limits_{k=1}^{4} C(D_k)P(Exam/D_k)}$$

TABLE 2–2. EVALUATION OF FOUR HYPOTHETICAL DIAGNOSTIC POSSIBILITIES

D_k	$C(D_k)$	$P(Exam\|D_k)$	$C(D_k)P(Exam\|D_k)$	$\dfrac{C(D_j)P(Exam/D_j)}{\sum\limits_{k=1}^{4}C(D_k)P(Exam/D_k)}$
1	0.5	0.6	0.30	0.65
2	0.3	0.4	0.12	0.26
3	0.1	0.1	0.01	0.02
4	0.1	0.3	0.03	0.07
		Sum	0.46	1.00

This is equivalent to using the diagram of Figure 2–3 as a target for dart throwing. If you hit the area labeled "exam," then what is the probability that the dart also lies in the area of diagnosis 1?

In essence this represents in a simplified manner the diagnostic function. Given a certain set of examination information that is consistent with a number of diagnoses, what is the most likely or most credible diagnosis? Logically, it is that diagnosis that has the greatest probability of association with the available information when compared to all the diagnostic possibilities.

Since the physician operates on the basis of observation, it is imperative that diagnostic skills be developed and studied. The formulation presented allows the use of modern computing devices to assist the physician in defining the degree of certainty associated with his diagnosis of disease. In addition, the signs and symptoms he elicits and discovers must be evaluated as to accuracy, precision, sensitivity, and specificity.

Accuracy and precision. By accuracy we mean that the word, test, or other notation truly describes an actual state of nature. We describe in this book a large number of methods and techniques for personal examination of patients. The terminology we use is generally accepted and, we hope, contains a minimum number of ambiguities. If physicians are to converse intelligently with each other or to learn from past experience, then the words that we use should have precision and accuracy of meaning, just as the tests that we evaluate in the clinical examination and the laboratory x-ray must be accurate and precise.

For example, the word inflammation is used by clinicians to describe skin areas that are red, hot to touch, swollen, and tender. This usage of the word seems accurate, since the word inflammation derives from the root meaning "to set on fire." But what of the use of the word inflammation by pathologists to describe infiltration, hyperemia, and stasis changes that they observe in tissue sections under the microscope? Such double meanings make application of the word imprecise, since we must know something about who is using it to determine what it means. We suggest, therefore, that terms be kept as simple and truly descriptive as possible, consistent with general understanding, and that the Anglo-Saxon roots of the English language be utilized in preference to terms derived from other tongues. If something is red, hot, and tender let us say that. If a patient has fever let us say that, instead of pyrexia. If a patient sweats let us say that, instead of diaphoresis. It should be a goal of the clinician to describe clinical findings with accurate terms used precisely. Unless clinical findings are so evaluated, there is little hope that modern logic theory will be of any aid to the clinician. A computer or sophisticated abstract manipulation will not make inaccurate and imprecise observations more accurate or more precise.

Sensitivity and specificity. Related to the two terms discussed above are the words sensitivity and specificity. Sensitivity relates to the capacity of a test to detect the presence of some given state of nature. Specificity refers to the capacity of a test to demonstrate one characteristic and nothing else. One thus can use a specific test to detect the absence of a given state of nature, i.e., to detect "normal persons." In order to illustrate the two terms, suppose we are concerned with the relationship of the presence of spider nevi to the occurrence of esophageal varices in patients with liver disease. From data collected at the University of Kansas Medical Center, the authors have obtained the following information from 565 patients with liver disease (Table 2–3).

We might ask the question, "How sensitive is the presence of spider nevi in detecting patients with esophageal varices?" This is equivalent to dividing the figure in box A by the total number of cases in boxes A and B or 95/160 or 57 per cent. We are also interested in how specific this test is, that is, in how many patients who do not have spider nevi also do not have esophageal varices. This is equivalent to D/C + D or 298/405 or 74 per cent.

Some tests are quite sensitive, detecting a subtle state of nature, but conversely may be of low specificity since they also "detect" a large percentage of normal persons. Some individuals describe those patients in box B of Table 2–3 as "false negatives"

TABLE 2–3. THE RELATIONSHIP OF SPIDER NEVI TO ESOPHAGEAL VARICES IN LIVER DISEASE*

		Spider Nevi		
		Present	Absent	
Esophageal Varices	Present	A 95	B 65	160
	Absent	C 107	D 298	405
		202	363	565

*From data collected at the University of Kansas Medical Center.

and those in box C as "false positives." We believe that these terms are ambiguous and internally inconsistent. They are usually used because the investigator does not know how many individuals are actually represented in box D.

Operational diagnoses. In order to achieve the aim of clinical medicine, that is, the pragmatic application of knowledge to the benefit of the ill person, we must collect information from the clinical examination in an accurate manner, describe it precisely, and evaluate its sensitivity and specificity. We believe that the dynamic and daily evaluation of signs and symptoms is the maneuver that produces the operational definitions upon which clinicians act, regardless of the diagnostic label attached to the patient. Diagnostic labels are important from the standpoint of description of groups of patients, the study of disease processes in these patients, and the overall evaluation of therapeutic management. Individual management of patients, however, rests with the signs and symptoms that each patient manifests, and the physician's actions are conditioned and directed by these manifestations. This is what we mean by operational diagnoses—they are the groups of signs and symptoms that the physician actually uses in making decisions about management and therapy of the ill person.

The Medical Record

Usage and function. The physician in his daily work deals with a great variety of problems. As Weed has said, "It is this multiplicity of problems. . . that constitutes the principal distinguishing feature between his activities and those of other scientists." Dr. Weed has long reasoned that clinical instruction of physicians should be based upon a system that assists them in defining and following patients' problems one by one while systematically relating and resolving them. Specifically he suggests as the core of this orderly approach "the problem-oriented record." This plan is no radical departure from tradition but clearly is a design for indexing and organizing initial and continuing observations required in the study of a patient. This plan has great appeal because of its real effectiveness as a learning device for the student. The complaint that the system adds too much burdensome detail is more apparent than real; in fact, many economies of all variety and improved effectiveness in patient care quickly accrue to conscientious adherents.

Persuasion that there is need for an orderly display of biomedical, emotional, and social data concerning a patient and his health problems is far more important than acceptance of any rigid format. Many modifications of the problem-oriented record will no doubt be created, but there are certain basic characteristics of this chart form as outlined by Dr. Weed, as noted in the following discussion.

Data base. This unit of information begins with elicitation and recording of the traditional *chief complaint* followed by suitable development of the *present illness,* giving consideration to the presenting complaint but also including current and active problems. Each problem needs to be recorded and served separately. Each problem is designated by its main symptom if new and unrefined, but by classical diagnostic terms if well documented. Data included under each numbered problem should be subdivided as follows: (1) Subjective (Subj.) — symptoms as presented by the patient. (2) Objective (Obj.) — certain and documented historical data such as previous records, x-ray and laboratory data, or surgery and biopsy reports. (3) Treatment (Rx) — includes such items as properly identified medications, diets, and physical therapy. (4) Significant negatives (Neg) — includes responses to questions posed regarding symptoms. An optional approach used by many physicians is that of simply eliciting the problems and then developing the usual and appropriate information concerning each item in the area devoted to the present illness, devoting only brief attention to previous, chronic, or resolved problems.

The *Past History, System Review, Social History, Family History,* and details of the *Patient Profile,* including typical and usual activities, are framed in the usual manner. The *Physical Examination* adds significantly to the data base.

Variable but locally determined *Baseline Laboratory Data* are collected and added to the collected information. This usually includes a blood count, urinalysis, VDRL, chest x-ray, electrocardiographic tracing, blood urea nitrogen, blood sugar, and perhaps blood cholesterol.

Problem list. This list is constructed by identification of all problems from the past and in the present. Plans for ideal patient care require that such a list be complete, including incidentals as well as more serious problems. Biomedical, emotional, and social difficulties assume equal status in programs of therapy for the total patient. Any manifestations of an illness requiring a plan for resolution deserve the status and listing of a problem. The total exhibition of all problems in the form recognized is essential in all health records.

Variable sophistication in the listed problems is to be expected and in fact is preferable of a problem in terms of a finished diagnosis before the data make such a conclusion valid. Replacing the complaint of "chest pain" with the term "myocardial infarction" or "ischemic heart disease" prior to development of valid documentation is premature; however, such refinement of the problems should promptly follow collection of information which makes this proper. The problems then will range from physical findings or symptoms through abnormal laboratory findings, physiological aberrations such as atrial fibrillation, to an etiological diagnosis such as rheumatic heart disease with mitral stenosis.

If a refined and listed diagnosis has several conspicuous signs or symptoms, they may logically be listed as a part of the problem. If, as observations proceed, one of these signs requires special attention, it may then be listed as a separate problem to make certain that suitable observations are made and progress is recorded. The attitude of the observer should be that of clarifying the record for any other secondary observer with a minimum of effort and confusion.

As quickly as warranted, problems are elevated from a less to a more sophisticated status until an acceptable final diagnosis is achieved, i.e., chest pain, myocardial infarction, ischemic heart disease with posterior myocardial infarction.

Initial plan. The initial plans should include the following three elements.

Diagnostic considerations. The differential diagnosis is placed here with clear indication of the diagnostic approach that will be used to identify the correct diagnosis. Each hypothesis or diagnostic possibility should be tied to a specific plan so that the strategy is clear. Lumping a long list of possibilities and covering this with a long list of general plan items is not acceptable.

Therapeutic plans. Even though symptom-oriented and noncurative, these parts of the orders are also linked to the numbered problems.

Education of the patient. This portion of the plan may be simple and meager, but discipline in total patient care requires it.

Progress notes. Pertinent information gathered from the patient, the laboratory, or consultations must be incorporated in a problem-oriented fashion in order to show the daily progress

(Text continued on page 86.)

A

UNIVERSITY OF KANSAS MEDICAL CENTER
RAINBOW BLVD. AT 39TH ST., KANSAS CITY, KANSAS 66103

DEPARTMENT OF MEDICINE

PROBLEM LIST

PROBLEM NUMBER	DATE ONSET	PROBLEM	DATE RESOLVED	PROBLEM NUMBER	DATE ONSET	PROBLEM	DATE RESOLVED

PROBLEM LIST

Chart continued on following pages.

Chart continued.

1

UNIVERSITY OF KANSAS MEDICAL CENTER

TIME:_____ DATE:_____ PLACE:_____

INFORMANT:_____ RELIABILITY:_____

REFERRAL SOURCE:_____ REFERRAL LETTER: YES NO

ADDRESS:_____

ANTICIPATED DISCHARGE DISPOSITION:_____
(REF. M.D., KUMC CLINIC, OTHER M.D.)

PATIENT

NAME:_____

AGE:_____ SEX:_____ RACE:_____

PROFILE

BIRTHPLACE:_____

RESIDENCE(S):_____ EDUCATION:_____

OCCUPATION(S):_____

MARITAL STATUS: M S W D RELIGION:_____ NUMBER OF CHILDREN:_____

AGES AND SEXES OF CHILDREN:_____

MILITARY EXPERIENCE, FOREIGN TRAVEL:_____

BRIEF DESCRIPTION OF LIFE STYLE (HOME SITUATION, AVERAGE DAY, ETC):_____

HABITS	MEDICATIONS	DIET ESTIMATED CALORIE INTAKE, BALANCE, MEAL DISTRIBUTION, IDIOSYNCRACIES, ETC.	ALLERGIES
TOBACCO:____	1.____		1.____
	2.____		2.____
ALCOHOL:____	3.____		3.____
	4.____		4.____
OTHER:____	5.____		5.____
	6.____		6.____
	7.____		7.____

PATIENT   **DATA BASE**   PROFILE

PRESENT ILLNESS	DATA BASE	PRESENT ILLNESS

CHIEF COMPLAINT:

HISTORY OF THE PRESENT ILLNESS:

BINDING LINE

Chart continued on following pages.

Chart continued.

3

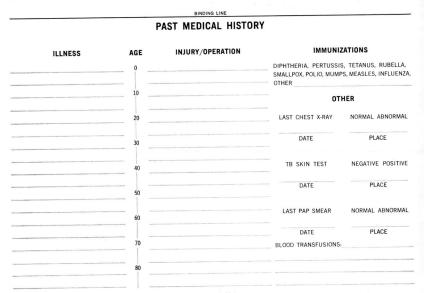

BINDING LINE

PAST MEDICAL HISTORY

ILLNESS	AGE	INJURY/OPERATION	IMMUNIZATIONS
	0		DIPHTHERIA, PERTUSSIS, TETANUS, RUBELLA, SMALLPOX, POLIO, MUMPS, MEASLES, INFLUENZA, OTHER

OTHER

LAST CHEST X-RAY	NORMAL ABNORMAL
DATE	PLACE
TB SKIN TEST	NEGATIVE POSITIVE
DATE	PLACE
LAST PAP SMEAR	NORMAL ABNORMAL
DATE	PLACE

BLOOD TRANSFUSIONS:

AGE markers: 0, 10, 20, 30, 40, 50, 60, 70, 80

FAMILY HISTORY

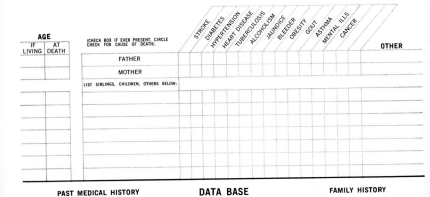

AGE IF LIVING	AGE AT DEATH	(CHECK BOX IF EVER PRESENT, CIRCLE CHECK FOR CAUSE OF DEATH).	STROKE	DIABETES	HYPERTENSION	HEART DISEASE	TUBERCULOSIS	ALCOHOLISM	JAUNDICE	BLEEDER	OBESITY	GOUT	ASTHMA	MENTAL ILLS	CANCER	OTHER
		FATHER														
		MOTHER														
		LIST SIBLINGS, CHILDREN, OTHERS BELOW:														

PAST MEDICAL HISTORY   DATA BASE   FAMILY HISTORY

SYSTEMS REVIEW	**DATA BASE**	SYSTEMS REVIEW

INSTRUCTIONS FOR COMPLETING REMAINDER OF THIS FORM:

1. Fill in blanks, where indicated.

2. Circle to indicate a positive or abnormal response or finding; elaborate and use drawings.

3. Underline to indicate a negative or normal response or finding.

4. Leave unmarked to indicate no response, question not asked, or examination not done.

GENERAL: WEIGHT: AT 18 YRS._____KG.
MAXIMUM____KG, MINIMUM____KG.
RECENT LOSS OR GAIN, WEAKNESS,
FATIGUE, FEVER, CHILLS, NIGHT SWEATS,
ANOREXIA, INSOMNIA,
SYNCOPE, OTHER.

SKIN: COLOR CHANGE, ITCHING, RASH,
MOLES, HAIR CHANGE, NAIL CHANGE,
OTHER.

HEAD: TRAUMA, HEADACHES, OTHER.

EYES: BLURRED VISION, GLASSES,
CONTACT LENSES, BLIND SPOTS,
SCOTOMA, REDNESS, ITCHING, BURNING,
DRYNESS, EXCESSIVE TEARING, PAIN,
GLAUCOMA, DATE LAST EXAM_____,
OTHER.

EARS: DEAFNESS, TINNITUS, DISCHARGE,
PAIN, OTHER.

NOSE: DECREASED SMELL, BLEEDING,
DRYNESS, DISCHARGE, OBSTRUCTION,
PAIN, OTHER.

MOUTH: BLEEDING GUMS, SORE TONGUE,
DENTAL PROBLEMS, PAIN, POST-NASAL DRIP,
OTHER.

THROAT: SORE THROAT, DYSPHAGIA,
PAIN, HOARSENESS, TONSILLITIS, OTHER.

NECK: STIFFNESS, DECREASED MOTION,
PAIN, OTHER.

BREASTS: DISCHARGE, LUMPS, PAIN,
BLEEDING, NIPPLE RETRACTION, OTHER.

RESPIRATORY: COUGH, SPUTUM,
PLEURISY, HEMOPTYSIS, WHEEZING,
DYSPNEA, EXPOSURE TO TB, OTHER.

CARDIAC: CHEST PAIN AT REST,
CHEST PAIN ON EXERTION,
PAROXYSMAL NOCTURNAL DYSPNEA,
ORTHOPNEA, EDEMA, PALPITATION,
CYANOSIS, MURMUR, OTHER.

VASCULAR: PHLEBITIS, VARICOSITIES,
CLAUDICATION, RAYNAUD'S, OTHER.

BINDING LINE

4

Chart continued on following pages.

Chart continued.

5

BINDING LINE

GASTROINTESTINAL: NAUSEA,
VOMITING, ANTACID USE, BELCHING,
DYSPHAGIA, HEARTBURN, HEMATEMESIS,
MELENA, CHANGE IN BOWEL HABITS,
HEMATOCHEZIA, LAXATIVE USE, ENEMA USE,
FISSURES, FISTULA-IN-ANO,
RECTAL ABSCESS, RECENT X-RAY STUDIES,
DIARRHEA, CONSTIPATION,
CLAY-COLORED STOOL, JAUNDICE,
DARK URINE, BLOATING, HEMORRHOIDS,
HERNIA, OTHER.

GENITO-URINARY: DYSURIA, URGENCY,
FREQUENCY, HESITANCY, SMALL STREAM,
INCONTINENCE, DRIBBLING, DISCHARGE,
STONES, POLYURIA, NOCTURIA,
HEMATURIA, VD, SEXUAL PROBLEMS,
OTHER.

GYNECOLOGIC: MENARCHE AGE_____,
CLIMACTERIC AGE_____,
POST-MENOPAUSAL BLEEDING,
IRREGULAR FLOW, LIGHT FLOW, HEAVY FLOW,
SPOTTING, DYSPAREUNIA,
VAGINAL DISCHARGE, CONTRACEPTION,
GRAVIDA_____PARA_____
AB_____OTHER.

MUSCULO-SKELETAL: MUSCLE PAIN,
CRAMPS, WEAKNESS, WASTING, TRAUMA,
TENDERNESS, FRACTURE, JOINT PAIN,
JOINT SWELLING, JOINT STIFFNESS,
KYPHOSIS, SCOLIOSIS, LORDOSIS,
THORACIC EXCURSION, OTHER.

NEUROLOGICAL: SEIZURES, TICS,
VERTIGO, DIZZINESS, TREMOR,
PARESTHESIAS, DYSARTHRIA,
INCOORDINATION, OTHER.

PSYCHIATRIC: NERVOUSNESS,
HYPERVENTILATION, DEPRESSION,
INSOMNIA, THOUGHT OF SUICIDE,
EMOTIONAL INSTABILITY, ILLUSIONS,
HALLUCINATIONS, DELUSIONS,
MEMORY IMPAIRMENT, OTHER.

ENDOCRINE: HEAT INTOLERANCE,
COLD INTOLERANCE, CHANGE IN HAIR DIST.,
BREAST CHANGE, VOICE CHANGE,
POLYDIPSIA, POLYURIA, OTHER.

HEMATOLOGIC: ANEMIA, EASY BRUISING,
EASY BLEEDING, BLEEDING GUMS,
LYMPHADENOPATHY, OTHER.

SYSTEMS REVIEW · **DATA BASE** SYSTEMS REVIEW

PHYSICAL EXAMINATION	**DATA BASE**	PHYSICAL EXAMINATION

VITAL SIGNS:

TEMP._____RESP._____WT. _____HT._____

	SUPINE	SITTING	STANDING
PULSE: REG., IRREG.			
BLOOD PRESSURE — RA			
LA			
LEG			

GENERAL DESCRIPTION:

BEHAVIOR DURING INTERVIEW:

SKIN: NORMAL; DRY, MOIST, COARSE, SMOOTH, RASH, SCARS, TELANGIECTASIA, NEVI, PETECHIAE, NAIL CHANGES, PIGMENTATION OR DISCOLORATIONS, NEEDLE TRACKS, ECCHYMOSES, HIRSUITISM, LOSS OF HAIR, OTHER.

LYMPH NODES: NORMAL; CERVICAL, SUPRACLAVICULAR, EPITROCHLEAR, AXILLARY, INGUINAL, FEMORAL, SPLEEN, OTHER.

EYES: NORMAL; BULB, SCLERAE, CORNEA, CONJUNCTIVAE, EYEBROWS.

PUPIL: SIZE R_____MM L_____MM. REACT TO LIGHT, ACCOMMODATION. VISUAL ACUITY, NYSTAGMUS.

FUNDI: DISCS, ARTERIES, VEINS, HEMORRHAGES, EXUDATES, MICROANEURYSMS.

OD(RIGHT)   OS(LEFT)

VISUAL FIELDS: NORMAL, ABNORMAL.

(SEE NEURO FOR E.O.M.)

OD   OS

EARS: NORMAL; PINNA, TOPHI, CANAL, TYMPANIC MEMBRANE, DISCHARGE, CERUMEN, OTHER. (SEE NEURO FOR HEARING)

NOSE: NORMAL; SEPTUM, MUCOSA, OBSTRUCTION, SINUS TENDERNESS, OTHER.

BINDING LINE

6

Chart continued on following pages.

Chart continued.

7

BINDING LINE

MOUTH AND THROAT: NORMAL; LIPS, GUMS, TONGUE, BUCCAL MUCOSA, TEETH, TONSILS, UVULA, PHARYNX, SALIVARY GLANDS.

NECK: NORMAL; THYROID, TRACHEA, VENOUS DISTENSION—(SEE C.V. EXAM) NUCHAL RIGIDITY, MASS, NODES, BRUITS.

BREASTS: NORMAL; MASS, TENDERNESS, DISCHARGE, RETRACTION, ULCERATION, ASYMMETRY, DIMPLING, OTHER.

RESPIRATORY: RESP. _____/MIN.; NORMAL; LABORED, SHALLOW, KUSSMAUL, PERIODIC, OTHER.

USE OF ACCESSORY MUSCLES:	NO	YES	GRADE 1-4
NORMAL; SCALENES			
STERNOCLEIDOMASTOIDS			
OTHER			

CHEST AND LUNGS:
  INSPECTION: NORMAL;
  PALPATION: NORMAL;
  PERCUSSION: NORMAL;
  AUSCULATION: NORMAL;

CARDIOVASCULAR:

PERIPHERAL PULSES: NORMAL;

	R	L	
CAROTID			
BRACHIAL			
RADIAL			0=ABSENT
FEMORAL			1=DECREASED / 2=NORMAL
POPLITEAL			3=HYPERACTIVE
DORSALIS PEDIS			B=BRUIT
POST. TIBIAL			

CAROTID PULSE: NORMAL;
  QUALITY:
  AMPLITUDE:
  RATE:
  RHYTHM:

JUGULAR VEINOUS PULSE: NORMAL;
  EXT. JUGULAR VEINS ARE DISTENDED
  TO_____CMS ABOVE ANGLE OF LOUIS
  AT_____DEGREES TRUNCAL ELEV. FROM SUPINE

HEART:

  INSPECTION: NORMAL;

  PALPATION: NORMAL;

  PERCUSSION: NORMAL;

  AUSCULTATION: NORMAL;

	S_4	$M_1 T_1$	S.E.C.	$A_2 P_2$	O.S.	S_3
AORTIC						
LSB						
APEX						

PHYSICAL EXAMINATION   **DATA BASE**   PHYSICAL EXAMINATION

PHYSICAL EXAMINATION	DATA BASE	PHYSICAL EXAMINATION

ABDOMEN:
  INSPECTION: NORMAL;
    SCAPHOID, FLAT, DISTENDED, OBESE,
    DILATED VEINS, SCARS, OTHER.
  PALPATION: NORMAL; RIGIDITY,
    TENDERNESS, REBOUND, GUARDING,
    MASS, FLUID WAVE, HERNIA, LIVER
    (SPAN AT MCL:_____CMS.).
  PERCUSSION: NORMAL; TYPANI,
    SHIFTING DULLNESS, OTHER.
  AUSCULTATION: NORMAL; BOWEL SOUNDS
    (HIGH-PITCHED, RUSHES, ABSENT, DISMISSED)
    RUBS, BRUITS, OTHER.

GENITALIA:
  MALE: NORMAL; TESTIS, SCROTAL MASS,
    EDEMA, TENDERNESS, PENILE LESION,
    DISCHARGE, OTHER.
  FEMALE: NORMAL PELVIC; LABIA, BSU,
    CLITORIS, INTROITUS, CERVIX, UTERUS,
    ADNEXAE, CUL DE SAC, DISCHARGE,
    PAIN WITH CERVIX MOVEMENT, OTHER.
  PAP SMEAR: DONE, NOT DONE
  VAGINAL MATURATION INDEX: DONE, NOT DONE.

RECTAL: NORMAL; SPHINCTERTONE,
    TENDERNESS, FISSURE, HEMORRHOID,
    MASS, OTHER.
  STOOL: ABSENT, PRESENT, COLOR _____
  BLOOD: GROSS, OCCULT NEGATIVE, POSITIVE
  PROSTATE: NORMAL, OTHER.

EXTREMITIES: NORMAL; EDEMA,
    CYANOSIS, VARICOSITIES, ULCERATION,
    CLUBBING, OTHER.

  BONES AND JOINTS: NORMAL; SWELLING,
    RESTRICTION, TENDERNESS, WARMTH,
    REDNESS, DEFORMITY, OTHER.

NEUROLOGICAL:
  MENTAL STATUS: NORMAL;
    APPEARANCE: DISORDERED, AVERAGE, NEAT, BIZARRE.
    PSYCHOMOTOR ACTIVITY: NONE, SLOW, AVERAGE, FAST.
    AFFECT: FLAT, AVERAGE, EXAGGERATED, LABILE.
    MOOD AND ATTITUDE: DETACHED, SAD, SUSPICIOUS, HOSTILE, DEMANDING, OBSTINATE,
      ANXIOUS, FRIENDLY, SEDUCTIVE, HELPLESS, COOPERATIVE.
    SPEECH AND ASSOCIATIONS: MUTE, DISORGANIZED, LOOSE, CIRCUMSTANTIAL, AVERAGE,
      LOGICAL.
    THINKING STYLE: CONCRETE, FUNCTIONAL, ABSTRACT.
    INTELLIGENCE: RETARDED, DULL - NORMAL, NORMAL, BRIGHT.
    MEMORY IMPAIRMENT: NONE, REMOTE, RECENT.
    JUDGMENT: POOR, AVERAGE, GOOD.
    DISORIENTATION: NONE, (TIME, PLACE, PERSON).
    INSIGHT: NONE; LITTLE, AVERAGE, GOOD.
    SUICIDE: NONE, IDEATION, THREAT, ATTEMPT, NO INFORMATION.

BINDING LINE

8

Chart continued on following pages.

Chart continued.

9

BINDING LINE

NEUROLOGIC: (CONT.)

CRANIAL NERVES: NORMAL

  I. NORMAL; ABNORMAL

  II. NORMAL; ABNORMAL (SEE EYE FOR V.F.'S)

  III, IV, VI. NORMAL; ABNORMAL (PUPILS, PTOSIS, EOM, NYSTAGMUS)

  V. NORMAL; ABNORMAL (3 DIVISIONS — CORNEAL, MASSETERS, TEMPORAL, PIN AND TOUCH)

  VII. NORMAL; ABNORMAL (BROW, MOUTH, NASO-LABIAL FOLD, TASTE)

  VIII. NORMAL; ABNORMAL (RINNÉ WEBER, WHISPERED VOICE)

  IX, X. NORMAL; ABNORMAL (SWALLOW, UVULA, GAG, PHONATION)

  XI. NORMAL; ABNORMAL (STERNOCLEIDOMASTOID, TRAPEZIUS)

  XII. NORMAL; ABNORMAL (PROTRUSION, TREMOR, FASCICULATION, ATROPHY)

REFLEXES:

STRETCH	R	L		SUPERFICIAL	R	L
JAW			0—ABSENT	ABDOMINAL		
BRACHIORADIALIS			1—DIMINISHED	CREMASTERIC		
BICEPS			2—NORMAL	PLANTAR		
TRICEPS			3—INCREASED			
KNEE			4—CLONUS	FRONTAL LOBE		
ANKLE				SUCK		

FRONTAL LOBE — CHECK IF PRESENT

	R	L
SUCK		
SNOUT		
PALMO-MENT.		
GRASP		

RELAXATION PHASE: NORMAL; PROLONGED

MOTOR:

  MUSCULAR STRENGTH: NORMAL; ABNORMAL (HEMIPARESIS, HEIMPLEGIA, PROX. WEAK)

  MUSCULAR TONE: NORMAL; ABNORMAL (SPASTIC, FLACCID, RIGID, COGWHEEL, CONTRACTURE)

  MUSCULAR VOLUME: NORMAL; ABNORMAL (ATROPHY, HYPERTROPHY)

  INVOLUNTARY MOVEMENTS: NOT PRESENT; PRESENT (TREMOR, DYSTONIA, ASTERIXIS, CHOREA)

COORDINATION:

  LIMB: NORMAL; ABNORMAL (F-N, F-F, H-K, RAPID ALTERNATING)

  GAIT: NORMAL; ABNORMAL (WALK, HEEL, TOE, TANDEM)

  ROMBERG: NORMAL; ABNORMAL

SENSORY:

  BASIC SENSATION: NORMAL; ABNORMAL (PAIN, TOUCH, TEMP, VIB., POSITION)

  CORTICAL SENSATION: NORMAL; ABNORMAL (2 POINT DISCRIMINATION, OBJECT IDENTIFICATION)

MENINGEAL SIGNS: NOT PRESENT; PRESENT (BRUDZINSKI, KERNIG, NECK RIGIDITY)

SCREENING LAB: This is data to be obtained within the first 24 hours, unless this information has been obtained recently. If the item relates to a problem, refer in the blank to that problem number, where the result is listed under objective data.

Hgb_____ Hct_____ Wbc_____ Diff._____ Sed Rate_____ BUN_____ BS_____ Ca_____

Uric Acid_____ Chol._____ VDRL_____ Urinalysis_____

Sickle Cell prep. (Blacks)_____ Tbc Skin Test: PPD Strength_____ Reaction_____ Cms.

EKG (MEN OVER 35); NORMAL; ABNORMAL

CHEST X-RAY: NORMAL; ABNORMAL

OTHER:

EXAMINER'S SIGNATURES:
Student
House–Staff
House–Staff
Senior Staff

PHYSICAL EXAMINATION   **DATA BASE**   PHYSICAL EXAMINATION

Chart continued.

INITIAL PROBLEM LIST:

INITIAL PLAN (For each active problem—include diagnostic impression and/or differential diagnoses):

10

in solution of the patient's problems. These notes, arranged in orderly fashion, include *subjective* statements by the patient, *objective* findings of the examiner, *assessment* by the physician or other examiner, and further *plans* now indicated in either the diagnostic or therapeutic category.

The illustrated history form is not necessarily ideal but serves as a prototype of the structuring desirable if a standard data base is to be made for each and every patient entering the health care system. Each patient is at some time entitled to such a recording of his health status. Obviously, for a minor problem of episodic character such an elaborate format does not seem quite appropriate, but for continuing care it does seem essential. For the less important and subsequent encounters this is not required; a simpler form can in these instances be supplemented.

BIBLIOGRAPHY

Bauer, J.: Differential Diagnosis of Internal Diseases. New York, Grune & Stratton, 1955.

Bird, B.: Talking with Patients. Philadelphia, J. B. Lippincott Co., 1955.

Bjorn, J. C., and Cross, H. D.: Problem Oriented Practice. Chicago, Modern Hospital Press, 1970.

Charvát, J., McGuire, C., and Parsons, V.: A review of the nature and uses of examinations in medical education. WHO Public Health Papers, 36:1, 1968.

Chesterton, G. K.: Practical Cogitator or the Thinker's Anthology. Boston, Houghton Mifflin Co., 1953.

Davis, R. E.: Teaching physical diagnosis: Emotions and privileges. J.A.M.A., 226:1114, 1973.

DeGowin, E., and DeGowin, R.: Bedside Diagnostic Examination. 2nd ed. New York, The Macmillan Co., 1969.

Engle, R. L.: Medical diagnosis: Present, past and future. II. Philosophical foundations and historical development of our concepts of health, disease, and diagnosis. Ann. Intern. Med., 112:520, 1963.

Engle, R. L.: Medical diagnosis: Present, past and future. III. Diagnosis in the future, including a critique on the use of electronic computers as diagnostic aids to the physician. Ann. Intern. Med., 112:530, 1963.

Engle, R. L., and Davis, R. J.: Medical diagnosis: Present, past and future. I. Present concepts of the meaning and limitations of medical diagnosis. Ann. Intern. Med., 112:512, 1963.

Feinstein, A.: Clinical Judgment. Baltimore, Williams & Wilkins Co., 1967.

Feinstein, A. R.: Scientific methodology in clinical medicine. Ann. Intern. Med., *61*:1162, 1964.

Graham, J. R.: Systematic evaluation of clinical competence. J. Med. Educ., *46*:625, 1971.

Harvey, A. M., and Bordley, J.: Differential Diagnosis. Philadelphia, W. B. Saunders Co., 1972.

Hockstein, E., and Rubin, A. L.: Physical Diagnosis. New York, McGraw-Hill Book Co., 1964.

Hurst, J. W., and Walker, H.: The Problem Oriented System. New York, Medcom Press, Inc., 1972.

Judge, R. D., and Zuidima, G. A.: Physical Diagnosis. Boston, Little, Brown & Co., 1968.

MacBryde, C. M.: Signs and Symptoms. Philadelphia, J. B. Lippincott Co., 1970.

Morgan, W. L., Jr., and Engel, G. L.: The Clinical Approach to the Patient. Philadelphia, W. B. Saunders Co., 1969.

Pickering, G.: Physician and scientist. Br. Med. J., *2*:1615, 1964.

Price, R. B., and Vlahcevic, Z. R.: Logical principles in differential diagnosis. Ann. Intern. Med., *75*:89, 1971.

Quarrick, E. A., and Sloop, E. W.: A method for identifying the criteria of good performance in a medical clerkship program. J. Med. Educ., *47*:188, 1972.

Robbins, L. C., and Hall, J. H.: How to Practice Prospective Medicine. Indianapolis, Methodist Hospital of Indiana, 1970.

Weed, L. L.: Medical Records, Medical Education, and Patient Care. Cleveland, The Press of Case Western Reserve University, 1969.

White, K. L., et al.: School of Medicine and North Carolina Memorial Hospital, The University of North Carolina, Chapel Hill, N. C. Chicago, The Year Book Publishers, Inc., 1960.

3
EXAMINATION OF THE SKIN

When you glance at a patient, or later examine him more carefully, you first see the skin. Therefore, look for any sign that will provide a clue as to the reason for the patient's visit. The experienced and observant physician learns to recognize and interpret cutaneous signs of internal and external disease. The ruddy face of a hypertensive patient, the brown face and hands of a patient with Addison's disease (Fig. 14–7) or porphyria (Fig. 3–1), the pale face of an anemic or chronically ill patient, the flushed, perspiring face of a feverish patient, and the yellowish tinge of the skin in a jaundiced patient are all important signs that provide valuable clues to the well trained physician.

The physician of the past observed and appreciated these signs since there were few laboratory tests available to assist him in the diagnosis of disease. The picture of the family doctor with his chin on his hand watching the patient is known to all. The modern physician makes a grave mistake if he overlooks the information that can be obtained from an adequate history and a careful examination of the largest organ of the body, the skin.

History taking, as it relates to the skin, can be a short procedure for the patient with a wart on his finger, or it can be extensive for the patient with generalized urticaria or diffuse pigmentation of the skin.

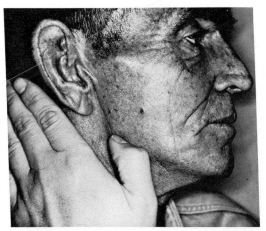

Figure 3–1. *Increased skin pigmentation of face of patient with porphyria cutanea tarda compared to normal hand.*

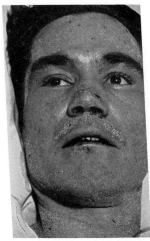

Figure 3–2. *Urea frost in patient with chronic nephritis.*

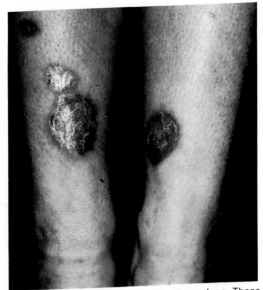

Figure 3–3. *Necrobiosis lipoidica diabeticorum on legs. These are reddish yellow indurated plaques.*

Although patients may not complain of symptoms involving the skin, these questions should be asked routinely:

"Have you had any skin troubles in the past?"

"Do you now have any 'breaking out' or rash on your skin?"

"Does your skin itch?"

"Do you have any sores that have not healed?"

"Does the sun have any bad effect on your skin?"

"Have you ever had any x-ray or radium treatments?"

"What is your occupation?"

If a skin disease or lesion is the chief complaint of the patient, the following facts of his past history must be obtained:

"Where did the skin disease first begin, on the arm, leg, ear, or somewhere else?" This question will often provide a clue to the cause of a dermatitis and emphasizes the fact that a certain area was the primary site. A generalized dermatitis rarely begins all over the body; it usually starts on an ear, foot, or some other part, before spreading.

"What have you been using as local treatment for this skin trouble?" There are two reasons for this question. First, local home therapy may have aggravated the disease, since "over-treatment dermatitis" is a common condition. Second, if the patient says he has been using calamine lotion for his rash, you would be thought woefully inadequate in the art of medicine if you prescribed a similar medication without explaining why.

"Are you taking any medicine by mouth or by shot for any disease? Are you taking any laxatives, vitamins, aspirin, or other drugs?" These questions should always be included in any medical history but are especially important in relation to skin disease, since drugs commonly cause skin eruptions. It is important to specifically mention laxatives, vitamins, and other commonly used medicines because people forget that these are drugs.

Always ask if there is a history of allergy in the patient or in the family, and ask, "Have you had any asthma, hay fever, or eczema?" There are two reasons for this question, also. Eczema is a

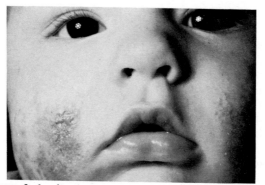

Figure 3-4. Atopic eczema of cheeks with crusted lesions.

common skin problem, and so knowledge of a previous history of eczema could assist in making a diagnosis. Also, allergic patients have a more sensitive or "itchy" skin, and do not respond as well to local therapy. It is helpful to know this fact in advance since you can thus predict, "Mrs. Jones, don't expect to be cured of your hand dermatitis in a few days. Some cases require several weeks, and even then the trouble can recur."

"Does this skin lesion itch? How severe is the itching?" A good index of the severity is whether the patient is awakened from sleep by the itching. If he is awakened by the itching, it should be labeled as severe. The presence or absence of itching in a generalized eruption is important in establishing a diagnosis. Patients with pityriasis rosea experience itching, but the rash of secondary syphilis, which can mimic pityriasis rosea, almost never itches. This fact is so important that if a rash resembling pityriasis rosea does not itch, a serologic test for syphilis should be performed.

"What cosmetic preparations, facial make-up, skin lotions, soaps, or hair preparations do you use?" The skin is affected by the chemicals applied to it, and one must consider the effect of cosmetics and soaps. The commonly used emollient, lanolin, irritates the skin of children with atopic eczema, and bathing too frequently causes the skin of the elderly to itch and crack.

EXAMINATION OF THE SKIN

In a careful and complete examination of the skin, these points must be emphasized.

1. Good lighting is necessary. Some faintly erythematous lesions are not visible without adequate light.

2. Examine the skin in its entirety. The clothes must be removed if there is any indication of a generalized eruption or if the eruption that is visible is puzzling. Do not take the patient's word that there isn't some rash elsewhere on the body. They may think that what they have elsewhere is unrelated to the visi-

ble skin lesion. This is a decision you must make after a complete examination.

3. Don't be afraid to touch the skin and the skin lesions. Palpate any nodules or papules, roll the lesions between your thumb and forefinger, scrape off any scale so that you can see the base, or stretch the skin to see if the lesion blanches.

4. Make a close-up examination of the lesions. Look for the primary lesion. Even in an extensive dermatitis, the primary lesion may be seen at the edge of a group or patch of lesions. Note the secondary or special type lesions. Use a hand lens to observe fine diagnostic points, such as Wickham's striae in lichen planus.

5. Examine the nails, the hair, and the mucous membranes of the mouth, nose, and anogenital area.

6. Special equipment and techniques can be used for examining specific skin lesions. These include examination by Wood's light (a specially filtered ultraviolet light that delivers about 3650 Å radiation) for tinea of the scalp, patch testing for contact allergens, scraping the skin for potassium hydroxide preparations of fungi, cultures of scrapings on Sabouraud's agar for fungi, and cultures for bacteria. The surgical removal of a skin lesion for histopathological study is a special procedure. Other laboratory procedures may or may not be indicated.

After a careful examination of the entire skin, these questions should be answered as you write your record.

1. General condition of the skin? Is the texture dry, moist, scaly, or greasy; is the consistency firm, flabby, or soft; is the color pale, red, or brown?

2. Location or distribution of lesions? "On the arm . . ."

3. Color of the lesion or lesions? "A red . . ."

4. Configuration of lesion or lesions? "Diffuse," "discrete," "well circumscribed."

5. Shape? "Flat," "oval," "irregular."

6. Size? "25¢ sized," "3 × 5 cm.," "extensive," "generalized," and so on.

7. Lesion type (primary or secondary)? "Papule," "scaly patch," "lichenified area," and so on.

8. Odor? Make a note of the odor of the lesions.

Additional information that should be entered on the record:

1. Arrangement of the lesions: "grouped," "single."

2. Relationship of lesion to the hair follicles: "around hair follicles," "at hair follicles," and so on (Fig. 3–5).

3. Examination of the scalp. You must part the hair with your fingers or a comb to adequately examine the hair and scalp.

4. Examine a hair or hairs separately. Hairs may be knotted, broken off, or brushlike on the ends.

5. Inspect the fingernails and toenails. Psoriasis can be confirmed by the presence of pits in the nail plate, or evidence of systemic disease can be confirmed by a change in nail plate growth (Fig. 3–6).

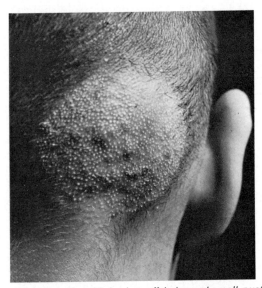

Figure 3–5. *Tinea capitis with broken-off hairs and small pustules of the scalp.*

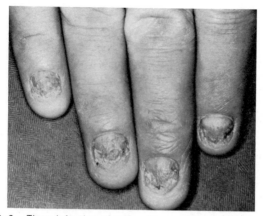

Figure 3–6. *Tinea infection of nails with crumbling of distal nail plate.*

6. Record the results of examination of the mucous membranes of the mouth, lips, nasal opening, and anogenital area.

7. Do not forget the ears and the auditory canals.

PRIMARY, SECONDARY, AND SPECIAL SKIN LESIONS

In order to accurately describe a skin lesion, you must learn a few simple terms. To the uninitiated, many skin eruptions may look alike, but most of them have characteristic *primary lesions.* Well defined *secondary lesions* result from scratching, infection, or overtreatment.

Primary Lesions

Macules are up to 1 cm. in size, circumscribed, flat discolorations of the skin (Fig. 3–7). Examples: freckles and flat nevi.

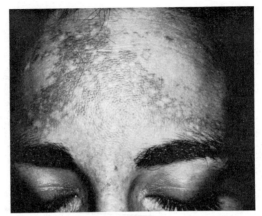

Figure 3–7. Chloasma of forehead demonstrating macular lesions.

Patches are larger than 1 cm., circumscribed, flat discolorations (Fig. 3–8). Examples: vitiligo, senile freckles, and measles rash.

Papules are up to 1 cm., circumscribed, elevated, superficial solid lesions (Figs. 3–9 to 3–14). Examples: elevated nevi, warts, and lichen planus.

A wheal is a type of papule that is edematous and transitory (Fig. 3–15). Examples: hives and insect bites.

Plaques are larger than 1 cm. and are circumscribed, elevated, superficial solid lesions (Fig. 3–16). Examples: mycosis fungoides and localized neurodermatitis.

Nodules are up to 1 cm. in size and are solid lesions whose depth may be above, level with, or beneath the skin surface (Figs. 3–17). Examples: nodular secondary or tertiary syphilis, epitheliomas, xanthomas.

Tumors are larger than 1 cm. and are solid lesions whose depth may be above, level with, or beneath the skin surface (Figs. 3–18 to 3–20). Examples: tumor stage of mycosis fungoides and larger epitheliomas.

(*Text continued on page 102.*)

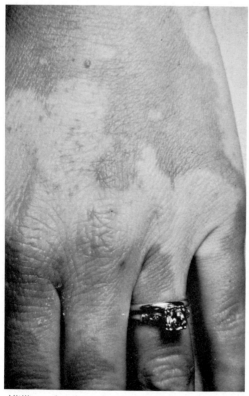

Figure 3-8. *Vitiligo, showing macular patches of depigmentation on the dorsum of the hand.*

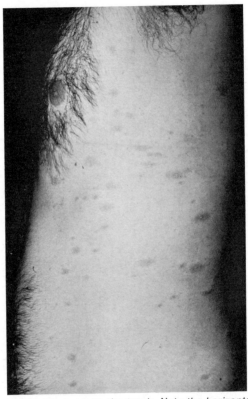

Figure 3-9. *Pityriasis rosea on the trunk. Note the horizontal orientation of the papulosquamous lesions.*

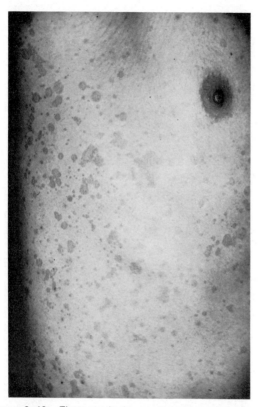

Figure 3-10. *Tinea versicolor, scaly lesions on the trunk.*

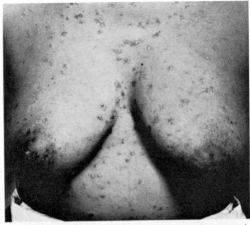

Figure 3-11. *Papulosquamous eruption on chest in secondary syphilis.*

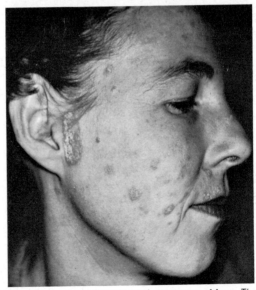

Figure 3-12. *Chronic discoid lupus erythematosus of face. The lesions are papulosquamous.*

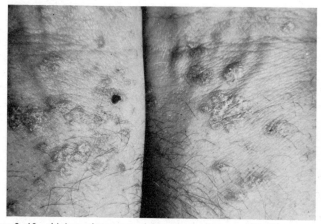

Figure 3-13. *Lichen planus papulosquamous lesions of the flexor aspect of the wrists.*

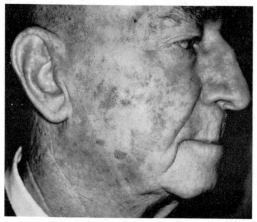

Figure 3-14. *Senile keratoses.*

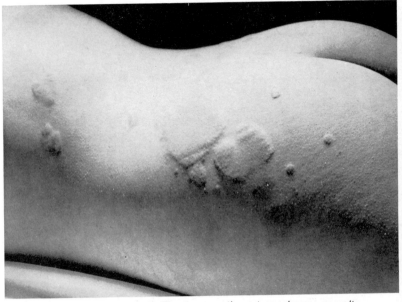

Figure 3–15. Urticaria. These are erythematous plaques or welts.

Vesicles are up to 1 cm. in size and are circumscribed elevations of the skin containing serous fluid (Fig. 3–21). Examples: early chickenpox, herpes zoster, and contact dermatitis.

Bullae are larger than 1 cm. and are circumscribed elevations containing serous fluid (Figs. 3–22 and 3–23). Examples: pemphigus and second-degree burns.

Pustules are varied in size, are circumscribed elevations, and contain purulent fluid (Fig. 3–24). Examples: acne and impetigo.

Petechiae are up to 1 cm. in size and are circumscribed deposits of blood or blood pigment in the skin (see Fig. 16–8).

(Text continued on page 108.)

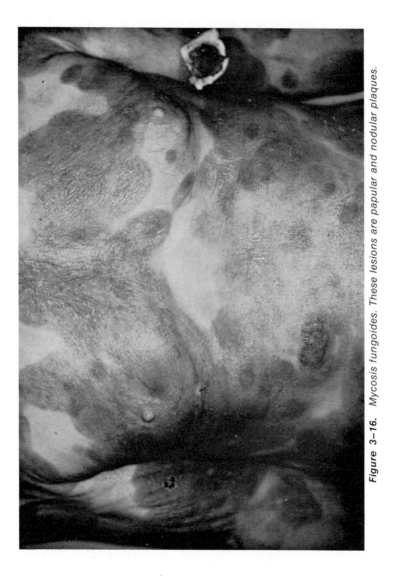

Figure 3–16. Mycosis fungoides. These lesions are papular and nodular plaques.

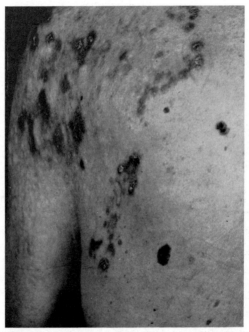

Figure 3–17. Tertiary lesions of syphilis demonstrating grouped and serpiginous papules and nodules.

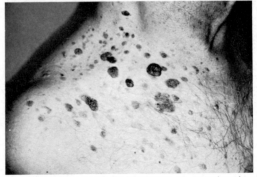

Figure 3–18. Multiple seborrheic keratoses on anterior shoulder area.

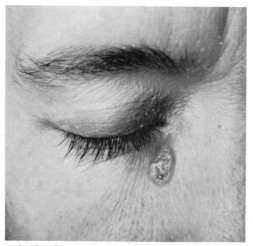

Figure 3–19. *Basal cell epithelioma. This is a small tumor.*

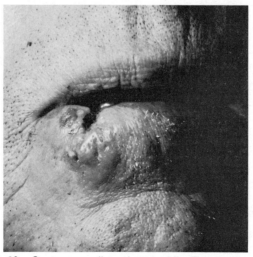

Figure 3–20. *Squamous cell carcinoma of lip. This is a large tumor.*

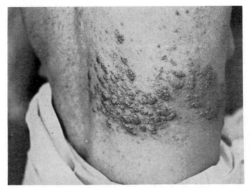

Figure 3–21. *Herpes zoster on lateral chest wall with groups of vesicles.*

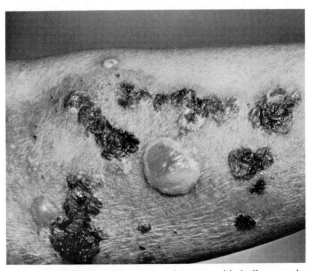

Figure 3–22. *Erythema multiforme on forearm with bullous and crusted lesions.*

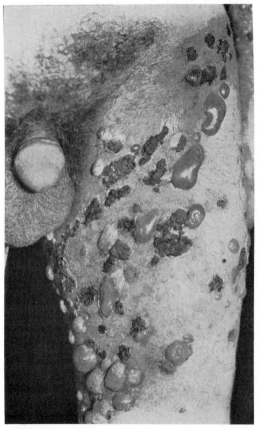

Figure 3–23. *Pemphigus vulgaris showing bullous and crusted lesions. (Domonkos, A. N.: Andrews' Diseases of the Skin. 6th ed. Philadelphia, W. B. Saunders Co., 1971.)*

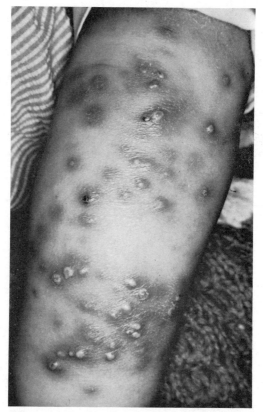

Figure 3-24. *Multiple folliculitis with pustules on forearm.*

Secondary Lesions

Scales (squamae) are shedding, dead epidermal cells that may be either dry or greasy (Fig. 3-25). Examples: dandruff and psoriasis.

Crusts are variously colored masses of skin exudates (see Figs. 3–22 and 3–23). Examples: impetigo and infected dermatitis.

Excoriations are abrasions of the skin. They are usually superficial and traumatic (Fig. 3–26). Examples: scratched insect bites and scabies.

Fissures are linear breaks in the skin that are sharply defined and have abrupt walls. Examples: congenital syphilis and athlete's foot.

Ulcers are irregularly sized and shaped excavations in the skin that extend into the dermis or corium (Figs. 3–27 and 3–28). Examples: varicose ulcers of the leg and tertiary syphilis.

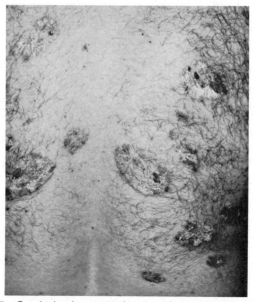

Figure 3–25. *Psoriasis demonstrating papulosquamous lesions on the back.*

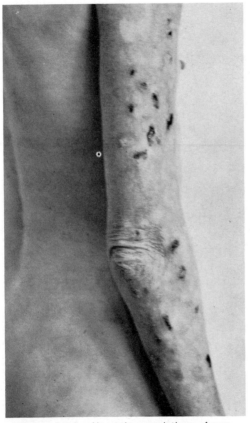

Figure 3–26. *Necrotic excoriations of arm.*

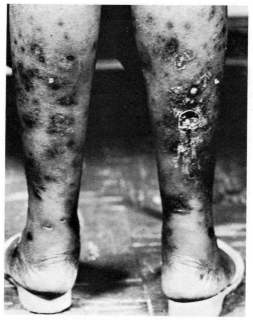

Figure 3–27. Tuberculous ulcers of legs.

Scars are formations of connective tissue that replace tissue lost through injury or disease.

Keloids are hypertrophic scars (Fig. 3–29).

Lichenification is a diffuse thickening and scaling with a resulting increase in the skin lines and markings.

Several combinations of primary and secondary lesions commonly exist on the same patient. Examples: papulosquamous lesions of psoriasis, vesiculopustular lesions in contact dermatitis, and crusted excoriations in scabies.

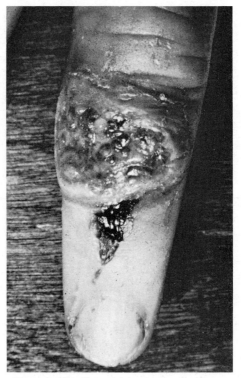

Figure 3–28. Sporotrichosis ulcer on finger.

Special Lesions

There are also some primary lesions, limited to a few skin diseases, that can be called specialized lesions.

Comedones or blackheads are plugs of whitish or blackish sebaceous and keratinous material lodged in the pilosebaceous

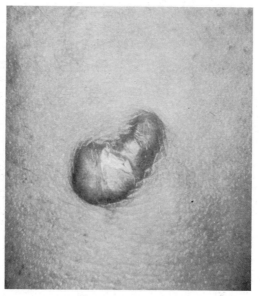

Figure 3-29. *Keloid.*

follicle. Blackheads are usually seen on the face, the chest, the back, and rarely on the upper part of the arms. Example: acne.

Milia or whiteheads are whitish nodules, 1 to 2 mm. in diameter, that have no visible opening onto the skin surface. Examples: on healed burn or superficial traumatic sites, healed bullous disease sites, or newborn babies.

Telangiectasias are dilated superficial blood vessels. Examples: spider hemangiomas and chronic radiodermatitis.

Burrows are tunnels in the epidermis. They may be very small and short (in scabies) or tortuous and long (in creeping eruption).

In addition there are distinct and often diagnostic changes in the nail plates and the hairs.

COMMON CLINICAL TERMS

Alopecia — Hair loss resulting from cessation of growth in the follicle.

Erythema — Redness of the skin.

Melanin — The dark amorphous pigment of the skin, hair, and melanotic tumors.

Nevus — A circumscribed new growth of the skin considered congenital or developmental in origin, which when present from birth is commonly designated a birthmark; more precise descriptions intimate the cell type is sebaceous nevus, melanotic nevus, vascular nevus.

Pruritus — Intense itching, frequently a symptom of many skin diseases.

Sclerosis — Induration or hardening of the skin from inflammation of the interstitial substance.

Telangiectasis — A condition characterized by dilatation of the capillary vessels and arterioles forming a variety of angioma.

COMMON CLINICAL SYNDROMES

The following dermatologic syndromes affect approximately 90 per cent of the patients seen in office practice dermatology. It may be more exciting and stimulating to the physician to be able to recognize some of the rarer problems in the field of dermatology (as is also true for any of the other fields of medicine), but the common problems also can provide stimulating diagnostic challenges.

Dermatologic Allergy

Contact dermatitis (dermatitis venenata) — A very common papulovesicular or oozing dermatosis caused by exposure of the skin to either *primary irritant substances,* such as harsh soap or caustic chemicals, or to *allergenic substances,* such as poison ivy or ragweed resin.

Poison ivy dermatitis — Rather easily distinguished from other forms of contact dermatitis by the linear configuration of the vesicles.

Atopic eczema (disseminated neurodermatitis) — An endogenous dermatitis that is quite chronic and occurs primarily in individuals where there is a personal or family history of atopy, such as previous atopic eczema, hay fever, or asthma. There are two clinical forms of atopic eczema, namely, *infantile eczema,* where the vesicular crusted lesions are primarily seen on the face, and *adult atopic eczema,* where the red, scaly, lichenified lesions are primarily seen on the cubital and popliteal fossae.

Nummular eczema—A variant of atopic eczema. The lesions classically are coin-shaped and occur primarily on the legs, arms, and buttocks, particularly in the winter time.

Drug eruption—Must be thought of when a patient presents with a rather generalized eruption, particularly with urticaria, morbilliform, or erythema multiforme-like lesions.

Fixed drug eruption—An example of a single lesion due to an allergy from an internally administered chemical. Most commonly this is a purplish red plaque or patch that keeps recurring in the same area following every drug ingestion.

Localized Pruritic Dermatosis

Localized neurodermatitis (lichen simplex chronicus)—The commonest example in this group of pruritic dermatoses. It is manifested clinically by a single patch or plaque of red, scaly, dry, thickened lichenified skin most classically seen at the nape of the neck or around the ankles, but can occur in the anal area, ear, wrist, or other areas. Many cases of localized neurodermatitis are the end result of vigorous scratching of a primary skin problem such as atopic eczema, contact dermatitis, lichen planus, or other pruritic skin problem.

Acne–Seborrhea Complex

Acne and seborrheic dermatitis (dandruff)—Both are inherent problems seen in persons with oily skin. These conditions are hereditary and develop after the age of puberty.

Acne—Can cause comedones, pustules, and deeper cystic boil-like lesions that can eventuate in severe scarring of the skin of the face, back, or chest. This common disease, while not life-threatening, can be very disturbing emotionally to a teen-age girl or boy who has now become very conscious of appearance. Unfortunately, acne is believed by many to be a symbol of uncleanliness; certainly that is not true. The condition is mainly internal.

Papulosquamous Dermatoses

The papulosquamous dermatoses group includes five or six common skin problems that are grouped together because of the similarity of the clinical lesions. These dermatoses can have varying clinical pictures, but for the most part they present as discrete papulosquamous lesions of the trunk. This group includes:

Psoriasis—A very common and tremendously annoying chronic skin problem of unknown etiology.

Pityriasis rosea—A rather common eruption that occurs most frequently in young adults and lasts approximately six weeks.

Tinea versicolor—A superficial fungus infection of the skin that responds nicely to Selsun scrubs.

Lichen planus—A rather chronic papular violaceous eruption that is thought to be related somewhat to emotional tension.

Secondary syphilis—Can mimic any of the other papulosquamous dermatoses, usually does not itch, and is quite rarely seen except in city health clinics.

Generalized drug eruption—Can mimic any of the other papulosquamous dermatoses and is usually diagnosed by a physician who has a high index of suspicion for such an allergic drug problem.

Dermatologic Infections

Bacteria—May cause skin infections such as impetigo, ecthyma, boils, carbuncles, infectious eczematoid dermatitis, and secondary bacterial infection.

Viruses—May cause skin infections such as herpes simplex, herpes zoster, chickenpox, warts, molluscum contagiosum, and several other viral skin problems.

Fungi—May cause skin infections such as superficial fungus infections of the feet, crotch, body, scalp, hands, and nails, and deeper fungus infections such as sporotrichosis, blastomycosis, and other deep infections.

Tumors of the Skin

Nevi(moles)—The commonest tumors of the skin, which can be dermal or junctional.

Malignant melanomas—Can arise from junctional nevi or sui generis, are fortunately extremely rare tumors of the skin.

Keratoses—*Actinic keratoses* and *seborrheic keratoses,* with their many variants, are the commonest tumors of the elderly skin.

In addition to the above commoner problems of the skin there are cases of *exfoliative dermatitis* from many causes, *bullous dermatoses*, various *pigmentary dermatoses*, skin diseases *related to internal disease*, such as the collagen diseases, and also conditions affecting the *hair*, *nails*, and *mucous membranes*.

BIBLIOGRAPHY

Fitzpatrick, T. B., and Walker, S. A.: Dermatologic Differential Diagnosis. Chicago, Year Book Medical Publishers, 1962.

Sauer, G. C.: Manual of Skin Diseases. 3rd ed. Philadelphia, J. B. Lippincott Co., 1973.

4
EXAMINATION OF THE NERVOUS SYSTEM

The neurological examination is a way of evaluating the integrity of those dynamic regulators of bodily functions—the central and peripheral nervous systems. The examination consists of observation of the responses of the patient to various kinds of stimuli. The stimuli may be natural, such as touch or pressure sensations on various parts of the body, as well as gravity, movement, visual and acoustic stimuli, and conversation or verbal commands, or they may be specially devised by the physician, such as hot or cold objects, pinpricks, or touch with a delicate object. The observed responses are also varied—different types of movement (occurring either spontaneously or in response to command), gait, tendon reflexes, "attentiveness" to stimuli, speech, verbal responses to questions concerning applied stimuli, spontaneously occurring speech, the correct solution of problems involving some use of symbols, or abstract thought.

The neurological examination described in the following pages is a somewhat arbitrary selection of stimulus-response combinations designed to sample the functioning of various parts of the nervous system. Almost any part of the neurological examination can be amplified if preliminary findings warrant the expenditure of more time. In this way you can include stimuli that may elicit other responses to demonstrate normal or impaired nervous system function.

Before conducting the examination you will have taken an appropriate history. In eliciting the history of nervous system disease, it is particularly important to derive a clear idea of the chronology of the illness. A relentlessly progressive course is characteristic of neoplastic disease and many diseases of unknown cause that we call "degenerative." An abrupt onset of a maximal neurological defect and subsequent recovery, or at least the achievement of a plateau, are characteristic in the history of vascular "accidents." Certain diseases are marked by a fluctuating course, i.e., remissions and exacerbations (e.g., multiple sclerosis and myasthenia gravis). The chronology usually provides the key to the nature of the disease, the neurological examination to the site of the disease process.

Certain symptoms are indicative of dysfunction of specific portions of the nervous system and should often be explored in detail. Headache (with attention to its frequency, location, precipitating events, severity, and accompanying symptoms), episodes of impairment of consciousness, seizures, loss or distortion of sensation in various areas of the body, dysfunction of one or more limbs, vertigo, blurred vision, diplopia, dysarthria, dysphagia, and urinary urgency are among these. The questions must be couched in the patient's own idiom; the details sought for will depend on the diagnostic suspicions aroused by the history of the illness.

BEHAVIOR AND CONSCIOUSNESS

The neurological examination usually begins when you introduce yourself and any associates to your patient. Identify yourself as a physician if the patient is not aware of this. A handshake is frequently the natural greeting. Careful observation is made of the patient's demeanor in response to this initial contact.

Note the general level of activity; the range of normal behavior in this situation is familiar to all—a smile, a return of the proffered handshake, and a few words of greeting are the usual response.

Hyperactivity. Patients may be hyperactive in response to stimuli. They may jump when spoken to or when touched, move excessively rapidly, respond with excessive speed. These findings, frequently associated with fine tremor, suggest heightened neuromuscular excitability—an important manifestation of anxiety, apprehensiveness, or one of many metabolic abnormalities (e. g., hyperthyroidism, sedative withdrawal, or intoxication with stimulants).

Hyperactivity also occurs in delirium; in this state the individual is hallucinating and is in poor contact with his surroundings. Hyperactivity is seen in a wide variety of intoxications, both exogenous (e. g., after ingestion of large amounts of belladonna alkaloids, marijuana, or any of a number of other drugs) and endogenous (e.g., in the course of septicemia and uremia).

Another type is seen in manic or hypomanic excitement. Here the patient has no tremor or startle reaction when touched, but is overly talkative and jocose. The patient is usually constantly moving, talking, laughing—frequently in a pleasant, witty fashion, but also frequently in an obtrusive, annoying, and inappropriate way.

Actively agitated behavior also occurs in the course of schizophrenia. These patients are characteristically intermittently hyperactive, with other periods of quiet, even withdrawn, behavior. There is no evidence of neuromuscular excitability, tremor, or consistent startle reaction. Bizarre, inexplicable behavior is characteristic.

Hypoactivity. Varying degrees of depressed response to the environment are more common than hyperactivity. The patient may move slowly, look at the examiner, make no reply to the introduction, or make no move to take the proffered handshake. The pattern of response may derive from any of several causes:

1. Certain cultural backgrounds discourage spontaneity of expression, particularly on introduction to a stranger. These

variations of response that are not of physical origin are usually comparatively minor, are reversible as the patient feels more secure, and are elucidated by a perceptive social history. Occasionally, illiteracy itself is mistaken for some defect in attention or awareness.

2. Patients with emotional depression are slowed in their general activity and responsiveness. They usually show evidences of sadness, with or without agitation, and may weep. If they do not cooperate well on examination, it is with accompanying manifestations of preoccupation and worry, but not with drowsiness. They frequently voice concern about supposed physical illnesses, and indeed frequently have anorexia, constipation, insomnia, and inability to concentrate. A striking tendency to be self-accusatory and self-deprecatory occurs in their stream of talk.

Since suicide is an ever-present danger, even in patients who deny considering it, the patient must be adequately protected and the diagnosis of depression kept in mind in patients with unusual, confusing, or inconsistent clinical findings.

3. Malingerers may simulate drowsiness or depressed states of consciousness. Since such states are acted performances, they are usually accompanied by bizarre signs unrecognizable as parts of physical disease, and they are "overacted."

4. Catatonic schizophrenia is manifested by a slowing of all responses, and is occasionally difficult to differentiate from organic diseases. Catatonia, however, usually involves some active negativism. Rather than being slow to answer questions, or shake hands, the patient withdraws, often turns his head away, firmly closes his eyes, or puts his hand behind him. He may appear greatly agitated, or terrified. Behavior indicating reaction to hallucination and gesturing that appears privately symbolic are common.

5. The best understood of the states that cause an impaired response to the environment are those that probably result from lesions to the ascending reticular activating system (RAS). The state of responsiveness of the patient must be described in detail, as it usually indicates the functional state of the RAS. This sys-

tem may suffer permanent damage, e.g., from trauma or tumor; or it may be temporarily affected, e.g., by anesthetics or sedatives. It may be affected to various degrees, producing varying depths of impaired consciousness.

The term "semi-stupor" refers to the state in which patients fall asleep unless constantly stimulated. "Coma" refers to states in which the patient cannot be aroused. It is important to record whether the patient is comatose to the point at which verbal commands produce no response or at which severe painful stimuli do not produce response; such observations are essential, not only for the initial diagnosis but also in order to follow the patient's course toward improvement or increasing illness.

It is, of course, essential to note other aspects of the behavior of the comatose patient; many of these are described elsewhere in the text. Are the patient's extremities flaccid to passive movement, or do certain ones exhibit resistance? Extension of the arms and legs suggests a process that has damaged the neuraxis in the high brain stem (decerebration); resistance to passive movement on one side of the body suggests a contralateral lesion above the spinal cord (spasticity). Persistent deviation of the head, body, or eyes to one side suggests an irritative lesion in the contralateral cerebral hemisphere.

Coma may result from various causes. The following are the most common with a few comments concerning their identifications.

INTOXICATIONS. The most frequent are those resulting from ingestion of sedative drugs. Respirations are shallow and usually slow; the skin is pale and cold; and, in the advanced stage, blood pressure is depressed. The extremities are flaccid and areflexic. In other kinds of intoxications, other autonomic manifestations (hypertension, tachypnea) may be apparent.

MENINGITIS OR ENCEPHALITIS. The patient is febrile and tachypneic, and usually has a stiff neck. Seizures and focal neurological signs are frequently present. Depression of consciousness may be of any degree from drowsiness to deep coma. Examination of the spinal fluid frequently provides the diagnosis.

HEAD INJURY. Neurological signs, tachypnea, shock, signs of scalp injury, and evidences of other bodily injuries are frequently present. Spinal fluid is frequently bloody.

DIABETIC ACIDOSIS. Tachypnea, flushing, and warm, dry skin are present. Coma is of varying depth. Levels of blood sugar and plasma ketones are elevated.

HYPOGLYCEMIA. Respirations are slow and deep; skin is cool and moist.

CEREBRAL OR SUBARACHNOID HEMORRHAGE. Coma is frequently deep, with stiff neck and focal neurological signs. The spinal fluid is usually quite bloody.

POSTICTAL COMA. The comatose state is usually not prolonged (not over an hour), and the patient can usually be aroused by painful stimuli.

INCREASED INTRACRANIAL PRESSURE. Deep coma from this cause occurs late in the course of the condition, is usually associated with unequal size of pupils, papilledema, and an increase in muscular tone. Rapidly increasing intracranial pressure is frequently associated with increasing drowsiness.

HIGHER FUNCTIONS

In the fully awake, conscious patient, the next task in the neurological examination is an evaluation of what may be called the higher functions—speech, understanding, reading, calculation, and writing.

In certain persons this part of the examination need not be performed. In a college graduate, for example, who has given a detailed, articulate history full of astute observations and evidences of perfectly preserved memory, further testing is superfluous. In many cases, however, a sampling of the functions is necessary, and indeed it is imperative in any patient whose complaints include symptoms referable to the head, to behavior, or to altered states of consciousness.

Before assessing more isolated disturbances of speech and symbolic function, it is important to ascertain both the educational level of the patient and his orientation. Testing for the latter should be introduced by some preliminary polite questions, e.g., "Do you have any trouble with your memory? Do you mind if I ask you some simple memory questions, such as . . . ?" Some minor mistakes in dates are not significant. Gross mistakes in time (particularly in identifying the season of the year or errors by several years) and mistakes by the patient in knowing roughly where he is (e.g., "the hospital") or in establishing the identity of those around ("Dr. X," or even "doctors and nurses") are usually indicative of gross brain dysfunction. Disorientation does not completely nullify the value of specific findings in the field of speech or symbolic function, but it does diminish the reliability of those findings as indicators of localized brain dysfunction.

Spontaneous Speech

The spontaneous speech of the patient as he relates the history, for example, must be listened to with care. Observe whether the volume of speech seems normal, reduced, or increased in amount. Listen to the articulation of words, the syllabic structure of words, and the structure of sentences and sentence series, as well as the power of the voice and inflection.

Three kinds of gross speech disturbance are described in the following paragraphs; others are described later.

Lesions of the tongue muscles or of the nuclear or peripheral nerve supply to the tongue. These result in an articulation defect. The speech is difficult to understand and resembles that of one who is trying to speak with an object in his mouth. This speech is occasionally confused with aphasia, or disturbance of speech resulting from a cerebral hemisphere lesion; but it is apparent on careful listening that, unlike aphasia, this speech has no disturbance in syllabic word formulation, word or phrase sequence, sentence structure, or grammar. Disturbances of speech caused by nuclear or peripheral nerve damage are frequently associated with the deficiency that results from soft palate weakness—nasal speech.

Aphasias. Two major types of spontaneous speech disturbances occur as a result of lesions of the dominant cerebral hemisphere. In over 95 per cent of the population, whether right-handed or left-handed, the dominant hemisphere for speech is the left. Speech disturbances resulting from cerebral hemisphere lesions are termed aphasia.

Motor or expressive aphasia results from lesions in the more anterior portions of the dominant hemisphere, in the region of the inferior portion of the "motor cortex," or its subcortical projections. In this syndrome, spontaneous speech is markedly reduced in amount; in acute stages, or with severe damage, patients may be unable to formulate any language, although they can phonate. Usually, however, they are not able to *imitate* the phonation of even simple sounds, such as those described below. When the disease is slightly less severe they can say only a few words or phrases, frequently those with emotional connotations (e.g., profanity), expressive of their frustration at being unable to speak. As the patient recovers, speech returns, but with severe distortion of language structure. Single words, particularly polysyllabic words, are stumbled over and frequently distorted, so that wrong syllables are inserted. Frequently, there are long periods of hesitation and repetition of single words or syllables as the patient tries to continue. Sentence structure is affected. The small "connecting" words, both prepositions and verbs, tend to be omitted, giving what has been called a "telegraphic style." As recovery continues, these abnormalities of spontaneous speech become less and less pronounced; the patient may be left with only moderate difficulty with polysyllabic words or with the correct formulation of sentences.

To further examine the patient with motor or expressive aphasia, the special sign of apraxia of mouth and tongue may be elicited. In the more acute and severe cases, the patient cannot imitate simple tongue or mouth movements demonstrated to him, e.g., extruding the tongue, moving it from side to side, and opening and closing the mouth. In less severe stages he may be able to do these tests, but he cannot say "ah," "e," or consonant sounds, e.g., "ba" or "pa" on command. He cannot whistle.

Sensory or "receptive" aphasia. This results from lesions of the dominant (usually the left) hemisphere in its posterior temporal portion. Maximal deficits of this nature result from lesions that are temporoparietal and extend to the subcortical white matter.

Spontaneous speech is not reduced in amount and may be increased. There are numerous mistakes in the use of words and in language structure. Frequently, conglomerations of syllables that are similar in sound to the desired word are used with some rapidity, producing a rather strange effect similar to that of humorous "double-talk." When these distortions of language become severe, they result in an incomprehensible jargon, called paraphasia. In contradistinction to the patient with motor, or expressive, aphasia, the patient with relatively "pure" sensory aphasia is usually unaware of his deficit. This speech distortion is occasionally mistaken for psychiatric disease—for the neologisms of schizophrenia or the flight of ideas of manic psychosis. Neologisms, however, are not characterized by approximations in sound to the desired word; they usually, furthermore, have some apparent symbolic meaning and appear in the context of grossly distorted behavior. Manic flight of ideas is not usually accompanied by malformed words.

The other major sign of sensory aphasia is impaired understanding of auditory stimuli. Despite abundant spontaneous speech, the patient cannot accurately reproduce spoken words. This deficit varies in severity from the rare inability to identify even nonverbal sounds (e.g., the tinkle of ice in a glass, the jingle of keys) to the more common inability to understand spoken commands.

Before leaving the subject of spontaneous speech, five additional types of speech disorder that accompany nervous system disease will be described.

Cerebellar disease. Here the speech is staccato and jerky. It displays a disorder of rhythm that is probably derived from the same mechanism as the intention tremor of the extremities and trunk, which it frequently accompanies. This speech is often referred to as "scanning."

Parkinsonism and similar diseases of the basal ganglia.
Speech in these disorders becomes progressively more low
pitched, devoid of inflection, and weaker in volume. In the advanced states it is a monotonous, faintly audible speech, often
barely above a whisper.

Diffuse brain diseases. Particularly in those diseases that involve the frontal lobes (notably general paresis), the patient
stumbles over the pronunciation of the polysyllabic words. This
defect may be apparent in spontaneous speech, but it can be
highlighted by listening to the accuracy with which a patient
repeats a test phrase, such as "rural electricity," "Methodist Epis-
copal," or (if one's prejudices warrant), "God bless the Com-
monwealth of Massachusetts." The patient with frontal lobe
disease will frequently garble the pronunciation of these words.
Here one is probably demonstrating an early aphasia.

Athetosis. With athetosis, and frequently with spasticity,
resulting from various types of damage to the central nervous
system occurring in the prenatal period or in the first months of
life, the speech is often severely dysarthric. The speech may
sound similar to that produced by a tongue weakened by a lower
motor neuron lesion, but the sound is probably the result of impaired coordination of the tongue muscles.

Stuttering and stammering. Prolonged hesitation before
producing single words, or the involuntary repetition of a word
or syllable, is not usually associated with known organic disease
of the central or peripheral nervous system. Occasionally the
search for words by a patient recovering from aphasia will simulate stuttering; they are in all probability, however, of markedly
different etiology.

Further Testing of the Patient for Aphasia and Apraxia

The patient is requested to "Do this. Put one hand on your
head or one finger on an ear." If the patient cannot imitate these

acts, it is futile to test with language further; the patient may be generally confused, may be unable to understand the words "Do this," or may have a marked disturbance of movement on a conceptual, not a motor, basis. This we call apraxia, and it is usually associated with a parietal lobe lesion in the dominant hemisphere. Patients with apraxia make clumsy, grossly inappropriate movements with their hands, both on verbal commands and on attempting to imitate actions of the examiner.

Ask your patient to do these simple tasks: "Put one hand on top of your head." "Open your mouth." "Lift up your arm." If he can accomplish these tasks, he is asked to repeat words, beginning with single, simple words and progressing to phrases and then to simple and more complex sentences. The patient with sensory aphasia, in the early stages of these tests, fails to repeat the word, phrase, or sentence, looks quizzical, gives a phonetic approximation of the requested words, or says he cannot remember.

There are three pitfalls in the testing of these "higher functions."

1. The demonstration of a deficit may be highly dependent on the difficulty of the task. The fact that an individual can repeat a simple phrase or sentence, for example, does not mean that he is free from sensory aphasia; he may fail completely on a sentence with two clauses.

2. Fluctuation of response is the rule in patients with aphasia deficits and other manifestations of cerebral hemisphere dysfunction. A patient may, for example, be able to speak a few sentences coherently on one occasion, and on another he will be almost mute. This variability occasionally leads the unwary examiner to an incorrect underestimation of the patient's disability and occasionally to a diagnosis of malingering or other psychiatric disease. Anxiety and fatigue tend to depress the patient's performance.

3. The patient frequently attempts to conceal aphasia and other deficits of higher function. Various protective devices are used—the patient may refuse to perform tests because of fatigue, "nervousness," or indignation over his intelligence being

tested. An aphasic patient will frequently say he cannot hear. It is important for the examiner to be sympathetic but persistent in his attempt to achieve a thorough examination.

It is doubtful whether expressive or receptive aphasia ever occurs in completely pure fashion, although it is not uncommon for one or the other element to be preponderant. Frequently, however, the patient displays "global" aphasia; in this syndrome marked diminution in speech (and other characteristics of expressive aphasia) is present, as are the defects of receptive, or sensory, aphasia.

Other Tests of Higher Functions

If any type of aphasia, memory, or judgment disorder is present, it is important to test the patient in a few more detailed ways in order to elicit signs of localized cerebral hemisphere dysfunction.

1. Ask the patient to point to his right or left ear, knee, or shoulder. Ask him to point to his thumb, little finger, then the examiner's thumb, little finger. Right-left confusion and difficulty identifying fingers are signs of dysfunction of the parietal lobe of the dominant hemisphere.

2. Ask the patient to perform simple arithmetical problems involving two columns or long multiplication (if education warrants). Specific dysfunction in the use of numbers (acalculia) is another sign of parietal lobe disease of the dominant hemisphere.

3. Ask the patient to write from dictation. Writing is a highly complex function and may be impaired by a number of purely motor disorders. Impairment of grammar, omission of words, gross confusion in spelling with repeated letters, or simple inability to remember what was dictated (agraphia or dysgraphia) are signs of damage to the "language center," the posterior temporal and parietal area of the dominant hemisphere.

4. Ask the patient to name objects upon visual presentation.

Inability to do this (anomia) may be an early sign of temporal lobe disease of the dominant hemisphere.

5. If the patient has a deficit of motor function, inquiries such as "Do you have any difficulty using your arm or leg?" should be made. Injuries to the nondominant parietal lobe tend to produce a deficit in awareness of the contralateral side of the body, and particularly in awareness of any deficit in the function of that side (anosognosia).

6. The patient should be asked to draw a daisy, a bicycle, or the face of a clock with the hands pointing to nine o'clock. With lesions of the nondominant parietal lobe, half of the object is frequently omitted, the two halves are superimposed, or the axis of the picture is markedly rotated (constriction apraxia). This sign is frequently accompanied by spatial disorientation, the patient being unable to remember directions and their relations.

Judgment and Abstraction Ability

With diffuse cerebral disease, patients will often show subtle changes in behavior, such as lapses in taste, inexplicable arbitrary decisions, poor emotional control, or rapid changes in emotional states. Often this history can only be obtained from an observant relative, the patient himself denying the symptom. In more advanced stages of the disease of the frontal lobe, the patient may be inappropriately facetious with the examiner. Urinary incontinence may occur in these patients, even when they are fully awake and ambulatory; they frequently give no explanation or apology. Bilateral cerebral hemisphere disease may also produce sudden outbursts of apparently unmotivated weeping, or more rarely, laughing ("forced laughing or crying").

A few simple tests of abstraction ability should be carried out if dysfunction is suspected. (1) The patient can be given a series of objects, e.g., "carrot, bean, lettuce," and asked what they have in common or "how they are alike." The patient with diffuse brain disease will often not understand this concept and will describe each object separately. Often this behavior persists even after an example is given. (2) The explanation of a proverb is asked for. The patient may be asked if he has heard the saying "Don't count your chickens until they are hatched." If he assents, he is asked "what it means." The brain damaged person will usually rephrase the proverb, using the same words, and be unable to generalize to such terms as "plans."

MOTOR FUNCTION

Somatic muscle function is the major observable reaction of the organism to the environment. The status of the "motor systems" can be divided into six parts: evaluation of strength, inspection of muscle substance, evaluation of muscle tone, evaluation of types of coordination, testing of gait, and spontaneous abnormal movements.

Strength. Before evaluating muscle strength, it is essential to know whether there is any medical contraindication to muscle testing, in or out of bed. It may be mandatory to keep certain joints immobilized or to keep the patient at complete rest.

If a full examination is permissible, muscle strength in the arms and legs can be evaluated by the following tests:

1. The patient's arms are held outstretched, above the horizontal, and the patient is instructed to resist all movements. Attempt to depress the whole arm, bend the elbow, bend the wrist joint, and bend the interphalangeal joints—testing, among others, the deltoid, triceps, and wrist extensor and flexor muscles. Homologous muscles are tested first on one side, then on the other. Look for asymmetry in muscle strength or focal muscle weakness, e.g., in one muscle or in the distal muscles of the extremities as opposed to the proximal.

2. Ask your patient to remain with arms outstretched with eyes closed for a few minutes. Any impairment in the strength of shoulder girdle muscles that has been suspected becomes apparent by a downward drifting of the affected arm. (This test can also demonstrate other abnormalities—an upward drift of one arm is usually associated with cerebellar disease; a change to-

ward the vertical axis of the hand is frequently associated with sensory loss). The patient is then asked to grip with maximum strength with each hand, testing the flexors of the fingers and wrists, and to relax his grip and spread his fingers rapidly. Persistent involuntary contraction indicates the unique phenomenon of myotonia.

Observe the patient standing. Various abnormalities may be identified at this time. The patient with basal ganglion disease (characteristically, paralysis agitans) stands bent forward with arms flexed (Fig. 4–1); whereas weak abdominal muscles produce a grossly protuberant abdomen and lordosis. The patient may tend to fall forward or backward (basal ganglion disease) or to one side (unilateral cerebellar disease). Gross forward-back-

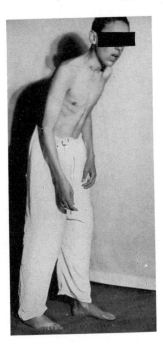

Figure 4–1. *Stance in postencephalitic Parkinson's disease.*

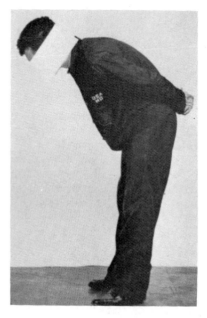

Figure 4-2. Camptocormia, one of the postures in hysteria. (Abse, D. W.: Hysteria and Related Mental Disorders. Baltimore, Williams & Wilkins, 1966.)

ward tremor of the trunk may occur with midline cerebellar disease (titubation). Finally, the hysterical patient may display a variety of abnormalities. For example, he may be unable to stand, although normal muscle function has been demonstrated in bed, or he may show a marked flexion of the spine called "camptocormia" (Fig. 4–2).

Then ask the patient to stand with heels and toes together, eyes open. With severe cerebellar disease, patients will frequently stagger and fall in this test. If the patient performs successfully, he is asked to close his eyes; if he now becomes markedly unsteady and falls, a loss of proprioceptive sensation is suggested (Romberg's sign).

Have the patient stand on one foot, then on the other, and then hop five times in place. The patient cannot lift himself off the floor if there is weakness of the gastrocnemius, a powerful muscle difficult to test adequately in other ways. Hopping also is difficult with ataxia, even in the early stages (the patient being unable to maintain his balance), or with spasticity, which is discussed on page 135.

Leg and truncal muscles are tested with the patient supine and prone.

With the patient in the supine position, test the abdominal muscles by having him flex his neck against resistance while the midline abdominal wall is palpated. Integrity of the abdominal muscles is demonstrated by the ability of the patient to rise to a sitting position. The iliopsoas muscles are tested by having the patient flex the hip against forceful resistance. The anterior tibial is tested by having the patient dorsiflex the foot. The thigh adductor muscles are tested by having the patient draw the leg to the midline. The peronei are tested by eversion of the feet.

In the prone position, the gluteus maximus is tested by having the patient elevate the leg from the horizontal against resistance.

Intercostal muscles are evaluated by observing the depth of respiration.

Inspection of body of muscle. Visual inspection of the body will reveal whether there seems to be a normal soft tissue mass surrounding the bony frame. (It cannot, of course, be determined how much of this soft tissue is muscle and how much is fat or fibrous tissue.) Generalized loss of soft tissue and, more importantly, localized areas of wasting should be carefully noted, as they may indicate the location of the motor neuron or peripheral nerve affected. If soft tissue wasting is seen, look for fine contractions of small parts of the affected muscles while at rest (fasciculations). These abnormal contractions often indicate disease of the anterior horn cell.

Muscle tone. By "tone" is meant the resistance of the muscle to passive movement. There is normal "feel" when you stretch the voluntary relaxed muscle in an awake, cooperative patient. Abnormal tone is measured against this norm and occurs as hypo- or hypertonicity.

DECREASED MUSCLE TONE — HYPOTONICITY. The commonest cause of decreased tone is a lesion somewhere along what Sherrington termed the "final common path" of the motor impulse. This path includes the anterior horn cell of the spinal cord, the anterior (motor) nerve root, the peripheral nerve, the neuromuscular junction, and the muscle itself. Disease of any of these structures will cause weakness and decreased tone—a combination called "flaccidity." The determination of the site on the "final common path" responsible for flaccidity is made by searching for other signs. Almost all flaccidity is accompanied by depressed tendon reflexes—exceptions being affections of the neuromuscular junction (notably myasthenia gravis) and some muscle diseases in which reflexes are normal. Fasciculations (brief, nonrhythmic twitches occurring erratically in various parts of a muscle), in the presence of flaccidity, usually point to anterior horn cell disease. Unilateral sensory loss plus flaccidity indicates peripheral nerve or nerve root disease.

Sudden lesions of the nervous system at levels rostral to the anterior horn cell can also produce flaccidity, e.g., transections of the spinal cord (producing paraplegia and bilateral sensory loss) or lesions of one side of the diencephalon (producing hemiplegia).

Cerebellar disease can produce mildly impaired muscle tone in those limbs also showing ataxia.

INCREASED MUSCLE TONE—HYPERTONICITY. One common pattern of increased resistance to passive movement is termed spasticity. It affects, commonly, the antigravity muscles—specifically, the flexors of the elbows and the extensors and adductors of the legs, sparing others. Muscle resistance is also phasic—strong at first, then giving way suddenly. In this syndrome, the deep tendon reflexes are exaggerated, and the pathological reflexes described on page 145 are present. This syndrome indicates affection of one of several "upper motor neuron" descending tracts, rostral to the level of the anterior horn cell. Common sites for disease are the corticospinal tracts (cerebral cortex, internal capsule, cerebral peduncles, medullary pyramids, and lateral columns of spinal cord).

The other major type of increased muscle tone is rigidity,

which tends to affect muscles without regard to their relation to gravity. The most striking clinical example is parkinsonism or paralysis agitans. Muscle resistance is characteristically intermittent when the muscle is palpated while being tested—an effect called "cogwheel rigidity." Reflexes are unaffected. The syndrome is characteristically associated with a tremor (described on page 140), a paucity of spontaneous face and body movement, and diminished "associated" movements—such as arm swing while walking. These later phenomena are referred to as "akinesia." There is frequently an associated gradual change in posture (described on page 132). Lesions are generally in the basal ganglia, particularly the substantia nigra.

Striking increases in extensor tone are seen in a few other situations:

1. With lesions of the high brain stem, the patient is usually unconscious; the arms and legs are held in striking extension and the arms are pronated. This posture is known as decerebrate rigidity.

2. With long-standing spinal cord transections, legs again may be held in extensor rigidity.

Coordination. Normal movement is highly dependent on the ability to smoothly contract the proper muscles to the degree needed, and to simultaneously relax the opposing muscles. Impairment in these abilities produces incoordination, which may be derived from disease of the cerebellum or its connections, corticospinal tract disease (spasticity), or sensory loss.

Cerebellar disease. Cerebellar disease results in failure to grade muscle contraction properly and in failure to contract the antagonist muscle so as to stop the desired movement. These failures result in an overshooting of the target, followed by a second muscle contraction to compensate for the error. This contraction is also frequently inaccurate and is followed again by a compensatory contraction. This sequence of events results in a number of clinical signs.

Intention tremor. Instruct the patient to touch your finger, and then touch his own nose. As the pointing finger approaches the target it displays a coarse tremor. You can accentuate this sign by moving your target finger, or by removing it to a distance, forcing the patient to stretch.

With the patient supine (or sitting), intention tremor can also be demonstrated in the leg. Have the patient lift a foot high in the air and touch your finger. Then have him touch the heel of the elevated foot to the opposite leg and run the heel down the shin. Intention tremor can be watched for in the course of this maneuver; it is manifested by a to and fro movement of the foot as it is drawn down the leg.

IMPAIRED CHECK SIGN: REBOUND SIGN. The patient flexes the elbow against resistance. When the arm is released, the biceps pulls the forearm back excessively, a compensatory extension occurs, then another contraction, producing an oscillation or "rebound." In the normal individual most of the contraction is isometric, so that little or no movement occurs. Similar testing can be performed on the deltoid muscle (outstretched arms) and others.

IMPAIRED SUCCESSION MOVEMENTS: ADIADOKOKINESIS. Instruct the patient to alternately pronate and supinate the hand, to evert and invert the foot, or to flex and extend the metacarpophalangeal joint. Patients with cerebellar disease perform these acts slowly and clumsily, failing to fix the more proximal joint in the extremity. With more severe disability, succession movements are impossible.

Cerebellar incoordination restricted to the arms and legs indicates disease of the cerebellar hemispheres. Ataxia of gait or of the trunk and titubation (described on page 139) indicate disease of the cerebellar vermis.

DISEASE OF THE MOTOR CEREBRAL CORTEX OR THE CORTICO-SPINAL TRACT. These disorders produce a clinically important sign that can be called impairment of coordination—slowness and clumsiness in finger movement, as tested by having the patient rapidly approximate each finger to the thumb. This deficit does not necessarily imply impairment of strength, and can exist in the almost complete absence of other signs of spasticity. Corticospinal tract disease does not cause incoordination of movement at the more proximal joints (e.g., elbow, wrist) nor any incoordination in the legs.

SENSORY LOSS.   Incoordination of movement can be produced in arms or legs by impaired sensation, with resultant clumsiness of movement and some ataxia of limb movement. Sensory loss can usually be distinguished from cerebellar disease, however, by the absence of the jerky to and fro tremor and by the absence of the impaired check phenomenon characteristic of cerebellar disease. Sensory impairment results in a slow, uncertain, searching type of voluntary movement.

Gait.   First ascertain that testing gait is compatible with the patient's physical condition, and be sure to protect the patient carefully from falling.

Gait should be tested with instructions to:

1. Walk naturally.
2. Walk "as if you are in a hurry."
3. Turn rapidly at the end of walking.
4. Walk heel to toe along a real or imaginary straight line.

The speed and fluidity of movement, the associated movement (e.g., arm swing), and the accuracy of foot placement are all observed.

The following are some common types of gait disturbance.

"FOOT-DROP" GAIT.   This is caused by weakness in dorsiflexing the ankle. To overcome this handicap, the patient elevates the affected foot higher than normal and the foot tends to point downward—a "steppage" gait. Such a gait occurs commonly in conditions causing flaccid weakness of the peripheral muscles of the leg, e.g., in peripheral neuropathy.

SPASTIC GAIT.   This is associated with spastic weakness as described on page 135. Movement is slowed, and flexion of the knee and hip joints is slowly and imperfectly performed. There is a lack of fluidity of movement. The affected leg (or legs) tends to remain adducted; in the more severe hemiplegia, the patient has to swing the affected leg around (circumduct), since he cannot flex and elevate it. In minimal or questionable spastic gait disturbance, it is particularly important to observe the patient attempting speed, as this accentuates the defect.

PARKINSONIAN GAIT. The patient shows a loss of arm swing on the affected side. The gait is short-stepped, and in severe cases, the patient has marked difficulty in starting to walk. The trunk develops a forward list, eventually forcing the patient, with his difficulty in stepping, to have to run forward "to catch up" with the center of gravity. The affected arm is characteristically held in semiflexion at the elbow and wrist.

CEREBELLAR GAIT. The patient shows either or both of the following abnormalities: (1) He cannot accurately place one foot in front of the other, and leg movement is jerky and uncoordinated; he tends to fall to one side. The abnormality becomes pronounced on heel to toe walking or hopping. (2) He may be unable to stabilize his trunk in the vertical posture, so that it tends to jerk back and forth. This motion is called "titubation."

SENSORY DEPRIVATION GAIT. The patient with sensory loss in the legs, particularly loss of position sense, tends to stagger, but usually not to the extent of the patient with cerebellar deficit; the former can frequently compensate by vision and is particularly handicapped with eyes closed. The foot placement has more of a "searching" nature, rather than being jerky.

WEAKNESS OF PELVIC AND ABDOMINAL MUSCLES. The patient is lordotic with a protuberant abdomen, and he walks with a wide-based "waddle" because he is unable to keep the pelvis horizontal on each step. This handicap is frequently combined with weakness of the proximal muscles of the legs, so that the patient tends to drag his legs rather than to lift them.

GAITS ASSOCIATED WITH HYSTERIA. A wide variety of abnormal gaits are displayed by hysterical patients; in one common variety the patient walks very slowly, weaving about and balancing on each step; in another the posture remains severly bent with no other disturbance of nerve, muscle, or joint function (camptocormia, see Fig. 4–2).

Abnormal movements. The most common disorders of movement are those that result from cerebellar disease (incoordination and intention tremor) and those caused by disease of the corticospinal tracts (spasticity). These abnormalities are not, in general, apparent when the individual is at rest. A few other motor disturbances are apparent on testing motor function, notably certain tremors, which may disappear at rest.

TREMORS SEEN ON MOVEMENT. One of these is a fine rapid tremor of the outstretched fingers, and sometimes of the head or feet — the frequency being about 6 per second. This phenomenon is almost always associated with heightened neuromuscular excitability and is seen in a variety of conditions mentioned previously. Anxiety is a common cause, as is withdrawal from sedatives such as alcohol, short-acting barbiturates, meprobamate, and many others. It also occurs in intoxication with stimulants and in hyperthyroidism. Rare causes are tetanus, tetany, or rabies. A frequent accompanying neurological sign is hyperreflexia. In the case of the withdrawal and stimulant intoxication states, distractibility, rapid speech, signs of an overactive sympathetic nervous system (sweating, dilated pupils), easy and excessive startle reaction, and, in severe cases, hallucinations occur. Seizures are frequent and may be expected in the states of excessive neuromuscular excitability.

Slower rhythmical tremor of the outstretched hands, of greater amplitude, is seen in three conditions.

BENIGN FAMILIAL TREMOR. In this condition, the tremor involves the head and hands, but only rarely the lower extremities. It is usually not apparent at rest. It exists on any type of innervation of the hands, but it is not markedly accentuated by tests of coordination (unlike the tremor of cerebellar disease). There are no other neurological signs, and a family history of a similar disturbance is usually readily elicited.

PARALYSIS AGITANS, OR PARKINSONISM. The tremor has about the same rate as, or is slower than, that of benign familial tremor. It is usually present both at rest and on innervation but is not accentuated by intentional movement. There is frequently a paradoxical reduction in the tremor during intentional movement. The tremor is most common and usually most severe in the fingers, but it may later involve all extremities and the head and neck. The other abnormalities of muscle tone have been described.

TREMOR OF HEPATIC DISEASE. With any type of diffuse, severe liver disease, a tremor may be seen when the patient holds the arms outstretched with the hand maximally dorsiflexed at the wrist. There is an intermittent diminution of extensor tone at the wrist, causing the hand to fall momentarily—only to be again raised (asterixis). This produces, in the severe stages, the appearance of a tremor of the hands that has a particular "wing beating" or "flapping" nature. The sign is frequently present in minimal form. In a rare disease, hepatolenticular degeneration (Wilson's disease), this sign is present in severe form, combined with signs of cerebellar dysfunction and of other types of motor dysfunction (e.g., basal ganglion disease).

TREMORS SEEN "AT REST." It is frequently quite difficult to ascertain that the limbs and extremities are truly at rest. During sitting and standing, there is much unconscious postural innervation of many muscles, and the signs of cerebellar dysfunction may be quite apparent; this is not a "rest" situation.

The actual difference between "tremor at rest" and "tremor on movement" is, of course, highly pragmatic and relative, since the body is being continuously subjected to various efferent stimuli, e.g., from the skin, joints, viscera, and special sense organs. It is only when certain of these are removed—those connected with the necessity for making sitting and standing postural adjustments—that we say the body is "at rest." In this latter state, then, several involuntary movements may occur, many of which may become accentuated by movement and almost all of which may become accentuated by emotional tension.

The tremor of paralysis agitans, described previously, is unique in that it is usually present at rest and is somewhat diminished by movement. It is frequently phasic in nature, waxing and waning over a period of several seconds.

MOTOR TICS. Rapid, arrhythmic contractions of a whole muscle or group of muscles that produce a gross movement of trunk, head, or limb may occur repetitively. Common examples are a jerking of the head to one side and a twitch of the shoulder or of the face. These stereotyped movements are frequently of psychogenic origin; they can also be residuals of encephalitis. In general, the more severe and persistent the motor tic, the more suspicious one should be that it is of organic origin. Postencephalitic tics are frequently bizarre in appearance and are associated with fixed abnormal postures of portions of the body and with muscle rigidity as described on page 135.

CHOREA. Rapid, nonrhythmic movements of skeletal musculature are called "chorea." These movements are asymmetrical and vary constantly in the location and strength of the muscular contraction. Some cause, for example, a minimal twitch of a finger joint; others, a fairly gross movement of the neck or shoulders. Facial grimacing and tongue movements are common. Chorea is usually seen in one of two syndromes: Sydenham's chorea, a syndrome of children and young people, which has a variable relationship to rheumatic fever, and Huntington's chorea, occurring in adult life, a hereditary degenerative disease of the cerebral cortex and basal ganglia.

ATHETOSIS. Slow, writhing movements of the extremities and trunk are called athetosis. These almost invariably appear in ths early years of life and are the result of damage to the basal ganglia in the paranatal period.

TORTICOLLIS. Involuntary rotation of the head to one side, frequently accompanied by other neck movement (flexion or extension of the head), is called torticollis. The head deviation is, characteristically, intermittent. The etiology is unknown.

DYSTONIA MUSCULORUM DEFORMANS. Gross, slow, long-sustained truncal movements occur in this entity, which occurs almost solely in children and young adults. The movements usually include torsion of the trunk, torticollis, and occasionally sustained pronation-supination movements.

REFLEX EXAMINATION

Deep tendon reflexes. Muscle contraction in response to a sudden stretch produced by striking the tendon (deep tendon

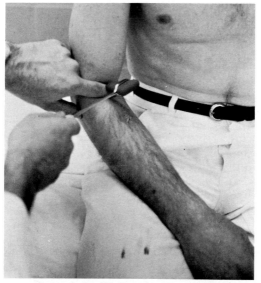

Figure 4-3. Eliciting the biceps reflex.

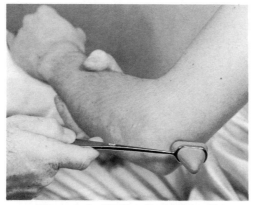

Figure 4-4. Eliciting the triceps reflex.

reflex, or DTR) can be theoretically produced in any striated muscle. Certain of these reflexes are customarily selected because of their availability and usefulness in localizing nervous system disease.

The extremity in which the reflex is to be examined must be relaxed, the patient preferably supine. The limb must be properly positioned. (The elbow should be semiflexed for the biceps reflex, the knee flexed for the quadriceps.) The extremity must frequently be supported, e.g., a hand under the knees in testing the quadriceps, or supporting the sole of the foot in testing the patellar reflex. The latter reflex, if sluggish or absent, can be elicited in different positions—with the patient kneeling on a chair, back to the examiner, feet hanging over the edge—or with the patient prone, knees flexed.

Two useful tendon reflexes that are frequently overlooked are the pectoralis and the adductor. The pectoralis, a reflex of the cervical 5, 6, 7 segments, is elicited with the patient supine. Place your index finger over the tendon just anterior to the axilla, then tap your finger with the reflex hammer which should produce sharp adduction of the arm. To elicit the adductor

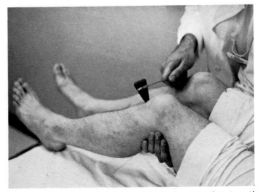

Figure 4–5. *Eliciting the quadriceps reflex in a recumbent patient. The examiner's arm supports the thighs slightly until the tendons relax.*

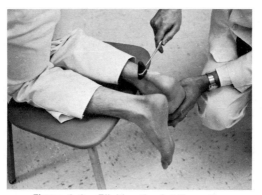

Figure 4-6. Eliciting the Achilles reflex.

reflex, a reflex of lumbar 1, 2, 3 segments, place your finger on the powerful adductor tendon just medial to the thigh; the response is adduction of the leg when the finger is tapped.

In all tendon reflexes except the patellar, the finger is placed over the tendon to be struck, and a sharp blow with the reflex hammer is administered. The homologous reflex on the opposite side is immediately tested for comparison, each performed two or three times.

Superficial reflexes. The reflexes examined are the abdominal and, in the male, the cremasteric. Abdominal reflexes are tested by stroking, from midline outwards, the four quadrants of the abdominal wall and observing the localized muscular contraction of the abdominal muscles. A sharp stimulus should be used.

The cremasteric reflex is tested by stroking the inner medial surface of the thigh with a sharp instrument and watching for elevation of the ipsilateral testicle, the normal response.

Pathological reflexes. The Babinski response is sought for by stroking the plantar surface of the foot with a sharp object, on the lateral border, from heel to the ball of the foot and then medially (Fig. 4–7). The normal response is a plantar deviation

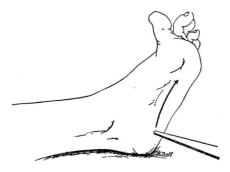

Figure 4–7. Diagram of method of producing Babinski reflex.

of the foot and toes. The Babinski response, which indicates impaired function of the corticospinal tracts, consists of an upward movement of the great toe and "fanning" of the other toes. It is frequently quite difficult to differentiate an early Babinski sign from a normal withdrawal response, and it is extremely important to do so since the Babinski response is one of the most important of neurological signs. Lessening the "tickle," by stroking the side of the foot or forcefully running one's finger distally down the anterior surface of the lower leg, may make the Babinski response unequivocal.

It must be remembered that reflex activity varies with the physiological state of the organism. Many normal persons are persistently hyporeflexic. Normally brisk reflexes gradually disappear under deep sedation, in hypokalemia, and in other types of metabolic disturbance. With heightened neuromuscular excitability, the reflex level gradually rises so that reflexes become extremely active, and clonus may appear (a repetitive, self-sustaining series of contractions upon muscle stretching). Such states occur in many metabolic derangements (uremia, hypocalcemia), intoxications with stimulants, and withdrawal from sedatives. Such states frequently precede convulsive seizures.

Three generalized types of tendon reflex abnormality are of particular diagnostic importance:

1. Moderately slow muscular contraction with delayed relaxation is characteristic of myxedema or hypothyroidism.

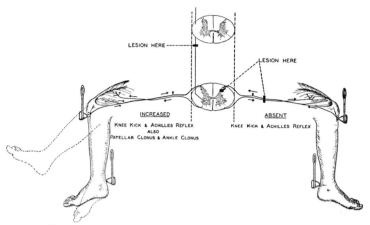

Figure 4–8. *Diagram illustrating lesions affecting reflexes.*

2. Excessive swinging of the lower leg when the knee jerk is tested while the leg is hanging free over the side of the table and the patient is sitting (pendulous reflex) is usually diagnostic of cerebellar disease.

3. Excessively brisk contraction with slow or subnormal postreflex muscle relaxation is the mark of corticospinal tract disease.

Another unique reaction, to percussion of muscle instead of tendons, is myotonia — a sustained, slow muscle contraction best elicited in the thenar eminence of the hand.

Several localizing patterns of deep tendon reflex abnormality are possible and of diagnostic significance.

Absence or depression of one or more reflexes unilaterally in the presence of normal reflexes elsewhere. This pattern indicates a break in the reflex arc at the segment of that reflex. It indicates localized disease of the spinal cord, of the anterior or posterior nerve roots, or of the peripheral nerve and is usually accompanied by signs of flaccid weakness as described on page 135 (Fig.

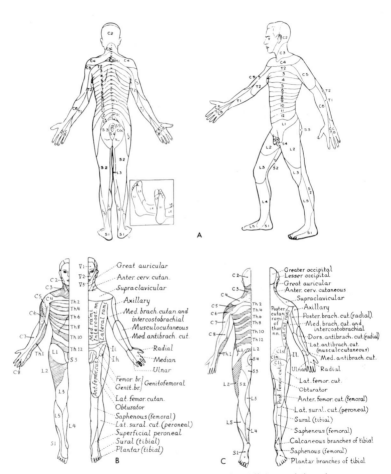

Figure 4–9. A, B, and C. Sensory supply of the skin by peripheral nerve segments. (Truex, R. C.: Strong and Elwyn's Human Neuroanatomy. 4th ed. Baltimore, Williams & Wilkins, 1959.)

4–8). Figure 4–9*A* indicates the spinal segments and peripheral nerves supplying the tendon reflexes most frequently tested.

Exaggeration of deep tendon reflexes on one side of the body. This sign usually indicates disease of one or more of the "upper motor neuron" tracts, particularly the corticospinal tracts, somewhere above the level of the anterior horn cell. It is the common reflex pattern in, for example, hemiplegia from cerebral thrombosis and hemorrhages, cerebral hemisphere tumors, and asymmetrical lesions of the brain stem. This pattern is frequently associated with spastic weakness as described on page 135. Localization of the site of the upper motor neuron damage is a complex matter; in general, the more the lesion is restricted to the motor cortex itself, the more restricted hyperreflexia can be. For example, if the lesion is restricted to the motor cortex, hyperreflexia may be restricted to one arm or leg, whereas in more caudal lesions, in the brain stem or spinal cord, the arm and leg both tend to be hyperreflexic. With spinal cord lesions, hyperreflexia tends to be bilateral. For accurately locating the lesion, however, other accompanying signs are used.

Exaggeration of reflexes caudal to a certain level on the trunk. With partial or complete transections of the spinal cord, the tendon reflexes below that level become hyperactive. This occurs, for example, in thoracic cord lesions.

SENSORY EXAMINATION

No part of the neurological examination is more difficult than the evaluation of the patient's appreciation of sensation. Four of five somewhat artificial types of stimuli are selected to sample the patient's reception of the many and varied stimuli of the external world. Even the norms of reaction to these selected stimuli are difficult to establish; they vary in certain respects with age and with states of awareness.

Customarily sampled in even the most cursory neurological examination are the sensation to pinprick (often miscalled "pain," which is, in fact, a much more complex phenomenon), to light touch, to vibratory sense, and to joint movement sensation (position sense). The extent to which other stimuli are used in testing the patient will depend largely on the results of testing with the previous ones. If suspicion of sensory loss to pinprick or light touch is present, then the patient should be carefully tested for normal perception of hot and cold. If these modalities are normal, but vibratory or joint sensation seems to be impaired, other tests should be done to evaluate "discriminatory" sensation—two point discrimination, perception of objects by touch, perception of "form" symbols from touch patterns, and weight discrimination.

Test Objects and Testing Techniques

Pinprick. In this discussion, because of general usage, "pain" will be used synonymously with "pinprick" despite the inaccuracy of this identification, as was previously noted. Either an ordinary sharp pin or a tailor's marking wheel can be used. The latter is preferred by some since it can more easily deliver a series of stimuli of nearly uniform intensity in series, as it is run over the skin in the desired direction, in order to elucidate an area of disturbed sensation. Stimuli with these objects must be carefully kept below injurious intensity, even when the skin appears analgesic.

In evaluating patterns of pain sensation, a few rules should be observed.

1. The patient should be asked, when two areas are stimulated, "Do these feel the same?" rather than "Do these feel different?" The latter question tends to promote excessive introspection in some patients that will result in false and fluctuating reports of sensory responses. It is wise, if differences in pain are reported from two areas, to deliberately *intensify* the pinprick stimulus to the area reported as less sensitive. If there is a true organic lesion, this area will still be less sensitive than the normal; if the difference was merely a perception of minor stimuli strength, then the hypalgesia will change sides with this maneuver.

2. If an area of altered sensation is found, it is easier to elicit its boundaries by starting within the hypalgesic area and moving outward to normal areas in various directions. This rule applies to other skin sensations, such as temperature and light touch.

3. Statements by the patients that the pin is felt less on one side than the other must not always be taken to mean that the side with the lesser sensation is the abnormal area. Although this is usually the case, occasionally the area with affected sensation will be *hyperalgesic;* in this case the homologous area on the other side with *normal* sensation will be reported by the patient as less sensitive. This confusion can be avoided by asking the patient to identify the "normal" feeling area, which most patients can readily do.

Light touch. A camel's-hair brush, a wisp of cotton, or porous paper is used. Any pressure is avoided. Allowance must be made for the thickness of the skin, especially on calloused surfaces where this modality cannot be easily evaluated.

Temperature. This modality need be tested only if there has been some other sign of sensory disorder. Glass or metal tubes filled with hot and cold water are usually used for testing, but it is difficult to maintain striking temperature differences for more than a few minutes. If more prolonged testing is desired, a piece of ice wrapped in paper or cloth can be used; results with this cold stimulus can usually be considered representative of all temperature stimuli.

Vibratory sense. The best testing instrument is a large aluminum tuning fork that vibrates at 128 cycles per second. The low frequency and the aluminum are desirable because they provide a long duration of vibratory sensation. The tuning fork is struck vigorously and placed over a bony prominence; the patient is asked whether he feels the vibration.

Responses should be "controlled" by, on occasion, *not* striking the tuning fork. Inattentive patients or those with severe sensory loss may report feeling the vibration at these times; these results cast doubt on the validity of the response and indicate the need for telling the patient to be "sure" he feels the vibration.

Vibratory sense is frequently diminished in the elderly, i.e., in the eighth decade and beyond, and prematurely in patients with certain diseases, notably diabetes mellitus and pernicious anemia. In any except aged adults, however, some vibratory sense with the tuning fork should be felt to the tips of the extremities. Abnormality indicates posterior column disease.

Joint sensation. The normal individual immediately appreciates even a few degrees of movement of the interphalangeal joints. Have the patient close his eyes and tell you when he first knows his finger (toe, wrist, ankle) is being moved and in which direction. In most patients, this should first be demonstrated with the eyes open. Grasp the joint lightly on its lateral surfaces (to avoid giving up-down pressure clues) and slowly move it until the patient responds. Several random tests are performed on each joint. If finger and toe sensation are quickly and accurately perceived, no further testing is needed; if they are defective, wrist and ankle movement (affected only by more gross lesions) are tested.

Discriminatory Sensation

There are several examinations that are thought to test the ability of the central nervous system to integrate and interpret the "simple" kinds of sensation (i.e., touch, pinprick, and temperature). Three points can be made about these tests before they are described.

1. In the presence of an obvious loss of touch sensation, they cannot be interpreted. These are tests of normal function of the parietal lobe of the brain (contralateral to the extremity tested), and one can think of the parietal lobe as using the crude touch sensations as material out of which patterns are built. If the material is absent or is grossly diminished in amount (as in peripheral neuropathy or spinal cord lesions), then the patterns cannot be built, and neither can parietal lobe function be tested.

2. These tests are usually used only in the hand. Whereas sensation from all parts of the body can be, and is, integrated into patterns, it is in the hand that sensory discrimination is most

delicate and is most essential for rapid and accurate use of the part.

3. These tests should be used when there is impaired function of the extremity, but only when there is also no accompanying gross sensory loss. A clue in the motor examination that discriminatory sensation may be impaired is pseudoathetosis. This term refers to a slow drifting up and down of the fingers of the outstretched hand, giving the effect of a searching movement.

The tests are as follows:

Stereognosis. The blindfolded patient is asked to identify a small object (e.g., comb, key) placed in his palm. Not only the accuracy of the patient's answer is assessed, but also the dexterity with which he manipulates the object. The patient with astereognosis will move the object clumsily, may say quite simply that he does not know what it is, or will give an erroneous answer. He will usually attempt to aid the one hand with the other. Another delicate test of the same nature is that of requiring the patient to identify the denomination of a coin.

After testing the hand suspected of impaired sensation, it is wise to test the other hand in order to compare the speed and accuracy of responses.

Palm writing. A number is slowly written with a blunt object (e.g., dull pencil) in large script on the patient's palm. Again, the accuracy and speed with which the numbers are "read" are compared for the two palms.

Two point discrimination. The distance between which two points can be identified as two separate stimuli varies widely from one part of the body to another. The test is usually performed on the fingertips, where the normal nervous system can identify stimuli placed a few millimeters apart as separate. In the palm of the hand, the distance will be somewhat greater, but on the trunk, the distance must be a matter of inches before the nervous system can distinguish between the stimuli.

Texture and weight. The ability to define the "feel" of surfaces is also an elaboration or integration of touch impulses. Swatches of felt, silk, and toweling are placed in the patient's hand and he is asked to identify them, or at least to distinguish rough textures from smooth. Similarly, the ability to differentiate weights can be tested. Two or more metal measuring weights, e.g., 200 and 500 gm., can be placed in the patient's palm in sequence; he is then asked which is heavier.

Double simultaneous stimulation. The normal adult can easily recognize the fact that a pinprick or touch stimulus is being applied to two widely separated parts of his body, e.g., both hands or both feet. With damage to the parietal lobe, however, the phenomenon of extinction may occur. The patient notices no, or only questionable, diminution in sensation in the extremities contralateral to the diseased parietal lobe when each hand or foot is tested separately. When bilateral homologous parts of the body are tested simultaneously (e.g., both hands, both feet), the patient is aware *only of the stimulus to the site opposite the normal hemisphere,* and he "extinguishes" the stimulus contralateral to the damaged hemisphere.

The lighter the touch, the more sensitive is this test. It is, furthermore, not an all or none result; a patient may frequently show extinction on 50 per cent of the trials; if the extinction is consistent to the same side, it is highly diagnostic. The test for extinction has proved to be a valuable screening test for hemisphere sensory dysfunction; double simultaneous stimulation is also used to elicit early and minimal visual field defects.

Patterns of Sensory Dysfunction

All modalities of sensation cannot be examined in every patient. It is important, therefore, to search in patients for patterns of sensory impairment that are commonly met with clinically. Several of these are described in the following paragraphs.

Single Peripheral Nerve Sensory Loss. The areas subserved by the separate peripheral nerves are indicated in Figures 4–9*B* and *C*. In general it will be noted that in the hand and arm, the border between these areas divides the lateral from the medial side of the hand, arm, leg, and, to a lesser degree, of the foot. It is important from a practical point of view to run the sensory stimulus (pin, hair) from, for example, the little finger to the thumb across the fingertips or from the ulnar to the medial side of the hand in searching for differences of sensation. Similarly, lateral and medial portions of the foot and leg must be compared.

Difficult differential diagnostic problems arise concerning certain sensory patterns caused by nerve root lesions as compared to single peripheral nerve lesions. In the hand, the eighth cervical dermatome area of sensory distribution is similar to that of the ulnar nerve, and the sixth cervical to that of the median nerve. The sciatic nerve distribution is similar to that of the L_5, S_1, and S_2 nerve roots combined. The correct diagnosis is made by (1) carefully delineating the area of sensory loss (it is different with peripheral nerves as opposed to nerve roots), (2) noting the presence of and type of pain (nerve root pain is darting and extends, characteristically, from the spine to the peripheral portions of the extremity), and (3) analyzing the accompanying reflex and motor disorders in terms of correspondence to a nerve root or peripheral nerve distribution. Disturbed sensation in the thumb and index finger can be caused, for example, either by a C_6 nerve root lesion or a median nerve lesion, but the former commonly causes depression of the biceps tendon reflex (C_5, C_6), while this reflex (whose efferent segment is carried by the musculocutaneous nerve) is unaffected in median nerve lesions.

Polyneuropathy. Frequently, all the peripheral nerves are affected in one or more extremities, usually in their distal portions only. This syndrome, which occurs in a wide variety of clinical conditions—notably with many systemic diseases (vitamin B deficiency, diabetes mellitus, and many exogenous and endogenous intoxications)—gives rise to characteristic patterns of sensory abnormality. The patient complains of paresthesias ("tingling" or "electricity" feelings) in the distal parts of the extremities affected; these sensations are frequently unpleasant or even painful in a continuous, aching way. Using both the pin and cotton wisp, begin at the fingertips and progress proximally, requesting the patient to note any change. The characteristic

TABLE 4–1. COMPARISON OF POLYNEUROPATHY
WITH CONVERSION HYSTERIA

	Polyneuropathy	Hysteria
Level of sensory change	Graduated	Sharp
Type of sensory loss	Partial	Frequently complete
Associated reflex loss	Usually present	Absent
Limbs affected	Symmetrical	Usually one limb or two on same side
Comparison of levels of pin sensation and touch sensation	Different	Identical

finding is an increase in the intensity and "clarity" of both pinprick and touch sensation at a level, in one or more extremities, that tends to be the same around the circumference of the extremity. This type of sensory loss is frequently called "glove" or "stocking." The level of sensory change may be anywhere from the base of the fingers to the wrist—or even, more rarely, at the shoulder in the upper extremity and at homologous levels in the foot and leg. It is very common for this type of sensory loss to be fairly symmetrical in both legs, in both arms, or in all four extremities.

A similar type of sensory loss is found in psychiatric states—"conversion hysteria"—in the absence of organic pathology. The differences in these two conditions are summarized in Table 4–1.

The peripheral nerve syndrome comprises sensory loss to *all* modalities (either in the single peripheral nerve or polyneuropathy pattern), flaccid weakness of the extremity, as described in a previous section, and a depressed or absent tendon reflex in the affected portion of the extremity.

Spinal cord sensory syndromes. The tracts carrying various types of sensation diverge in the spinal cord; characteristic, then, of spinal cord lesions is *dissociation* of one type of sensory loss from another. The types of this dissociated loss are as follows:

Damage to the dorsal column of the spinal cord. This is commonly seen in certain metabolic diseases and in spinal cord compression and is characterized by diminution of vibratory and position sense with preservation of pinprick and touch sensation. The sensory loss is almost inevitably symmetrical in two or in all four extremities. The gait is frequently wide-based because of the impaired position sense.

Unilateral spinal cord lesion. It is rare for the spinal cord, small as it is, to be affected on one side solely, but occasionally a lesion (particularly trauma) will affect only one side.

Because the fibers carrying pain and temperature sensation cross to the spinothalamic tract on the opposite side soon after entering the spinal cord, the clinical picture will be that of diminution of pinprick and temperature sensation on the opposite side of the body, below the level of the lesion.

Because the corticospinal tracts do not cross at the spinal cord level, there will be clinical signs of their affection, *ipsilateral* to the lesion. These signs will be spastic weakness of greater or lesser degree, as described on page 135, with hyperactive reflexes and a Babinski sign.

In lesions affecting one side of the cord, signs of nerve root dysfunction are also common because of the proximity of these structures. Irritation of nerve roots produces sharp pain, and damage to nerve roots produces sensory loss — usually in a clearly segmental distribution, radiating from the trunk distally.

Central core of spinal cord. The fibers carrying pain and temperature sensation cross the spinal cord to the contralateral spinothalamic tract either at the segment of entry or a few segments higher. Lesions in the center of the spinal cord, such as syringomyelia, therefore cause loss of pinprick and touch sensation bilaterally. The loss is restricted to the segments involved. Touch and vibratory sensation tend to be preserved (the opposite occurs in disease of the dorsal column.) Painless burns of the extremities are the common early symptoms of these lesions. They are most frequent in the cervical spinal cord, resulting in a characteristic pattern of symmetrical loss of pinprick and temperature sensation in both arms.

SEVERE COMPRESSION OF SPINAL CORD.   The sensory pattern in this lesion is an exception to the rule that dissociated sensation is manifested by cord lesions. The characteristic finding is a change in the quality or quantity of sensation at a certain level, both anteriorly and posteriorly. These levels tend to be best defined in the trunk (thoracic cord lesions), but, of course, they can occur at any segment. When the level is in the cervical cord, the line between normal and impaired sensation will characteristically divide the lateral from the medial half of the hand. It cannot be overemphasized that the level is frequently only partial; the patient feels the stimulus *less clearly* below a certain level than above. This sensory finding is frequently accompanied by some spastic weakness and hyperreflexia below the level.

Brain stem syndromes.   Sensory disturbances caused by brain stem lesions consist of impaired sensation of one whole side of the body. Facial hypalgesias (sensory loss) or paresthesias (distorted sensations) characteristically occur and may be either ipsilateral or contralateral to the bodily sensory loss. Combinations of cranial nerve, corticospinal tract, and cerebellar dysfunctions are, of course, usually associated with brain stem syndromes.

Thalamic syndrome.   A characteristic distortion of sensation occurs with lesions of the thalamus. Diminution of sensation, in moderate degree, occurs over the side of the body contralateral to the lesion. Spontaneous pains throughout that side of the body are present, frequently precipitated by light tactile stimuli or emotional excitement.

Cerebral hemisphere lesions.   Diminution of sensation in one half of the body, contralateral to the lesion, is the common manifestation of hemisphere lesions. The more the lesion is localized to the cerebral cortex, the more the sensory disturbance shows two particular characteristics:

1. Localization to one part of the body, e.g., right arm or right face and arm.

2. Loss of discriminatory sensations (as described previously) with comparatively intact pinprick and touch sensation.

CRANIAL NERVES

Olfactory nerve. The sense of smell is tested with any aromatic substance that can be easily carried, e.g., coffee or oil of wintergreen. It is important not to use substances actually irritating to the mucosa (e.g., spirits of ammonia), since they stimulate trigeminal nerve endings in the nasal mucous membranes. Each nostril is tested separately.

Optic nerve. The examination of the eye includes evaluation of visual acuity, pupillary reactions, extraocular movements, corneal sensation, the optic fundus, and the visual fields. Some of these subjects will be discussed in Chapter 7, Examination of the Eyes.

Visual acuity. Visual acuity may be rapidly checked using a Snellen chart at 20 feet, testing each eye separately and recording the smallest type read. When loss of vision is severe, the patient should be asked to count the examiner's fingers, or to recognize motion, or just to distinguish between light and dark.

Pupillary reactions. The normal reaction has been discussed. A few important abnormal pupillary reactions are the following:

Argyll Robertson pupils. This abnormality, usually seen in syphilis of the central nervous system, is characterized by pupils that are small, unequal in size, irregular in outline, and poorly reactive or nonreactive to light, with normal reaction to accommodation.

Adie's pupil. This phenomenon, of unknown cause, may be unilateral or bilateral; unequal pupils may then occur; the affected pupil is large and reacts to light and darkness by extremely slow constriction and dilatation. It is not associated with disease, but it frequently occurs with absent reflexes.

Unilateral dilated fixed pupil. This is the characteristic pupil of third cranial nerve (oculomotor) palsy—usually associated with ptosis and a laterally deviated eye.

Visual fields. If you stand directly in front of the patient and he fixes his gaze on your nose, a good evaluation of the vis-

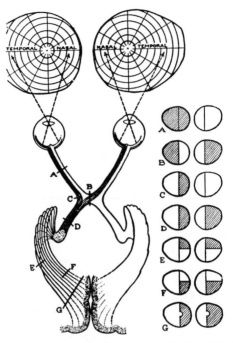

Figure 4-10. *Optic pathway showing how lesions at various points appear on the field of vision. (Homans, J.: A Text-book of Surgery. 5th ed., 1940. Courtesy of Charles C Thomas, Publisher, Springfield, Illinois.)*

ual fields can usually be accomplished by confrontation. A small white object is brought from the peripheral quadrants of the field medially to the central field, the patient being instructed to respond when he sees it. Each eye, of course, must be tested separately. A valuable refinement of the test is the use of double simultaneous stimulation. Here the patient fixes gaze with both eyes on your face while you hold both hands in the lateral (temporal) portion of the patient's visual fields. Move the fingers of each hand separately and then together, asking the patient to point to the hand that moved. Minimal or questionable visual field defects on one-sided testing are frequently made definitive by the consistent "extinction" of the impaired field on bilateral simultaneous testing. Furthermore, the test can be made sensitive by reducing the amount of finger movement used as a stimulus.

Common visual field defects are:

1. Impaired field in one eye, normal in the other; diagnostic of a lesion anterior to the optic chiasm.

2. Bitemporal restriction of the visual field; diagnostic of a lesion at or near the optic chiasm.

3. Complete homonymous hemianopsia (whole temporal field in one eye, whole nasal in the other); diagnostic of lesion posterior to the optic chiasm, usually in the optic tract or occipital cortex.

4. Homonymous quadrant defect (homonymous defect as above, but restricted to upper or lower quadrant); diagnostic of, respectively, temporal or parietal lobe brain lesion.

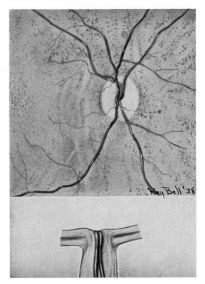

Figure 4–11. Normal fundus of the eye.

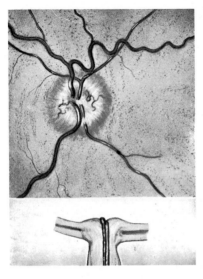

Figure 4–12. *Moderately "choked" disc.*

OPTIC FUNDI. The technique of examination will be described in Chapter 7. Inspection of the optic disc may reveal one of two abnormalities of particular interest in neurological disease.

Papilledema or papillitis. In early stages the disc borders are blurred and veins are engorged and tortuous. In later stages, hemorrhages occur, the borders of the disc are indistinguishable, and actual elevation of the disc can be measured on the ophthalmoscope. With the presence of normal visual acuity and such a funduscopic picture, the diagnosis is probably papilledema; with markedly impaired acuity, it is papillitis.

Optic atrophy. The disc is chalky white, extremely sharply defined, and avascular.

Many types of abnormalities of the retina and blood vessels are, of course, possible; appropriate manuals should be consulted.

Extraocular movements — III, IV, VI nerves. The position of the eyelids is observed. If one eyelid droops, ptosis is present, and this is usually caused by impaired function of the third cranial nerve (or its nucleus), of the sympathetic nervous system (Horner's syndrome), or of the neuromuscular junction (myasthenia gravis). This differential diagnosis is made by observing the severity of the ptosis and the size of the pupil. If ptosis is extreme, Horner's syndrome is ruled out. In Horner's syndrome the pupil in the affected side is smaller than the other; in third nerve lesions it is larger; in myasthenia it is normal.

The position of the globes is observed next; several abnormal patterns are commonly seen:

1. One eye may be deviated medially; even on effort it can-

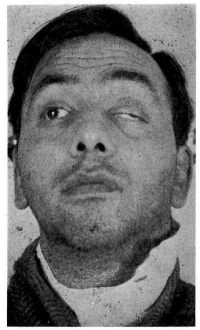

Figure 4–13. *Patient with left oculomotor nerve palsy due to intracranial aneurysm. (Cogan, D. G.: Neurology of the Ocular Muscles, 1956. Courtesy of Charles C Thomas, Publisher, Springfield, Illinois.)*

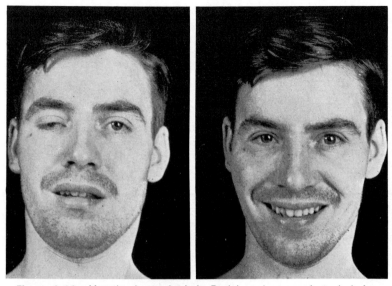

Figure 4–14. *Myasthenia gravis. Left: Facial weakness and ptosis before neostigmine. Right: Fifteen minutes after administration of 1.5 mg. neostigmine. (Cogan, D. G.: Neurology of the Ocular Muscles, 1956. Courtesy of Charles C Thomas, Publisher, Springfield, Illinois.)*

not be moved laterally. This syndrome indicates weakness of the lateral rectus muscle or dysfunction of the abducens nerve or its nucleus (sixth cranial nerve). This cranial nerve is commonly affected peripherally by increased intracranial pressure from any cause and by diabetes mellitus.

2. One eye may be deviated laterally and cannot be moved by effort. As indicated, this sign is one of medial rectus muscle, or oculomotor nerve, dysfunction.

3. The eyes may both be medially deviated (convergence). Here either the function of both lateral rectus muscles is impaired, or if the convergence can be overcome, a convergence spasm, probably a hysterical symptom, is present.

4. The eyes may be divergent (severe lesion of the midbrain and the convergence center).

5. Both eyes may be deviated to the right or left. Such forced conjugate deviation can occur from cerebral or pontine lesions. Cerebral lesions may stimulate eye movements to the contralateral side temporarily (as is seen, for example, in seizures) or to the ipsilateral side permanently when due to destructive lesions.

Eye movements are then tested through their full range while the patient is interrogated concerning diplopia. Lesser degrees of muscle weakness, not leading to overt deviations of the eyes, may be detected. Impaired upward gaze is a sign of midbrain disease. It should be emphasized that myasthenia gravis frequently manifests itself by ophthalmoplegia and must be suspected in any kind of extraocular muscle weakness unless clearly ruled out (usually by means of an intravenous edrophonium test). Also to be looked for are disconjugate gaze, the eyes moving independently, and monocular nystagmus—a definite sign of pontomedullary disease. Jerky eye movements are indicative of cerebellar disease.

Nystagmus refers to rhythmical, conjugate, involuntary eye

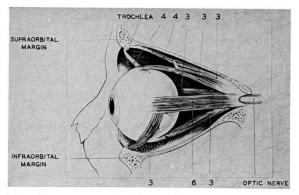

Figure 4–15. *The nerve supply of the ocular muscles. Numbers refer to the cranial nerves. (Corning, H. K.: Lehrbuch der topographischen Anatomie. 5th ed. Wiesbaden, J. F. Bergmann, 1914.)*

movements that may be horizontal, vertical, or rotary. Nystagmus is commonly seen in disease of the vestibular portion of the eighth cranial nerve, either peripherally or in the nuclei of the brain stem, and in dysfunction of the pontomedullary region, whether this be transient, as in intoxications with barbiturates (one of the common causes), or long-lasting, as in multiple sclerosis or tumors of the brain stem. These latter two conditions frequently also produce other cranial nerve palsies. Nystagmus with unilateral preponderance is usually associated with disease of the labyrinthine system, whereas slow, coarsely swinging nystagmus is frequently associated with disease of the vestibulocerebellar connections.

Fifth cranial nerve. The trigeminal nerve is a mixed nerve containing both motor and sensory fibers.

The motor root of the trigeminal nerve innervates the muscles that close the jaw. When affected unilaterally, the opened jaw deviates to the side of the lesion. Ask the patient to clench the jaws shut, then check for atrophy of the masseter and temporalis muscles by observation and palpation.

There are three sensory roots to the trigeminal nerve. The ophthalmic (first) division of the nerve provides sensation of the anterior scalp, the superior portion of the face, and the cornea. Decreased sensation in this portion of the face is usually accompanied by a decreased corneal reflex. With the patient's gaze deviated away, touch a wisp of cotton to the cornea; a prompt blink should result. The maxillary (second) division of the nerve supplies the midportion of the face, the upper jaw, the oral cavity, and the nose. The mandibular (third) division supplies the lower jaw and the teeth of the lower jaw. Sensation to pinprick and touch can be tested inside the oral cavity, which is entirely supplied in its anterior part by the trigeminal nerve. Disturbed sensation is frequently confined to one division, either when the lesion is peripheral to the ganglion or, more rarely, in the sensory nucleus of the trigeminal nerve itself. Trigeminal neuralgia is a severe painful affliction of the face that occurs without demonstrable impairment of sensation.

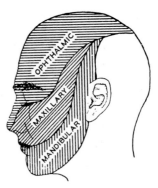

Figure 4-16. *The branches of the trigeminal nerve.*

Seventh cranial nerve. Weakness of one side of the face may be evident on inspection—a sagging cheek, a drooping lower eyelid, and failure to close the eyes. Ask the patient to open his eyes widely (while wrinkling of the frontalis muscle is observed), to show his teeth, to puff out his cheeks with air, and to whistle. (The latter requires considerable strength of the perioral muscles). Occasionally, facial asymmetry may be misdiagnosed, in that prior facial palsies may produce late contractures of the facial muscles on the weak side, which will lend an appearance of sagging to the normal side. If both upper (i.e., frontalis and periocular muscles) and lower parts of the face are involved, the lesion is usually in the facial nucleus or facial nerve; if just the lower part of the face is involved, the lesion is usually in the "upper motor neuron," i.e., in the corticobulbar tract in the hemispheres or brain stem. If a portion of the facial nerve that accompanies the chorda tympani is affected, the patient will also have lost taste on the anterior two-thirds of the tongue. Taste is tested by the careful application of concentrated solutions of sugar, vinegar, salt, or quinine to the extended tongue by means of an applicator. The patient must, of course, keep the tongue extended. In case of delayed appreciation of the sensation, due to a unilateral lesion, the opposite side can be used as a normal control.

Occasionally fasciculations are seen in the facial muscles. They are commonly the result of fatigue, but if severe and persistent, they are a sign of irritation of the facial nucleus, and thus of medullary disease.

Eighth cranial nerve. The auditory nerve has two branches, the cochlear and vestibular nerve. Diseases of the cochlear nerve cause altered hearing, usually deafness, frequently associated with tinnitus, or some variety of abnormal spontaneous auditory sensation in the head. The degree of hearing loss can readily be tested by holding a watch at varying distances from either ear. The distance at which the ticking can no longer be heard will depend upon the watch, but this simple method will demonstrate a difference in hearing on the two sides. It is important to determine whether the deafness is due to a conduction defect from a disease in the middle ear, or is a result of altered nerve mechanisms in the cochlea or the cochlear nerve. Audiometry should be employed.

WEBER'S TEST. When a vibrating tuning fork is held against the forehead, the sound is better heard in the normal ear if the disease is due to auditory nerve damage, but it is better heard in the affected ear if there is an obstruction in the middle or external ear.

RINNE'S TEST. A tuning fork is first held in front of the ear and then placed on the mastoid process. If the sound is not heard when the tuning fork is held near the ear, but is heard when it is placed against the mastoid process, the lesion is probably in the middle ear or external auditory canal and not in the nerve itself.

The vestibular nerve plays an important role in balance and appreciation of body position in space. Disease of the vestibular branch of the auditory nerve may cause nystagmus and vertigo.

True vertigo is a sensation of "whirling" and must be differentiated from faintness, ataxia (a motor disturbance), and loss of consciousness. Patients with labyrinthine disease will usually display their hypersensitivity to movement by resisting sudden head movement of any kind. If you rapidly move the patient's head, he may stagger, display obvious signs of discomfort, or become nauseated.

Nystagmus, if not found by the ordinary test of having the patient look in different directions, should be sought for with the patient's head hyperextended, turned to each side, and rapidly changed in position.

Ninth and tenth nerves. The function of these cranial nerves is evaluated together. Dysfunction is manifested by:

1. Nasal speech (due to failure to elevate the soft palate).

2. Observed immobility of the soft palate, with the tongue depressed and the patient attempting to phonate. If one side only is affected, the palate rises (the normal side only), producing an asymmetrical curtain-like effect.

3. Impaired gagging when the pharyngeal wall is stimulated.

4. Impaired sensation to touch on the posterior part of the tongue and the pharyngeal walls.

5. Accumulation of mucus in the mouth. Pharyngeal weakness produces defective swallowing, and secretions therefore accumulate. The patient may actually regurgitate food or fluid through the nose.

6. Orthostatic hypotension. The glossopharyngeal nerve carries the stimuli from the carotid sinus that aid in maintaining blood pressure upon assumption of the upright posture. The ninth and tenth nerves are affected by masses in the neck, by lesions of the medulla oblongata (neoplastic, vascular, or degenerative), and occasionally by metabolic disturbances affecting other cranial nerves.

7. Hoarseness. All muscles of the larynx except the cricothyroid are supplied by the recurrent laryngeal nerve (a branch of the vagus), and lesions of the tenth nerve therefore cause vocal cord paresis and hoarseness. Irritative lesions of the tenth nerve can cause a "brassy" cough.

Eleventh nerve. Atrophy of the sternocleidomastoid muscle can be observed in the neck when the head is turned away from the side of the suspected lesion; weakness can be assessed by the ease with which this movement is opposed, and the muscle can be palpated. When both muscles are weak and atrophied, the neck is noticeably slender, and the patient has difficulty flexing the head.

Atrophy of the upper portion of the trapezius muscle may also be apparent by inspection for symmetry.

Twelfth nerve. When atrophy of the tongue occurs, increased wrinkling of the tongue surface becomes apparent. With advanced atrophy the protruded tongue deviates to the affected side. If the lesion is nuclear, fibrillations of the tongue muscle can be observed as minute twitches on the mucosal surface.

Speech disturbance, in bilateral affection, may occur moderately early and is characterized by articulation deficits. There is no impairment, as has been discussed in an earlier section, of language structure. The speech sounds as if the patient is burdened by an object in his mouth; this effect results, of course, from the impaired mobility of the tongue. Swallowing is frequently impaired because the tongue cannot manipulate the bolus of food properly and place it in the proper relationship to the pharyngeal wall.

ANCILLARY EXAMINATIONS OF THE NERVOUS SYSTEM

Mobility of the spine. In various neurological syndromes, there may be marked muscle spasm preventing movement of the spine.

1. With meningeal irritation of any type, and occasionally with posterior fossa brain tumors, there may be marked nuchal rigidity. When the examiner attempts to flex the neck with the patient supine, the knees will involuntarily flex also.

When the examiner attempts to extend the leg of a patient who is lying on his back with the thigh flexed, extension of the knee is limited by muscle spasm and pain. This sign is called Kernig's sign and is usually present in cerebrospinal meningitis.

Brudzinski's sign is often present in meningitis and is of

considerable diagnostic value. In reality there are two Brud-zinski signs. The first is elicited by passive flexion of one leg, which causes a similar flexion of the leg that is not touched. The other sign is elicited by raising the patient up by his neck. A positive sign may consist of flexion of the legs, the knees, the hips, or, at times, of all four extremities. The first of these signs is often referred to as the "contralateral reflex," whereas the second is referred to as "Brudzinski's neck phenomenon." The second sign is more common than the first.

2. With compression of the fifth lumbar or first sacral nerve roots, there is frequently a limitation of the ability to raise the leg while it is in a fully extended position. With the patient supine, the examiner lifts each of the patient's legs in turn, the knee remaining fully extended. The normal range is at least 60 or 70 degrees; in the youthful, to 90 degrees. With nerve root compression, severe pain will be felt on the ipsilateral side, in the low back, or in the sciatic notch region. Some individuals will have a degree of limitation that results from tight "hamstring" muscles.

Palpation and percussion of the head and spine. The entire scalp should be firmly palpated. Small irregularities of the underlying skull are frequently present in normal individuals. Occasionally, however, bony defects or abnormal protuberances may be palpated. These may or may not be tender.

Points in the scalp or in the posterior portion of the neck that are painful to deep palpation may be present in patients with vascular or muscle tension headaches.

In patients in whom there is a question of a spinal cord lesion, firm palpation and percussion of the spinous processes of the vertebrae must be carried out. Localized tenderness often indicates the site of a diseased vertebra.

Auscultation of the head. In all patients with a headache, in those complaining of a "noise in the head," and in those with cranial nerve dysfunctions, the head should be carefully examined with a stethoscope. It is particularly important to listen with the bell stethoscope over the closed eyes to search for a bruit that may indicate an intracranial vascular lesion of some nature, most frequently a malformation.

It is also important to auscultate the area overlying the carotid arteries at the base of the neck in patients with symptoms referable to the head. Substantial bruits here also may indicate abnormalities of the underlying vessels.

COMMON CLINICAL TERMS

Apraxia—Inability to carry out purposeful movements in the absence of paralysis.

Ataxia—Impaired coordination of the limbs or trunk manifested by loss of smooth synergy between agonist and antagonist muscles.

Diplopia—Double vision.

Dysarthria—Speech impairment due to impaired movements of the tongue.

Flaccidity—Weakness of skeletal muscle associated with diminished resistance of the muscle to passive stretch.

Hypalgesia—Diminished sensation to pain or pinprick.

Paraplegia—Paralysis of both lower extremities.

Paresthesias—Abnormal sensations referred to the surface of the body, having qualities of a tickling or tingling character.

Ptosis—Drooping of the eyelid.

Spasticity—Impaired function of skeletal muscle associated with increased resistance of the muscle to passive stretch that varies with the limb position and also associated with increased tendon reflexes.

COMMON CLINICAL SYNDROMES

Akinetic mutism—Awake patient with normal attentiveness and motor power as tested by eye movements but without spontaneous speech or movement.

Aphasia—Impaired form of speech formulation associated with greater or lesser difficulty in articulating words and the ability to understand spoken speech, due to a lesion in the frontal-temporal portion of the dominant hemisphere.

Capsular hemiplegia—Spasticity of one arm and leg associated with diminished sensation on the same side of the body.

Chorea—Ceaseless occurrence of rapid, jerky, but coordinated movements, performed involuntarily.

Homonymous hemianopsia — Visual field defect characterized by loss of nasal field on one side, temporal field on the other, due to a lesion in the appropriate cerebral hemisphere behind optic chiasm.

Internuclear ophthalmoplegia — Impaired conjugate lateral movements of the eyes without specific paralysis of a single extraocular muscle with accompanying monocular nystagmus.

Lateral medullary syndrome — Dysfunction of several of the following: Sensation on one side of the face, ability to swallow, lateral eye movement, ipsilateral cerebellar control, sensation on the opposite side of the body, usually due to infarction of a lateral portion of the medulla and adjacent portion of the cerebellum.

Parkinsonism — Unilateral or bilateral bradykinesia or slowing of spontaneous movement accompanied by rhythmic tremor, flexion posture of the body and rigidity of muscles, with reflexes remaining normal.

Posterolateral column syndrome of the spinal cord — Bilateral spasticity of the lower extremities and/or the upper extremities (depending on the cord level) and associated diminution of vibratory sense to that level, with normal preservation of pinprick and touch sensation.

Transverse myelitis — In the acute stage, loss of sensation below a segmental level with loss of reflexes and loss of bladder and bowel control. In more slowly progressing lesions, diminished sensation below the segmental level with hyperreflexia and spasticity and impaired control of bowel, bladder, and sexual function.

BIBLIOGRAPHY

Adams, R. D., Denny-Brown, D., and Pearson, C. M.: Diseases of Muscle. A Study in Pathology. 2nd ed. New York, Harper & Row, 1962.

Alpers, B. J., and Mancall, E. L.: Clinical Neurology. 6th ed. Philadelphia, F. A. Davis Co., 1971.

Baker, A. B., and Baker, L. H. (eds.): Clinical Neurology. Hagerstown, Maryland, Harper & Row, 1971.

Brain, W. R.: Diseases of the Nervous System. 7th ed. London, Oxford University Press, 1969.

Brock, S., and Krieger, H. P.: The Basis of Clinical Neurology. The Anatomy and Physiology of the Nervous System in Their Application to Clinical Neurology. 4th ed. Baltimore, Williams & Wilkins Co., 1963.

Brodal, A.: The Cranial Nerves, Anatomy and Anatomico-Clinical Correlations. Springfield, Illinois, Charles C Thomas, 1959.

Cogan, D. G., and Williams, H. W.: Neurology of the Visual System. Springfield, Illinois, Charles C Thomas, 1966.

DeJong, R. N.: The Neurologic Examination. Incorporating the Fundamentals of Neuroanatomy and Neurophysiology. 3rd ed. New York, Hoeber, 1967.

Denny-Brown, D.: The Basal Ganglia and Their Relation to Disorders of Movement. London, Oxford University Press, 1962.

Mayo Clinic: Clinical Examinations in Neurology. 3rd ed. Philadelphia, W. B. Saunders Co., 1971.

Merritt, H. H.: A Textbook of Neurology. 4th ed. Philadelphia, Lea & Febiger, 1967.

Steegmann, A. T.: Examination of the Nervous System. A Student's Guide. 3rd ed. Chicago, Year Book Medical Publishers, 1970.

Vinken, P. J., and Bruyn, G. W. (eds.): Handbook of Clinical Neurology. Amsterdam, North-Holland Publishing Co., 1969.

Walsh, F. B., and Hoyt, W. F.: Clinical Neuro-ophthalmology. 3rd ed. Baltimore, Williams & Wilkins Co., 1969.

5
EXAMINATION OF THE HEAD AND NECK

Inspection and palpation are the most productive maneuvers in examination of the head and neck. Percussion and auscultation, except in certain vascular lesions, are not often applicable to examination of this area of the body.

THE HEAD

Upon observing a patient, note the position of his head. An exaggerated forward thrust may be the result of an abnormality of the cervical vertebrae. Patients with the Klippel-Feil syndrome have a characteristic position of the head due to fusion of the cervical vertebrae (Fig. 5–1). Tilting of the head may result from an attempt to compensate for defective vision or to diminish the discomfort of a furuncle or abscess on the neck.

Head movements are often suggestive of certain diseases. In Parkinson's disease a slight but constant tremor of the head occurs, whereas, in contrast, patients with a habit spasm make sudden, unexpected movements of the head, often accompanied by facial grimaces. In aortic insufficiency a common finding is constant jerking of the head forward and backward synchronously with the heart beat. This is de Musset's sign, named after

175

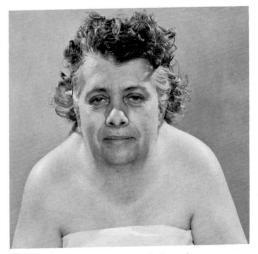

Figure 5–1. *Klippel-Feil syndrome.*

the poet who suffered from aortic insufficiency and showed this phenomenon. Sudden, jerky movements of the head may be observed in chorea.

The size and shape of the head should be noted. In hydrocephalus, the large head with the bulging forehead is quite striking (Fig. 5–2). An equally striking picture is the tower skull or steeple head (Fig. 5–3). This deformity, seen in oxycephaly, is due to premature synostosis of the coronal and sagittal sutures. Patients suffering from oxycephaly show marked exophthalmos with heavy eyelids, resulting in a dull, vacant expression. Prominent frontal bosses and some exophthalmos are present in Apert's syndrome. The skull in rickets often has a flattened or squared appearance. Paget's disease produces a characteristic enlargement of the cranial vault so that the shape of the head resembles that of an acorn (Fig. 5–4). Asymmetry of the head and face occurs in a few rare genetic disorders.

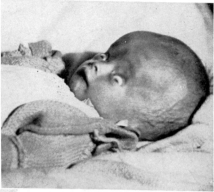

Figure 5-2. Hydrocephalus.

Figure 5-3. Steeple head. (Mitchell, A. G., and Nelson, W. E.: Textbook of Pediatrics. 5th ed. Philadelphia, W. B. Saunders Co., 1950.)

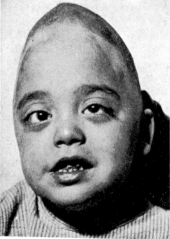

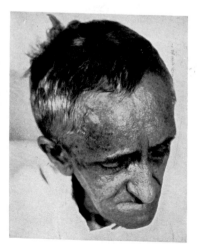

Figure 5-4. Head in Paget's disease of the bone.

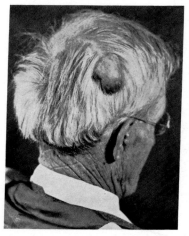

Figure 5–5. Sebaceous cyst of the scalp.

The forehead in congenital syphilis may show bilateral anterior bosses and, at times, posterior bosses as well. This latter condition gives the skull such a distinctive appearance that it has been described as a cross-bun skull. The bosses are commonly referred to as Parrot's nodes. Tumors originating in the skin or subcutaneous tissue of the forehead may produce striking changes. Sebaceous cysts of the scalp are common and may be either singular or multiple (Fig. 5–5). Tumors of the frontal bone, such as osteoma, cause a marked prominence of the forehead. A bulging prominent rounded mass, usually partially collapsible and pulsating, in the glabellar or lower midforehead is typical of an encephalocele; dermoid cyst or ectopic brain in the same location due to the same developmental abnormality may present a similar round mass, but the aperture of the bony defect cannot be felt as in the case of encephalocele. Gardner's syndrome of multiple osteomas, fibromas, epidermoid cysts, and intestinal polyposis may be suspected if multiple osteomas involve the skull. Frontal sinusitis often produces marked swelling of the forehead, accompanied by intense frontal headache and fever.

Percussion of the skull is seldom rewarding. However, auscultation is sometimes of value. Cranial bruits may be heard on auscultation of the skull. Loud bruits that are heard by the examiner are usually heard by the patient; however, the patient may hear bruits that are inaudible to the examiner. In both cases, the bruit is synchronous with the heart beat, and occlusion of the carotid artery by strong digital pressure causes the bruit to disappear. Listen to the head with the patient standing and lying on his back, on his abdomen, and on both sides. Bruits may be heard within the head in the Sturge-Weber syndrome, in which large angiomas involve the leptomeninges. The presence of a port-wine nevus on the face should alert the physician to listen over the same side of the skull.

In carotid cavernous fistula, which is usually the result of a fractured skull, palpation of the eyeball reveals a systolic thrill, and auscultation reveals a systolic murmur over the eyeball and temple on the side of the injury. Cranial bruits have been described in arteriovenous fistulas of the cerebral vessels, vascular malformations, brain tumors, intracranial saccular aneurysms, angiomas of the scalp, glomus jugulare, carotid body tumors, and Paget's disease. Systolic cranial bruits may also be heard in coarctation of the aorta, in hypertensive cardiovascular disease, and in toxic goiter because the sound may be transmitted via the carotid arteries to the cranial vessels.

Face

Pallor, cyanosis, argyria, and jaundice are all readily seen in the face. The patient with aortic insufficiency is usually pale; the patient with mitral valve disease, ruddy or flushed. Girls in their teens who have mitral lesions often have beautiful complexions with high coloring. Patients with heart failure may be cyanotic, as are persons with congenital heart defects in which blood is shunted from the right to the left side of the heart. When seen in the acute stage, carbon monoxide and cyanide poisoning produce a cherry red complexion. Marked flushing of the cheeks, "hectic flush," is common in pulmonary tuberculosis.

The facial features as well as the size and shape of the head are quite distinctive in acromegaly (Fig. 5–6). The features of acromegalic patients are so striking that anyone who has carefully observed such a patient will immediately recognize a subsequent case, often without being able at first fully to explain his reasons for the diagnosis. Here again, as is frequently the case in medicine, the visual sense rapidly registers and recalls a complex set of findings without conscious reasoning. The massive face with its craggy eyebrows, prominent nose, and massive lower jaw form a characteristic and unforgettable picture.

The appearance of the face in leprosy is often pathognomonic. Here again, the experienced physician makes an instantaneous diagnosis because he has seen the condition before. The characteristic appearance of the leper's face is due to subcutaneous infiltration over the forehead, cheeks, and chin, combined with a flattening and broadening of the nose (Fig. 5–7).

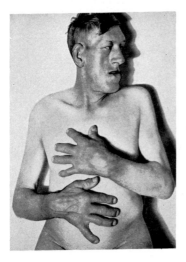

Figure 5–6. Acromegaly.

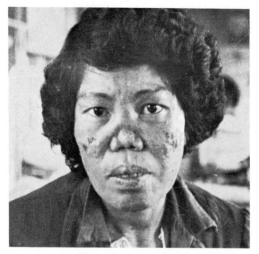

Figure 5-7. *Leprosy.*

The resemblance to a lion's face is striking and gave origin to the term "leonine facies." The telltale signs of bald eyebrows, elongated ear lobes, and premature wrinkling of the face are so pathognomonic that the lay public in indigenous areas can readily recognize those diseased.

The facial expression produced by adenoid enlargement is characteristic—the mouth hangs open and the chin recedes somewhat. The impassive, sphinxlike expression of patients suffering from paralysis agitans is so striking that the "parkinsonian mask" is recognized as one of the cardinal signs of this disease. This expressionless face, with its elevated eyebrows and facial immobility, was not mentioned by Parkinson himself but may be a very early sign of the disease. Hippocrates' delineation of the facies indicative of approaching death (the Hippocratic facies) remains after more than two thousand years a classic description: "a sharp nose, hollow eyes, collapsed temples; the ears cold, contracted and their lobes turned out; the skin about the fore-

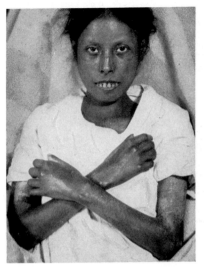

Figure 5–8. *Scleroderma. The skin is very tight over the hands and also over the face. The patient is trying to smile and show all her teeth.*

head being rough, distended, and parched; the color of the whole face being green, black, livid, or lead-colored."

The skin of the face may be markedly thinned and tightened in scleroderma. This tightening may be so severe that the patient is unable to close his lips over the teeth or to smile (Fig. 5–8).

The changes in the skin from radiodermatitis commonly caused by repeated doses of superficial radiation for acne, hirsutism, or ringworm are quite characteristic. The skin is dry and inelastic like parchment, is hairless, does not sweat, and has a thin pinched appearance that is due to atrophy of subcutaneous fat. Patchy pigmentation, multiple papillomatoses, keratoses, and even skin cancers are frequently seen.

Facial hemiatrophy (Romberg's disease) produces a tight, thin, brown pigmented skin with atrophy of the subcutaneous fat, muscle, and bone in the affected area usually unilaterally and often in a segmental area of the tissue innervated by the trigeminal nerve (Fig. 5–9). The depressed atrophic area of the forehead and scalp is so striking as to appear to be excised as by tangential sword cut, thus the description "coup de sabre" (Fig. 5–10). Unilateral hypertrophy with overgrowth of bone and soft tissues causing definite asymmetry is usually caused by a neurofibroma, hemangioma, or lymphangioma.

A marked lateral shift and recession of the chin, giving the semblance of a very full cheek and jaw on one side compared to a smaller, more normal appearance of the opposite side, is due to diminished growth of the head and neck of the mandible, often seen in temporomandibular ankylosis. The mouth can be scarcely opened a few millimeters, if at all, and the larger side is actually the normal side.

In the Ehlers-Danlos syndrome, or pseudoxanthoma elasticum, the skin is flexible and elastic, allowing the face to be distorted if the skin is stretched (Fig. 5–11). Many individuals suffering from this disorder can touch the tip of their nose with

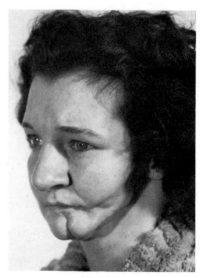

Figure 5–9. *Facial hemiatrophy (Romberg's disease). Atrophy in distribution of the mandibular division of the trigeminal nerve.*

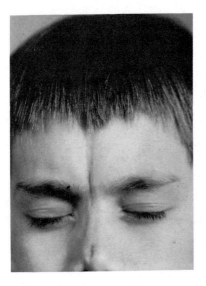

Figure 5–10. *Facial hemiatrophy, showing typical "coup de Sabre."*

their tongue. The skin of the face and neck of eunuchs is often deeply creased and wrinkled (Fig. 5–12). In early stages the phenomenon is particularly noticeable about the eyes.

In some patients suffering from tonic spasm of the muscles of the face, the eyebrows may be raised and the angles of the mouth drawn out, forming the so-called sardonic grin or risus sardonicus, a condition seen most frequently in tetanus. Chvostek's sign, a pathognomonic finding in tetany, is elicited by tapping sharply with the finger just in front of the external auditory meatus over the facial nerve at its point of emergence from the parotid gland. This maneuver results in a contraction or spasm of the facial muscles on the same side since it stimulates the hyperexcitable facial nerve. The most marked examples of tetany occur in hypocalcemic states such as that resulting from accidental removal of the parathyroid glands. Tetany may also be observed in a milder form when the patient becomes alkalotic after continued vomiting or prolonged hyperventilation.

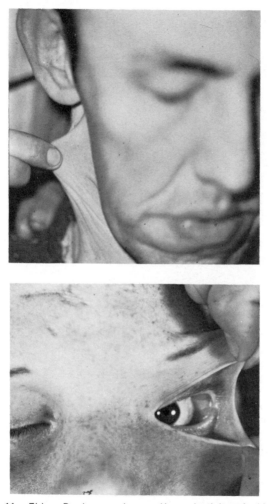

Figure 5–11. *Ehlers-Danlos syndrome. Hyperelasticity of skin. (Scheie, H. G., and Albert, D. M.: Adler's Textbook of Ophthalmology. 8th ed. Philadelphia, W. B. Saunders Co., 1969.)*

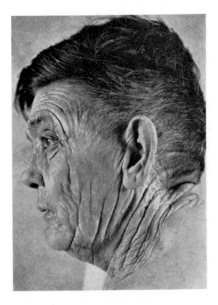

Figure 5–12. *The face and neck of a eunuch showing marked creases and wrinkles.*

Paralysis of the facial nerve, Bell's palsy, is almost always unilateral. The muscles on the affected side of the face are paralyzed and when the patient is asked to wrinkle his forehead, the affected side remains smooth. He is unable to shut his eye on the affected side (Fig. 5–13) and cannot move the affected half of the mouth if asked to show his teeth. The patient is also unable to whistle. Patients with involvement of the facial nerve from leprosy typically have paralysis of the orbicularis oculi muscles of one or both sides. This condition, called lagophthalmos, leads to blindness because of exposure of the cornea with subsequent drying, keratitis, ulceration, scarring, or perforation of the globe. The orbital branch of the nerve is frequently involved without complete palsy.

When involvement of the facial nerve is supranuclear or nuclear, there is accompanying hemiplegia or evidence of in-

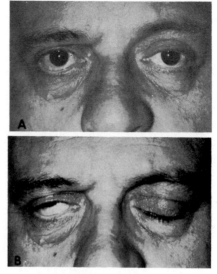

Figure 5–13. Bell's palsy of the right side. A, Eyes open in primary position. Note ptosis of left lid. B, Attempted lid closure. Note weakness of right orbicularis and upward rotation of right eye, or Bell's phenomenon. (Courtesy of Dr. David J. McIntyre.)

volvement of other cranial nerves. In most instances, however, only the nerve trunk itself is involved, and the signs are due to paralysis of the muscles supplied by the nerve. When the facial nerve is involved, after the chorda tympani has joined it, the sense of taste is lost over the anterior two-thirds of the tongue on the affected side. A bizarre sweating on eating in the distribution of the auriculotemporal nerve (Frey's syndrome) is seen fairly frequently as the result of peripheral injury to the facial nerve, most often postoperatively following removal of a parotid tumor.

Single or bilateral enlargement of the parotid glands occurs in mumps, in Mikulicz's syndrome (Fig. 5–14), in Sjögren's syndrome, and sometimes as a terminal event in severe infections. Parotid enlargement due to parotitis or abscess may occur with dehydration in postoperative or very ill patients, usually in the elderly, or may be caused by a stone in the parotid duct or gland. Tumors of the parotid gland are most often smooth, round or multinodular, nontender, and of rubbery hard consistency. If there is associated facial palsy and the mass is hard and fixed to deep structures, the tumor is fairly sure to be a malignant one. Prominence in the parotid region which definitely enlarges and gets hard when the patient tightly clenches his teeth is due to hypertrophy of the masseter muscle. A small, round, inflammatory nodule just in front of the root of the helix and the tragus is most likely an infected preauricular sinus, which can be seen as a small dimple or sinus in the skin of the root helix (Fig. 5–15).

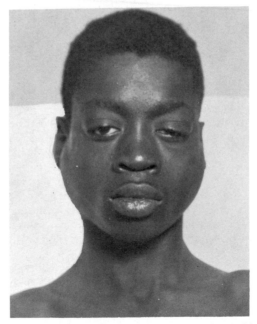

Figure 5–14. Mikulicz's syndrome. Note enlarged parotid glands.

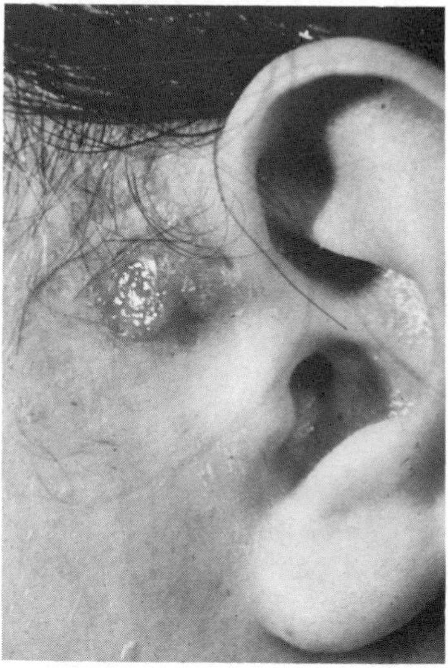

Figure 5–15. *Preauricular sinus. Note dimple at bottom of root helix and granuloma just anterior to it.*

Facial Bones

Swelling is often so marked after facial injury that visual evidence reveals only marked soft tissue edema and ecchymosis. Visual examination of the occlusion is very helpful to decide if the jaws are broken and displaced. Extraocular movements should be carefully appraised as well as gross vision and reaction of the pupils to light. A frequent finding in an involved orbit is the lack of free synchronous movement of the globe in various directions, but especially on upward gaze. Diplopia is an important finding. The lids may be so swollen that they may have to be forced open gently to allow examination. Anesthesia of the cheek and adjacent upper lip and nose usually means that the infraorbital nerve has been injured. Diminished sensation of the lower lip and adjacent chin means that the mental nerve is defunctionalized; this is usually the result of disruption of the inferior alveolar nerve running in its mandibular canal, which has been displaced by a fracture. Careful palpation for abnormal movements of the mandible with associated pain as well as careful symmetrical comparisons of the orbital rims, malar prominences, and zygomatic arches may disclose bony displacement. If the patient cannot open or close his jaw, the zygomatic arch may be impinging upon the ramus or coronoid process of the mandible. Palpation over the temporomandibular joints as the patient tries to move the jaws may reveal some displacement. Limitation of movement due to pain and cracking or snapping of the jaws indicates pathology in the joint. A deviated depressed nasal bone or cartilage may be felt to be out of place, but swelling of soft tissue often makes such abnormal bone relationships hard to detect.

Bloody and especially watery discharges from the nose and ears after severe injury are likely to contain cerebrospinal fluid which has escaped through meningeal tears with skull fractures. A gloved finger inserted gently into wounds of the scalp or careful palpation of hematomatous swellings may reveal a depressed skull fracture. A hematoma along the mastoid tip (Battle's sign) is indicative of temporal bone fracture. In all of these instances, a neurological appraisal is indicated.

Hair

In syphilis and diabetes, the hair may be scanty, or the scalp may show small, irregular patches of baldness. Occasionally there may be complete loss of hair or total baldness in these diseases. In some patients with pituitary insufficiency, and particularly in Simmonds' disease, the hair may be extremely sparse. In alopecia areata the patient suddenly loses patches of hair, leaving spots of baldness. Patients suffering from this disease often awaken in the morning to find a handful of hair on the pillow and a bald spot on the scalp where the hair fell out. Loss of hair in typhoid fever is common. Distinct patches of baldness may be the result of thermal or radiation burns and are common in ringworm infestation of the scalp.

In myxedema the hair is scanty and is invariably harsh, dry and lusterless—a sign suggestive of thyroid deficiency. In pediculosis capitis infestation, the hair is matted together and covered with nits. Close observation discloses numerous lice running about among the hairs. The exaggerated form of this condition is known as "plica polonica." Enlarged lymph nodes in the postauricular and mastoid area are often present in patients harboring such head lice. Loss of hair over the frontal area is seen in some genetic disorders such as myotonic dystrophy. Waardenburg's syndrome is characterized by a white forelock associated with deafness, heavy eyebrows, and a broad-based nose.

Lips

The lips may be deformed from birth, as is the case in cleft lip (formerly called harelip), which is due to failure of the nasolabial ridges to unite during fetal life (Fig. 5–16). The process may involve one or both sides of the upper lip, extend-

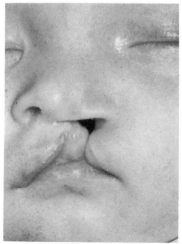

Figure 5–16. Cleft lip, unilateral complete.

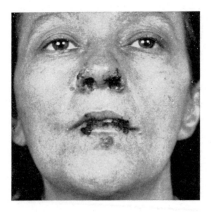

Figure 5–17. Herpes labialis et nasalis.

ing to the floor of the nose through the gum and palate, and may be complete all the way to the pharynx. The lips may reflect generalized edema, as in patients with nephritis, or may be part of a more localized tissue reaction, as in angioneurotic edema. Extremely dry lips are often seen in feverous patients, in diabetes mellitus, and in severe dehydration from any cause.

One of the commonest lesions on the lips is herpes labialis, the well known "cold sore" or "fever blister" (Fig. 5–17). This begins as a collection of small, painful vesicles and rapidly proceeds to form scabs. This eruption often is not limited to the lips but extends to the nose or cheek.

The upper lip, particularly, may be the seat of a chancre, which should always be suspected when a patient shows a large, persistent, firmly indurated, but relatively painless sore on the lip (Fig. 5–18). Adults who have suffered from congenital syphilis often show "rhagades," small linear scars running out from the mouth upon the cheeks (Fig. 5–19). In riboflavin deficiency, fissures in the corner of the mouth are common. Perlèche, a monilial infection of the labial commissures, particularly of children but also of adults, produces thickening and desquamation of the epithelium at the corners of the mouth and often results in fissures. Similar lesions may result from poorly

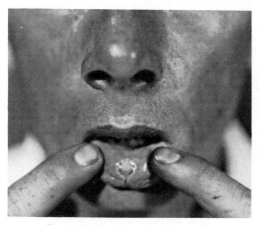

Figure 5–18. Chancre of lower lip.

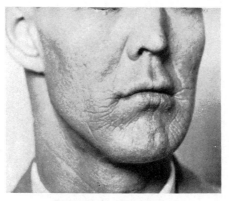

Figure 5–19. Rhagades.

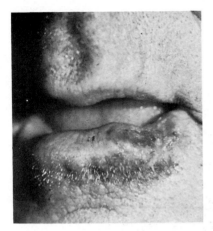

Figure 5-20. Carcinoma of the lower lip. Note ulceration. Palpation of the margins and depth will indicate greater involvement.

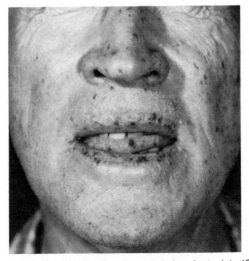

Figure 5-21. Osler-Weber-Rendu disease (telangiectasia). (Quick, A. J.: Hemorrhagic Diseases and Thrombosis. Philadelphia, Lea & Febiger, 1966.)

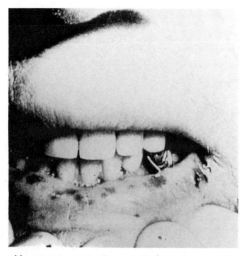

Figure 5-22. *Mucocutaneous pigmentation in Peutz-Jeghers syndrome. (Stauffer, J. Q.: Hereditable multiple polyposis syndromes of the gastrointestinal tract. In Sleisenger, M. H., and Fordtran, J. S.: Gastrointestinal Disease: Pathophysiology, Diagnosis, Management. Philadelphia, W. B. Saunders Co., 1973.)*

fitting dentures that channel saliva out through the commissures, resulting in maceration of the skin. White patches, called leukoplakia, are frequently found on the lower lips of heavy smokers and those exposed to the elements (sun and wind). In an old or middle-aged person, a firm, painless, slowly growing lip ulceration with hard borders is usually a carcinoma (Fig. 5-20).

Soft, collapsible, blue spots on the lower lips are varicose veins and raised, bluish red, tumorlike nodules often with a strawberry-like surface are hemangiomas or lymphangiomas. Common papillary warts are frequently seen on the lips of children who have been biting the warts on their fingers. Small, subcutaneous, red angiomas may be seen in patients with Osler-Weber-Rendu disease or hereditary telangiectasia (Figs. 5-21 and 15–4). Pigmented spots on the oral surface of the lips and the cheeks are a part of the Peutz-Jeghers syndrome and are associated with intestinal polyposis (Fig. 5–22).

Teeth and Gums

The teeth and gums often give important indications of systemic disease, and, conversely, the condition of the teeth and gums may affect the general health of a patient. The presence of pyorrhea alveolaris (Riggs' disease) is established by demonstrating retraction of the gums from the roots of the teeth and by pressing out small quantities of pus from the root sockets. In elderly persons, pyorrhea leads to marked loosening or loss of teeth. The teeth should be further examined for caries or cavities and for the presence of crowned teeth which may be devitalized. Perhaps the most striking appearance of the teeth occurs in congenital syphilis, first described by Sir Jonathan Hutchinson and since known as "Hutchinson's teeth" (Fig. 5–23). His original description follows:

The central upper incisors are the test-teeth .... The teeth are short and narrow. Instead of becoming wider as they descend from the

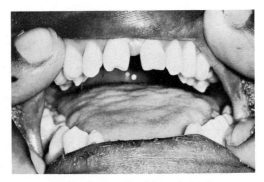

Figure 5–23. *Hutchinson's teeth.*

gum, they are narrower at their free edge than at their crowns, their angles having been, as it were, rounded off. In the center of their free edge is a deep vertical notch, made by the breaking away or non-development of the middle lobe of the tooth-crown. This notch taken together with the narrowness and shortness of the tooth, is the main peculiarity.

Hutchinson's triad, characteristic of congenital syphilis, consists of Hutchinson's teeth, interstitial keratitis, and labyrinthine disease causing deafness. Another type of tooth very characteristic of congenital syphilis is the "screwdriver tooth."

Imperfect dentition or crumbling, decayed teeth may call attention to dietary faults. In inveterate chewers of tobacco, the molars usually show a smooth, polished surface and sometimes may be ground down to the level of the gums. Incisor teeth that do not hit or meet and occlude with the teeth of the opposite jaw may have minute saw-toothed cutting edges. The presence of minute amounts of fluorine in drinking water results in teeth that are pitted and stained yellow, brown, or black (Fig. 5–24). This condition is called "mottled enamel" or "fluorosis."

The lead line in chronic lead poisoning is an important diagnostic sign, and its recognition by astute physicians has saved many patients with severe abdominal pain from unnecessary surgical operations. It consists of a black, finely stippled line occurring on the gums just below the point at which the teeth

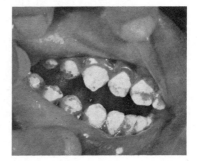

Figure 5–24. *Mottled enamel due to fluorine in water.*

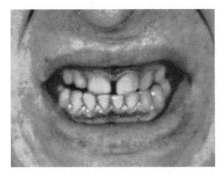

Figure 5-25. Lead line.

emerge or at the border of teeth and gums (Fig. 5–25). Henry Burton, who first described this phenomenon, wrote, "The edges of the gums attached to the necks of two or more teeth of either jaw, were distinctly bordered by a narrow leaden-blue line, whilst the substance of the gum apparently retained its ordinary colour and condition." Examination of this line with a

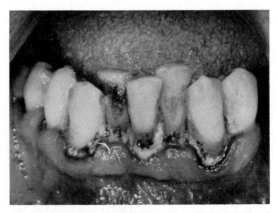

Figure 5-26. Bismuth line and local irritation of the gingiva in a patient receiving bismuth therapy. (Glickman, I.: Clinical Periodontology. 4th ed. Philadelphia, W. B. Saunders Co., 1970.)

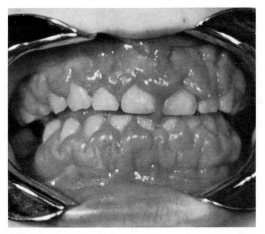

Figure 5–27. Hyperplasia of the gums in acute monocytic leukemia.

hand lens shows that it consists of innumerable dots, placed close together in a row.

Other heavy metals, especially bismuth, may produce a similar line. Chronic mercury poisoning causes spongy gums in which the teeth tend to loosen.

In scurvy the gums are soft, tender, and spongy; the teeth are often so loose that they can be plucked out with the fingers.

Hyperplasia of the gums may be the result of various diseases or medications, such as acute monocytic leukemia (Fig. 5–27) or the excessive use of diphenylhydantoin (Dilantin). At times the etiology is obscure. Fibroma of the gums presents a striking picture and occurs frequently in patients with tuberous sclerosis. A hard tumor at the gingival margin of the lower teeth and supported on a relatively narrow stalk is "epulis," a giant cell fibroma that is the result of an inflammatory reaction and is benign (Fig. 5–28). A long ridge of bone felt along the inside of the mandible in the floor of the mouth, most prominent from canine (cuspid) to the second molar, is called a torus mandibularis

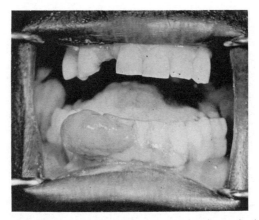

Figure 5–28. *Epulis, a hard fibrous tumor growing from gingival margin.*

and has little pathological significance. In the midline just behind the symphysis a projection of bone toward the frenulum of the tongue is the genial tubercle which sometimes protrudes enough in the edentulous patient to interfere with the wearing of a lower denture. Neurofibromas may involve the gums in von Recklinghausen's disease.

Normal occlusion is the correct meshing of the maxillary and mandibular teeth (Fig. 5–29). Malocclusion may indicate a fracture of the jaw or midface or may be the result of a congenital or developmental anomaly. Underdevelopment of the mandible associated with median cleft palate (Pierre Robin syndrome) does not allow the teeth to occlude anteriorly and, conversely, marked forward growth of the jaw as in acromegaly produces an overbite with malocclusion. For a normal bite the upper jaw is of a slightly greater arch spread than the lower one, so that the upper teeth overlap the lowers slightly and the upper teeth are slightly behind the lowers by the width of a third of a molar tooth, making the cusps interdigitate. A sudden change in the bite will be most disturbing to the patient and may produce

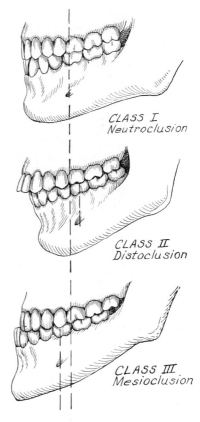

Figure 5-29. Occlusion. Class I, neutroclusion; note relationship of cusps of opposing first molars. Class II, distoclusion; note incisor protrusion and maxillary molars a bit forward of mandibular molars. Class III, mesioclusion; note forward position of all mandibular teeth. (Dingman, R. O.: The management of facial injuries and fractures of the facial bones. In Converse, J. M. (ed.): Reconstructive Plastic Surgery. Vol. II. Philadelphia, W. B. Saunders Co., 1964.)

pain in the temporomandibular joints or cause headache (Costen's syndrome).

Osteomyelitis and tumors of the mandible may produce marked distortion of the gums and the teeth of the lower jaw. Many tumors of the jaws relate to cysts or new growths of the teeth, the mandible being involved more often than the maxilla. Cancer of the alveolar process, buccal cheek, floor of the mouth,

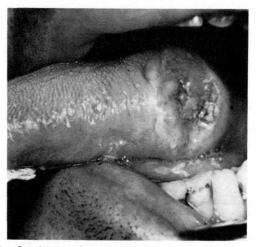

Figure 5–30. *Carcinoma of tongue, a common site of origin. Grasping the tongue and pulling it out facilitates the examination. Palpation is important to determine extent.*

or tongue (Fig. 5–30) can and does involve either jaw and should be carefully palpated to determine fixation and the depth of involvement. "Eyes" on the end of the palpating finger are more important in these instances than the eyes in the head of the examiner.

Tongue

The old-time physician always looked carefully at the patient's tongue, and many stories were told of his uncanny ability to diagnose disease from the tongue's appearance. His modern successor should never omit this time-honored but simple procedure, since in certain diseases the tongue shows a characteristic appearance.

In scarlet fever the tongue may be red, may be covered with a slight fur, and may show enlarged reddened papillae, giving rise to the term "strawberry tongue." This tongue is especially striking because there is commonly an area of pallor around the mouth. In typhoid fever the tongue is heavily coated and furred and is often covered with brownish sores. The tongue in pernicious anemia and sprue has a striking appearance—pale, smooth, glossy, and atrophic (Fig. 5–31). In the early stages of pernicious anemia, however, the tongue, although sore, may appear normal. In sprue the tongue, though commonly pale and smooth, may at times be red, inflamed, or fissured. The tongue in pellagra is at first rough and swollen; later it becomes smooth and very red and often shows glossitis. Excessive smoking may produce mild glossitis with brownish gray discoloration of the tongue and a smoker's bad breath.

The tongue in Ludwig's angina may be acutely inflamed, painful, and so swollen that it protrudes, preventing the patient from closing his mouth. In leukoplakia the tongue is covered

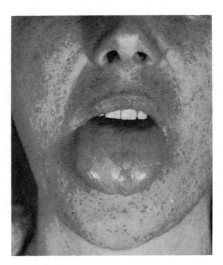

Figure 5–31. Tongue in pernicious anemia.

with firm, white, indurated lesions resembling firmly attached crusts (Fig. 5–32). The condition is common in smokers, and may become malignant. In myxedema and cretinism the tongue may be enlarged and protrude from the mouth, but it is not painful. A congenital tumor of the lymphatics or blood vessels, often an admixture, produces a very large tongue (Fig. 5–33), often with a strawberry-like surface. With upper respiratory tract infections, such a tongue may swell rapidly, appear bluish black, and be bathed in copious pink, blood-tinged saliva. The tongue may protrude in children with Down's syndrome. Amyloidosis may also cause the tongue to be enlarged and biopsy reveals the characteristic deposits of amyloid material. In dehydrated patients the tongue is small and dry.

Carcinomas of the tongue (see Fig. 5–30) produce marked induration with destruction and ulceration. Tuberculosis of the tongue is sometimes seen as a granulomatous ulceration in the midline of the back of the tongue, whereas cancer is rarely, if ever, in the midline.

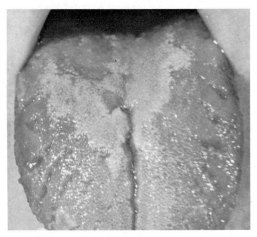

Figure 5–32. *Leukoplakia of tongue.*

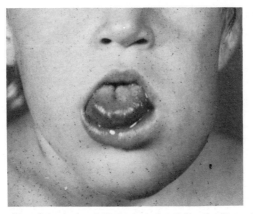

Figure 5-33. *Lymphangioma of the tongue involving the floor of the mouth, chin, and left cheek.*

The geographic tongue, although striking in appearance and a cause of great worry to the patient, is quite harmless in itself (Fig. 5–34). It is commonly seen in nervous persons. The patient shown in the illustration was suffering from mild hyperthyroidism. The appearance of the geographical tongue changes daily, the "map" commonly passing through a cycle of changes.

A curious-looking tongue is the so-called scrotal tongue, which presents grooves and markings much like those on the surface of the scrotum (Fig. 5–35). This condition may be related to vitamin B deficiency and is often relieved by treatment with vitamin B complex. The tongue in Addison's disease shows at times small, irregularly shaped, round or oval areas of black or brown pigmentation.

Marked furrowing of the tongue is in most instances congenital. Food particles often collect in the deep furrow, undergo fermentation, and produce tenderness.

Ulcers on the frenulum under the tongue are often seen in children with whooping cough. The paroxysms of coughing cause protrusion of the tongue, and the frenulum is constantly forced against the sharp edges of the lower incisor teeth, resulting in erosion. Sublingual ulcers may also appear in histoplasmosis. Aphthous ulcers (chancre sores) are small, painful, shallow craters with an inflammatory base occurring usually along the margins of the tongue. They may be multiple and involve also the buccal cheek, palate, or floor of the mouth. A virus is often the cause and the ulcers more commonly occur after frequent sucking of candy. Scarring of the tongue is often seen in epileptics who bite their tongues during convulsions.

The veins on the under surface of the tongue give us a good indication of the venous blood pressure, according to May. When a person is erect or sitting, the veins are collapsed unless

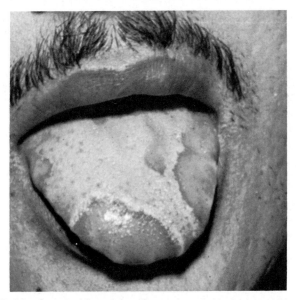

Figure 5–34. Geographic tongue. (Domonkos, A. N.: Andrews' Diseases of the Skin. 6th ed. Philadelphia, W. B. Saunders Co., 1971.)

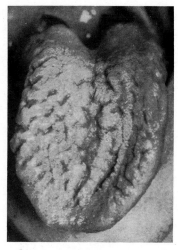

Figure 5–35. *Scrotal tongue. (Courtesy of Dr. Hayes Martin.)*

the venous pressure is abnormally high, i.e., more than 200 mm. of water.

Clusters of small, dilated varicose veins along the under surface of the tongue may reach a large size and occupy the whole under surface of the tongue. Their round shape and black color have suggested a resemblance to caviar, and are without any pathological significance (Fig. 5–36). A ranula or cystic swelling in the floor of the mouth under the tongue and alongside the molar teeth is due to a blocked sublingual gland. The cyst is usually single, moderately tense, and filled with thick clear mucus (Fig. 5–37).

In lesions of the central nervous system in which the nucleus of the hypoglossal nerve is involved, the tongue is not protruded in the midline but deviates away from the normal side and toward the side on which the lesion is located. In parkinsonism, rhythmic movements of protrusion and retraction of the tongue are not uncommon and spastic athetoid movements may

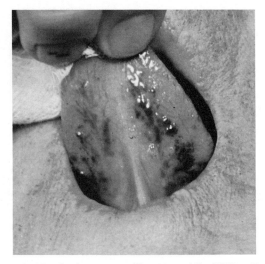

Figure 5–36. *Caviar tongue. (Courtesy of Dr. William Bean.)*

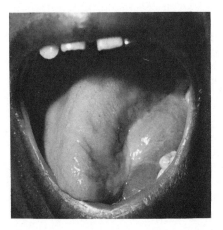

Figure 5–37. *Ranula, a cystic swelling on floor of mouth in sublingual gland region.*

be prominent in patients with cerebral palsy. Excessive salivation is common in these children. In contrast the mouth is dry, and the tongue may stick to the hard palate in dehydration, excessive radiation therapy, and in the xerostomia of Sjögren's syndrome.

In myasthenia gravis the tongue may show an abnormal fatigability like that of the eyelids and of other voluntary muscles. Thomas Willis, who first described myasthenia gravis, has left a classic description:

> I have now a prudent and honest Woman in cure, who for many years has been obnoxious to this kind of bastard Palsey not only in the Limbs but likewise in her Tongue; this person for some time speaks freely and readily enough, but after long, hasty or laborious speaking, presently she becomes as mute as a fish, and cannot bring forth a word, nay, and does not recover the use of her Voice till after an hour or two.

Breath

The breath may give important clues in diagnosis. The breath in alcoholic intoxication is of characteristic odor and in uremia the breath may have a urinous odor. In diabetes mellitus, particularly when there is marked acidosis, the breath has a sweetish "fruity" odor because of the acetone. Many patients with severe diabetes breathe out so much acetone that the atmosphere becomes saturated with it, and the odor is noted by the physician the moment he enters the room. This acetone or ketotic breath may also occur in starvation and in infants and young children who, as the result of illness, have not eaten for 24 hours or longer. The mousy, amine odor noted on the breath of patients with severe parenchymal liver disease is quite characteristic. Sometimes referred to as fetor hepaticus, it is often described as a "musty smell." Children with phenylketonuria may have a breath odor reminiscent of new-mown hay.

In oral sepsis the breath may have a disagreeable odor. This condition is known as halitosis, a term quite as well known to the general public as to the physician.

The most disagreeable breath of all is that of the patient

with a lung abscess. The infection, in such cases, is largely due to putrefactive organisms, and as a result the patient's breath has the odor of decaying vegetable or animal matter. Such patients announce their presence to their neighbors and also their diagnosis to an alert physician. Nearly as bad is the odor of an ulcerating necrotic cancer of the oral cavity, especially after heavy radiation.

The odor of patients with certain diseases was stressed by an earlier generation of physicians. Many of these odors are fairly characteristic but are difficult to describe. The odor in diphtheria may be characteristic. In smallpox the odor is extremely disagreeable. A "mousy odor" has been described in typhus fever, a slight, sweetish, fetid odor in measles, and an acid sweat smell in rheumatic fever.

Buccal Cavity

In severe anemias the mucous membrane of the mouth is pale. Koplik's spots, which are small bluish white spots surrounded by a small red margin, appear on the area of the mucous membrane of the cheek opposite the molars, near the opening of the parotid duct, and are pathognomonic of measles. They appear before the skin eruption, and thus permit an early diagnosis of this disease.

The buccal mucous membranes are frequently pigmented in patients with Addison's disease.

Mucous patches, white, sharply circumscribed areas that are 0.5 to 1 cm. in diameter and are a characteristic sign of secondary syphilis, are seen on the mucous membranes of the mouth near the bases of the gums. They may be present on the palate or anywhere on the mucous membrane of the buccal cavity.

General redness of the throat or pharynx may indicate pharyngitis, the early stage of diphtheria or scarlet fever, or any other infection.

Tumors, benign and malignant, do occur in both hard and soft palate as well as in the labial sulci and buccal gutters. A very hard, bony, midline tumor of the hard palate is the torus palatinus, quite benign, but likely to interfere with the wearing of an upper plate. A mixed tumor of accessory minor salivary glands may be found in the hard or soft palate as a discrete, round, rubbery hard mass. Cancer of the palate is uncommon and usually appears as a red ulcerating mass or nodule. Among chewers of tobacco, carcinoma of the buccal gutter, starting as white leukoplakia patches and later an ulcerating mass fixed to the mandible, is very common, especially so in Southeast Asia where betel nuts are mixed with slaked lime and tobacco and held as a "quid" in the buccal cheek by most adults.

Paralysis of the soft palate is seen occasionally as a sequel of diphtheria. In the days before the use of diphtheria antitoxin, such paralysis was common. This complication was described by Aretaeus the Cappadocian, who noted that many patients with diphtheria feared to drink water because it would "return by the nostrils."

Perforation of the palate was formerly a common occurrence due to syphilis, but is now more frequently seen in patients with carcinoma or after radiation therapy. Sometimes palatal perforations are of congenital origin. A contracted upper dental arch with cross bite (where one dental arch has moved inside or outside the other and the teeth do not occlude) is very common after cleft palate repair. The palate is usually high and arched in Marfan's syndrome and in Turner's syndrome.

The tonsils may be the seat of acute follicular tonsillitis or diphtheria. In the former condition the process begins as numerous small abscesses in the tonsillar crypts, the abscesses coalescing later to form a large grayish patch on the surface of the tonsils. In diphtheria there is a dirty grayish membrane that spreads over the surface of the tonsils and frequently spreads to the fauces and uvula. Removal of this membrane leaves a bloody surface beneath. The careful physician has learned by experience that a streptococcal sore throat may closely resemble diphtheria, and therefore he always takes a throat culture. The tonsils may be absent in persons with agammaglobulinemia or ataxia-telangiectasia.

Vicent's angina, an infection of the tonsil and gums, is usually unilateral and causes necrosis with a dirty yellow exudate that leaves a bleeding surface when removed. Vincent's angina has been mistaken for both diphtheria and syphilis.

A peritonsillar abscess (quinsy) may follow acute tonsillitis. The patient with this disorder commonly has a high fever, dysphagia, and rigidity of the neck. The rigid neck, combined with spasm of the buccal muscles producing "locked jaws," has led to the false diagnosis of tetanus. In such cases the physician may be unable to see the abscess, since the patient cannot open his mouth wide enough, but may feel the swelling by inserting a finger into the mouth. Indeed, digital oral examination should be done on any patient presenting evidence of oral disease.

A retropharyngeal abscess may be seen on inspection in children suffering from tuberculosis of the cervical vertebrae. This swelling may produce a peculiar barklike cough which the French have called "cri du canard" (cry of a duck). The swelling can often be better felt than seen.

In inflammation of the pharynx or fauces, the uvula is enlarged, pendulous, and semitranslucent. An enlarged uvula frequently produces a shallow, irritating cough, which is worse at night when the recumbent position allows the uvula to fall down on the base of the tongue. Uvular pulsation synchronous with the heart beat may occur in aortic insufficiency, as described by Muller. A swollen uvula and soft palate are not uncommon the day after a prolonged alcoholic bout.

Palpation of the oropharynx, hypopharynx, and naso-pharynx is quite possible and may reveal important findings in the diagnosis of certain tumors and inflammations. It is well to hold the tongue forward by having the patient grasp his tongue with the aid of a dry piece of cloth or gauze and pull it out. The examining gloved finger is swept gently around in every direction, even well up and behind the soft palate.

THE NECK

Examination of the neck should always be done in an unhurried and careful manner. Familiarity with the landmarks

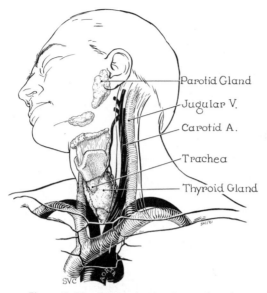

Figure 5–38. *Anatomic structures of neck.*

of the muscles, vessels, and bony or cartilaginous structures, as illustrated in Figure 5–38, facilitates the examination.

The first maneuver is that of inspection of the neck for asymmetry, unusual pulsations, tumors, or limitation of motion. By simple extension and lateral deviation of the neck, tension of the sternocleidomastoid brings into view the boundary of the anterior and posterior triangles. Enlargement of the thyroid, unusual swelling of the lymph nodes, or abnormality of the vascular structures may immediately become apparent. The necks of patients with Turner's syndrome or the Klippel-Feil syndrome have characteristic fanlike folds of skin extending laterally from the neck to the shoulders. This abnormality is described as a "webbed neck" (see Figs. 5–1 and 15–14).

Both normal and abnormal structures should be further

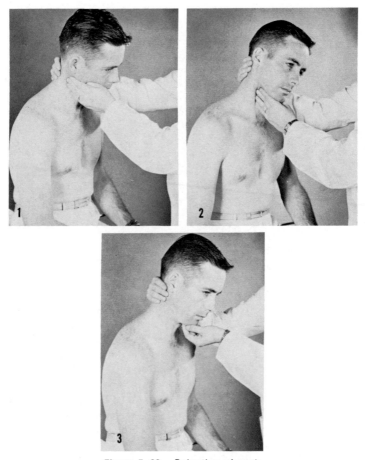

Figure 5–39. Palpation of neck.

studied by palpation. First, attention should be given to the identification of the hyoid bone, thyroid cartilage, and thyroid, the sternocleidomastoid muscle, mastoid process, cricoid cartilage, and the carotid arteries. Palpation of the lymph nodes should be carried out as indicated in Figure 5–39, using the tips of the fingers and gentle pressure. Fixation and positioning of the patient's head can be accomplished by placing one hand behind the occiput while palpating with the other hand. Slow, gentle, sliding or rotary motions with the palpating fingers, first in the anterior triangle, then in the posterior triangle, and finally in the submental region, will be more likely to reveal slightly enlarged lymph nodes than will heavy palpation.

Palpation of the submandibular structures is aided if a gloved finger is placed in the mouth. The floor of the mouth and the submandibular salivary glands and lymph nodes can be felt easily. Stones in the salivary ducts can be felt only in this manner.

Palpation of the thyroid deserves individual consideration. Usually the normal thyroid is palpable as a firm, smooth mass which moves upward with swallowing. In the patient with a short, obese neck, it is extremely difficult or impossible to identify.

When enlargement or nodularity of the thyroid is noted, careful outlining of the structures with the palpating fingers is required. This is most easily and accurately done if you stand behind the patient. The fingertips of both hands should rest firmly on the structures of the thyroid, with the trachea separating the hands, as indicated in Figure 5–40, *1*. The patient is then asked to swallow. As he does, the thyroid slips between the fingers, permitting evaluation of the two sides for size, contour, firmness, and tenderness. For more exact evaluation of each lobe and pole of the thryoid (Fig. 5–40, *2*), retract the sternocleidomastoid and palpate the lobe or nodule with the other hand. If the lower pole is not palpated, it probably is beneath the sternum and may be revealed by percussion.

General enlargement of the thyroid gland is a striking feature of Graves' disease. Auscultation of the thyroid gland in

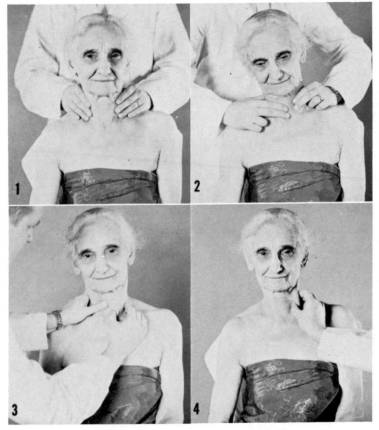

Figure 5–40. *Palpation of thyroid gland.*

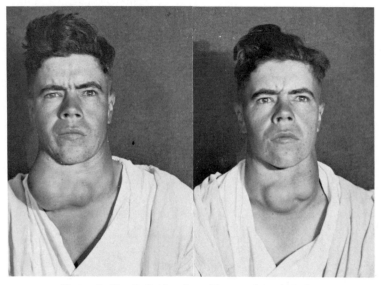

Figure 5-41. Colloid goiter with myxedema in twins.

Graves' disease may reveal a systolic bruit, which must not be confused with a cardiac murmur transmitted along the carotid artery. It should also be remembered that a bruit may be heard over the carotid artery if the bell of the stethoscope is applied with too much pressure. A systolic thrill, synchronous with the bruit, is felt in some patients. A thyroid bruit or thrill is almost pathognomonic of Graves' disease and occurs only rarely in colloid goiters and other thyroid abnormalities. Cysts of the thyroid gland, unaccompanied by any marked, generalized enlargement, are common.

Thyroglossal duct cysts or sinuses are residua of the tract of descent of the thyroid gland from the base of the tongue. The thyroid gland may be present anywhere along this tract, but most frequently there is, over or just below the midbody of the hyoid bone, a midline swelling or a nodule that moves upward on the initiation of swallowing (Fig. 5–42). This is a cyst that is likely to be infected. If it had been an abscess that ruptured, a draining sinus or fistula may communicate with the foramen cecum of the tongue.

If you now return to the front of the patient, further information may be gained by displacing the trachea as shown in Figure 5–40, *3*. It may be helpful to palpate the upper pole of the thyroid between the thumb and forefinger as indicated in Figure 5–40, *4*.

A branchial cleft cyst may produce marked swelling in the neck, sometimes presenting as such a tense firm mass that it is difficult to differentiate it from a solid tumor mass. These cysts are characteristically in the upper lateral neck just anterior to the sternomastoid muscle, but can occur as low as the sternal notch. Instead of cysts they may be sinuses of fistulous openings (Fig. 5–43) which may communicate by way of an epithelium-lined tract all the way to the tonsil. Those masses or sinus tracts

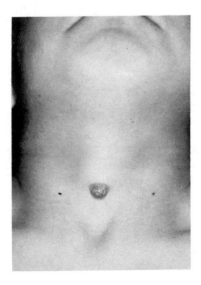

Figure 5–42. Thyroglossal duct cyst. It is at the midline and moves upward with swallowing.

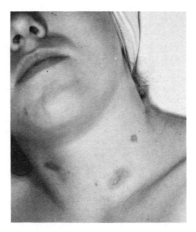

Figure 5-43. *Branchial cleft sinuses, just anterior to sterno-mastoid muscle. There is a nevus higher up on the left.*

do not move upward on swallowing. The cysts contain a thick, yellow, turbid mucus.

In aortic valve insufficiency, the carotid arteries often pulsate with unusual force and violence. Indeed, the diagnosis is frequently suggested by this sign alone. Throbbing carotid arteries are, however, occasionally seen in other conditions—notably, severe anemia, hyperthyroidism, and arteriosclerosis, especially when the latter is associated with arterial hypertension. Careful inspection of the carotid arteries may show clearly an irregularity of the heart beat, such as that due to premature contractions or to atrial fibrillation. Indeed, these two conditions may often be diagnosed by simple inspection of the carotid pulse without palpating the radial pulse or listening to the heart.

Pulsation above the right clavicle may be due to elongation of the innominate artery. It is seen especially in hypertensive and arteriosclerotic patients and may be falsely diagnosed as an aneurysm of the innominate artery. Aneurysm of the carotid artery may produce a striking enlargement which pulsates with each heart beat.

The pulse in the jugular veins should be studied carefully.

When there is obstruction to the flow of blood into the large thoracic veins, the jugular veins are markedly distended. This is seen particularly in intrathoracic tumors. In cardiac failure the veins of the the neck are usually engorged. More sophisticated features of the venous pulsations in the neck are described in Chapter 9, which deals with examination of the heart.

Auscultation of the supraclavicular fossa and posterior triangles of the neck may reveal a low-pitched venous hum. A venous hum has no particular significance except that it may be confused with other sounds. It is obliterated by light pressure on the neck veins at a point superior to the area where it is heard.

Auscultation of the carotid arteries is a necessary maneuver for detection of carotid artery obstruction, which is frequently associated with extensive atherosclerosis. Points of auscultation should be below and above the clavicle, over the innominate and subclavian arteries, then over the carotid, and finally over the bifurcation. A systolic bruit should arouse suspicion of carotid insufficiency. If a diastolic as well as a systolic component can be heard, the findings are quite convincing. Differentiation must be made from a transmitted aortic murmur.

The differentiation of tumors or enlargements in the neck tests the skill of the clinician. The physical findings of palpation are by far the most significant. Pathological changes in the cervical lymph nodes, inflammatory or neoplastic, are very common, and may be difficult to diagnose and delineate from other soft tissue tumors, or inflammatory or degenerative processes. The presence of enlarged nodes in the upper anterolateral neck, if of short duration with tenderness and redness, indicates lymphadenitis, secondary to a severe cold, tonsillitis, pharyngitis, or an infection of the skin of the face, scalp, or neck. Multiply enlarged cervical nodes, sometimes fluctuant, often adherent and matted together, and usually nontender, and even draining sinuses to the overlying skin are usually the result of chronic granulomatous processes, such as tuberculosis (Fig. 5–44), syphilis, or one of the mycoses. An abscess or sinus from an infected branchial cleft cyst may produce a similar picture.

Malignant disease in cervical nodes occurs as a primary

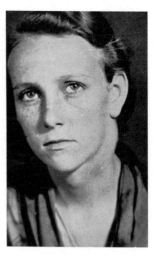

Figure 5–44. *Tuberculosis of cervical lymph glands.*

process in the lymphomas (Hodgkin's disease, lymphatic leukemia, or lymphosarcoma); the involvement is nearly always multiple, but with discrete nodes early and, later, a multinodular matted mass of large nodes. Hodgkin's disease often produces a marked bilateral enlargement of cervical nodes, which form a mass about the neck resembling a horse collar (Fig. 5–45). Lymphosarcoma produces softer nodes than does Hodgkin's disease. The masses in both are relatively nontender.

The secondary involvement of lymph nodes in the neck from a primary malignant lesion of some epithelial structure is one of the commonest and most important findings that leads to the location of a primary site (Fig. 5–46). Obvious carcinoma of the skin of the face, neck, and scalp or nevi that have undergone recent change in the same regions are easy to find, but the examiner, having looked carefully in these areas as well as in the lining of the anterior oral and nasal cavities, must search in more hidden sites, paying particular attention to the base of the tongue, tonsillar fossae, nasopharynx and hypopharynx, para-

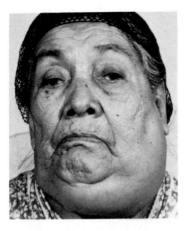

Figure 5–45. *Cervical lymph nodes in Hodgkin's disease.*

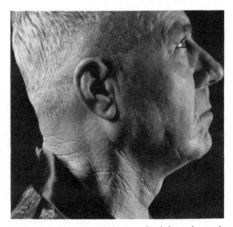

Figure 5–46. *Metastases in multiple cervical lymph nodes from primary carcinoma of the parotid.*

nasal sinuses, larynx, and thyroid. Such areas require special and unusual examination techniques, but the important point is that the hidden primary site must be diligently sought. Secondary malignant disease in cervical nodes most often is found in the upper deep nodes just anterior to the sternomastoid muscle, and just below the angle of the jaw above the horn of the hyoid bone. These nodes are very hard unless secondarily broken down and fluctuant and are usually nontender except when growing rapidly. Metastases from the thyroid gland and larynx may first present in nodes of the mid lateral or lower neck. A firm, discrete mass in the supraclavicular region is commonly a metastasis from the lung or breast, and, on the left side in the region of the thoracic duct, may be secondary spread from the gastrointestinal tract. Such a node is commonly referred to as Virchow's node, after the man who described it.

Primary tumors of the other soft tissues are less frequent. Lipomas, which are usually superficial, soft, round, multilobular, nontender, and movable, may occur anywhere in the neck (Fig. 5–47). Neuromas may be soft and pedunculated or firm

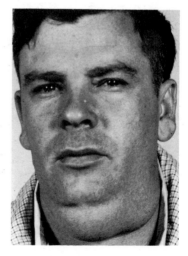

Figure 5–47. Lipoma of subcutaneous tissue of neck.

subcutaneous nodes, sometimes multiple and widespread, as in von Recklinghausen's neurofibromatosis. A diffuse, soft, multicordlike, nontender mass that feels like a bag of worms beneath the skin is the characteristic finding in plexiform neuroma. A primary muscle tumor, rhabdomyosarcoma, which may involve any of the neck muscles, is rare but occurs more frequently in children. Soft, collapsible, rapidly growing, light-transmitting tumors of the neck in infants are relatively common and may be large, involving any or all of the soft tissue structures (Fig. 5–48). These are lymphangiomas or cystic hygromas which contain lymph in large or small locules diffusely invading all adjacent structures. An admixture with vascular forming elements may be present in lymphangiomas or the vascular tumor may be entirely of blood vessel origin. A hemangioma is readily recognized by a bluish or red discoloration of the skin. Such tumors, if of any depth, are collapsible and sometimes pulsating. Carotid body tumors (Fig. 5–49) or chemodectomas, are round, firm, nontender, pulsating masses of the carotid bifurcation just posterior to the horn of the hyoid. They are movable in the horizontal, but not the vertical plane.

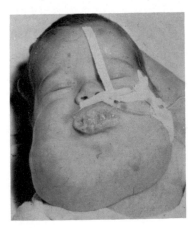

Figure 5–48. *Lymphangioma of neck, extensive, transluminant.*

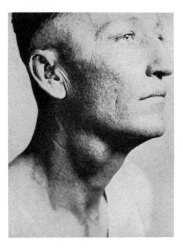

Figure 5–49. Tumor of carotid body.

Torticollis, or wryneck, produces a characteristic deviation of the head toward the affected side, caused by a tight band or cord in the sternocleidomastoid muscle (Fig. 5–50). This condition is said to be congenital, but it frequently is the result of contracture in an organizing hematoma in the muscle stretched or torn during delivery.

Poliomyelitis may cause atrophy of the trapezius or sternomastoid. Injury to the spinal accessory nerve from trauma or surgical operation can cause the same picture of these paralyzed fibrotic muscles. Marked rigidity of the neck occurs with meningitis, so much so that the head is thrown backwards and the neck cannot be flexed to bring it forward. The child shown in Figure 5–51 had boardlike rigidity of the neck, and could be raised nearly to the sitting position by lifting with the hand at the back of the head.

Injuries to the neck or inflammatory processes may produce muscle spasms. Irritation of the nerve roots may be the cause of spasm or pain from injury to the cervical spine, or be present with arthritic changes in the vertebrae. A "stiff neck" is common

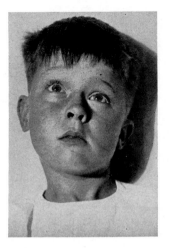

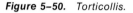
Figure 5–50. *Torticollis.*

after unusual exercise, trauma to muscles, myositis such as with a common cold, or with emotional tension.

A cervical rib can, at times, be palpated in the neck. Although this finding may be incidental and found more often on routine x-ray examination, it can be the cause of vascular change or referred pain in the upper extremity.

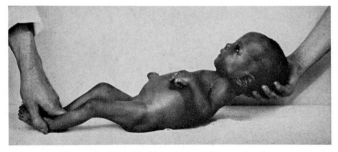

Figure 5–51. *Rigidity of neck in meningitis.*

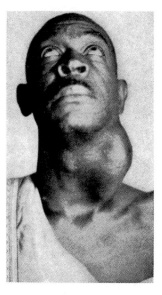

Figure 5-52. *Aneurysm of left carotid artery.*

An aneurysm of the carotid or innominate artery is usually obvious because of the gross pulsatile excursion of its mass (Fig. 5-52). An enlarged lymph node overlying the carotid artery can produce a transmitted pulse beat to the examiner's finger.

A very important finding in aortic aneurysm is the well known Oliver sign, or tracheal tug. No one has described this sign more accurately or in fewer words than Oliver himself: "Place the patient in the erect position, and direct him to close his mouth, and elevate his chin to the fullest extent, then grasp the cricoid cartilage between the finger and thumb, and use gentle upward pressure on it, when if dilation or aneurysm exist, the pulsation of the aorta will be distinctly felt transmitted through the trachea to the hand."

COMMON CLINICAL TERMS

Bell's palsy—Idiopathic unilateral facial muscle paralysis due to facial nerve dysfunction. (Fig. 5–13)

Dysphagia—Difficulty in swallowing.

Lumpy jaw—Subcutaneous granulomatous nodules about the mandible and adjacent neck due to actinomycosis.

Opisthotonos—Extreme hyperextension of spine seen most commonly with meningitis. The back may be so arched that the occiput of the extended head approaches the heels.

Rhinolalia—Nasal escape of air through nose in speaking due to incompetence of the soft palate. Causes a nasal type of speech often with articulation errors, snorting, and grimacing.

Rhinorrhea—Discharge from nose; serious connotation if watery after head injury.

Scrofula—Old term for tuberculous cervical lymphadenopathy, frequently with draining sinuses. (Fig. 5–44)

Trismus—Inability to open jaws usually caused by spasm of the muscles of mastication, commonly occurring in tetanus, dental abscess, injury to mandibule or temporomandibular joint.

Xerostomia—Dryness of the mouth from lack of normal secretion.

COMMON CLINICAL SYNDROMES

Apert's syndrome (acrocephaly)—Narrowing of skull anteroposteriorly with a mounding upward and widening horizontally. Fingers and toes fused (syndactyly).

Carotid sinus syndrome—Dizziness, fainting, sometimes convulsive seizures that result from overactivity of the carotid sinus reflex. May occur if carotid body stroked or palpated during physical examination.

Graves' disease—Exophthalmic goiter. Protruding eyeballs, lid lag, enlarged thyroid, tremor of hands, overanxiety, elevated metabolism, flushed face.

Meniere's syndrome (endolymphatic hydrops)—A disorder of the labyrinth of the inner ear characterized by tinnitus, vertigo, and fluctuating hearing loss of the sensorineural type.

Mikulicz's syndrome—Diffuse enlargement of the salivary and lacrimal glands, usually bilateral, with lymphoid infiltration of the glandular parenchyma associated with systemic diseases such as the lymphomatous or chronic granulomatous processes. (Fig. 5–14)

Paget's disease of bone — Deforming sclerosing overgrowth of bone; may be any bone but commonly skull. (Fig. 5–4)

Turner's syndrome — Retarded growth and sexual development, webbing of neck, low posterior hairline, deformity of elbow; associated with abnormality of sex chromosomes.

BIBLIOGRAPHY

Ackerman, L. V., and del Regato, J. A.: Cancer—Diagnosis, Treatment, and Prognosis. 4th ed. St. Louis, The C. V. Mosby Co., 1970.

Cochrane, R. G., and Davey, T. F.: Leprosy in Theory and Practice. 2nd ed. Baltimore, Williams & Wilkins, 1969.

Dingman, R. O., and Natvig, P.: Surgery of Facial Fractures. Philadelphia, W. B. Saunders Co., 1964.

Locke, C. E.: Intracranial arteriovenous aneurysm or pulsating exophthalmos. Ann. Surg., *80*:1, 1924.

Marie, P.: Two Cases of Acromegaly. Translated by Proctor S. Hutchinson. London, New Sydenham Society, 1891.

Martin, H., and Koop, C. E.: The precancerous mouth lesions of avitaminosis. Am. J. Surg., *57*:195, 1942.

Martin, J. D., Jr., and Mabon, R. F.: Pulsating exophthalmos, review of all reported cases. J.A.M.A., *121*:330, 1943.

May, A.: The tongue sign for high venous pressure. Am. Heart J., *26*:685, 1943.

Morgan, W. S.: Mikulicz's disease and Sjögren's syndrome. N. Engl. J. Med., *251*:5, 1954.

Naffziger, H. C.: Progressive exophthalmos associated with disorder of the thyroid gland. Ann. Surg., *108*:529, 1938.

Oliver, W. S.: Physical diagnosis of thoracic aneurysm. Lancet, *2*:406, 1878.

Parrott, J.: La syphilis héréditaire et le rachitis. Paris, Masson et Cie, 1886.

Poppen, J. L.: Cranial bruit—its significance. Surg. Clin. North Am., *35*:881, 1955.

Rogers, B. O.: Rare craniofacial deformities. *In* Converse, J. M.: (ed.): Reconstructive Plastic Surgery. Vol. III. Philadelphia, W. B. Saunders Co., 1964, pp. 1213–1305.

Squires, B. T.: Pattern of the human tongue. Lancet, *1*:647, 1955.

Stark, R. B.: Cleft Palate—A Multidisciplinary Approach. New York, Harper and Row, 1968.

Sydenstricker, V. P., Geeslin, L. E., Templeton, C. W., and Weaver, J. W.: Riboflavin deficiency. J.A.M.A., *113*:1697, 1939.

6
GENERAL PRINCIPLES OF THE EAR, NOSE, AND THROAT EXAMINATION

Seat your patient comfortably in a chair in an erect position with both feet in contact with the floor. Then sit on the subject's right with a lighted incandescent 150-watt lamp placed eight inches above and ten inches behind the patient's right ear. Wear a headmirror as close to the left eye as possible and focus the beam of light into the various cavities to be examined, so that your hands are free for manipulating instruments.

THE EAR

The ear, the organ of hearing and balance, is divided into three portions: (1) the external ear, or auricle, with the external auditory canal; (2) the middle ear, the tympanic cavity that connects with the mastoid cells and nasopharynx and contains the eardrum membrane and the auditory ossicles; and (3) the internal ear with the cochlea and static labyrinth, containing the semicircular canals, the utricle, and the saccule. All three portions play a role in the hearing function. The auricle, or external ear, plays the least important role. It is relatively much smaller than in other animals, and it cannot change its position to hear sounds better because its musculature is rudimentary. It simply serves to dampen sounds that arise from behind the head. The external auditory canal carries sound to the middle ear where it strikes the tympanic membrane, setting it into vibration. The effective sound waves are then transmitted by the auditory ossicles to the oval window, resulting in motion of the labyrinthine fluids, which in turn stimulates the cochlear nerve.

The sensory nerve supply of the auricle comes from the great auricular nerve and the lesser occipital nerve, both of which are branches of the cervical plexus; from the auriculotemporal branch of the mandibular nerve, which is a branch of the trigeminal nerve; and from Arnold's nerve, a branch of the vagus nerve. In the middle ear, the chorda tympani, a branch of the facial nerve, passes deep to the eardrum membrane between the malleus and the incus. The middle ear and the adjoining

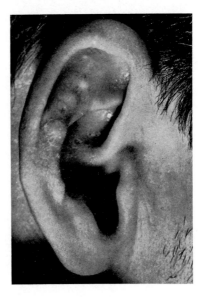

Figure 6–1. Tophi of ear. (Courtesy of Dr. E. P. Pendergrass. In Hopkins, H. U.: Leopold's Principles and Methods of Physical Diagnosis. 3rd ed. Philadelphia, W. B. Saunders Co., 1965.)

mastoid area are also supplied by branches from the trigeminal, facial, glossopharyngeal, and vagus nerves. In the internal ear or cochlea, the end organ of hearing is supplied by the cochlear division of the auditory nerve; the static labyrinth, the end organ of equilibrium, is supplied by the vestibular branch of the same nerve.

The patient who requests an ear examination usually presents because of pain, defective hearing, tinnitus, discharge, or vertigo. It should be recalled that the middle ear is supplied by branches of four cranial nerves and that diseases of other organs supplied by these nerves, such as the teeth, tonsils, tongue, pharynx, or mouth, may cause referred pain in the ear.

The ear should be carefully examined in cases of suspected

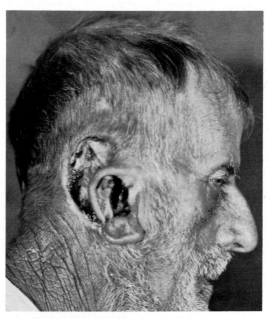

Figure 6–2. Carcinoma of the ear.

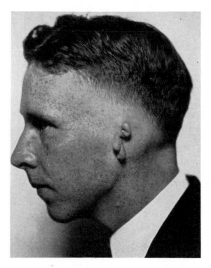

Figure 6–3. Developmental deformity of the ear.

gout for tophi, which are hard, nodular deposits of sodium biurate upon the cartilage (Fig. 6–1). The deformed so-called "cauliflower" ears of the professional pugilist are well known. The deformity is due to hemorrhage or infection between the cartilage and perichondrium, with subsequent fibrosis and loss of cartilage. Cutaneous tuberculosis or lupus vulgaris may attack the ears and erode large areas; carcinoma may cause much destruction and distortion of the auricle (Fig. 6–2). Keloids following trauma are sometimes seen. Developmental deformities are rarely encountered (Fig. 6–3), but when seen are often associated with malformations of the genitourinary tract.

For the examination of the external auditory canal an ear speculum or an otoscope should be employed (Figs. 6–4 and 6–5). Before introducing the instrument, pull the auricle slightly upward, backward, and outward to facilitate introduction. Be sure that there is no debris or particles of cerumen in the canal and, if necessary, remove them with a swab. One of the most

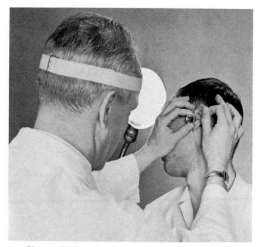

Figure 6–4. *Employment of the speculum.*

common conditions seen is excessive or impacted cerumen, which may obstruct the ear and seriously impair the hearing. Furunculosis, acute or chronic external otitis due to microorganisms (yeast or fungi), causes excoriation of the walls of the canal or external meatus with pain, tenderness, itching, and some diminution in hearing. Unless there is an obstruction in the canal, the eardrum membrane can be seen without difficulty. Note whether the membrane is intact, whether the normal translucency is present, and whether the drumhead is retracted, as in middle ear adhesions, or bulging laterally, as in acute otitis media. If there is a recent or healed perforation of the drumhead, it is usually visible.

Tests for hearing include the whispered and spoken voice, a ticking watch, tuning forks, and the more accurate electrically calibrated audiometer. When testing the patient's hearing be sure that the patient closes, with his finger, the ear that is not being tested. The distance from the ear at which a watch is nor-

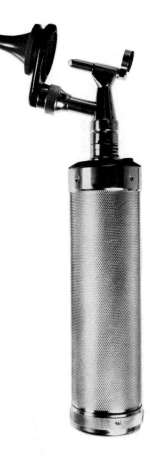

Figure 6–5. Otoscope.

mally heard varies but averages 5 to 15 inches. The voice and watch tests are reliable only when the examiner has had much practice with people of both normal and impaired hearing. Other tests of hearing are described in Chapter 4.

Chronic otitis media, one of the common causes of hearing loss, may present a variety of findings. Some patients hear better during clear, dry weather than they do when it is damp and rainy. This is not true of conductive hearing loss of chronic otitis media, but is true in neurosensory hearing loss. Thomas Willis, in the seventeenth century, described a woman "who, although she was deaf, whenever a drum was beaten in the room, heard every word clearly," and mentions a deaf man "who, passing close to a bell-tower when one of the numerous bells rang, could hear one's voice very easily, but not otherwise." This phenomenon, frequently observed since, is known as "paracusis willisii," and is often seen in otosclerosis.

The unit of hearing employed in audiometry is the decibel, which is the least change in intensity that can be detected by the ear. It is not an absolute value, but instead compares the relationship between two sound intensities.

THE NOSE

In diseases associated with difficulty in respiration, notably pneumonia and, to a lesser extent, heart disease, the nostrils dilate with inspiration and contract with expiration.

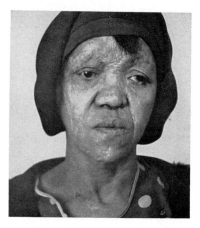

Figure 6–6. Saddle nose.

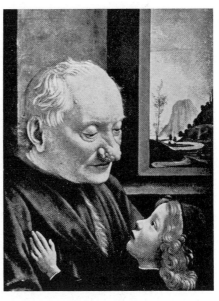

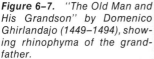

Figure 6-7. *"The Old Man and His Grandson" by Domenico Ghirlandajo (1449–1494), showing rhinophyma of the grandfather.*

Erosion of the nasal bones in syphilis may result in the typical "saddle nose" (Fig. 6–6). In rhinophyma the nose is red, large, and bulbous. Ghirlandajo and Holbein have immortalized rhinophyma on canvas (Fig. 6–7), and Cyrano de Bergerac was a well known example. Lupus erythematosus produces the characteristic "butterfly" lesion on the nose with the wings extending out over the cheeks (Fig. 6–8). The lesion, sometimes called Cazenave's disease, consists of disc-like patches covered with scales or crusts that fall off leaving dull white cicatrices.

Acne rosacea produces a marked reddening of the tip of the nose, which instantly suggests that the owner of the nose has a weakness for alcoholic beverages. Often, however, these persons are teetotalers, or even rabid prohibitionists, and resent the insinuation.

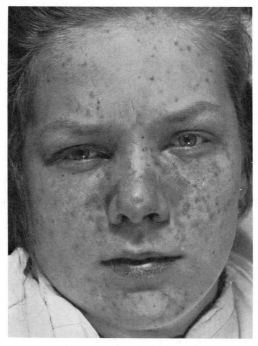

Figure 6–8. Lupus erythematosus.

Tumors originating within the nose, nasopharynx, or nasal sinuses may produce marked deformity of the face. Figure 6–9 shows the marked asymmetry of the face produced by a sarcoma of the maxillary bone.

One should never neglect to look into the nasal fossae (Fig. 6–10). The nasal interior is examined by means of a bivalved speculum, which must be introduced without making contact with the sensitive septum. Once inserted, it is spread and pulled laterally. A perforation of the nasal septum is due occasionally to syphilis, but it may be the result of nonspecific ulceration, chromium poisoning, or intranasal trauma.

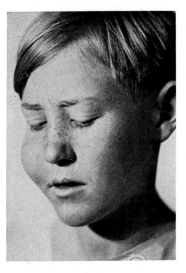

Figure 6–9. Sarcoma of maxillary bone.

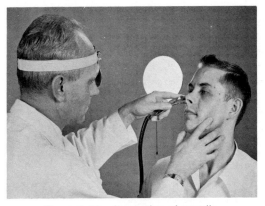

Figure 6–10. Inspection of nostrils.

Nosebleed may be an early symptom of typhoid fever, the result of high blood pressure or polycythemia, or result from erosion of the small vessels in the mucous membrane. Repeated picking of the nose, however, is the commonest cause.

THE PHARYNX AND LARYNX

The pharynx is examined, along with the teeth and buccal cavity, by manipulation of the tongue with a depressor. The nasopharynx is inspected by means of a small mirror introduced behind the soft palate after the tongue has been depressed. One must search for polyps, pus, tumor masses, and choanal atresia. A laryngeal mirror is used to examine the larynx. Grasping the tongue gently with a piece of gauze and pulling it forward, the examiner places the mirror, which has been slightly warmed, against the soft palate in front of the uvula. Some examiners, before inserting the laryngeal mirror, swab the posterior pharyngeal wall with 4 per cent cocaine to produce local anesthesia and facilitate the examination.

In addition to this method of examining the larynx, the indirect method, there is also the direct method, in which a laryngoscope powered by an electric battery is employed. The patient lies on his back, and the examiner, bending over him, introduces the laryngoscope into the patient's mouth, lifting the tongue and the epiglottis. Laryngoscopy may reveal paralysis of the vocal cords, acute or chronic laryngitis, neoplasm, tuberculosis, or a congenital anomaly.

COMMON CLINICAL TERMS

Anosmia — Loss of sense of smell.
Diplacusis — Sound out of phase in the two ears.
Dysphagia — Difficulty in swallowing.
Dysphonia — Difficulty in speaking.
Epistaxis — Bleeding from the nose.
Hematemesis — Vomiting of blood.

Hemoptysis—Coughing up of blood.
Hyperacusis—Unusual sensitivity to high intensity sound.
Hypoacusis—Diminished hearing.
Otalgia—Pain in the ear.
Vertigo—A false sensation of motion.

COMMON CLINICAL SYNDROMES

Kartagener's syndrome—Bronchiectasis; absence of frontal sinuses; dextrocardia.
Cri du chat syndrome—Cat-cry sound of the voice due to congenital anomaly of larynx.
Gradenigo's syndrome (abscess of apex of petrous portion of temporal bone)—Paralysis of sixth cranial nerve; ipsilateral paralysis of fifth nerve; homolateral otitis media.
Harada's syndrome—Sudden loss of vision and hearing due to hyperimmune response to retinal and cochlear pigment.
Meniere's syndrome (endolymphatic hydrops)—Tinnitus; vertigo; fluctuating hearing loss of sensorineural type.
Ramsay Hunt syndrome—Herpes zoster oticus.
Waardenburg's syndrome—Sensorineural hearing loss; white forelock of hair; depigmented patches on skin; increased intercanthal distance; one brown eye and one blue eye; hypertrichosis.

7
EXAMINATION OF THE EYES

The wise physician always examines both eyes of each patient regardless of the chief complaint.

Besides a wide variety of specific intrinsic eye diseases that do not affect general body health, a complete ocular examination, done regularly as part of each physical examination, will often reveal ocular signs of general systemic disease. These ocular signs may represent the initial and, occasionally, the only physically demonstrable evidence of disease. Some of the resulting ocular symptoms may prompt the patient's visit to the doctor.

A number of ocular complaints are of functional, or psychogenic, origin. Sudden blindness in one or both eyes is often claimed by the hysterical patient. However, this loss of light perception (amaurosis), lesser degrees of visual loss, and a variety of more vague ocular complaints should be labeled as functional only after careful systematic examination for and elimination of causative organic local, ocular, and general systemic disease.

APPRAISAL OF THE VISUAL ACUITY

The systematic examination of the eyes should begin, when possible, with an appraisal of the visual acuity. When indicated, the visual fields and color vision should be tested.

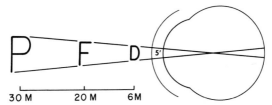

Figure 7-1. Diagram illustrating the relationship between object size, distance, and the minimum visual angle of five minutes.

By employing two factors, size of object and distance from the eye, it is possible to determine the minimum visual angle. Letters that subtend an angle of 5 minutes stimulate sufficiently disparate elements of the retina that they can be correctly identified by the normal eye (Fig. 7-1). A variety of visual acuity tests have been devised. The most common of these, the Snellen chart, is adapted for testing both the 20 foot distance vision and the 14 inch near-reading vision (Fig. 7-2). Either letters, numbers, or figures are used. For the testing distance selected, each element or space of the test figure subtends an angle of at least 1 minute, and the figure as a whole totals 5 minutes (Fig. 7-3).

Distance visual acuity is determined by utilizing light rays that are nearly parallel. Test figures that are closer than 20 feet (6 meters) give rise to divergent rays of light that require active accommodation of all but a few nearsighted (myopic) eyes, and thus these figures test more than just the acuity. When seated at 20 feet, the patient indicates the smallest line on the chart that he can read correctly. Visual acuity (V.A.) is expressed as a fraction. The numerator indicates the testing distance, in feet or meters, and the denominatior denotes the distance at which the identified figures subtend an angle of 5 minutes of arc. The visual acuity of the average anatomically normal eye is 20/20 (feet) or 6/6 (meters).

Patients who are unable to see the larger 20/200 letter may

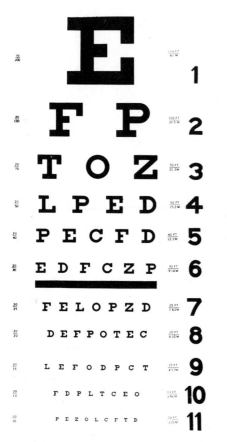

Figure 7–2. *Snellen chart. (Courtesy American Optical Company.)*

then be moved closer to the chart until this letter is identified. The numerator of the V.A. is then altered to note the distance from which this letter was seen, such as 5/200. If no letters are seen, the patient is asked to count a selected number of the examiner's fingers (F.C.), and the greatest distance at which this can be done accurately is recorded as F.C./test distance in feet.

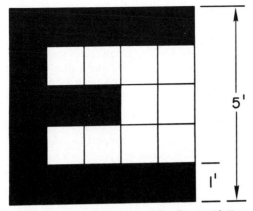

Figure 7–3. Construction of Snellen test letter.

Failing to count fingers, the patient is asked to identify the immobile versus the moving hand of the examiner (H.M.), and this is similarly recorded as H.M. /test distance in feet. The patient may have only light perception, and this is recorded as L.P./amount of visual field in which it is seen, such as L.P./temporal field only. The complete absence of light perception is called "amaurosis."

Patients with subnormal vision due only to errors of refraction (myopia, hyperopia, astigmatism) should show noticeable improvement when they are retested by having them read the chart through a pinhole perforated disc (P.H.) held in front of one eye while the other eye is occluded. Only paraxial parallel rays of light, not materially affected by these basic refractive errors, enter the eye through the pinhole. Any improvement over the initial uncorrected V.A. is added after the preface P.H.

EXAMINATION OF THE OCULAR MEDIA

Patients having deficient V.A. as shown by the pinhole test should receive a systematic eye examination to discover the cause. First, the clarity of the media of the eye (tears, cornea, aqueous, lens, vitreous) is determined with the hand flashlight and ophthalmoscope.

Only gross opacities of the cornea and lens can be identified with the flashlight. The most accurate initial evaluation of the ocular media is carried out with the ophthalmoscope. The *right* eye of the patient is examined with the examiner's *right* eye from a distance of 6 to 12 inches, with the ophthalmoscope held in the *right* hand (Fig. 7–4). Greater clarity and detail are possible if a 6 volt house current model is substituted for the conventional 2.5 volt battery powered instrument.

Any required distance spectacles lens should be worn by the examiner for maximum clarity in this examination. Rest your left hand on the patient's forehead where the thumb can be used to elevate the upper lid if it covers the pupil. This position is reversed for the examination of the left eye. All of these positions are more comfortably attained by bending over from positions to one side, rather than by standing or sitting directly in front of the patient. Place the plano (0) lens over the peephole of the scope by rotating the milled disc on the side of the ophthalmoscope head with the forefinger. The ophthalmoscope, used

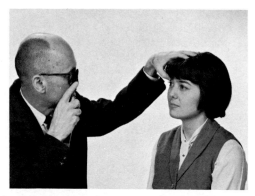

Figure 7–4. *Ophthalmoscopic (screening) examination of ocular media.*

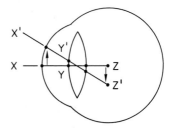

Figure 7–5. *Apparent displacement of opacities in ocular media with eye movement: Anteriorly placed opacities, X, move with eye to X'. Opacities in area Y–Y' move very little. Posteriorly placed opacities, Z, move to Z' in a direction opposite to the eye movement.*

in this manner, will illuminate the pupil of most normal eyes having clear media with a pink to orange-red reflected light. Any very high refractive error will reduce the brightness of this reflection, and *diffusely* clouded media, depending on its severity, will give a dull orange to black reflection. Significant *focal* opacities will appear as dark spots in the colored pupillary reflection.

Two simple methods are used to determine the location of these focal opacities. If the patient moves his eye upward slightly, the ophthalmoscopically visible opacities will (1) move upward if they are in the cornea or anterior chamber, (2) remain stationary or move much less than the eye if they are in the zone of the lens, or (3) move downward if they are in the vitreous (Fig. 7–5). After a + 10D* lens is placed in position over the peephole, move the ophthalmoscope slowly toward the eye, focusing in turn on the cornea, anterior chamber, lens, and vitreous until the magnified opacity is sharply outlined.

The tears. Tears that are excessively rich in mucus, pus, or other debris may interfere with vision. A deficient quantity of tears allows drying which disturbs the regular refracting surface of the cornea, and eventually results in opacity. There is a gradual reduction in tear production with aging. Acute tear defi-

---

*Measurements of lens strength are based on the metric system, and are expressed as the reciprocal of the focal length. A lens that has a focal length of 1 meter is said to have a strength of 1 diopter (1D). A 10D lens has a focal length of 1/10 or 0.1 meter. A 0.2D lens, on the other hand, has a focal length of 1/0.2 or 5 meters.

ciency occurs in some cases of inflammation (dacryoadenitis) and sometimes results from a tumor of the lacrimal gland.

Dry eyes follow a variety of chronic conjunctival inflammations. Trachoma destroys accessory lacrimal tissue and mucus-producing goblet cells, and secondary scarring may obstruct the ducts from the major palpebral and orbital lacrimal glands above their opening into the superior conjunctival fornix. Resultant breaks in corneal epithelium of pinpoint or larger size are most easily identified by staining them with fluorescein.

The cornea. Primary dystrophic deposits of several types of hyaline, degenerative collagen, and hyaluronidase-insensitive mucoid may occur at varying levels of corneal stroma in members of certain families in which other metabolic errors are unknown. In Hurler's disease (gargoylism), however, other systemic expressions of this genetic disturbance accompany the corneal clouding which is more intense peripherally. The swollen cytoplasm of fixed corneal corpuscles and the infiltrating macrophages, containing a mixture of glycoprotein and acid mucopolysaccharide, produce the clouding. Another congenital anomaly seen in dwarfed children, with cystinuria, results from the diffuse deposit of cystine crystals throughout the corneal stroma. Secondary aggregates of proteinaceous inflammatory debris and cells, known as keratic precipitates, or K.P., may dot the endothelial surface of the cornea in chronic iridocyclitis.

In band keratopathy, secondary deposits of gray to white calcium salts located subepithelially are usually most marked in the aperture area near the temporal and nasal margins of the cornea. Common etiologies include hypoparathyroidism, vitamin D intoxication, severe renal damage, and chronic intraocular inflammation (uveitis), with particular reference to sarcoidosis. Any secondarily vascularized focus in the cornea resulting from previous trauma or inflammation may subsequently contain lipid, particularly in persons with elevated blood cholesterol levels.

Generalized corneal edema, primarily of epithelium and endothelium, is characteristic of significantly elevated intraocular pressure (glaucoma) or pathologically depressed intraocular pressure (hypotony). *Focal* edema of the cornea is seen near chronic breaks in the epithelial barrier to tears and in the endothelial barrier to aqueous. Grayish white to light tan deposits resembling edema of the epithelium are occasionally seen after ingestion of quinoline products, notably the malarial depressants, and after chronic use of chlorpromazine. Blood pigments may enter and permanently stain the corneal stroma as a result of hemorrhage in the anterior chamber (hyphema) associated with damage to the corneal endothelium or increased intraocular pressure (glaucoma).

The anterior chamber. Both hyphema (blood) and hypopyon (pus) in the anterior chamber may cause visual loss. Bleeding in this area may result from blunt or perforating trauma. Spontaneous bleeding most often occurs from newly formed, fragile iris surface vessels (rubeosis) in long-standing diabetes or after retinal vascular occlusive disease, particularly of the central vein. Monocular spontaneous hyphema in early life may arise in a focal iridic or ciliary body expression (tumor) of juvenile xanthogranuloma (nevoxanthoendothelioma), with or without accompanying skin lesions. Spontaneous anterior chamber bleeding in an adult also occurs from malignant melanomas of the iris and ciliary body.

Hypopyon is most frequently seen in severe iris and ciliary body inflammations (iridocyclitis) and in frank intraocular infections (endophthalmitis). Iridocyclitis is an associated finding in several systemic disorders, such as ankylosing spondylitis in young male adults. Hypopyon associated with arthritic symptoms and urethritis suggests gonococcal infection and Reiter's disease. In some children, with chronic periarticular polyarthritis (Still's disease), iridocyclitis and band-shaped opacity (calcium deposits) of the cornea occur.

The lens. Any opacity of the crystalline lens (cataract) situated in the axial (pupillary) line may interfere with vision. This diagnosis is established by observation with the appropriate ophthalmoscopical lens (+ 10). Since the lens is of ectodermal origin, the occurrence of cataracts associated with dermatological anomalies and acquired disorders of the skin is not surprising. Only severe expressions of congenital ectodermal dysplasia or acquired exfoliative dermatitis are likely to be accompanied by a cataract. Similarly, disturbances in lens metabolism sufficient to produce cataracts occur only subsequent to profound metabolic alteration, as in hypoparathyroidism sufficiently marked to produce tetany.

The onset of regular types of cataracts due to aging is reportedly hastened by such metabolic disturbances as diabetes, and specific types of punctate opacity in the lens cortex are seen in relatively early life in some patients with myotonic dystrophy, mongolism, cretinism, or recurrent intraocular inflammation of the iris and ciliary body. Certain drugs produce lens opacities, and the benefits of their use must be measured against this potential hazard.

Previous blunt or perforating trauma or a retained intraocular foreign body may cause a variably dense cataractous change in one eye. A siderotic, brown to rusty change in color of a blue or lightly colored iris on one side suggests an iron-containing intraocular foreign body, even if a cataract is not present. If a soft tissue diagnostic x-ray of the eye is negative for a foreign body, further search for causes of hemorrhagic hemosiderosis of the iris or evidence of melanomatous new growth is indicated.

The continuing addition of new lens fibers throughout life results in a gradual enlargement of the lens and compression of the more central fetal and juvenile lens fibers, with resultant change in the index of refraction. A reduction in the angle of surface curvature accompanies the increase in size, which reduces the refractive strength of the lens. This results in increasing difficulty with near vision in relation to distance vision (presbyopia) by 40 to 45 years of age. Nearly all persons who previously had useful 20/20, or 6/6, vision, with or without spectacle help, will require additional spectacle assistance after this age to make up for the resulting loss of accommodation.

At any age, parasympatholytic agents, systemically administered or topically applied in adequate dosage, will temporarily produce inactivity of the ciliary muscle and pupillary sphincter.

The accommodative loss and visual blurring result primarily from the loss of ciliary muscle effect upon the lens through its zonular attachments, and vision is affected very little by the dilated (mydriatic) pupil. Certain systemic diseases, such as diphtheria, produce toxins that may permanently paralyze either the ciliary muscle or the pupillary sphincter muscle or both.

The vitreous body. A variety of disorders produce vitreous opacities. With advanced age or in high myopia, the vitreous may be unusually liquid, allowing free movement of opacities affected by gravity. Ophthalmoscopically visible showers of yellowish, refractile crystalline bodies that gradually settle in the fluid vitreous of an immobile eye after initial movement are called "synchysis scintillans." These are relatively more common after recurrent or chronic intraocular inflammatory disease or recurrent hemorrhage. Monocular, more or less stationary, round to irregular, white, calcium soap opacities (asteroid hyalopathy) may sometimes occur in clusters in nonliquefied, apparently normal vitreous. The appearance of these opacities is occasionally associated with late onset diabetes. Most patients with synchysis scintillans have reduced vision; it is common to find vitreous that contains asteroid bodies in an eye with normal visual acuity and no other external or internal evidence of disease.

The presence of blood in the vitreous, a disturbance which can result from any of several causes, may variably interfere with vision. Hemorrhage is a common complication of contusion and perforating trauma, but spontaneous hemorrhage more commonly occurs from new, thin-walled retinal surface vessels formed as a result of local vascular occlusive disease, long-standing diabetes, or certain blood dyscrasias. If hemorrhage is recurrent or of large magnitude, secondary organizing strands of scar tissue form. The contraction of these strands results in vitreous displacement and separation of the pars optica retina from the retinal pigment epithelial layer (retinal detachment). Two other causes of elevation and separation of the retina from the pigment epithelial layer are primary tumor of the underlying choroid, such as malignant melanoma, and the formation of a hole in the pars optica retina. This latter condition allows the proteinaceous debris and liquefied vitreous elements to accumulate between the pars optica retina and the pigment epithelial layer, leading to retinal detachment.

THE FUNDUS EXAMINATION

If all parts of the ocular media are sufficiently clear, a systematic examination of the fundus is possible by means of appropriate ophthalmoscopical lenses from a position close to the patient's eye (Fig. 7–6). If the patient requires a marked astigmatic correction, a clearer view will be obtained by examining the fundus through his corrective spectacle lens. The effect of simple myopic and hyperopic errors can be minimized by interposing the appropriate ophthalmoscopical lens to obtain a clear image. Blurring produced by the effort of accommodation can be minimized in the same manner. The examiner should wear his own spectacles and keep both eyes open during this examination.

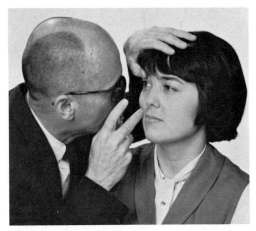

Figure 7–6. Technique of ophthalmoscopic fundus examination.

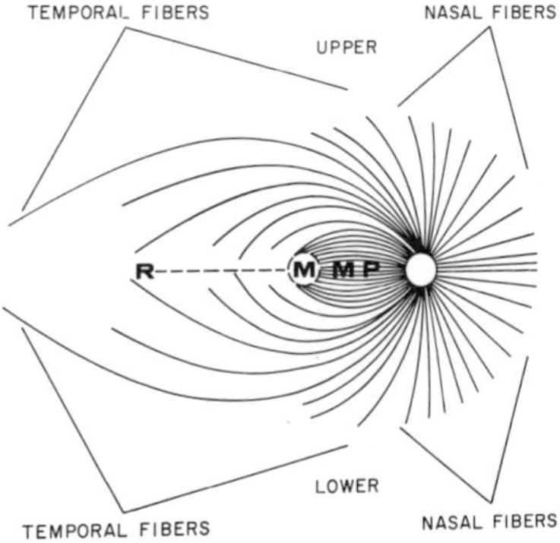

Figure 7–7. Diagrammatic illustration of retinal nerve fiber distribution, right eye. **R**, raphe at site of noncrossing fibers from upper and lower temporal quadrants; **M**, macula; **MP**, maculopapillary bundle.

While the patient is becoming accustomed to the light, the physiologically blind and, therefore, least light-sensitive area of the fundus, the optic nerve head (disc), should be examined. Pay particular attention to its shape and color and to the relationships of emergent vessels. The physiological disc is circular or slightly oval vertically. The color varies geographically, depending on the amount and distribution of the vascularized, axon- and glia-containing extension of the retinal nerve fiber layer interposed between the examiner's eye and the white, sievelike, scleral lamina cribrosa. Usually the temporal third, carrying only the thinner layer of maculopapillary retinal fibers, is paler than the pinker superior, medial, and inferior poles of the disc. These latter areas are crossed by a large number of arcuate retinal axons and by more supporting vascularized glial tissue from the remainder of the peripheral temporal and all of the nasal retina (Fig. 7–7). A fine, brown, serrated line of pigment epithelium is visible at the outer disc margin in some lightly pigmented fundi.

Most of the large retinal artery and vein branches are distributed over the nasal half of the disc and obscure some of the details of retinal nerve fiber anatomy. The point of their emergence from and disappearance into the disc is characterized by a "vessel cone" excavation associated with a variable exposure of the whiter, sievelike, scleral lamina cribrosa. This physiological excavation is decreased or absent with papilledema and is increased by optic atrophy and uncontrolled, long-standing glaucoma. Less often, congenital malformations may distort or cover this area in many ways, and "colobomatous" failure of the inferior fetal fissure of the nerve to close may increase the cone's width and depth remarkably.

When the fundus is heavily pigmented, the disc stands out in contrast, whereas a pale fundus shows a less precise disc outline. The outline of the disc varies in different refractive conditions. In uncorrected high astigmatism the disc has an elongated oval shape. This distortion is quickly corrected by interposing the proper spectacle lens. In marked hyperopia the disc appears small, and its margins are frequently blurred.

The peripheral retina and, finally, the most light-sensitive area of the retina, the macular zone, should be examined in turn and by a personally selected systematic routine so that all areas of the fundus are observed.

The periphery of the fundus can be better examined after the pupil is dilated. Before this is done question the patient regarding earlier attacks of acute glaucoma, and measure the intraocular pressure. (See the discussion of the technique of tonometry on page 284). Weak solutions of sympathomimetic agents, such as 2½ per cent phenylephrine (Neo-Synephrine), produce mydriasis by increasing the pupillary dilator tone and do not alter accommodation. At the completion of the examination, a parasympathomimetic agent, such as 1 per cent pilocarpine, should be used to produce reconstriction of the pupil, in order to minimize the possibility of the development of acute angle closure glaucoma.

Become familiar with normal retinal anatomy by regular observation of the retina of every patient. Only by this means will you be able to utilize the diagnostic information provided by deviations from this normal picture.

THE PUPILLARY REFLEX

Besides carrying the visual fibers, the optic nerve carries axons from the light-sensitive elements in the rod and cone zone of the retina. These large pupillomotor fibers follow the course of the smaller visuosensory fibers and undergo the same semidecussation at the chiasm. The *afferent* arc continues in the optic tract to a point proximal to the lateral geniculate body, where the fibers enter and synapse in the pretectum. Secondary fibers of ipsilateral and crossed types pass ventrocaudally around the aqueduct to synapse at the nucleus of Edinger-Westphal. *Efferent parasympathetic* fibers then travel with the third cranial nerve and its inferior division through the branch to the inferior oblique muscle to reach the ciliary ganglion. After synapse, the fibers innervate the pupillary sphincter and ciliary muscles by way of the ciliary nerves.

Although the size of the pupil is controlled by reciprocal action of the sympathetically innervated dilator and parasympathetically innervated constrictor muscle fibers, the dilator function is primarily tonal, and any significant alteration in pupillary size is accomplished by lesser or greater amounts of sphincter activity. Predominating dilator activity or lesser sphincter activity results in a larger pupil (mydriasis), whereas decreased dilator activity or increased sphincter activity results in a smaller pupil (miosis).

The term "pupillary reflex" refers to the physiological miosis produced by an adequate light stimulus. The *direct* reflex is miosis occurring in the eye stimulated by the light, and the *consensual* reflex is the miosis occurring in the other eye. The consensual reflex is usually less marked than the direct reflex.

Specific clinicopathological changes in the pupillary reaction are outlined in Chapter 4, Examination of the Nervous System, but remember that wide variations in pupillary size occur physiologically. In infancy the pupils are quite small. During childhood and early adult life they reach their largest size, becoming smaller again later in life. Eyes with lesser pigment usually have wider pupils than do dark eyes. Larger myopic eyes frequently have larger pupils than do smaller hyperopic eyes. During sleep and in some unconscious patients, the pupil is contracted. This contraction presumably results from a decrease in the usual inhibitory cortical influence on the nucleus of Edinger-Westphal and thus is a result of increased sphincter tone. Miosis also occurs with accommodation and convergence in the "near point reaction." This is best tested by alternate reference to a distant object and to near-reading material.

Pupillary size is materially affected by systemically and topically administered drugs, most of which alter the autonomic innervation of the dilator and sphincter muscles; a few act directly on the muscles or on the myoneural junction. Changes in pupillary size are occasionally very rapid and of small amplitude; this neurologically unimportant "hippus" is most common in neurasthenic persons.

About one in four persons has a slight physiological difference in pupillary size; a variation of 2 mm. or more is called "anisocoria" (Fig. 7–8). The cause of acquired anisocoria should always be sought. Congenital anisocoria is often overlooked for years, and examination of old photographs will reveal its presence.

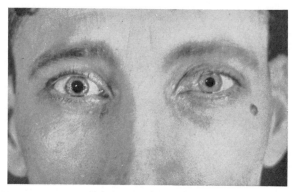

Figure 7–8. Anisocoria.

With extreme lateral gaze, the pupil of the abducted eye is frequently noticeably larger. Congestion of the vessels in the iris is one of the factors resulting in a smaller pupil in the inflamed eye of persons with iridocyclitis. Posterior adhesions (synechiae) of the iris to the lens at the pupillary margin produce one or more scallops, or flattened zones, and alter the reaction to light. Reaction is also altered (depressed) and another form of flattening of the pupillary margin occurs when the iris base is torn and displaced centrally from its attachment to the ciliary body (iridodialysis) following blunt or perforating trauma. Anomalous congenital and secondary inflammatory anterior adhesions (synechiae) of iris to cornea may displace and distort the pupil. Topically administered sympathomimetic agents initially affect the vertically oriented dilator fibers and result in a temporarily vertically oval pupil; this is followed by an even larger, round pupil upon full action of the drug.

EXTERNAL EXAMINATION

The palpebral fissure. The initial appearance of a patient may be altered materially by a change in the size or shape of the palpebral fissure in one or both eyes. The upper lid normally covers as much as 2 to 3 mm. of the cornea while the lower lid rides at or slightly below the inferior corneal limbus. Alterations in this "usual" appearance may reflect changes in the eyelid anatomy or position, the eye size or position in the orbit, or the size of the orbit (see Fig. 5–13).

The blink reflex. Observe the involuntary blink reflex and pay particular attention to its synchronous bilateral nature. Neurasthenic individuals and persons wearing contact lenses often show an *increased* frequency of *bilateral blinking. Increased monocular blinking* follows physical irritation, including abrasions and foreign bodies, of that eye. *Decreased monocular blinking* is common following any process that results in decreased sensitivity of the cornea, particularly when this decrease is associated with deficit of the first division of the trigeminal nerve. Local denervation follows some forms of intraocular surgery, such as cataract extraction, but may also result from scarring after trauma or after extensive inflammatory disease, particularly herpes simplex and herpes zoster. Corneal sensation is easily tested, and the response in the two eyes compared, by using separate, drawn out wisps of cotton from which the unsteady tips have been clipped with scissors. Approach each cornea from outside the visual line, temporally, while the patient fixes a distant object with the other eye. Touch the cornea gently but firmly outside the pupillary line, taking care to avoid the eyelashes and lid margin. Evaluate the amount of lid blink, head retraction, and patient comment for each cornea.

Decreased monocular blinking is also seen in patients with facial nerve deficit and resulting Bell's palsy of facial muscula-

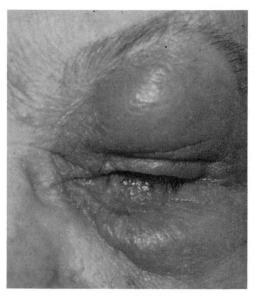

Figure 7-9. Effusion into eyelids.

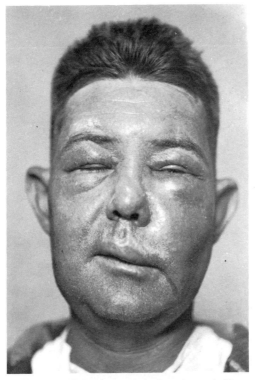

Figure 7–10. Edema of the face in nephritis.

ture, even though corneal sensation is normal. Contrary to expectation, it is the lower lid that droops from the eye, resulting in a large lacrimal lake and frequent tearing (epiphora). In spite of this full lacrimal lake, the cornea is frequently quite dry because of the individual's inability to completely close the lids voluntarily. Corneal drying and its complications, ulcer formation and scarring, occur in some cases even if the eye can be retracted upward beneath the upper lid in attempted closure

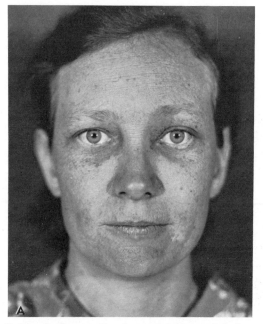

Figure 7-11. *Angioneurotic edema of right eye: A, before attack;*
(Illustration continued on opposite page.)

(Bell's phenomenon, illustrated in Figure 5-13) because this nonreflex movement is not carried out frequently enough. Measures to protect the cornea should be instituted early, before the complications of drying occur.

Decreased bilateral blinking is present in certain stages of general anesthesia. Unconscious patients in shock frequently present with unblinking, open eyes, which must be closed manually and kept closed to avoid the same types of corneal damage and visual loss already discussed.

The eyelids. Many minor blemishes, often due to contactants, first occur in the thin eyelid skin because of its limited keratinized layer, poor skin appendage development, and loose

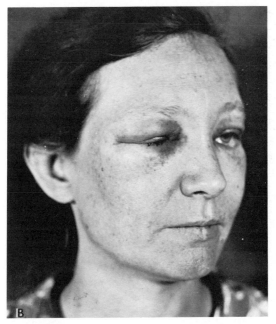

Figure 7–11 (Continued).   B, *during attack.*

attachment to underlying tissue planes. Firmer attachment of
thicker, more keratinized skin is present over the tarsus at the lid
margins and at the orbital margins. The presence of this thicker
skin accounts for the limitation of effusions into the lids at these
points (Fig. 7–9). Focal lid edema accompanies the inflammatory
feature of obstructions of the parafollicular glands of Zeis (hordeolum, or sty, illustrated in Figure 7–14).

Either bilateral or unilateral edema, frequently of marked
proportions, may accompany systemic trichinosis or other forms
of visceral larval migrans. Edema of the lids is also seen in acute
glomerulonephritis, in which facial edema may coexist (Fig. 7–
10). Migratory, painless, noninflammatory, and often recurring

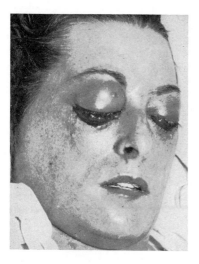

Figure 7-12. Exophthalmos in cavernous sinus thrombosis.

edema of the eyelids, conjunctiva, and other facial structures is often described as being numb in cases of angioneurotic edema (Fig. 7–11). Venous obstructive processes, particularly of the cavernous sinus (Fig. 7–12) or of the varicosity-prone valveless orbital veins, produce extensive orbital and lid edema that may close the aperture.

The aperture may be narrowed because of enophthalmos accompanying congenital anomalies or because of fracture of the orbital wall with displacement of the orbital contents into a contiguous paranasal sinus or cranial fossa. Congenitally small (microphthalmic) eyes or scarred contracted eyes inadequately supporting the upper lid may permit the aperture to narrow. True phimotic narrowing of both the vertical and horizontal aperture measurements occurs as a congenital anomaly. Unilateral or bilateral acquired selective depression of the upper lid (ptosis), often progressive during the waking hours, may be seen at any age, with or without other symptoms and signs of myasthenia gravis. Patients with bilateral ptosis frequently furrow the frontalis muscle and tilt their heads backward in order to see under the drooping lids. A light-sensitive inflamed eye is frequently voluntarily closed, partially or completely. The differential diagnosis of other causes of ptosis is outlined in Chapter 4, Examination of the Nervous System.

Falciform folds of skin may cover a portion of the lid from early life and are most often present on the nasal side of the upper lid (epicanthus). In Caucasians, the epicanthic folds disappear with growth of the skull and of the bridge of the nose, whereas permanence of the epicanthus is characteristic of Orientals, whose skin folds frequently cover the inner canthus and caruncle. Acquired folds of slightly discolored thin skin are common in later life and may cover the lash line. An infrequent pathological inflammatory process produces this effect in early life; this blepharochalasis may be so marked that it interferes with vision by hanging over and depressing the upper lid.

Irregular, yellow xanthelasmic plaques are most frequently seen near the nasal extremes of the upper and lower lids (Fig. 7–13). They may occur in persons with no demonstrable illness, but are more frequently seen in diabetics and in patients with

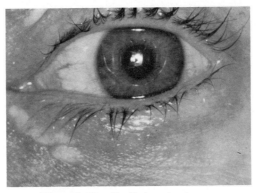

Figure 7–13. *Xanthelasmic plaques.*

primary hypercholesterolemia, in whom they occasionally enlarge to tumor size masses (tuberous xanthoma).

The lid margin regularity is frequently interrupted by an accumulation of seborrheic, greasy debris on and about the eyelash bases. This phenomenon may or may not be associated with a variable degree of inflammation. A similar blepharitis is produced less frequently by parasites, notably crab lice and their nits, which are attached to the eyelashes and grossly resemble dandruff.

Focal loss of eyelash and eyebrow pigment (poliosis) is occasionally seen. These white hairs may be present congenitally and are one prominent feature of the Waardenburg syndrome. Acquired poliosis in association with pigment loss in the contiguous skin (vitiligo) is a curious accompaniment of some granulomatous inflammatory disorders, such as the Vogt-Koyanagi syndrome.

The parafollicular gland of Zeis and the follicles about the eyelashes are easily obstructed by seborrheic and other types of debris. These structures then become infected and produce a sty

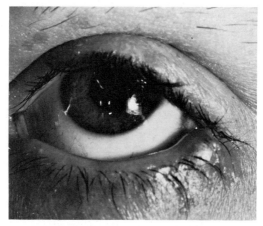

Figure 7–14. *Hordeolum (sty).*

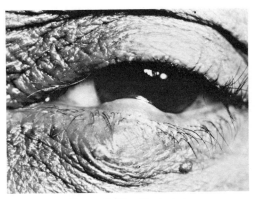

Figure 7-15. Chalazion.

(hordeolum), which is red and painful (Fig. 7-14). The lid margin may also reveal a mass due to an obstructed tarsal meibomian gland (chalazion) (Fig. 7-15), which is infrequently inflamed and seldom painful.

A widened palpebral fissure may reflect an unusual forward position of the eye that, nevertheless, allows adequate lid protection and normal function. This condition is usual in some Negroid groups in whom a shallow bony orbit is the rule. It is accentuated by the premature closure of suture lines in oxycephaly. Orbital congestion, seen in carotid cavernous fistula, not only causes forward displacement of the eye (proptosis) but may also result in orbital pulsations that are synchronous with the heart beat. Orbital congestion is also associated with cordlike, tortuous, dilated conjunctival vessels and occasionally with conjunctival edema (chemosis).

Any mass in the orbit may displace the normal-sized eye with resultant widening of the fissure. The most common lesion of this type is a congenital hamartoma (hemangioma), which may not be evident itself until later life when it enlarges or bleeds. Secondary inflammatory "pseudotumors" can also cause proptosis. Most orbital lesions produce proptosis with selective

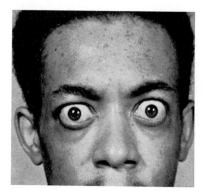

Figure 7-16. Extreme exophthalmos in hyperthyroidism.

exposure of the inferior portions of the eye and *apparent retraction of the lower lid.*

Selective retraction of the upper lid, with or without proptosis (Fig. 7-16), is more common in endocrine disturbances. It is probably the most common lid sign (Dalrymple's sign) in hyperthyroidism, in which it is often associated with lid fullness (Enroth's sign) and with lid lag on downward gaze (von Graefe's sign). Conjunctival edema and limitation of eye movement, particularly upward (gaze), are especially significant signs of endocrinopathic orbital disease in which proptosis (exophthalmos) may be present.

Widening of the palpebral fissure is seen after topical administration of sympathomimetic drugs as well as with irritative lesions of the cervical sympathetic chain or of its branches to the smooth muscle fibers of the upper lid.

The pathologically large eye in high myopia gives the impression of proptosis with a wide fissure and is particularly noticeable when it is monocular. Secondarily enlarged eyes (buphthalmos) that result from unsuccessfully managed congenital glaucoma have a similar appearance but are usually congested, often scarred, and occasionally show ectatic blisters lined with brownish black uveal pigment (staphyloma). These areas transilluminate well, whereas hemorrhagic and tumor masses do not.

By holding the lids apart, one can determine the position and patency of the lacrimal puncta. In conditions involving lacrimal sac obstruction, pressure over the distended sac produces a significant, visible reflux of tears and of any associated inflammatory debris into the precorneal lacrimal lake through patent canalicular channels and puncta.

The palpebral conjunctiva. The palpebral conjunctiva can be easily exposed by having the patient maintain both eyes open and looking down. You can then easily "flip the lid" by grasping the eyelashes of the upper lid and by pulling out and up while pressing in and down on the upper tarsal margin with the forefinger or thumb of the other hand (Fig. 7–17). The lower palpebral conjunctiva is most easily exposed by having the patient open both eyes and look up. Pull the lids down and simultaneously push inward over the inferior tarsal margin with the side of the index finger or thumb tip. The upper lid is returned to its normal position by having the patient look up. Simple release of traction allows reposition of the lower lid.

The conjunctiva over the posterior lid surface is pale pink, smooth, and firmly bound to the tarsus. The vertical, linear, yellow, meibomian acini in the tarsus usually show through the conjunctiva. Secondarily calcified, inspissated mucus that is caught in conjunctival infoldings on the posterior tarsal surface appear as yellow dots in adult life. These calcified bits of mucus are occasionally responsible for foreign body sensations when they touch the cornea, but seldom need excision.

The conjunctiva above the upper and below the lower tarsal margins has a redder color than does the conjunctiva over the posterior lid surface. In early life, the zone just above the upper and just below the lower tarsal margins shows a variable degree of lymphoid follicle formation. This reaction, normally absent from the posterior tarsal conjunctiva, is frequent, severe, and extensive in response to a variety of physical irritants, specific

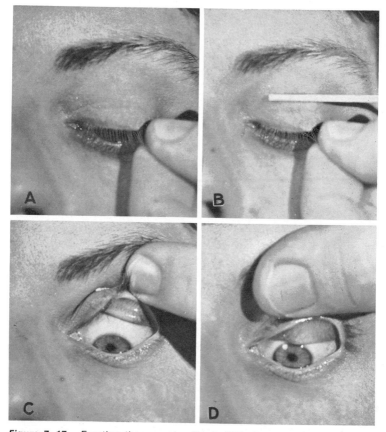

Figure 7-17. *Everting the upper eyelid: A, With the patient looking down, the lashes are grasped between the thumb and forefinger. The eyelid is pulled downward and away from the globe. B, Applicator stick makes pressure above tarsal plate. C, The eyelid is pulled quickly upward and everted. D, The thumb maintains eversion by pressing the eyelashes against the supraorbital tissues. (Scheie, H. G., and Albert, D. M.: Adler's Textbook of Ophthalmology. 8th ed. Philadelphia, W. B. Saunders Co., 1969.)*

allergens, and certain viruses. The follicle is rounded, slightly raised, translucent, and of slightly less coloration than the surrounding conjunctiva.

Trachoma, a viral disease, produces scarring associated with irregular vascularization of conjunctival surface vessels. The large, scarred, follicular changes may resemble the cobblestone-like papillae of vernal conjunctivitis, which show a central vascularized core from the beginning. When they are chronic, both diseases spread to involve the posterior tarsal conjunctiva and result in secondary corneal irritation and increased light sensitivity (photophobia) with resultant narrowing of the aperture.

The ocular conjunctiva. The bulbar conjunctiva covering the exposed surface of the sclera is pale and loosely attached except at the limbus. At the limbus the episcleral vessels are easily seen beneath the conjunctiva and represent branch extensions of the blood supply to the underlying ciliary body and iris. It is this ring of deeply situated pericorneal vessels that becomes engorged and gives rise to the reddish blue "ciliary flush" seen with iridocyclitis, endophthalmitis, and other intraocular

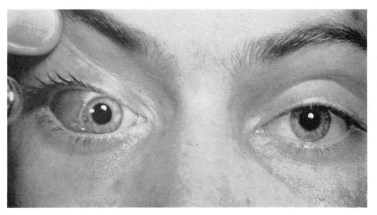

Figure 7-18. Subconjunctival hemorrhage of right eye.

congestive conditons such as glaucoma. In contrast, the "superficial" conjunctival vessels which are most numerous and widespread are found peripherally and over the posterior lid surface. Congestion of this group of vessels suggests conjunctival inflammation.

Both types of injection occur simultaneously with inflammation of the cornea and conjunctiva (keratoconjunctivitis), in which the underlying ciliary body and iris share the inflammation with the cornea. The loose attachment of the bulbar conjunctiva to the sclera permits large accumulations of transudative and exudative fluid (chemosis) in congestive and inflammatory diseases of the orbit, eye, and lids. These accumulations of fluid may result in prolapse of the conjunctiva between the lids. Minor extravasations of blood spread freely in this area (Fig. 7–18). They occur spontaneously more often than with known trauma, frequently beginning during sleep, and are usually painless.

DISEASES OF THE EYE

Conjunctivitis.   The normal conjunctival surface and tear lake contains only a few saprophytic organisms. A large proportion of "red eyes" reveal only vascular engorgement and a mild secretory response with 48-hour cultures free of bacterial pathogens. Many cases undoubtedly occur in response to physical irritants, specific allergens, or viral infection. Combinations of wind, dust, bright light, heat, cold, smoke, vaporizing agents, make-up, hair spray, and a variety of other agents can often be associated with the initial symptoms and signs. Except in cases of corneal involvement, pain is usually mild and of a scratchy foreign body type and is usually relieved temporarily by any eyewash used.

The most typical feature of conjunctivitis is the discharge produced which varies considerably with the cause and severity of the disease. In certain bacterial infections, the organism can be identified in the epithelial cells found free in the discharge or scraped free with a spatula. Extracellular pathogens are identified less easily in a smear, and their presence should be determined by appropriate culture techniques. Diseased epithelial cells, organisms, inflammatory cells, and increased mucus from conjunctival goblet cells make up the purulent exudate of bacterial infections. A limited serous secretion that contains little cellular debris accompanies some viral infections. Excessive and, often, ropy masses of mucus are more characteristic of vernal conjunctivitis, and cytologic examination of this debris may show significant eosinophilia.

Chronic pseudomembranous exfoliation of conjunctival epithelium and profuse discharge are seen in association with the stomatitis that is characteristic of erythema multiforme. This disease and pemphigus commonly result in scarring and shrinkage of the conjunctiva with obliteration of the cul-de-sac and fusion of lid and bulbar tissue (symblepharon). Acute pseudomembranous changes, however, seen with nasopharyngeal disease of the same nature, suggest beta hemolytic streptococcic and diphtheritic infections.

Most conjunctival inflammations are mild, and bacteriological diagnosis often is inconclusive. As a result, many forms of conjunctivitis are classified on the basis of their clinical course rather than on the basis of the etiological agent. Acute catarrhal conjunctivitis is diagnosed when an acute inflammation causes only a seromucinous discharge. Conjunctivitis should not be diagnosed unless there is significant discharge. This will eliminate unnecessary treatment of infected eyes between attacks of acute infection, the "red eyes" accompanying senile degenerative conditions, and reactions to physical irritants. Similarly, the asymptomatic "folliculosis," so common to the fornix conjunctiva of adolescents, will not be turned into a symptomatic iatrogenic inflammation by unnecessary treatment. "Purulent conjunctivitis" is diagnosed when the discharge contains pus; the most prolific producers are the pneumococcus and gonococcus.

Preauricular lymphadenopathy is not common with catarrhal and mild purulent conjunctivitis. Slight tender enlargement of the preauricular and less frequently the submaxillary gland is a common accompaniment of epidemic keratoconjunctivitis (E.K.C.) and adenovirus disease. Severe enlargement, occasionally with suppuration, occurs in the preauricular lymph nodes as part of the oculoglandular syndrome of Parinaud. In this condition, the possibility of a conjunctival infection with Leptothrix should be considered, particularly if the patient has had close association with dogs and cats. Oculoglandular tularemia often presents with ulcerative change in the conjunctiva at the innoculation site of this disease. Lymphogranuloma venereum and tuberculosis are less frequent causes of this syndrome.

Although pain is rarely severe and is frequently absent, itching occurs along with nasal congestion in allergic "hay fever" patients. Itching is particularly prominent in both acute and chronic vernal conjunctivitis.

Degenerations and new growths. In adult life, a slightly yellowish, mildly elevated mass of tissue is frequently noted over the nasal limbus and, less frequently, temporally. It is usually asymptomatic unless it is exposed to physical irritants, of which ultraviolet light, smoke, and dust are noteworthy. This mass, or "pinguecula," is composed of hyalinized collagen and senile elastotic material in the subepithelial stroma; no fat is present as the color might seem to imply. Arising in the same area and often containing pinguecular tissue in its base, a fibrovascular wedge of connective tissue covered by conjunctival epithelium may grow over adjacent clear cornea. This "pterygium" produces corneal opacity where it is attached at its apex. It is seen in persons exposed to considerable sunlight. It causes symptoms under essentially the same conditions as the pinguecula, but it can also disturb vision when it extends to cover any portion of the pupillary zone.

Single or multiple cysts of unruptured goblet cells are common in all areas and are usually asymptomatic except in a cosmetic sense as blemishes. Dyskeratotic plaques and frank squamous cell carcinomas are unusual and resemble their appearance on other mucous membrane surfaces.

Disorders of the cornea. The normal adult cornea usually measures 11 mm. vertically and 12 mm. horizontally. Smaller (microcornea) and larger (megalocornea) sizes may be present anomalously at birth or result secondarily from stretching due to uncontrolled congenital glaucoma. Congenital, yellowish white, round or oval dermoid growths occasionally are seen at the junction of corneal and limbal tissue.

Any process resulting in chronic edema of the cornea may, in time, stimulate the entry of new vessels either from the contiguous superficial conjunctival plexus or the deeper ciliary plexus. Superficial vascularization usually follows superficial inflammations associated with tissue loss (ulcer). Both normal corneal anatomy and pathological change in this small area are best seen with focal illumination and with some form of magnification such as a loupe; epithelial breaks may be more clearly outlined by the application of fluorescein from moistened, dye-impregnated paper strips. The morphological description of the epithelial break is important in the case of the "dendritic ulcer" of herpes simplex, since effective therapy depends on manual removal of the contiguous virus-containing cells or the destruction of the same cells with appropriate medication.

Punctate dots and larger zones of stromal and epithelial opacity may be secondarily vascularized in cases of herpes zoster, particularly when there is involvement of the nasociliary branch of the ophthalmic division of the trigeminal nerve (Fig. 7–19). Ocular involvement in this disease is a serious matter, since visual loss and loss of the eye are complications. Eye involvement should be assumed even without symptoms if the ophthalmic division of the fifth cranial nerve is affected, and the patient should be repeatedly examined, preferably with the help of the special instrumentation available to the ophthalmologist. Even after the healing of skin lesions, a neuroparalytic (anesthetic) cornea is a prime base for repeated infection and ulceration, which can eventually result in scarring and visual loss.

To remain optically clear, the cornea must remain moist. Significant reduction in tears and mucus allows drying and breakdown of the epithelial barrier to infection and its complications. Although a gradual reduction in the number of tear-producing acini in the lacrimal glands occurs with aging, certain

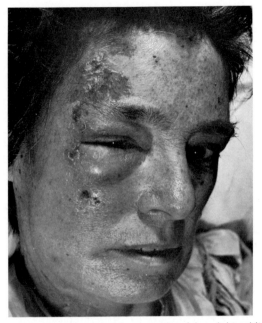

Figure 7–19. *Herpes of forehead involving right orbit.*

postmenopausal women develop a severe shortage of tears, along with salivary gland deficiency and dry mouth. The resulting red eyes are often overlooked because of the painful and disabling arthritis that occurs as another feature of Sjögren's syndrome. The shortage of tears can be demonstrated by inserting a 5-millimeter-wide strip of Whatman no. 40 filter paper into the lacrimal lake by bending a few millimeters over the lower lid margin between the palpebral and bulbar conjunctival surfaces away from the cornea. At least 15 mm. of filter paper will be wet in 5 minutes by normal tear formation in this Schirmer test. Dry conjunctiva and cornea also occur in severe malnutrition in infancy, particularly when there is accompanying vitamin A deficiency.

Any severe and persistent inflammation of the anterior choroid, ciliary body, or iris may stimulate an inflammatory response in the deep stroma of the cornea (keratitis profunda) and may eventually result in the formation of new vessels and scars. The anterior uveal inflammation of congenital syphilis first produces this "salmon patch" type of inflammatory vascularization in the peripheral cornea in childhood (Fig. 7–20). When the inflammatory phase of this interstitial keratitis subsides, diffuse scarring and empty "ghost" vessels may be seen in the posterior cornea. There is a variable reduction in vision if the axial pupillary portion of the cornea is involved. Severe cases produce gross scarring and marked loss of vision that is not correctable with a spectacle lens (amblyopia).

In later adult life, intracellular and extracellular fat is deposited near the end of Bowman's and Descemet's membranes. A 1- to 2-millimeter-wide, partial to complete ring of

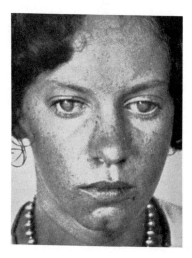

Figure 7–20. *Interstitial keratitis.*

grossly white debris that is separated from the sclera by a narrow clear zone of cornea can be seen with the aid of a pocket flashlight. This "arcus" or "annulus senilis" has no significant relationship to altered fat metabolism. Earlier in life, occasionally in adolescence, a noninflammatory ectasia and thinning of the central cornea (keratoconus) may occur. Progressive change in this bilateral disorder of unknown etiology is associated with the development of marked degrees of astigmatism and eventual central corneal opacity.

Disorders of the sclera. In the infant the thin sclera allows enough of the underlying uveal pigment to be seen to produce a grayish blue cast. This color change may be accentuated by anomalous delayed condensation of the sclera from about the third month of development. The resulting "blue sclera" is seen in association with brittle bones in osteogenesis imperfecta and with dislocation of joints and deafness in the syndromes of van der Hoeve and de Kleyn. The sclera is secondarily thinned and the eye enlarged in uncontrolled congenital glaucoma, resulting in a similar discoloration. A change in color, to dark blue or black, accompanies the focal ectasias of thinned sclera seen terminally in both congenital and acquired adult glaucoma; these "staphylomas" are most frequently noted either near the limbus over the scleral sulcus or at the equator beneath the insertions of the rectus muscles, where the sclera is normally thinnest.

In later life fat deposits in the episclera give it a slightly yellow cast. The sclera is commonly stained yellow in the course of jaundice; the pigment is most noticeable in the fornices away from the limbus. The limbal zone is selectively colored more yellow than the fornices following ingestion of the malarial depressant quinacrine (Atabrine). In "melanosis oculi," the uvea and, to a variable extent, the overlying sclera show excessive brownish black pigmentation. This color change may also be seen in association with the nevus of Ota in the skin of the eyelid and face. A recessive inherited disorder of phenylalanine and tyrosine metabolism (ochronosis) may cause the deposit of black "ochre" pigment focally and diffusely in the episclera where it can be seen easily through the conjunctiva in association with alkaptonuria and discolored (black) cartilage. Grayish blue to light tan translucent zones are frequently seen in the sclera of elderly persons and are caused by deposits of calcium sulfate.

True inflammation of the sclera (scleritis) is an unusual primary process. Secondary scleritis and episcleritis may occur in connection with severe internal inflammations of the contiguous choroid or of the ciliary body or with external inflammations of the orbital tissues. Certain rheumatoid conditions and polyarteritis nodosa are occasionally complicated by severe uveitis and scleritis. Secondary softening and thinning of the sclera rarely results in perforation of the globe (scleromalacia perforans). Inflammatory disease of the more vascularized episclera is much more common. Numerous allergic, infectious, and toxic conditions may show this nonspecific reaction. Circumscribed (nodular) episcleritis has a significant statistical relationship to cranial arteritis and granulomatous inflammations, particularly sarcoidosis, in which the zone near the insertions of the rectus muscles is more commonly involved.

Disorders of the uvea. The melanin-pigmented vascular coat of the eye (uvea) is made up of the choroid, ciliary body, and iris segments. Pathological changes are frequently common to all three parts, but either the *posterior uvea* (choroid) or the *anterior uvea* (ciliary body and iris) may be individually involved. Inflammatory processes may be confined to the choroid (choroiditis), but the iris and ciliary body usually share inflammatory response, in which case the proper diagnostic term is iridocyclitis instead of iritis or cyclitis. Metastatic inflammatory diseases of the retina that spread to the underlying choroid (retinochoroiditis), such as toxoplasmosis and inclusion body disease, are uncommon in the anterior uvea. However, in fulminating infections, the iris and ciliary body may share the congestive inflammatory reaction even if not directly infected. Similarly, the iris and ciliary body respond to primary infections and ulcers of the cornea.

The exact etiology of most forms of uveitis is obscure. Even when the eye is lost, pathological examination may show only the results of the inflammation without a precise cause being identified. Because the infection is located inside the eye, diagnosis is based on the clinical morphological appearance of the reaction; it is here that the specialist's instrumentation, with slit lamp microscope and gonioprism, may be helpful for details of description and signs that would not be observed by more gross examination techniques. Diagnosis by association is taken as second best. General systemic immune reactions may be evaluated by skin and serological tests in an effort to confirm impressions gained from the history and physical examination. Positive x-ray evidence may confirm a clinical impression of ankylosing spondylitis obtained from a careful physical examination of a young male with recurrent iridocyclitis.

Aside from the physician's desire to successfully treat intraocular inflammatory disease and to prevent its extension and the loss of vision, the etiological background of a retinochoroiditis in a female of childbearing age has added significance. Like the spirochete of syphilis, the protozoan, Toxoplasma, is able to cross the placental barrier. Infected offspring, if they survive the extensive cerebral damage and resulting convulsions, often have severe central visual loss due to the development of dense macular retinal scars.

In addition to such general symptoms as blurred vision, photophobia, and local pain, every physician should learn the specific clinical signs of acute iridocyclitis. Acute iridocyclitis, acute conjunctivitis, and acute angle closure glaucoma may produce much the same history and present with a red eye, but they require widely divergent forms of treatment.

Even without the help of the slit lamp microscope, a variety of clinical symptoms and signs may be recognized in acute iridocyclitis. Pain is usually the primary complaint. It is deepseated, aching, and occasionally throbbing like that of a headache or toothache, with which it is often confused. Moderately severe cases are sensitive to light (photophobia) and often show increased lacrimation. Blurring of vision is common and results from tearing and a variable amount of ciliary muscle spasm, which also accounts for most of the pain. The "ciliary flush" of deep pericorneal vascular engorgement gives rise to a ring of redness in the limbal zone. The more peripheral conjunctival vessels are not involved unless there is coexisting conjunctivitis or unless previous heat or irritating medication has been applied. Miosis of the pupil occurs with inflammations of moderate severity, and the pupillary margin may be irregular due to adhesions (synechiae) between the posterior iris surface and the anterior lens capsule. Complete synechiae of this type produce a pupillary block to aqueous flow and result in one form of inflammatory secondary glaucoma.

Severe iridocyclitis, endophthalmitis, and corneal disease are associated with the production of a sufficient number of inflammatory cells that they will settle out in the inferior recess of the anterior chamber angle in the erect patient. This hypopyon can be seen grossly with a pocket flashlight. Keratic precipitates (K.P.) of inflammatory debris may be seen on the posterior corneal surface in chronic iridocyclitis. They are also more common on the inferior cornea where they may be seen at the time of an acute exacerbation of a previously unrecognized indolent chronic inflammation.

Most cases of iridocyclitis are unilateral. However, acutely devastating visual impairment accompanies the severe, bilateral panuveitis that follows perforating trauma to one eye, particularly trauma to the area of the ciliary body. This sympathetic ophthalmia is a constant threat even in properly repaired and managed cases of perforating trauma. Its precise etiology is unclear, and fortunately it is an infrequent disease. In the Vogt-Koyanagi syndrome, bilateral uveitis often accompanies depigmentation of the skin (vitiligo) and hair (poliosis) of the scalp, eyebrows, and lashes. Tinnitus and deafness may also be present. The posterior choroidal inflammation may be so severe that exudative retinal separation (detachment) results.

A variety of hamartomas, inflammatory tumors, and primary and secondary neoplasms occur in the uvea, where they are most commonly located posteriorly.

Hemangiomas may occur singularly within the uvea or as one of many widespread expressions of hemangiomatosis. They are most frequently identified in association with other parts of the vascular encephalotrigeminal syndrome (Sturge-Weber), of which the venous hemangiomas of the skin of the face and scalp are externally visible. A significant number of eyes, so involved, are also glaucomatous, and the congenital nature of this disorder may be suspected from the presence of an enlarged (buphthalmic) eye on the same side as the facial hemangioma. Neurofibromatosis of a localized or generalized extent may involve the ciliary nerves in the epichoroid, between the choroid and sclera, or produce visible nodules in the iris.

The most common malignant primary intraocular tumor in man, malignant melanoma, occurs initially in the uveal tract. It is far more frequent in the posterior uvea (choroid), where it elevates and displaces the overlying retina and, depending on its position, interferes with vision. Except when situated in the extreme anterior choroid and posterior ciliary body region, it is ophthalmoscopically visible as a variably pigmented, elevated, subretinal mass. It may metastasize to any organ or group of organs, but most often involves the liver. Metastases may be delayed many years after removal of the eye and tumor.

Unlike metastatic inflammation, which usually localizes in the retina, metastatic tumors transferred to the eye from any other source almost always localize in the uvea and are much more frequent in the posterior uvea. These tumors generally extend around the perimeter of the eye rather than forward toward the retina and vitreous. They are identified ophthalmoscopically as variably *depigmented* subretinal masses that tend to show a flat retinal separation, as opposed to the bullous hyperpigmented growth more characteristic of the primary malignant melanoma. The most common sources of metastasizing cells are carcinoma of the breast in the female and carcinoma of the lung in the male.

Congenital deficiencies (colobomas) of any or all parts of the uvea follow incomplete closure of the inferior fetal fissure. They are ophthalmoscopically visible as poorly pigmented or nonpigmented areas most often below and nasal to the optic nerve head, which may share in the colobomatous defect. Iris colobomas, also most often inferiorly placed, appear as inverted, tear-shaped, pupillary distortions.

Disorders of intraocular pressure.   The outer scleral and corneal tunic alone is not sufficiently rigid to maintain the rounded shape of the eye. The pressure produced by the intraocular contents keeps the eyeball "inflated" to make it an effective optical instrument. Solid structures, such as the crystalline lens, are normally of constant volume for any given short period. The lens does swell, however, with the absorption of aqueous following traumatic rupture of its capsule or as a result of changed osmotic relationships incident to the development of a thin capsule about a mature cataract.

The physiological volume changes inside the eye are altered only slightly by the actual blood volume in the vascular bed of the uvea and other structures. In the maintenance of normal intraocular pressure, as well as in its physiological and pathological variations, the major factor is the amount of aqueous humor in the eye. Much as is the case with cerebrospinal fluid, there is a selective production of aqueous across the blood-aqueous barrier, i.e., through the vessel walls beneath the inner surface of the ciliary processes.

Once formed, the aqueous passes behind the iris, around the lens, and through the pupil into the anterior chamber. It exits near the iris base through the trabecular spaces in the scleral sulcus at the corneal periphery. A selective outflow into the scleral and episcleral venous systems is accomplished at the junction of the trabecular spaces and canal of Schlemm. This inflow and outflow system normally maintains an intraocular pressure averaging approximately 20 mm. of mercury. There is no significant relationship between the intraocular pressure and the systemic blood pressure. However, the normal intraocular pressure is particularly attuned to normal peripheral blood pressure in the retinal arteries, arterioles, and capillaries in order to prevent pulsatile collapse and to permit a steady visual image.

Ophthalmoscopically visible spontaneous diastolic pulsatile collapse occurs physiologically in the major venous channels on and near the disc in some persons and has no ill effect upon vision. Spontaneous arterial or arteriolar pulsatile collapse, however, is pathological, produces a variable loss of vision, and suggests one of two general etiological conditions. Rarely, the exceedingly high intraocular pressures seen with angle closure glaucoma, of either the acute or secondary type, will collapse retinal arteries and arterioles. If not promptly relieved, this condition results in variable amounts of retinal infarction, edema of the retina and papilla, and subsequent atrophy of both structures. More commonly, marked reductions in the retinal arteriolar pulse pressure will allow normal intraocular pressure to produce pulsatile collapse. This condition is seen in some cases of occlusive disease of the ipsilateral internal carotid artery, of the ophthalmic artery, and of the ophthalmic artery's central retinal artery branch at some point posterior to the branching at the disc. The commonest cause of this condition is atherosclerosis. Partial and intermittent total occlusion of these vessels is responsible for symptomatic, periodic, monocular visual loss of variable duration.

When the retinal arteries and arterioles near the disc are observed ophthalmoscopically, these pressure relationships can be studied. By passive pressure with the finger through the lid or with a calibrated, spring-loaded ophthalmodynamometer (Fig. 7–21) on the paralimbal sclera after administration of a topical anesthetic, pulsatile arterial collapse or "blink" can be produced with pressures just exceeding the intraocular diastolic blood pressure. Total arterial collapse or "blanching" occurs when the intraocular pressure exceeds the peripheral systolic blood pressure in the retinal vessels. This type of examination (ophthalmodynamometry) is used to observe alterations in known values for peripheral blood pressure in cases in which obesity and other factors make evaluation of the blood pressure by other means difficult or impossible. Ophthalmodynamometry is more often of value, however, in the identification of lateralizing asymmetry on the two sides. Reduced perfusion pressure may be sufficient to produce the "blink" and "blanch" on the side of occlusive disease of the internal carotid artery, ophthalmic artery, or central retinal artery proximal to the visible retinal branches.

A physiological range of intraocular pressure change occurs throughout the waking and sleeping hours. This diurnal varia-

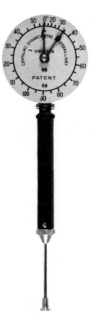

Figure 7-21. *Ophthalmodynamometer.*

tion frequently amounts to as much as 6 mm. of mercury. Initial intraocular pressure readings of between 12 and 25 mm. of mercury are generally considered to lie within the normal range. Intraocular pressures of 10 mm. of mercury or less are said to be pathologically low, and the condition is called hypotony. Intraocular pressures of 30 mm. or more are pathologically elevated, or glaucomatous. Because of such factors as instrumental margin of error, variation in patient cooperation during the pressure determination, and certain anatomical considerations such as variation in scleral rigidity, borderline pressures at either extreme should be retaken by several means and on several occasions.

Tonometry. Two quantitative methods, *indentation* tonometry and *applanation* tonometry, are used to determine the intraocular pressure. By digital palpation through the closed upper lid, one can determine only very gross elevations and reductions in the intraocular pressure. The "stony hard" eye of acute congestive angle closure glaucoma and the "mushy soft" eye of advanced hypotony will be made apparent by this means; but less marked, and still clinically significant, alterations in pressure may easily be overlooked.

You should acquaint yourself with and regularly use the more quantitative indentation tonometer. In this instrument, a variably weighted plunger impinges against the anesthetized cornea through the center of a footplate curved to fit the average anterior corneal surface. The upper end of the plunger touches, but is not attached to, a short, curved lever arm that supports a pointer set to be read against a measured scale. The scale reading obtained can be transposed, by chart, into millimeters of mercury. A reading of 0 on the scale is produced when the lower end of the plunger is lined up flush with the curve of the footplate. This reading may be obtained by placing the tonometer against an unyielding surface with the same curvature as the footplate. A steel button for this purpose is supplied with each tonometer, and the instrument should be pretested for accuracy before each corneal application. Depending on the weight used, the plunger will indent the cornea in inverse proportion to the resistance met.

The proper technique of tonometer application should be followed in detail if the results are to be clinically significant. First, the corneas are anesthetized by the instillation of one or two drops of 0.5 per cent proparacaine hydrochloride (Ophthaine) or tetracaine (Pontocaine). Place the patient in a recumbent position and have him look straight upward with both eyes open. Steady fixation is facilitated by having the patient look at his own fingertip placed in an optimal position to obtain vertical alignment of the eyes. A right-handed examiner stands or sits on the patient's right and has the patient use his left hand for finger fixation. While the patient maintains fixation with the eye not being tested, gently but firmly elevate first the upper lid with your left thumb, avoiding any pressure on the orbital contents

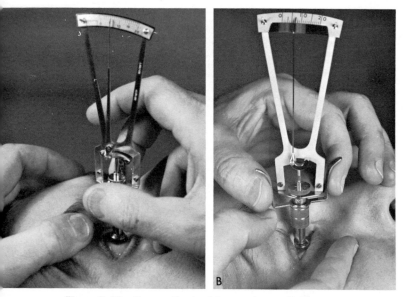

Figure 7-22. *Two methods of tonometer application.*

or eye. This is possible if the lid tissues are fixed between the thumb and the frontal bone at the orbital margin. In similar fashion, depress the lower lid with the forefinger of your left hand or the fourth or fifth finger of your right hand (Fig. 7–22). Apply the tonometer in as nearly a vertical position as possible, and read the scale.

Most good corneal applications show a pointer excursion of about one-half scale reading due to variations in intraocular pressure with each heart beat. If a reading between 3 and 8 on the scale marker is recorded, the instrumental margin or error is considered negligible, and the transposed intraocular pressure, in millimeters of mercury, is recorded on the patient's record. If the reading is more than 8, the eye is pathologically soft. If the reading is less than 3 with the initial 5.5 gm. plunger weight, add an additional 7.5 gm. weight to the upper plunger stem below the curved lever arm and reapply the tonometer to the cornea. If this weight does not give an acceptable reading range, it may be removed and the 10 gm. weight substituted. The intraocular pressure of the right eye is then taken in the same manner. As with other physical examination procedures, improvement in technique and accuracy of results come with practice.

The intraocular pressure may also be measured when the patient is seated erect in front of a slit lamp microscope and the ophthalmologist determines the pressure necessary to *flatten* a measured area of corneal surface, "applanation." This method not only has confirmatory value for indentation tonometry, but it theoretically removes the need for considering the anatomical variable of sclera rigidity.

Reduction of aqueous production and of intraocular pressure, sometimes of pathological proportions, occurs with inflammation of the ciliary body, in shock conditions, in diabetic coma, and after the use of certain drugs, such as the diuretic acetazolamide. Hypotony allows the outer tunic to develop folds, which can often be seen as opaque lines in the posterior cornea. After death, the eyes usually collapse, particularly anteriorly, under the weight of the closed lids.

GLAUCOMA. During life, a pathological elevation of intraocular pressure called "glaucoma" may occur, and in many areas of the world is the most common cause of blindness. Most types of glaucoma can be successfully treated by some means before significant visual loss occurs. The major problems center around awareness of the frequent occurrence of this disorder and its diagnosis. All practitioners of medicine should be aware of the possibility of glaucoma and regularly perform the diagnostic test. Glaucoma may occur at any time from birth to advanced age.

Because of our inexact knowledge, some forms of glaucoma are classed as "primary." A large variety of intraocular and a smaller number of systemic diseases are responsible for one or another type of complicating "secondary glaucoma." The use of an angled prism or mirror in several types of thick contact lenses permits a direct view of the iridosclerocorneal "filtration angle." With good illumination and moderate magnification, the individual anatomical structures of this area can be identified. This "gonioscopic" study permits further classification of primary and secondary glaucomas into the "open angle" type, in which the trabecular tissue is visible, and the "angle closure" type, in which the trabecular tissue is covered by the iris, which may or may not be adherent to the trabecular tissue.

The much publicized but clinically infrequent "acute primary angle closure glaucoma" is characterized by sudden elevations of intraocular pressure. Although all degrees of pressure elevation may occur and spontaneously resolve, the classic attack results in a "stony hard" eye with an immobile, or fixed, dilated pupil and an edematous hazy cornea inside a ring of limbal "ciliary flush" injection. The anterior chamber is shallow.

After the examiner has cleared the cornea with glycerin drops, the gonioscopic view of the filtration angle shows that the iris covers the trabecular tissue and variable amounts of the posterior corneal surface. The clinical symptoms include severe, aching pain, which is often confused with headache or toothache and is generally referred over the areas of the head supplied by the first division of the trigeminal nerve. Variable degrees of visual loss, nausea, and vomiting are present. When the eyes are not included in the physical evaluation of the patient, abdominal pain accompanying this vomiting is occasionally confused with pain from acute abdominal emergencies.

Acute primary angle closure glaucoma must be quickly differentiated from other more frequent causes of a "red eye" in order to prevent improper therapy and resulting blindness and disability. Treatment is primarily surgical and must be performed promptly before secondary adhesions (synechiae) develop between the iris and trabecular tissues. In the surgical procedure known as "iridectomy," a communicating hole is placed at the iris base to allow free movement of aqueous from the posterior chamber behind the iris base into the anterior chamber without going through the pupil. Permanent angle closure may result not only from delayed diagnosis in this type of primary glaucoma, but also from a number of types of secondary glaucoma.

Primary, chronic, open angle galucoma is the most common type. Clinical and research methods of examination, which center around repeated tonometry of the eye under various types of stress, point to the "pore area" that joins the finer trabecular spaces with the canal of Schlemm as the primary focal site of *increased resistance to aqueous outflow.* Very infrequently, *increased aqueous production* is also responsible for increased intraocular pressure; this condition is called "hypersecretion glaucoma."

Continuous application of the tonometer for 4 minutes gradually decreases the intraocular pressure. Recordings taken repeatedly during this period, as aqueous is squeezed out of the eye, form a pressure deterioration curve that can be compared with an established normal. "Tonography," so performed, is one of several clinical examination procedures that help to identify the type of glaucoma present. Since the incidence of chronic primary open angle glaucoma is approximately 2 per cent of the adult population, regular performance of tonometric examination cannot be overemphasized. Unlike victims of most other types of glaucoma, only a small proportion of these patients experience symptoms of the disease before irreparable visual loss has occurred. Even when retinal nerve fiber atrophy has occurred and significant visual field defect is present in the periphery, the central maculopapillary bundle is generally preserved, and the central visual acuity test remains disarmingly normal.

There are no dependable ophthalmoscopical signs in cases of degeneration and atrophy of the transparent retina with the light-absorbing pigment epithelial layer and blood-filled uveal coat behind it. However, at the optic nerve head, where vascularized, glial-supported axons course over the white, sievelike, scleral lamina cribrosa, the ophthalmoscopical signs of atrophy are *pallor* and *loss of substance.* Eventually, this weakened portion of the scleral tunic is pushed physically outward (posteriorly). This glaucomatous excavation, or "cupping," begins, and is often most marked, where the major vessel trunks are noticeably displaced nasally and acutely angulated over its margins. A different ophthalmoscopical lens is frequently required to bring the distally located vessels in the base of the excavation into focus.

Successful treatment of chronic primary open angle glaucoma is absolutely dependent on patient cooperation. Most cases respond well to medical therapy that reduces the resistance to aqueous outflow or limits aqueous production. Occasionally both mechanisms of treatment are necessary. The stress of additional aqueous production on the inadequate outflow channels can be avoided by cautioning the patient against ingesting large quantities of any fluid in a short time. Positive therapy consists of using topically applied eye drops of a solution of a salt of pilocarpine. The percentage of pilocarpine that is required for control is determined by trial and error. The weakest concentration that gives round-the-clock control when instilled at 4- to 6-hour intervals is prescribed.

Pilocarpine and similar drugs that increase the aqueous outflow by a variety of mechanisms are occasionally inadequate. The diuretic acetazolamide and a variety of other compounds, in proper dosage, selectively limit aqueous production. They are most often prescribed as supplementary glaucoma controls for short periods. The failure of all forms of medical therapy to control intraocular pressure occasionally necessitates the surgical creation of a fistula to the subconjunctival space (trephine, iridencleisis).

The outstanding clinical signs of *infantile glaucoma*, regardless of its etiology, are edematous clouding of the cornea and stretching of the outer sclerocorneal tunic. Corneal measurements exceeding 12 mm. and general eyeball enlargement (buphthalmos) are seen in association with congestive signs. Children with this disorder have noticeable photophobia and become agitated in bright light. In terms of its secondary effects upon the eye, this disease is usually well advanced at the time of diagnosis. The treatment is usually surgical, and the nature of the procedure used depends on the type and location of the obstruction to aqueous flow. Many cases are controlled by opening the intraocular channels to the trabecular spaces near the canal of Schlemn (goniotomy).

A large number of intraocular and a smaller number of systemic diseases may be complicated by "secondary glaucoma." Most cases may be explained by a mechanical obstruction to aqueous outflow, although the focus of obstruction may vary considerably. In the course of aqueous flow, the pupillary zone is the first site of frequent blockade. In inflammatory disease annular adhesions, known as posterior synechiae, develop between the pupillary margin and the anterior lens surface. The continued formation of aqueous forces the base of the iris forward against the trabecular tissue. This peripheral, circularly arranged doming of the iris toward the cornea is called "iris bombé." If not relieved promptly by the surgical formation of a secondary escape hole through the iris (transfixion), so that aqueous can get into the anterior chamber, the acute secondary angle closure glaucoma will become chronic, and the eye may be lost.

Occlusive, inflammatory, and organizing hemorrhagic membranes may block the pupil without involving the anterior lens capsule. In this case the entire iris surface is domed forward, often touching the posterior corneal surface and obliterating the anterior chamber. Transfixion or iridectomy is again necessary to prevent permanent adhesions (anterior synechiae) between the anterior iris surface and the trabecular tissue. Anterior synechiae may follow a variety of other circumstances without preceding pupillary block. The most outstanding causes of this complication are postinflammatory membranes that arise following recurrent acute and chronic iridocyclitis, and organized neovascularized membranes that follow a variety of retinal hemorrhagic disorders, such as diabetes and vascular occlusive disease.

Secondary open angle glaucoma most commonly complicates acute anterior uveitis, in which aqueous is continually formed but cannot escape because the trabecular channels are blocked by protein-rich debris and inflammatory cells in the recesses of the filtration angle. Liquefied lens protein, escaping through the thin capsule of a mature or hypermature cataract, may excite an inflammatory reaction, with the same end result. Massive, "eight-ball," anterior chamber hemorrhage from any cause may block the trabecular outflow channels. Severe obstruction to venous return from the orbit, seen in carotid-cavernous fistula, cavernous sinus thrombosis, and varicosities of orbital veins, may cause secondary open angle glaucoma.

Treatment of most of the secondary glaucomas begins, ideally, with prevention by proper management of the etiological process. Even after diagnosis, many cases will spontaneously resolve after successful treatment of the primary causative process.

Abnormalities of ocular motility. Nearly all eye movements are controlled by *involuntary* reflexes, even though they may be started and later secondarily modified by *voluntary* controls.

The visual act, or impulse, actually supplies the *primary* involuntary optomotor reflex for extraocular muscle function and eye movement. In order to maintain the best visual acuity, both eyes are turned to keep the image of each successive object of regard focused on each macular center (fovea). This is the involuntary visual fixation reflex, or fusion reflex. In reading, for example, reflex shifts in fixation result in a series of small jerks, or saccades, while the maculae briefly fixate each word or letter group. Large voluntary movements to the beginning of the next line are more easily seen by the examiner. The repetitious slow following and quick refixation movements of the eyes of persons watching the passing scenery from a moving vehicle are produced by another version of this reflex. The person observed is unaware of this optokinetic nystagmus just as he is in the examining room when he looks at alternately colored stripes or figures on a slowly rotating drum or on a passing strip of paper or cloth.

The optokinetic nystagmus is a physiological response and may be elicited both horizontally and vertically. Distinct reduction or absence of the response on one side has a localizing value in certain lesions of the central nervous system. This physiological response is particularly valuable in the case of a hysteric or malingerer who claims total loss of vision. The reflex is present after the sixth to eighth week of life and serves as a worthwhile test of *cortical* visual function from then on. The intact *subcortical* reflex to a light stimulus, on the other hand, is marked by pupillary miosis and does not indicate any visual perceptive function.

In the optokinetic nystagmus test, a drum or tape is moved slowly in front of the patient, the speed being kept constant in each direction. Any asymmetrical depression of optokinetic response is assigned to that side of the patient, right or left, from which the drum rotation or tape movement originated when the response was defective. This corresponds to the side toward which the rapid jerk, or recovery phase, was directed. Clinical experience shows that lesions of the corticopontine gaze pathway produce depression of the optokinetic response. False positive tests are unusual. Noticeable depression or absence of response when the figures pass from the patient's right toward his left suggests a contralateral, left, parietal lobe lesion or an ipsilateral, right, pontine lesion.

Additional "static reflex" ocular movement follows changes in head position with respect to gravity through proprioceptive impulses from shoulder and neck muscles and the otolith apparatus. Statokinetic reflexes produce eye movements in response to impulses arising from the semicircular canals when the head changes position in space.

One should remember that *voluntary ocular movements*, not individual extraocular muscles, are represented in the cortical oculogyric centers of each hemisphere at the posterior end of the second and third frontal convolutions. Stimulation of the left frontal oculogyric center results in a simultaneous and equal (conjugate) deviation of *both eyes* to the right. Destruction of the left frontal oculogyric center, from any cause, results in a paralysis of conjugate movement of the eyes away from the disabled side, toward the right. The integrity of the individual extraocular muscles involved in right gaze is demonstrated by clinical application of the intact subcortical statokinetic reflex. Quick, passive turning of the head to the left stimulates the ampulla of the left horizontal semicircular canal and results in a conjugate deviation of the eyes to the right, followed by a quick return to their original position. This "doll's head" eye motion is useful in comatose patients, since it establishes an intact vestibular-optic system.

The cerebral association of the two retinal images into a single, clear mental picture is called "fusion." Images of an object that fall on slightly dissimilar (disparate) retinal visual receptors in the two eyes may still allow fusion and, in addition, give the sensation of depth, or stereopsis. If the disparate points stimulated are sufficiently far apart to prevent fusion, double vision (diplopia) results. This is easily simulated by passively pressing one eye out of line while observing a fixed distant object.

DEVIATIONS OF GAZE. Observe the alignment of the two eyes first, *while the fusional reflex is operating*, and then ask the patient to fixate, with both eyes open, a distant finite object, such as a light source, straight ahead. The "uncover-cover" test is performed by covering one eye while observing the other eye for the slightest movement to fixate the light source. If no movement occurs, both eyes should be uncovered and allowed to refixate the light; then the second eye is covered while the nonoccluded eye is observed for any movement to fixate the light. If no movement is seen, the same test is repeated with the fixation object at 14 to 18 inches. If no deviation is discovered in these "primary positions," the same test is repeated in at least six other secondary, "cardinal positions" of gaze, which represent the zones of principle action of the six extraocular muscles of each eye (Fig. 7–23).

Until you become thoroughly familiar with this examination, deviations should be recorded on a blackboard or paper and should be compared with the schema in Figure 7–23 for interpretation. With practice, you will be able to face the patient and identify the cause of any demonstrated deviation without this intermediary recording step, remembering that the patient's and the examiner's muscle fields are reversed.

If definite movement is noted in one or all of these primary or secondary positions, synonymous diagnostic terms (tropia, manifest deviation, strabismus, squint) may be used. *Eso*tropia, *eso*deviation, and *internal (convergent)* strabismus (or squint) refer to the condition in which the deviating eye is observed to be looking *in* toward the nose and to come out to fixate the light when the other eye is covered (Fig. 7–24). Similarly, *exo*tropia, *exo*deviation, and *external (divergent)* strabismus (or squint) are applied to the condition in which the nonoccluded eye is observed to be looking *out,* laterally, and to come in to fix the test light. If one eye is observed to ride above the other and to come down to fix the light, it is described as *hyper*tropic. In such vertical deviations, the eye that is higher is labeled the higher, or hypertropic, eye.

No matter what nomenclature is used, deviations demonstrated by this method are of two general etiological types. When the amount and type of deviation is the same in all of the cardinal directions of gaze, it is considered nonparalytic, or comitant, and is assumed to arise from abnormal supranuclear innervation. Deviations of this type are materially improved or eliminated by general anesthesia of sufficient depth. Diplopia is seldom

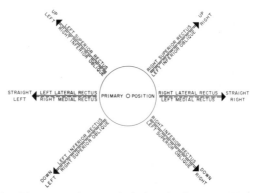

Figure 7–23. *Diagrammatic recorded plot of primary position and the six "cardinal positions" of gaze in relation to the zones of primary function of the six extraocular muscles of each eye.*

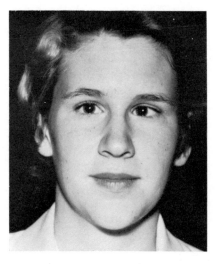

Figure 7–24. *Manifest accommodative esotropia. (Schaffer, D. B.: Pediatric Ophthalmology. In Scheie, H. G., and Albert, D. M.: Adler's Textbook of Ophthalmology. 8th ed. Philadelphia, W. B. Saunders Co., 1969.)*

a problem. Comitant internal (convergent) strabismus appears in the family history of over half the cases. Most cases are first noted between the second and fourth year of life, show small degrees of deviation, and are associated with moderate to severe farsightedness (hyperopia). The deviation in these patients is generally much improved or completely corrected by wearing the full farsighted spectacle prescription determined after the use of cycloplegic drops. Some patients in whom the deviation in near vision is more marked than that in distance vision require additional spectacle correction (bifocals).

Conversely, comitant external, or divergent, strabismus is more marked or seen only with initial distance fixation. This condition has no statistical relationship to hyperopia, and spectacles lenses worn for it may increase the deviation by reducing accommodative effort. The age of onset of divergent strabismus spans a much longer period, and the condition is often progressive until a constant plateau is reached. A small group of exotropias are associated with poor vision in the deviating eye resulting from high refractive errors or local disease, such as cataract, corneal scar, retinal separation, or intraocular tumor.

When the strabismus is much more marked in one of the cardinal directions of gaze than it is in the remainder, it is said to be "noncomitant." Most deviations in this group are due to paresis or paralysis of the extraocular muscles, although other structural changes in the orbit may be responsible for deficient muscle function. The amount of deviation is most marked in the field of action of the affected muscle or muscles for some time after the paralysis first occurs. Since each field of action is primarily represented by a separate muscle in each eye (see Fig. 7–23), repetition of the test in that field, first with one eye and then with the other eye fixing the test light, will usually show that the greatest deviation occurs when the eye with the paretic muscle is used for fixation. This is a clinical application of Hering's law that there is equal innervation of the muscles of each eye concerned in the same directional movement.

When gross *primary* failure of movement is present in one eye, the effect of this innervational surplus upon the nonparetic yoke muscle of the other eye can be seen as an additional *secondary* deviation, or "overshoot." This phenomenon may be observed by watching the normal eye while it is behind an occluder and the eye with the paretic muscle is used for fixation. These objective findings can be amplified by an examination in which the subjective "red lens" diplopia field technique is used. The diagnosis of extraocular muscle palsy due to specific neurological deficit is discussed as part of Chapter 4.

Noncomitant strabismus may arise from a variety of other nonneurological conditions. We have noted that focal inflammatory edema accompanying orbital pseudotumors, certain endocrine orbital changes, and orbital new growths may involve and variably reduce the function of the extraocular muscles. Acute loss of function is seen following trauma accompanied by serous or hemorrhagic effusions into the muscles or by actual rupture of the muscle fibers; occasionally muscle fibers are caught in a fracture site. Sometimes concomitant test results do not fit any one or any single group of functionally related extraocular muscles and vary noticeably from examination to examination. When this happens, even if ptosis is absent, the physician should consider the diagnosis of myasthenia gravis.

When no tropia has been demonstrated, and the eyes are in the primary position, looking straight ahead, electromyographical studies show that the extraocular muscles are still receiving innervational impulses. These influences are not clinically elicited in the presence of a clear visual image made possible by the fusional reflex. By simply changing the color or the shape and color of the image presented to one eye, or by occluding one eye, a relatively fusion-free situation is created, and the nature of these innervational influences can be measured. The specialist will often first use the method of changing a spotlight source to a line of white or colored light by placing a plain or colored "Maddox rod" prism over one eye. He then asks the patient to describe the relative position of the spot of light seen with one eye and the line of light seen with the other eye. This subjective test may be used to confirm and quantitate the routine, objective, "alternate-cover" screening test.

In the alternate-cover test, ask the patient to fixate a distant light source with one eye while the other eye is occluded. Move the occluder from one eye to the other rapidly enough to avoid fusional binocular vision. Observe the eye that has just been uncovered for any movement to fix the test light. The test is repeated with near (14 inches) fixation. Any movements observed are classed as "heterophorias" and are subclassified, like the tropias, into esophoria, exophoria, and hyperphoria. The horizontal phorias, unless of rather marked degree, seldom produce symptoms. Vertical phorias are infrequently associated with inability to read for sustained periods and general ease of fatigue with sustained close work, driving a car, and movie or television viewing.

It is worth repeating what was said at the beginning of this chapter: regardless of the chief complaint, the wise physician always examines both eyes of each patient anatomically and functionally.

COMMON CLINICAL TERMS

Amblyopia—Subnormal visual acuity *not* correctable by spectacle or contact lenses; cf. ametropia.

Ametropia—Subnormal visual acuity caused by some form of refractive error (hyperopia, myopia, astigmatism), which is correctable by spectacle or contact lenses.

Ectasia—Abnormal outward bulging of some portion of the corneoscleral tunic; to be differentiated from **staphyloma**, a common form of ectasia lined internally by uveal pigment from the iris, ciliary body, or choroid.

O.D. (oculus dexter)—right eye; **O.S. (oculus sinister)**—left eye; **O.U. (oculus uterque)**—each eye.

Phosphene—The sensation of light, often in flashes, produced by mechanical or electrical stimulation of the retina, central visual pathways, or cortex.

Photopic vision—Cone vision in a light-adapted eye.

Scotoma—A circumscribed area of visual loss within the visual field; to be differentiated from **sector defect, quadrantanopia, hemianopia,** and other forms of focal or generalized constriction of the field periphery.

Scotopic vision—Rod vision in a dark-adapted eye.

Uvea—The melanin-pigmented vascular coat of the eye including the iris, ciliary body, and choroid.

Vergence—Opposing movements of the two eyes toward one another (convergence) or away from one another (divergence); cf. version.

Version—Movement of the two eyes in the same direction, such as dextroversion (to the right) and levoversion (to the left).

COMMON CLINICAL SYNDROMES

Adie's syndrome (tonic pupil)—A disorder of unknown etiology, not related to systemic diseases, occurring as a female sex-linked trait and manifested in the second and third decades. A *slightly enlarged pupil* shows delayed and often diminished direct and consensual constriction and dilation in response to light stimulation and convergence effort. There may be associated reduced or absent tendon reflexes, particularly of the knee and ankle. Unlike the normal pupil, the affected pupil constricts following the instillation of 2.5 per cent methacholine drops. Full reaction is produced by miotics and mydriatics.

Argyll Robertson pupil—One that is of unusually small size (miotic) and reacts little or not at all to light but retains a relatively greater response to accommodation. The condition may be unilateral or bilateral and is usually but not always due to syphilis, in which case variable signs of central nervous system syphilis usually coexist. Atropine drops produce a reduced degree of dilatation.

Ehlers-Danlos syndrome (fibrodysplasia elastica)—A syndrome present at birth, usually transmitted as autosomal dominant but sometimes recessively inherited, characterized by thin, atrophic, fragile, and hyperelastic skin and often associated extreme laxity and repeated subluxation of joints. Eye findings include a variable mixture of lens subluxation and breaks in the lamina vitrea and Bruch's membrane, with the ophthalmoscopical appearance of vessel-like (angioid) streaks. Complicating hemorrhage from the underlying choriocapillaris beneath the pigment epithelium or retina may result in varying degrees of loss of vision. The hyperelastic skin may appear in large epicanthic folds (see Fig. 5–11), and ptosis is common. The cornea may be thin and conical. Glaucoma is frequently present.

Gradenigo's syndrome (temporal syndrome)—A syndrome due to extradural abscess or infection of the petrous portion of the temporal bone. Along with signs of auditory deficit if infection originated in the inner ear or as a complication of meningitis, ipsilateral involvement of the sixth cranial nerve produces lateral rectus paresis or palsy with esotropia in gaze to the affected side.

Grönblad-Strandberg syndrome (systemic elastodystrophy)—Usually manifested in youth or early middle age and of familial recessive inheritance, this syndrome of pseudoxanthoma elasticum (yellow fleck skin changes) in symmetrical folds of neck and about joints is associated with a variety of other results of fibrinoid degeneration of collagen tissues, such as focal arteriosclerosis and aneurysm formation. Focal Bruch's membrane degeneration in the eye results in thinning and breaks with appearance of vessel-like (angioid) streaks and complicating hemorrhage beneath the pigment epithelium and retina.

Horner's syndrome (cervical sympathetic deficit)—Mild ptosis, pseudoenophthalmos, and miosis due to interruption of the first neuron from the hypothalamus to and including the superior cervical ganglion. If the syndrome is congenital, the involved iris will show less pigmentation. There may be a reduction in tears accompanying anhidrosis of the face.

Sjögren's syndrome—Of unknown etiology, commonly associated with endocrine dysfunction, this syndrome occurs almost exclusively in women over 40, often beginning at time of menopause. It may respond to small doses of stilbestrol. There is dryness of the mouth and other mucous membranes, including the conjunctiva, with secondary blepharoconjunctivitis. The cornea will show secondary abrasions and occasional ulceration and visual impairment if changes are central. Scleroderma-like skin changes and arthritic changes are common.

Sturge-Weber syndrome (vascular encephalotrigeminal angiomatosis)—A syndrome characterized by vascular nevi of the face, scalp, extremities, trunk, and leptomeninges. The eye on the affected side is glaucomatous and often enlarged. *Choroidal hemangioma* often associated with nevoid marks of episclera and conjunctival telangiectases. Whether the disorder is inherited is debated.

Von Hippel-Lindau syndrome (retinocerebral angiomatosis)—A syndrome of angiomas, most often in cerebellum and walls of fourth ventricle, and visceral cysts variably in the kidneys, adrenals, ovaries, liver, and spleen. The patient may show epilepsy, psychic disturbances, or dementia as well as a variety of complications of retinal hemangiomas such as vitreous hemorrhages, new-formed iris vessels, and secondary glaucoma. The disorder is a dominant trait and is familial in at least 20 per cent of patients.

BIBLIOGRAPHY

Adler, F. H.: Physiology of the Eye. 4th ed. St. Louis, The C. V. Mosby Co., 1965.

Cogan, D. G.: Neurology of the Visual System. Springfield, Illinois, Charles C Thomas, 1966.

Duke-Elder, W. S.: System of Ophthalmology. Vols. 1 to 9. London, H. Kimpton, 1958–1966.

Scheie, H. G., and Albert, D. M.: Adler's Textbook of Ophthalmology. 8th ed. Philadelphia, W. B. Saunders Co., 1969.

8
EXAMINATION OF THE CHEST, LUNGS, AND PULMONARY SYSTEM

Inspection, palpation, percussion, and auscultation are all of value in examination of the chest. Correlation of historical and physical findings with information obtained from chest x-ray and certain physiological measurements results in increased accuracy, sensitivity, and specificity. Indeed, certain auscultatory sounds and changes in resonance, when limited to small areas or when produced by changes deep within the thoracic cage, may be detected only after the examiner has been alerted by changes seen in an x-ray study. Similarly, a simple spirometric tracing may provide clues to the presence of abnormal airway function, suggesting added steps in evaluation. Such abnormality might be overlooked in a purely physical examination because certain noises and wheezes can be heard only after the patient has been exercised, made to cough, or placed in recumbent position for an extended period.

TOPOGRAPHICAL ANATOMY

The signs that are demonstrable by physical examination of the chest relate to the lung, pleura, heart, mediastinal structures,

301

and the chest wall itself. Therefore, certain anatomical reference points on the chest should be noted.

The suprasternal notch marks the top point of the manubrium. The sternal angle, the point at which the manubrium and body of the sternum join, is also the location of the anterior attachment of the second rib: other rib levels may be identified from this reference point. Figure 8–1 illustrates the following lines and areas:

Midsternal line — a vertical line drawn through the center of the sternum and xiphoid.

Midclavicular line — a vertical line parallel to the midsternal line and extending downward from the midpoint of each clavicle.

Anterior axillary line — a line extending downward from the anterior axillary fold.

Posterior axillary line — a similar line originating at the posterior axillary fold.

Midaxillary line — a vertical line originating at a point midway between the anterior and posterior axillary lines.

Midspinal line — a line in the center of the back as defined by the spinal processes.

Midscapular lines — vertical lines on the posterior chest that are parallel to the midspinal line and that extend through the apices of the scapulae.

Infrascapular area — the region of the posterior thorax lying below the scapular area.

Interscapular area — the region of the posterior thorax lying between the scapulae.

The location of an identifying mark, percussion abnormality, auscultatory sound, or other change should be recorded or communicated as: "5 cm. to the left of the midsternal line at the level of the fifth rib."

The right lung is made up of an *upper*, a *middle*, and a *lower* lobe. The left lung is divided into an *upper* and a *lower* lobe. Each lobe is subdivided into two or more segments, each receiving its own subdivision of the bronchial tree, pulmonary artery, and pulmonary vein, and each is functionally separate from adjacent

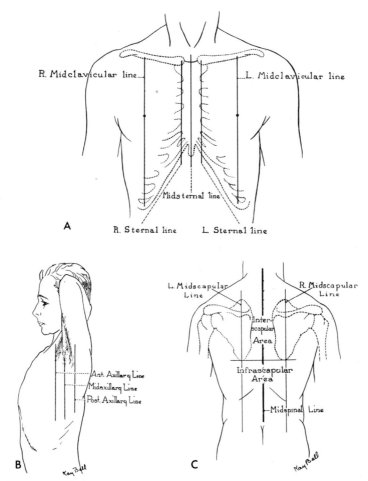

Figure 8-1. Reference lines on the chest wall: A, anterior view; B, axillary view; C, posterior view.

TABLE 8–1. THE BRONCHOPULMONARY SEGMENTS

Right Lung	Left Lung
Upper lobe	*Upper lobe*
1. Apical segment	Superior Division
2. Anterior segment *dorsale*	1 *and* 3. Apical posterior segment
3. Posterior segment *Vent</.le*	2. Anterior segment
	Inferior Division
Middle lobe	4. Superior lingular segment
4. Lateral segment	5. Inferior lingular segment
5. Medial segment	
	Lower lobe
Lower lobe	6. Superior segment
6. Superior segment	7 *and* 8. Anteromedial basal segment
7. Medial basal segment	9. Lateral basal segment
8. Anterior basal segment	10. Posterior basal segment
9. Lateral basal segment	
10. Posterior basal segment	

segments. Table 8–1 lists the 18 bronchopulmonary segments that make up the right and left lungs.

The topographical relationship of the lung segments to the chest wall is of fundamental importance, since pathological changes result in physical findings elicited on areas of the thorax overlying specific lung segments. Figure 8–2 shows the topographical projection of each lung segment on the chest wall. Solid lines mark the divisions between major lobes. Dashed lines indicate the individual segments.

HISTORY

A brief outline of important factors in the history and general evaluation follows. Often a symptom such as dyspnea must be personally observed by the examiner if interpretation of the patient's complaint is to be valid. At other times the environmental and occupational histories provide the only clue that more detailed observations are indicated.

Smoking. Cigarette smoking causes or aggravates certain diseases of the respiratory system; therefore, you should record the number of cigarettes used per day and the number of years of smoking. Malignant tumors of the bronchi seldom occur in patients who do not smoke. Chronic bronchitis and pulmonary emphysema occur more frequently in heavy smokers. Tobacco stains on the patient's fingers or teeth may add substance to the findings in the history.

Occupational history. A number of important pulmonary disorders are caused by exposure to specific occupational hazards. A brief outline of these diseases is given in Table 8–2. The history should include a chronological listing of all the jobs the patient has held as well as an evaluation of any unusual air pollution encountered.

GENERAL EVALUATION

Dyspnea. By definition, dyspnea is the patient's subjective awareness of insufficient ventilation. Throughout the examination you should evaluate a complaint of dyspnea by observing the patient's respiratory movements. During and after exercise, the sensation of breathlessness may be physiological and normal. Observation will indicate that the increased level of ventilation is appropriate and in keeping with that you would experience with similar exercise. Apprehensive or neurotic patients may complain of being short of breath, whereas observation of their respiratory movements reveals nothing other than an occasional sighing respiration. Many lung diseases result in increased levels of ventilatory air exchange or in labored breathing when there is mechanical impairment to respiratory movements, impedance to diffusion of respiratory gases across the lung membranes, or maldistribution of the gases or blood flow in the lung. Decreased oxygen supply to the body tissues, accumulation of carbon dioxide, or acidic shifts of blood pH cause the minute ventilation of the lung to increase.

Text continued on page 309.

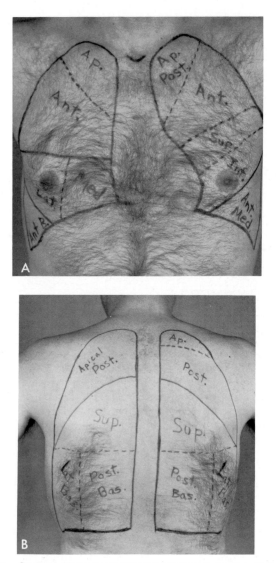

Figure 8–2. Outline of lung segments projected on thoracic wall: A, anterior view; B, posterior view;

Illustration continued on opposite page.

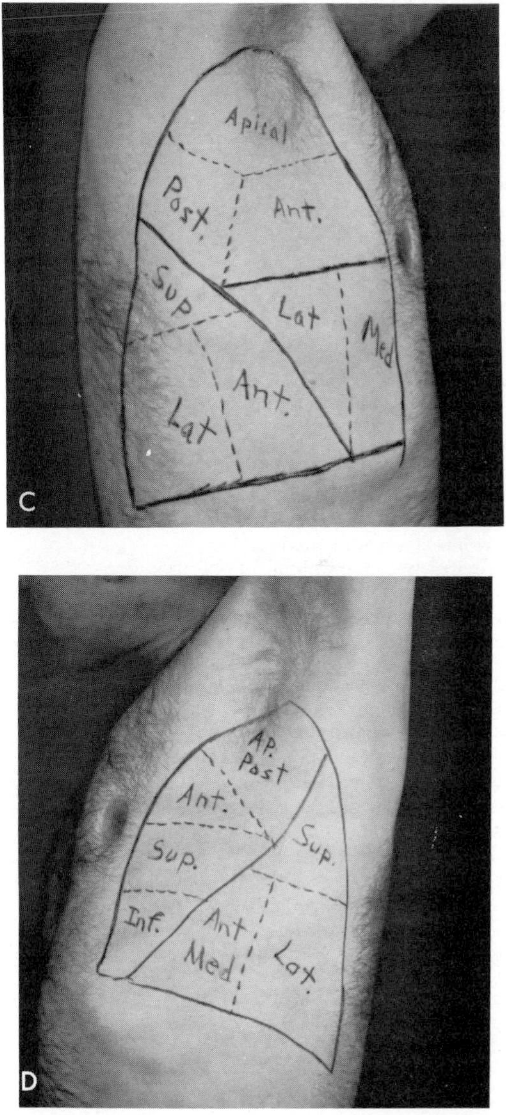

Figure 8–2 (Continued) C, right lateral view; D, left lateral view.

TABLE 8-2. SOME OCCUPATIONAL CAUSES OF PULMONARY DISEASE

Silicosis—inhalation of SiO_2
    Mining of coal, lead, and zinc.
    Working in iron foundry.
    Sand blasting.
Asbestosis—inhalation of asbestos
    Mining and processing asbestos.
    Boiler manufacturing.
    Insulation installers.
Bauxite pneumoconiosis—inhalation of aluminum oxide
    Mining and manufacture of aluminum products.
Talc pneumoconiosis—inhalation of magnesium silicate (talc)
    Rubber tire and shoe manufacturing.
Graphite pneumoconiosis—inhalation of graphite
    Mining and processing of graphite.
Siderosis—inhalation of iron oxide
    Foundry workers, electric welders.
Byssinosis—inhalation of cotton dust
    Cotton mill workers.
Beryllium pneumoconiosis—inhalation of beryllium
    Mining and processing beryllium compounds, radio tube manufacture, atomic energy research.
Various other metals—inhalation of metallic fumes such as manganese, vanadium, or osmium.
Silo filler's disease—inhalation of nitrogen dioxide
    Workers in recently filled silos.
Hypersensitivity pneumonitis
    An increasing number of lung diseases caused by exposure to organic dust material are being recognized. The reaction may be caused either by the material itself or by products of mold and fungi which have proliferated in the organic medium. Some of these are:
        Farmer's lung
        Maple bark stripper's disease
        Hemp worker's disease
        Bagassosis (sugar cane workers)
        Sequoiosis
        Pigeon breeder's disease

Cough.   Observe your patient carefully for the presence of a cough. Since coughing and sputum production are not socially acceptable, patients learn to handle such activity quietly and personally, even to the extent that they are hardly aware of the symptoms themselves. Often, questioning a family member or close associate of the patient provides a clue to the severity, persistence, and duration of cough. Ask the patient to breathe deeply three or four times in rapid succession. This will often initiate a paroxysm of coughing if secretions are present in the tracheobronchial tree. Certain patients whose lungs secrete an excessive amount of distasteful sputum, as a result of chronic bronchitis or bronchiectasis, sequester these secretions in the lung and continually avoid situations that incite coughing. Often the history or the observation of a cough provides the only early, tangible clue to the presence of chronic bronchitis.

Sputum.   Observation of the patient's sputum is mandatory. He may be unaware of its character because he swallows it rather than spits it out. During the examination, have your patient produce a sample for you to look at.

Patients who have a bronchopulmonary disease should be given a glass or plastic jar in which to collect a 24-hour sample. Note the quantity, color, viscosity, and odor of the sputum. Saliva, which is unacceptable for diagnosis, is recognizable by its clear, watery appearance. Translucent, grayish white, tenacious, and mucoid sputum is commonly seen in patients who have pulmonary emphysema. Yellow or green pus that occurs in globs or that completely colors the sputum is an important indication of inflammatory changes in the tracheobronchial tree. The odor of purulent material is usually obvious. Either a lung abscess or bronchiectasis may lead to the production of a large volume of purulent, foul sputum that separates into distinct layers upon standing.

HEMOPTYSIS.   The expectoration of sputum that is either streaked or grossly contaminated with blood is called "hemoptysis." Many diseases, such as carcinoma of the lung, bronchial tumor, or bronchiectasis, can cause hemoptysis, which may be the only physical sign evident until the disease state has become advanced. Prior to the current era of drug control, tuberculosis was the major cause of hemoptysis. Currently, tumors of the lung or bronchus and chronic bronchitis are the most frequent causes of hemoptysis in patients living in the United States. It is estimated that at least one-fourth of all patients with chronic bronchitis have hemoptysis at some time during their illness.

Classically, lobar pneumonia is accompanied by the production of bloody, rust-colored sputum. Infarction of the lung following pulmonary embolism may result in the expectoration of bloody sputum, although this sign is not invariably present. Abnormally high pressure in the pulmonary circulation may also result in episodes of hemoptysis. The red, frothy sputum seen in pulmonary edema which accompanies left heart failure and the recurrent bloody sputum seen in mitral stenosis are both classic examples of hemoptysis. Less common causes include arteriovenous fistulas, hamartomas, and telangiectasia of the lung.

Cyanosis. Cyanosis, a bluish discoloration of the skin, is associated with hypoxemia, or deficient oxygenation of the blood. There must be approximately 5 gm. of reduced, or unoxygenated, hemoglobin in the capillaries of the tissue before cyanosis becomes evident. By simple calculation it is obvious that anemic patients may never appear cyanotic, since even at very low blood oxygen tensions there is not enough reduced hemoglobin to produce cyanosis. Similarly, patients with polycythemia may appear cyanotic even though the oxygen tension in their blood remains relatively high. Patients in shock, in which the major portion of the cardiac output is shunted away from the extremities, may have localized cyanosis of the arms and legs. Cyanosis is best detected in the vascular bed of the lips, tongue, ear lobe, and nails. Direct measurement of blood oxygen tension and saturation demonstrates that visual perception of cyanosis is not a sensitive indicator of low oxygen tensions in the blood or tissues. Rather, you should recognize that when cyanosis is present, serious reduction of oxygen tension has occurred.

Cyanosis that accompanies pulmonary problems indicates either alveolar hypoventilation or an alteration of the normal balance between ventilated and perfused portions of the lung. Diseases of or injury to the central nervous system, the intercostal or phrenic nerves, or the muscles of respiration as well as the administration of depressant drugs or anesthetic agents may result in hypoventilation.

Obstruction to the flow of air in the conducting airways, such as there is in asthma, bronchitis, or pulmonary emphysema, may cause cyanosis. Cyanosis may also occur in lobar pneumonia or in atelectasis of the lung because blood continues to pass through portions of the lung in which the alveoli are no longer ventilated.

EXAMINATION OF THE CHEST

Examination of the chest is best accomplished when the patient is standing or is comfortably seated in an erect position

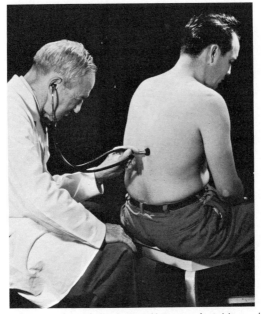

Figure 8–3. *Auscultation of the lungs. Note comfortable positions of examiner and patient.*

(Fig. 8–3). Complete evaluation is impossible when the patient is lying in bed, since the chest may not expand symmetrically and percussion and auscultatory sounds may be damped. Female patients should be provided with a sheet or shoulder drape. Very ill, postoperative, and unconscious patients present special problems, and you may need an assistant to hold the patient in position during part of the examination.

Inspection

Skeletal deformities, including kyphosis and scoliosis (see Chapter 14, Examination of the Back and Extremities), should be carefully evaluated, since they may alter the mechanics of respiration or affect the transmission of sound through the chest. A barrel chest (Fig. 8–4) may be associated with pulmonary em-

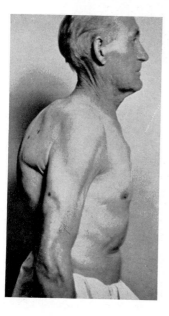

Figure 8–4. Barrel chest with kyphosis.

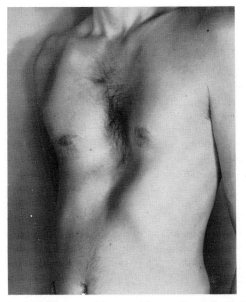

Figure 8–5. *Funnel chest in a 20 year old man. (Ravitch, M. M.: Disorders of the chest wall. In Sabiston, D. C., Jr. (ed.): Davis-Christopher Textbook of Surgery. 10th ed. Philadelphia, W. B. Saunders Co., 1972.)*

physema; however, modern procedures for diagnosing emphysema indicate that the barrel chest deformity may just as often be associated with the degenerative skeletal changes that accompany aging. A funnel chest, in which the lower sternum is displaced posteriorly, is readily apparent on inspection (Fig. 8–5). Funnel chest may cause displacement of the heart, mediastinal structures, and the lungs to abnormal locations and lead to findings that are incorrectly interpreted as representing disease state. Chicken breast, in which the sternum bulges forward like the keel of a ship, produces striking changes in the configuration of the chest but seldom alters lung physiology (Fig. 8–6).

Observe the chest wall carefully, noting any surgical scars

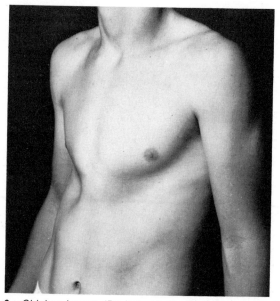

Figure 8–6. *Chicken breast. (Ravitch, M. M.: Disorders of the chest wall. In Sabiston, D. C., Jr. (ed.): Davis-Christopher Textbook of Surgery. 10th ed. Philadelphia, W. B. Saunders Co., 1972.)*

and the character and pattern of the subcutaneous blood vessels. The latter may provide a clue to mediastinal disease, since collateral circulation frequently develops on the chest wall following obstruction of the superior vena cava or the azygos veins by a tumor (Fig. 8–7).

Respiratory patterns. Carefully note the rate, depth, symmetry, and pattern of respiratory movements, keeping in mind that the patient is continually altering intrathoracic pressure in order to do work on the lung structures. These changes in pressure within the thorax cause air to flow into and out of the lung alveoli by way of the conducting airways. During normal inspiration, the diaphragm moves downward, and the thoracic cage

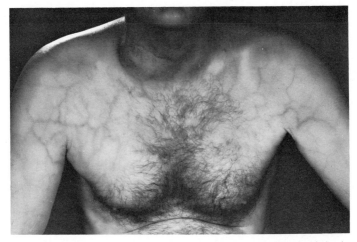

Figure 8-7. *Obstruction of superior vena cava in carcinoma of the lung. Note dilated jugular vein with visible veins over chest and shoulders.*

moves upward and outward. These movements increase the intrathoracic volume, which in turn decreases the intrathoracic pressure. As a result, air flows into the lungs. Exhalation occurs when the muscles of respiration are relaxed and the elastic thoracic cage is allowed to spring back into its rest position. Normally inspiration occupies a shorter period of the respiratory cycle than does the longer, passive, effortless expiration.

The flow of air into and out of the lungs can be related to changes in intrathoracic pressure, as shown in Figure 8-8. The graph illustrates a series of simultaneous measurements of the instantaneous airflow rate, the volume of air moved into or out of the lung, and the change in intraesophageal pressure (which approximates the change in intrathoracic pressure) during normal, quiet respiration in a normal patient. Small pressure changes of between 4 and 5 cm. of water in the thorax are sufficient to produce a tidal flow of air from the alveoli to the outside.

Each breath has a *tidal volume* of about 600 cc. of air. At rest,

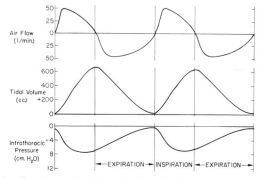

Figure 8–8. *Tracings showing relationship between airflow rate, total volume exchange, and intrathoracic pressure change in a normal person during quiet respiration.*

therefore, a respiratory rate of 8 to 10 breaths per minute causes the exchange of between 5 and 6 liters of air per minute. This amount of air, the *minute volume*, provides the quantity of oxygen needed and carries away the carbon dioxide produced by the body at rest.

An abnormally rapid rate of respiration, or *tachypnea*, may increase the minute ventilation. On the other hand, if the depth of breathing is decreased, tachypnea may only compensate for the reduced quantity of air exchanged with each breath. Certain patients with fibrosis of the lung, pulmonary edema, pleural disease, or rib cage fixation may breathe rapidly and shallowly. They thereby avoid having to stretch the lungs to a large size, a mechanically inefficient maneuver for them. Other patients may increase the minute ventilation to accommodate an increased gas exchange that is necessitated by exercise, fever, hypermetabolic states, or anxiety.

KUSSMAUL RESPIRATION. Minute ventilation may also increase during metabolic states that result in acidosis. In decompensated diabetes with profound acidosis, for example, respiration is increased in rate and depth; this "air hunger" is called

"Kussmaul respiration." Acidosis caused by either renal disease or drugs may result in a similar picture. Diseases of the central nervous system, such as meningitis, may increase minute ventilation, or conversely, respiration may be slowed by a hemorrhage or a brain tumor that increases intracranial pressure. A number of anesthetics and other drugs may also depress ventilation levels.

FORCED EXPIRATION.   As has been stated, expiration is normally quiet and passive. This is not so when a disease process limits the free outflow of air. In asthma, chronic bronchitis, and pulmonary emphysema, it may be necessary to increase positive pressure within the thorax considerably in order to expel air. The effort necessary to increase the intrathoracic pressure is reflected by a prolonged phase of expiration and by the visible use of accessory muscles of the neck, shoulder girdle, and intercostal areas. Associated findings include bulging of the supraclavicular spaces and fixation of the abdominal muscles. Frequently the patient purses his lips or phonates during expiration since these maneuvers reduce the work of breathing by helping to hold the airways open. Such variations are best detected after the patient has been asked to exercise a bit.

FORCED INSPIRATION.   During normal inspiration there is but slight retraction of the intercostal and supraclavicular spaces. If the lung has become mechanically rigid as a result of fibrosis or pulmonary edema, the greater negative intrathoracic pressure required to increase inflation of the lungs will be evidenced by retraction of the intercostal and supraclavicular structures. Blockage of the large airways, trachea, or larynx results in similar changes.

Deviations from the regular, rhythmical movements of respiration should be noted. Anxious patients may voluntarily interrupt their breathing pattern, vary its rate and depth, or sigh frequently.

CHEYNE-STOKES RESPIRATION.   Cheyne-Stokes respiration is one of the most striking types of respiratory irregularity. Hippocrates was familiar with this phenomenon and described the case of "Philiscus who lived by the wall," whose "respiration throughout was like that of a man recollecting himself." A tracing from a patient with Cheyne-Stokes respiration is shown in Figure 8–9. No one has described this type of respiration better than Cheyne himself, who in describing a patient wrote, "His breathing was irregular; it would entirely cease for a quarter of a minute, then it would become perceptible, though very low, then by degrees it became heaving and quick, and then it would gradually cease again. This revolution in the state of his breathing occupied about a minute, during which there were about 30 acts of respiration." This respiratory pattern occurs when the medullary respiratory center loses its usual fine sensitivity to fluctuations in carbon dioxide tension or to afferent stimuli. It is associated with brain tumor, cardiac disease, chronic nephritis, meningitis, pneumonia, or diseases that are accompanied by profound intoxication. Though a sign of grave prognostic import, it does not always signify a fatal termination.

BIOT'S RESPIRATION. Another striking variation, most commonly seen in meningitis, was first accurately studied by Biot (Fig. 8–10). He described it as follows: "This irregularity of the respiratory movements is not periodic, sometimes slow, sometimes rapid, sometimes superficial, sometimes deep, but without any constant relation of succession between the two types, with pauses following irregular intervals, preceded and often followed by a sigh more or less prolonged." This respiratory ir-

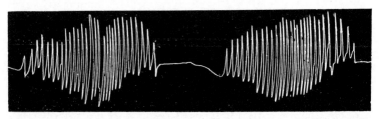

Figure 8–9. *Cheyne-Stokes respiration. (Conner, L. A., and Stillman, R. G.: A pneumographic study of respiratory irregularities in meningitis. Arch. Intern. Med., 9:203, 1912.)*

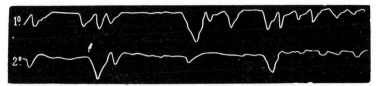

Figure 8-10. *Biot's respiration. (Biot, M. C.: Contribution à l'étude de phénomène respiratoire de Cheyne-Stokes. Lyon Méd., 23:517; 561, 1876.)*

regularity is reminiscent of the total cardiac irregularity of atrial fibrillation.

ASYMMETRIC CHEST EXPANSION. Normally, both sides of the thorax expand equally and at the same time. Note carefully any lag or incomplete expansion of one side. A lag may point to pleural effusion (which may also result in a bulging of the intercostal spaces), unilateral pleural thickening, foreign body, tumor in the airway, or changes in the neuromuscular apparatus. Patients who have acute pleural inflammation that stems from pneumonia, pleuritis, or infarction of lung may splint one side of the thorax to decrease the pain. The patient with acute pleurisy may lie on the affected side to limit the pain of the respiratory movement.

BRONCHIAL OBSTRUCTION. When a bronchus is obstructed, atelectasis, or collapse of the lung tissue, occurs behind the site of obstruction. If a sufficient volume of lung tissue has collapsed, the trachea and the apex beat of the heart shift to the affected side. Respiratory movements diminish and lag behind the normal side. In addition, the intercostal spaces are usually narrowed.

OTHER OBSERVATIONS. At times diaphragmatic activity with respiration is visible.

Under certain circumstances, empyema, or a collection of pus in the chest cavity, may be detected by inspection of the chest. Large accumulations of pus that have followed certain infections may rupture into a bronchus and be drained as sputum. Such accumulations may also perforate the chest wall, leaving a sinus tract that drains pus (Fig. 8-11).

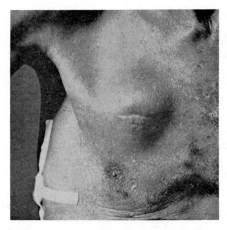

Figure 8–11. *Empyema necessitatis. Bandage shows site of attempted thoracentesis.*

Palpation

Palpation of the thorax is a useful adjunct to inspection. Any difference between the excursions of the two sides of the chest that is apparent on inspection is more evident when the hands are placed upon the chest and the difference in movement is both seen and felt. To do this, stand behind the patient and place the thumb of each hand just to the side of the spinal processes in the midthoracic region. At the same time extend the tips of the fingers to the midaxillary line on both sides (Fig. 8–12). As the patient inhales deeply, evaluate the degree and symmetry of chest expansion.

In patients with advanced pulmonary emphysema, the lung is overdistended with air, and the thorax assumes a position approaching full inspiration. Thus there may be very little difference in circumference between the full inspiratory and the full expiratory positions.

Palpate each rib and all portions of the chest wall with firm pressure. At the same time question the patient about pain and watch for signs of discomfort. Musculoskeletal changes and rib pain are often misinterpreted by both patient and physician as originating from within the thorax. With acute pleural inflammation, such as pleurisy or lung infarction, deep palpation of the rib interspaces will elicit pain which does not occur when similar pressure is applied to the ribs adjoining the interspace.

Note the position of the trachea by placing the index finger firmly into the suprasternal notch and locating the tracheal rings in relation to the sternum. A shift of the trachea to either side is a sensitive indicator of shift in position of mediastinal structures which may be produced by tumor, pleural effusion, or pneu-

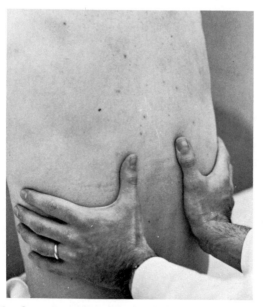

Figure 8-12. *Correct position of the hands for testing posterior expansion of the lungs.*

mothorax. When there is *pneumothorax* (air in the chest cavity) due to rupture of a subpleural lung bleb, a lung tear following trauma, or perforation of the chest wall, intrathoracic pressure may build up and produce *tension pneumothorax*, a medical emergency. This causes a shift of the mediastinum toward the opposite side. Pleural effusion and empyema may also push mediastinal structures to the opposite side (Fig. 8–13). When atelectasis, or collapse of lung tissue, has been caused by a mucous plug, tumor, or foreign body obstructing the bronchus, the mediastinal structures shift toward the affected side. Locate the apex beat of the heart and compare its position with the position of the trachea as further evidence of any mediastinal displacement.

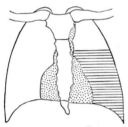

LEFT PLEURAL EFFUSION
HEART PUSHED TO RIGHT

Figure 8-13. *Effect of pleural effusion on cardiac dullness.*

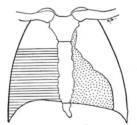

RIGHT PLEURAL EFFUSION
HEART PUSHED TO LEFT

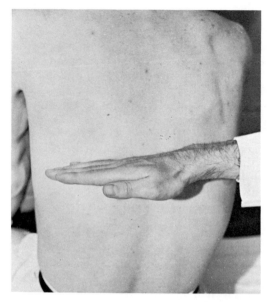

Figure 8-14. *Palpation for tactile fremitus using the ulnar surface of the hand.*

Tactile fremitus. The evaluation of tactile fremitus is an important palpatory procedure in examination of the chest. To elicit fremitus, place both hands upon the chest symmetrically, one on either side, and ask the patient to repeat the words "one, two, three" or "ninety-nine" in a deep, full voice. Move your hands to various parts of the chest, keeping them symmetrically placed, and compare the vibrations produced in the chest wall by the sound. Changes in fremitus are best sensed by the edge of the hand (Fig. 8-14).

Fremitus occurs when sound vibrations that originate in the larynx pass down the bronchi and cause the lungs as well as the chest wall to vibrate. The spoken tones, however, must have the same fundamental frequency as the lungs and the chest wall.

This phenomenon is similar to that which occurs when a certain note struck on a piano causes the vibration of another object nearby. The object has the same fundamental frequency as the note. Fundamental frequency of the female voice is often higher than that of the lungs; therefore, fremitus may be markedly diminished or even absent in women. In children, although the voice is high in pitch, it corresponds to the fundamental frequency of the small lungs; thus fremitus can usually be elicited in children. Normally, the intensity of the vibration varies in different parts of the chest, but fremitus can usually be felt more clearly on the right. The intensity of fremitus vibrations will change with level of inflation of the lung.

Fremitus increases when the lung consolidates as in pneumonia. It is much stronger over the consolidated area than over other parts of the chest.

Fremitus is decreased or may disappear when a pathological condition interferes with the transmission of sound waves from the lungs to the surface of the chest. Two conditions that commonly diminish tactile fremitus are effusion of fluid into the pleural space between the lungs and the chest wall or thickening of the pleura. Figure 8–15 is a trace recording that illustrates normal fremitus and diminished fremitus on the side of a

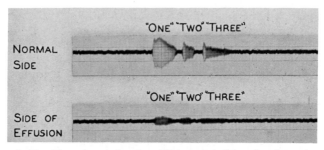

Figure 8–15. Phonogram showing differences in intensity of vocal sounds on the normal side of the chest compared with the side of pleural effusion in the same person.

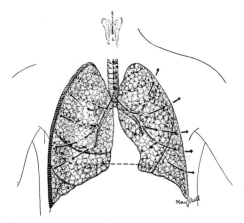

Figure 8–16. *The voice sounds producing fremitus pass readily through the chest wall on the normal left side, whereas on the right, transmission is interfered with by the thickened pleura.*

pleural effusion. Figure 8–16 indicates the findings that may be expected when sound vibrations are unable to penetrate through a thickened pleura.

An infiltrating tumor mass lying between lung and chest wall may also diminish or abolish fremitus. Fremitus is absent or markedly diminished on the affected side when there is atelectasis of an entire lung as a result of bronchial obstruction or when unilateral pneumothorax results in the collapse of a lung.

Percussion of the Chest

Percussion, best described by Auenbrugger (see Chapter 1), is the technique of striking the chest wall and then perceiving the character of the vibrations that are heard by the ear and felt by the fingers. The tactile sensation was first stressed by Piorry. It is commonly described as "the sense of resistance" felt by the fingers during percussion. Over areas of dullness, sound waves are of shorter length and greater frequency than over resonant areas, a difference readily perceived by the sense of touch. The experienced examiner usually depends equally upon the tactile sensation and upon the sound produced by percussion. The sense of resistance is greater in areas that are dull and greatest in areas that are "flat."

Direct percussion is that in which the chest wall is tapped lightly with the tip of the middle finger. In *mediate percussion* the distal parts of the middle and index fingers of one hand are pressed firmly against the chest wall; then the middle finger of the other hand is used to strike sharply the fingers on the chest wall. Percussion causes the air-filled thorax and its contents to vibrate. Fluids and tissues that do not contain air, however, are not set in vibration by the ordinary percussion stroke. These, then, act as damping bodies that alter the percussion note.

The character of the percussion note is determined by three factors: the ability of the chest wall to vibrate, the vibratory response of the lung, and the damping effect of solid organs or pathological masses. The limitations of the percussion method must be clearly understood in order to avoid the pitfalls of overrefined techniques; otherwise you may percuss your own ideas into the chest. Bear in mind that lesions that are more than 5 cm. away from the chest wall or are smaller than 2 or 3 cm. in diameter will not alter the percussion note. Free fluid in the pleural cavity may not be detected by percussion unless the volume exceeds 200 to 250 ml.; however, minimal pleural effusion produces alterations of percussion and fremitus long before it becomes large enough to be seen in a chest x-ray film.

Normal percussion sounds

RESONANT.   Percussion over the normal lung produces a resonant tone that is quite characteristic. This tone is loud in

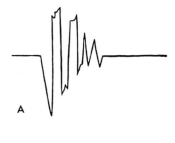

Figure 8–17. A, Resonance (lung); B, flat note (liver).

comparison with that obtained over a pleural exudate, higher in pitch than that of emphysema, and longer in duration than that of a pleural exudate. The tracing in Figure 8–17 shows that it is not a pure tone but contains numerous overtones that determine its quality and timbre. It should be emphasized that the term "resonant" is a relative term, since there is no absolute standard of resonance. What is normal lung resonance in one person may be abnormal in another. The person with a thick, muscular chest or a large amount of subcutaneous fat will show less resonance than one who has a thin chest wall with poorly developed muscles. Variations in resonance are noted in different parts of the chest of the same person.

DULL. A dull percussion note occurs when resonance is impaired. The degree of impairment varies and when complete the note is said to be "flat." A dull note is sometimes called a "soft" note, which emphasizes that it is not as loud as a resonant tone. The dull note is higher in pitch than a resonant note and is shorter in duration.

TYMPANITIC. A tympanitic percussion note may be differentiated from resonant and dull notes by its more distinguishable pitch and its purer tone. Its vibrations are simpler, are

more regular, and have a musical quality. In contrast to a resonant note, there is an almost complete absence of overtones, and
the pitch is usually higher. A tympanitic note is normally obtained on percussion of the stomach and intestines.

Percussion of the normal chest. Whenever possible, percussion of the chest should be carried out while the patient is sitting
or standing. Percuss downward from the apices, at first over the
front and then over the back of the chest. Always compare symmetrical points on the chest, percussing first a point on one side
and then the corresponding point on the other side. Strike with
equal force on the two sides of the chest and compare the degree
of resonance. A heavy stroke on the diseased side of the chest
may set enough normal tissue vibrating to mask the diseased
area and may actually produce more resonance than that obtained with a light stroke over the normal side. Light percussion
is usually better than heavy. Auenbrugger's description is still
pertinent: "The tone is clearer in thin persons, more indistinct
in fleshy individuals; indeed in obese individuals the sound is almost suppressed because of the mass of fat. It is especially the
anterior portion of the thorax which is most resonant; indeed
from the clavicle to the fourth true rib. For there the breasts and
the pectoral muscles increase the mass and a more indistinct
sound results."

The upper borders of the lungs, the pulmonary apices, extend anteriorly 3 to 4 cm. above the upper margins of the
clavicles and extend posteriorly to the level of the seventh cervical vertebra (see Fig. 8–2). The percussion note is normally
resonant up to these limits. The percussion note of each apex is
somewhat higher pitched than that obtained from lower parts of
the lungs.

As you percuss down the right anterior side of the chest, observe that the note is quite resonant until the fourth costal interspace is reached, where it is altered by the mass of the liver
underneath. At the sixth costal interspace the note becomes flat,
since the right lung no longer overlies the liver. This "liver
flatness" ordinarily extends to the costal margin. Verify that the
percussion note of the right lower border changes with respira-

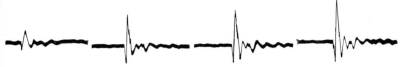

Figure 8–18. *Phonogram at base of right lung during inspiration. (Courtesy of Friedrich Müller.)*

tion. During inspiration the note at the border becomes louder and longer (i.e., more resonant) as the lung descends over the surface of the liver (Fig. 8–18).

As you percuss downward on the left side of the chest, observe that the percussion note is altered by the mass of the heart. First the resonance diminishes over the portion of the heart covered by the lung; then the diminished resonance gradually

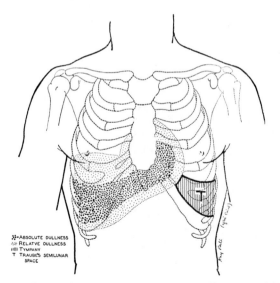

Figure 8–19. *Percussion outlines of normal chest. The areas of dullness are due to the heart and liver.*

becomes flat over the part of the heart not covered by lung. These changes are shown in Figure 8–19.

The lower border of the lung cannot be located accurately by percussion, since there is a gradual transition from the soft, resonant note over the lung to the loud, tympanitic note over the stomach.

The posterior aspect of the chest is less resonant than the anterior because the muscular development is greater and the note is more resonant in the interscapular area than over the scapulae themselves. It is more resonant at the midaxillary line on either side than at the midscapular line.

The mobility of the diaphragm on either side may be determined by percussion of the back. Instruct the patient to take a deep breath, and note the lower limit of lung resonance. Next, have him make a forced expiration, and determine the new limit of lung resonance. Normally, the difference between the level of lung resonance on forced inspiration and the level on forced expiration is from 4 to 6 cm. and is equal on the two sides (Fig. 8–20). If the excursion of the lung on one side is hindered or

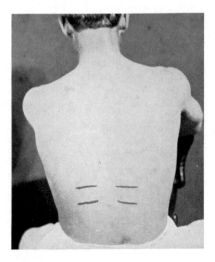

Figure 8–20. *Percussion limits of normal lung expansion at base.*

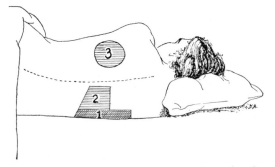

Figure 8–21. *Zones of dullness produced by position of patient: 1, zone of dullness due to deadening effect of mattress; 2, zone of dullness due to compression of chest by weight of body; 3, zone of dullness due to crowding of ribs. (Howard, T.: Percussion note of the back in the lateral position. J.A.M.A., 76:1229, 1921.)*

prevented by pleural adhesions or by effusion, the change in the level of resonance between deep inspiration and deep expiration is diminished or abolished, whereas on the normal side the customary difference remains. Paralysis of the phrenic nerve, most often a sign of mediastinal disease, causes similar changes. The diaphragm also fails to descend normally in pulmonary emphysema, in which the diaphragm is depressed and fixed on both sides.

When it is impossible to examine the patient upright, percussion must be carried out with the patient lying in bed. Errors may be made unless you remember that the position of the patient can influence the percussion note. This is especially true when the patient is lying on his side with his head propped up on a pillow. In this position the ribs are crowded together on the upper side, and this results in an impairment of the percussion note. There is also an area of impaired resonance on the side next to the bed (Fig. 8–21).

The areas of normal dullness vary greatly in different patients and also shift considerably when a patient who has been lying on one side turns to the other. The advice of Norris should be followed: "No examination of the lungs, however carefully performed, should be considered entirely satisfactory or final, if made in the recumbent position." Gross changes, such as the complete consolidation of a lobe in pneumonia, can usually be demonstrated in the recumbent position, but even then it is safer to turn the patient from side to side during the examination.

Abnormal findings on percussion. The areas of dullness produced by the heart and liver are the only normal exceptions to an otherwise dominant resonance. The following variations are abnormal:

HYPERRESONANCE. At times, part or all of an entire side of the chest may give a hyperresonant, or almost tympanitic, note. Hyperresonance occurs when the amount of air in the lung or chest cavity is greatly increased, as it is in pulmonary emphysema or pneumothorax. When these conditions occur, the areas of normal dullness over the heart may disappear completely. When one entire lung is consolidated, the other lung, now carrying on all the respiratory function, may show hyperresonance. In pneumothorax the hyperresonant percussion note over the affected side is due to undamped vibration of the chest wall. In pulmonary emphysema the percussion note may sometimes be tympanitic, particularly when the chest wall is thin and has poorly developed muscles.

DULLNESS AND FLATNESS. Dullness, or impaired resonance, results from any condition that interferes with the production of normally resonant vibrations within the lung or that interferes with the transmission of these vibrations to the outside. Consolidation of the lung parenchyma, therefore, results in a dull percussion sound. The most common causes of consolidation are lobar pneumonia and neoplasm, but any disease which excludes air from the alveoli of the lung may give rise to a similar finding. When either a bronchial tumor or a mucous plug results in atelectasis of a significant portion of a lung, resonance may be impaired.

Any pathological process that interferes with the transmission of the percussion stroke from the chest wall to the underlying lung parenchyma also causes dullness. The most common

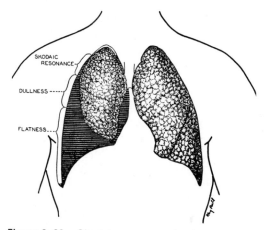

Figure 8–22. *Skodaic resonance in pleural effusion.*

examples are pleural fibrosis, pleural effusion, and empyema. When pleural effusion is extensive and displaces a major part of a lung, the percussion note is flat, and the resonance of the area immediately above the level of flatness may also be impaired. Still farther above the area of dullness, the chest may be resonant or even tympanitic on percussion. This phenomenon is called "skodaic resonance" after Josef Skoda, who noted that "when the lower portion of the lung is entirely compressed by any pleuritic effusion, and its upper portion reduced in volume, the percussion sound at the upper part of the thorax is distinctly tympanitic" (Fig. 8–22). In lobar pneumonia, skodaic resonance may be elicited over normal lung tissue that is just above an area of consolidation.

Resonance may be impaired on one side of the chest in patients with chest deformities such as scoliosis. When a patient has a marked curvature of the spine with convexity to one side, the ribs on the opposite side are pressed closely together. The percussion note over the compressed side is commonly higher in pitch and is impaired.

SHIFTING DULLNESS. Dullness that shifts when the patient changes position is considered by many to be the crucial test for free fluid within the pleural cavity. To test for free fluid, determine the level of dullness in the midclavicular line, first with the patient lying down and then after he has been sitting up for a few minutes. The time lapse allows free fluid to shift to the dependent parts of the chest. Shifting dullness, when present, is a reliable sign of pleural effusion.

Correct evaluation of pleural effusion is vital to accurate diagnosis. Pleural effusion may accompany heart failure, liver disease, or renal disease, as well as when disease affects the lungs and pleurae. If effusions caused by heart failure and cirrhosis are unilateral, they are more likely to occur on the right side than on the left. Pleural effusion may be the only finding in such diseases of the pleura as pleural tuberculosis, carcinomatous infiltration, and mesothelioma. It may also be an indication that pneumonia has become complicated by empyema. In order to accurately explain the cause of a pleural effusion, thoracentesis with bacteriological, cytological, and chemical analyses of the fluid may be necessary. In other instances pleural biopsy may be indicated. The usual, rapid response of pleural infections to appropriate antibiotic management makes a correct, early diagnosis of utmost importance.

Auscultation

Two methods are available for listening to the sounds produced by the lungs. *Immediate auscultation* consists of placing the ear directly against the chest wall, whereas in *mediate auscultation* the examiner utilizes a stethoscope. The mediate method is universally employed, but you should become familiar with the immediate method as well. The occasion may arise when, through unforeseen circumstances, you do not have a stethoscope with you. Moreover, the stethoscope may frighten a child who would not object to the examiner placing his ear against the chest. Again, just as you always have your fingers for percussion, so you always have your ears for auscultation.

Auscultatory sounds. Sounds are produced by vibration and are classified as either tones or noises. Sounds produced by oscillations of uniform frequency are called "tones." The pitch of the tone depends upon the frequency of vibration. The simplest example of a tone is the sound produced by a tuning fork vibrating at a regular rate. A noise, in contrast, has no regular rhythmical vibrations, but consists of a jumble of sound waves of different frequencies. A noise does not have a single, true pitch.

Tones have a musical quality and three principal characteristics:

1. The *intensity* or loudness of a tone depends upon the amplitude of its vibrations.

2. The *pitch* or tonality depends on the frequency of vibration—the higher the frequency, the higher the pitch.

3. The *quality* or timbre of a tone is a characteristic that eludes exact definition. No one can precisely describe the difference in quality of the same note when sounded by a tuning fork or a violin. Oscillographic studies show that a violin note has not only a fundamental tone but also numerous overtones that produce its characteristic timbre (Fig. 8–23).

The ease with which these vibrations are transmitted depends upon the elasticity, mass, and density of the transmitting media. Bone transmits sound better than soft tissue, since the vibrations are carried better through a uniform medium than through one of varying density. Sounds may be amplified when they are conducted, or transmitted, by a structure that has the same natural frequency of vibration as the sound it is transmitting. Ordinarily, the alveoli that surround the bronchial structures have a filtering effect, selectively transmitting lower frequency sounds and damping high frequency sounds in their passage to the chest wall. This explains the observation that when the alveoli become filled with fluid or exudate, higher frequency sounds which originate in the larger conducting

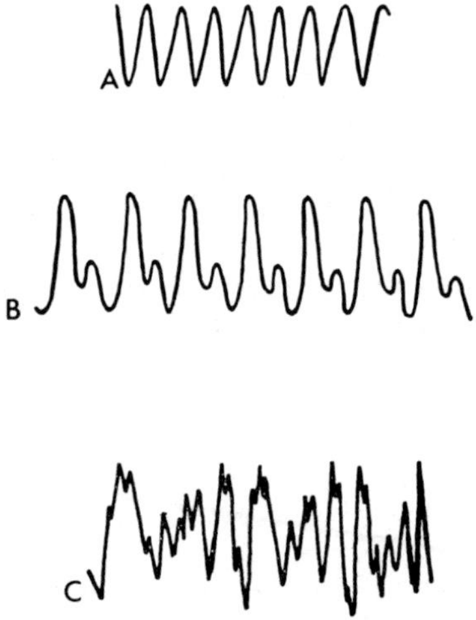

Figure 8-23. Recordings of vibration waves from different sources: A, tuning fork; B, violin (note fundamental wave with faint overtone); C, human voice. (Recorded with cathode-ray apparatus.)

airways are able to pass through lung to the chest wall. Ordinarily such sounds are only heard immediately over the trachea or the mainstem bronchi. A thickened pleura or pleural effusion reduces the transmission of all sounds because the vibrations are partially reflected at air-fluid or dense tissue interfaces.

Stethoscopes. The early monaural stethoscope devised by Laennec is now of historical interest only. The binaural stethoscope of today is made in a variety of models, but two fundamental design principles predominate. The Ford type (Fig. 8–24A) has a bell-shaped chest piece. The Bowles type (Fig. 8–24B) has a shallow bell chest piece covered by a diaphragm. A combination form is shown in Figure 8–24C. In recent years a number of light-weight, combination stethoscopes have become available (Fig. 8–25).

Unfortunately most stethoscopes are poor acoustical instruments. None transmit frequencies above 3000 cycles per second (c.p.s.) and many begin to decrease transmission at frequencies above 1000 c.p.s. All have amplification peaks. While certain

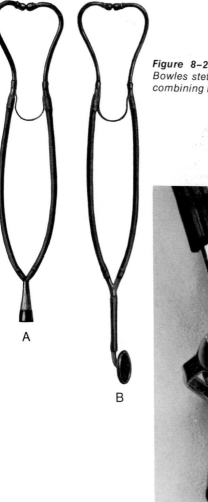

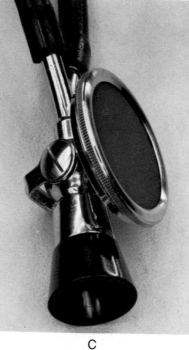

Figure 8-24. A, *Ford stethoscope;* B, *Bowles stethoscope; and* C, *stethoscope combining Ford and Bowles chest pieces.*

A

B

C

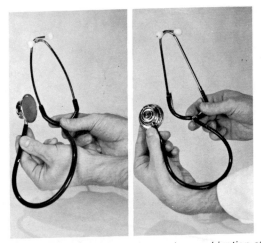

Figure 8–25. *Two views of a currently popular combination stethoscope.*

models with a diaphragm "seem" to transmit higher frequency sounds, they do so by selective filtering out of lower frequency components of the sound. At higher frequency ranges the level of sound transmission may vary as much as 50 decibels between various brands or models. To date there is no evidence that new design has produced an acoustically superior instrument although it has provided convenience. Choice becomes an individual matter, but the physician should be aware of the limitations of his tool.

Fortunately the frequency requirements for examination of sounds from the lungs and chest wall are less rigorous than those originating within the cardiovascular system. The sounds of respiration fall within the range of 80 to 800 c.p.s. and most of the sound transmitted to the ear is less than 500 c.p.s. Most instruments will transmit this range of frequencies with reasonable fidelity.

With any type of instrument, care must be taken to fit the chest piece of the stethoscope firmly against the chest wall in order to avoid factitial noise. The tubing employed for the stethoscope should be thick-walled, have a bore diameter equal to that of the chest and ear pieces, and be as short as is conveniently possible. A ³/₁₆ inch bore and a length of 6 to 18 inches is satisfactory. The length of the tubing may be quite critical in certain types of stethoscopes.

The most important point in the use of a stethoscope is to be familiar with the instrument you use. Familiarity with one type of stethoscope invariably gives rise to a certain partisanship. After deciding upon the model you prefer, take care to adjust the ear pieces to fit your ears.

Frequent errors in auscultation of the chest. It is often said that the beginner hears too much rather than too little; he has not yet learned to disregard sounds that are of no diagnostic importance and to concentrate upon the sounds that are significant. The ability to distinguish between important and unimportant sounds is acquired only by practice. Unfortunately, no short cuts exist.

The ideal conditions for auscultation are found in a soundproof room. Since ideal conditions are rarely present, you must learn to concentrate your attention upon what you hear through the ear pieces of the stethoscope and to be oblivious to other sounds within the room. Make sure that the sounds you hear are coming through the tubes of the stethoscope. Next, determine that the sounds come from the interior of the chest, i.e., the lungs and pleurae, and not from the skin or muscles. The following are the most common sources of error:

1. Breathing heavily on the tubing of the stethoscope produces a soft roaring sound. This error can be prevented by changing the position of the tubing.

2. The bell must be firmly and flatly applied to the chest wall. If one side is slightly elevated, a soft, muffled roaring, like that heard when a sea shell is applied to the ear, may result. A similar sound may be audible if the ear pieces of the stethoscope do not fit properly or if the stethoscope is used with the ear pieces reversed. A more common error results when the bell of the stethoscope is allowed to rub upon the skin of the chest. This

may produce sounds that simulate a pleural or pericardial friction rub. Familiarize yourself with these sounds by rubbing the bell of the stethoscope over the skin.

3. Sounds produced by friction of the stethoscope on hairs. A single hair under the bell of the stethoscope may produce crackling sounds almost indistinguishable from râles. The frequency and intensity of these sounds may be increased by rubbing the chest piece over the hairs. In patients with extremely hairy chests, it is difficult to avoid such extraneous sounds. A time-honored method of avoiding sounds produced by hairs is to wet them with water, soap, or petrolatum and to press them flat against the skin. At times it may be advisable to shave the skin in certain areas.

4. Sounds produced by muscles, tendons, and joints may lead to confusion and error. Patients who are chilled or nervous or who tense their muscles may produce in these muscles a characteristic set of soft sounds. In patients who are chilled, these sounds are of minimal intensity, are of great frequency, and disappear when the patient becomes warmer. They are frequently present when the patient ceases breathing for a few moments. The deeper, louder muscle sounds, which are heard particularly over the pectoral and trapezius muscles, are more intense when the patient breathes deeply, and have a loud, creaking, leathery quality. Location of such sounds over the pectoral or trapezius muscles stamps them as muscular in origin. Occasionally, they may be heard over all parts of the chest.

Muscle sounds may be confused with râles, but generally they are crumpled, muffled, and indistinct. Muscle sounds are not affected by coughing, which commonly changes the character and intensity of râles, and are usually more evanescent than true râles. In doubtful cases it may be necessary to withhold judgment until a second or third examination is made. Sounds that originate in the joints and fasciae usually disappear when the patient relaxes completely.

Normal breath sounds

VESICULAR BREATH SOUNDS. The sounds heard over normally functioning lung tissue are called *vesicular breath sounds*.

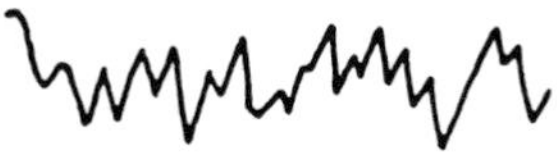

Figure 8–26. Tracing of vesicular breath sounds. (Recorded with cathode-ray apparatus.)

Their pitch is relatively low, with dominant frequencies in the range of 200 to 300 c.p.s. (Fig. 8–26) and almost none above 500 c.p.s.

The sounds are thought to be produced by the repetitive rushes of air into and out of alveoli being ventilated. The vesicular sound and its intensity closely follow the rushes of air into various alveolar areas of the lung as demonstrated by radioactive scanning with tagged gases, such as xenon, incorporated into the respiratory gas mixture. The sounds are loudest during inspiration and vary in intensity from the upper to lower portions of the lung during various phases of the respiratory cycle. The alveoli in lower portions of the lung are closed during certain low expansion phases of the respiratory cycle. Little or no sound is heard during exhalation. Vesicular breath sounds are normally heard over the greater part of the thorax but are modified where the trachea or large bronchi lie close to the chest wall. They increase in intensity as ventilation of the lung tissue increases; they disappear when the lung tissue is no longer ventilated, as in atelectasis (Fig. 8–27). Vesicular breath sounds are diminished and distant in pulmonary emphysema, in which there is an abnormally large amount of air that damps the sound. They are diminished or absent when pleural thickening or pleural effusion interferes with the passage of sound to the surface of the chest (Figs. 8–28 and 8–29).

BRONCHIAL, OR TUBULAR, BREATHING. This type of breathing was first described by Laennec as "the sound which inspiration and expiration make audible in the larynx, the trachea and the large bronchial trunks situated at the hilus of the lungs. This sound, heard on applying the stethoscope over the larynx or the cervical portion of the trachea, has a character quite distinctive. The respiratory murmur, especially during inspiration, lacks the soft crepitation which accompanies the aeration of the air cells; it

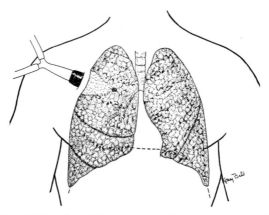

Figure 8–27. *Obstruction of bronchus abolishes vesicular breathing over area of atelectasis.*

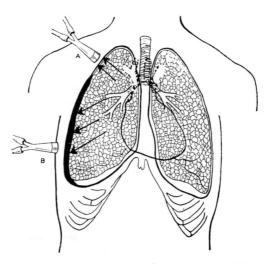

Figure 8–28. *Effect of thickened pleura on transmission of breath sounds. Vesicular breathing heard at* A, *but not at* B.

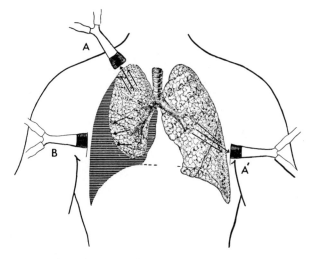

Figure 8–29. *Effect of pleural effusion in transmission of breath sounds. Normal sounds heard at A and A', but not at B.*

is more dry in a certain measure, and one perceives distinctly that the air passes into an empty and rather wide space."

Bronchial and tracheal breath sounds are produced by a turbulence of air passing over the walls of the bronchi and trachea respectively. Detailed studies have shown that tracheal breathing and bronchial breathing are similar but not identical. In bronchial breathing, expiration is louder, longer, and of higher pitch than inspiration, in contrast to vesicular breathing in which inspiration is louder. The higher frequency of bronchial breath sounds as compared with vesicular sounds is demonstrated in the tracing of Figure 8–30.

It must be emphasized that vesicular breathing alone is heard over most of the area of the lungs. Bronchial breathing is normally heard only over the trachea, primary bronchi, a limited area at the right apex, and the right interscapular area. When bronchial sounds are heard elsewhere, they are patholog-

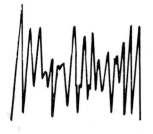

Figure 8–30. Bronchial breath sounds. (Recorded with cathode-ray apparatus.)

ical. The most common cause of abnormal bronchial breathing is consolidation of the lung (Fig. 8–31). When consolidation occurs, the damping action of air-containing alveoli is diminished, allowing the underlying, higher frequency bronchial sounds to be heard without alteration. Tuberculosis and lobar pneumonia are classic examples of diseases in which bronchial breath sounds appear. If a sufficiently large area of pulmonary infarction occurs after pulmonary embolization, bronchial breathing may be heard over the affected area. In pleurisy with

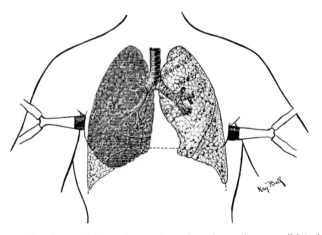

Figure 8–31. Bronchial breath sounds are heard over the consolidated right lung. Normal breath sounds are heard over the left lung.

effusion, distant bronchial breathing may be heard above the fluid level because of alveolar compression.

The absence of breath sounds, like abnormal transmission, indicates the presence of a pathological condition. A tumor or mucous plug that is obstructing a bronchus may result in the disappearance of normal vesicular breath sounds. In pneumothorax or large pleural effusion, breath sounds disappear on the affected side. When pulmonary emphysema interposes a large amount of air between the source of the sound and the chest wall, the breath sounds become distant.

Occasionally a crunching or clicking sound (xiphisternal crunch) is heard in a limited area over the xiphoid process at the end of the sternum. It may appear or disappear, depending upon the phase of respiration. Its occurrence does not indicate the presence of a pathological condition, and it should not be confused with other sounds related to the heart, pericardium, or lung.

Abnormal sounds over the lungs

Râle is the name commonly given to the noisy murmur caused, in those who are dying, by the air forcing its way with difficulty through the sputum which the lungs are no longer able to expel. For the lack of a more generic term, I take the word in a wider sense and designate as râles, all noises produced during respiration by the passage of air through all such liquids, as may happen to be present in the bronchi or lung tissue. These noises also accompany coughing when it is present; but it is always more convenient to investigate them by means of respiration (Laennec).

Generically the French word râle means noise. Since the time of Laennec there have been a number of explanations offered for the various pathological sounds heard over lung areas and an even greater variety of classifications. Many descriptive terms have been introduced that characterize râles as they appear to the imaginative listener. Only recently has better understanding of sound phenomena and physiological events of the respiratory cycle allowed more rational, though less euphonious, classification.

Râles are never detected over healthy lung tissue. They always indicate the presence of a pathological process in the lungs or pleurae. The sounds that Laennec lumped together under the term "râle" are classified today as (1) râles, (2) rhonchi, or (3) wheezes.

RÂLE. The term "râle" is used to describe crackling sounds that originate in the smaller bronchi or alveoli. They are due to "the explosive opening of airways in the territories of the lung deflated to residual volume." Slow motion analysis of the sound patterns has demonstrated that these crackling sounds recur in constant, repetitive cycles from one respiratory cycle to the next. They often change with position because pressure gradients within the lung also change to alter the dynamics of the small airways and alveoli. Over the years the term râle has been modified by many adjectives—dry, moist, high-pitched, sonorous, sibilant, crepitant, atelectatic—to name just a few. Such terms may have meaning to the observer, but they are seldom effective symbols for communicating the observation to others or for recording the results of the patient's physical examination. Instead it is more important to record whether the râle has a high, medium, or low pitch. Loudness should be estimated. Timing of the sound in relation to the respiratory cycle is important because some râles occur only during inspiration. The distribution of the râles in the chest and their persistence during the examination are important characteristics.

The râles of left heart failure, which commonly occur in more dependent parts of the lung, may disappear after coughing and then reappear, and may be accentuated by mild exercise. Râles associated with inflammatory exudates may be missed if the involved portion of the lung is not being ventilated during quiet respiration. They can be enhanced by asking the patient to inspire deeply several times or by instructing him to cough gently at the end of expiration. In the latter case, the râles appear with the following inspiration. Râles may be irregularly dispersed throughout the lung in bronchitis or bronchopneumonia, or may be well localized in an area of lobar or segmental pneumonia. Persistent râles occur in patients with bronchiectasis even at times when the patient is not acutely ill. They may be the only physical findings in patients with localized tuberculosis.

RHONCHUS. The term "rhonchus" is usually applied to sounds that come from the larger air passages. It has been described as a snoring or rattling sound, and it often has its onset early in the respiratory cycle. It may be present on inspiration, expiration, or both. Coughing may clear the mucus, fluid, or exudate that caused the rhonchus; thus, when a rhonchus is noted during an examination, ask the patient to cough and note whether the sound disappears. Rhonchi often occur in patients whose cough reflex is impaired. The occurrence of rhonchi may be the only clue to the presence of a bronchial tumor or foreign body that is partially obstructing an air channel.

WHEEZE. A "wheeze" is a high-pitched, piping or whistling sound resulting from partial airway obstruction. It has a musical quality, occurring with either inspiration or expiration. Wheezes are usually louder and more persistent during expiration, when the air passages are functionally narrowed. The pitch of a wheeze is determined largely by the linear velocity of the air jet which has broken into turbulent flow pattern in the airways and is not related to the size of the airway in which it is produced. In patients who have diseases that obstruct the airways, such as asthma or pulmonary emphysema, wheezing may be undetected unless the patient is instructed to exhale forcefully—as though he were trying to blow out a candle across the room. During attacks of asthma, the wheezing sounds may be so loud that they can be heard without a stethoscope.

PLEURAL FRICTION RUB. Pleural friction rubs were heard by Hippocrates, who observed that in pneumonia, "the lung is congealed to the ribs and squeaks like a leather strap." Little can be added to this succinct description except to note that a friction rub may be loud or soft, distant or close, and of high or low pitch.

The pleural surfaces are normally smooth and moist, and no sound is produced when the visceral pleura slips over the parietal pleura during respiration. However, when the surface of the visceral pleura is roughened by an inflammatory or neoplastic process, a rubbing sound is produced. The intensity of the sound varies with the type and degree of change. It is rough and harsh when the pleural surface is markedly roughened, and is softer and fainter if the pleura is only slightly or moderately roughened. The movement of the visceral over the parietal pleura is greatest at the lateral and posterior bases of a lung and decreases superiorly with little or no motion at the apex of the lung. For this reason a pleural friction rub is best heard when at the base of a lung and on the lower parts of the axillary lines, while it is not so marked on the upper parts of the lung and is rarely heard over the apex.

Pleural friction rubs vary greatly in intensity, ranging from a loud creaking noise that sounds close to the ear to a soft, almost inaudible rub or click. The presence of fluid in the pleural cavity may modify or abolish a pleural rub. In pulmonary infarction a pleural rub may occur briefly and then disappear as pleural effusion follows.

Friction rubs are heard during both inspiration and expiration. On rare occasions, they are heard during expiration alone. The sounds usually vary in intensity, disappearing for a short while only to reappear with increased intensity. Obviously, they disappear if the patient holds his breath. As a result of the tissue changes that accompany a friction rub, movement often causes severe pain, and the patient splints one side of his chest to avoid discomfort. In acute pleurisy accompanying a viral or bacterial infection, the pain at the onset may produce so much splinting of the chest wall that the sound of a friction rub will be missed unless the patient is forced to breathe deeply. Later the friction rub may disappear when effusion separates the roughened pleural surfaces. Occasionally, muscle sounds are mistaken for a pleural friction rub.

HAMMAN'S SIGN. This is a crunching, crackling sound that occurs synchronously with the heart beat when either interstitial or mediastinal emphysema is present. *Interstitial emphysema* is caused by the escape of air into the connective tissues of the lungs and mediastinum and may occur following surgery or trauma. At other times it results from a ruptured alveolus that allows air to escape. This occurs most commonly in patients who have severe, uncontrolled asthma or cough. The auscultatory crunching is usually heard most clearly when the patient is in a left lateral recumbent position with his breath fully expelled. The intensity of the sound varies with the patient's position. A pneumothorax may accompany interstitial emphysema.

VOCAL RESONANCE. The evaluation of vocal resonance (a term used interchangeably with *vocal fremitus* and often confused with *tactile fremitus*) is an important auscultatory procedure that has survived from classical physical diagnosis.

When a normal person speaks or whispers "one, two, three" or "ninety-nine," the voice sounds are heard through the chest as a soft confused murmur. The sound is loudest over the upper parts of the chest and over the areas in which the trachea and large bronchi are nearest the surface. Its intensity in various parts of the chest is comparable to that of tactile fremitus. It is more marked in thin-chested persons than in fat or muscular individuals and is more marked in those with deep voices; thus it is more apparent in men than in women.

Increased vocal resonance. The voice sounds are loudest over any area of consolidation in the lungs. This phenomenon is known as *bronchophony* and *pectoriloquy*, terms coined by Laennec.

Pectoriloquy is defined as the sound of the spoken word as heard through the chest wall. Laennec was the first to note this phenomenon: "Holding the stethoscope below the middle of the right clavicle, I had the patient speak; his voice seemed to come out directly from his chest and pass completely through the central canal of the stethoscope. This transmission of the voice took place only in a space about an inch square. In no other part of the chest could I find the same thing."

Laennec's differentiation between bronchophony and pectoriloquy is unclear, and much confusion persists regarding these two terms. A practical solution is to use the term bronchophony when the sounds are loud and clear but the words themselves are not distinguishable, and to use pectoriloquy to denote the occasions when the words are clearly understandable.

Vocal resonance may be tested by either speaking or whispering. Most observers find whispering of greater value. A small area of whispered pectoriloquy may be present in a patient with pneumonia before bronchial breathing can be detected and before an x-ray shows an area of consolidation. Both bronchophony and pectoriloquy indicate consolidation of lung tissue. "Bronchophony has clinically the same importance as bronchial breathing, and all that was said concerning the causation of bronchial breathing holds for bronchophony" (Edens). Bronchophony literally means the sound of the voice as heard over a large bronchus.

Egophony is a particular form of bronchophony that was classically described by Laennec, who coined the word from the Greek roots meaning "goat voice."

Egophony resembles pectoriloquy in that it also consists of loud resonance of the voice beneath the stethoscope. It is only rarely, however, that the voice appears to enter the tube of the instrument, and it very seldom passes right along it in the evident manner which characterized perfect pectoriloquy. The voice is higher pitched and sharper than the patient's natural voice and has, so to speak, a silvery tone; it produces the illusion that someone is speaking in the patient's chest. It possesses moreover, one constant characteristic from which it has seemed to me suitable to name the phenomenon; it is quavering and jerky, like the bleating of a goat and, as may be judged from the foregoing description, it is also similar in timbre to the noise made by that animal. This characteristic is subject to only slight variations, which the reader may picture to himself exactly if he calls to mind the effect produced by a chip placed between the teeth and the lips of a person speaking, the sound of the voice when transmitted through a cracked reed, or the stammering nasal tone of a Punch and Judy showman. This last comparison is often strictly accurate, especially in the case of men with a rather deep voice (Laennec).

Egophony is most commonly heard over pleural effusions of moderate size, usually near the inferior angle of the scapula. It is often heard over an area in which skodaic resonance is present or, occasionally, over an area of pulmonary consolidation. You can imitate egophony by counting "one, two, three . . ." and, while continuing the count, suddenly closing both nostrils with the fingers. This change to a marked nasal quality, popularly and falsely called "talking through your nose," closely resembles the change in vocal resonance that is noted when the stethoscope passes over an area in which true egophony is present.

Diminished vocal resonance. This abnormality results from the same pathological conditions that lead to diminished vocal fremitus as appreciated by tactile sense. Among them, occlusion of a bronchus, atelectasis, fluid in the chest, and thickening of the pleura are the most common.

COMMON CLINICAL TERMS

Apnea — The absence of breathing.

Cheyne-Stokes respiration — Cyclic irregularity of respiration in which the rate and depth increase markedly following a period of apnea, and terminating in another.

Clubbing — Enlargement of terminal phalanges, frequently associated with certain pulmonary and cardiac diseases.

Cyanosis — Bluish discoloration of skin and mucous membranes associated with severe arterial oxygen desaturation.

Dyspnea — The sensation of difficult breathing.

Friction rub — A grating sound or sensation, heard or felt arising from rubbing together of inflamed serous surfaces.

Hemoptysis — Expectoration of blood by coughing.

Orthopnea — The inability to breathe comfortably while supine.

Stridor — Difficult respiration characterized by high-pitched crowing sounds during inspiration.

Tachypnea — An increased rate of respiration.

COMMON CLINICAL SYNDROMES

Acute bronchitis — This is an acute infectious process of the bronchi characterized by cough and the production of purulent sputum. Râles or wheezes may be heard on auscultation, but there is no lung consolidation. The occurrence of fever is variable.

Atelectasis — Atelectasis occurs when an area of lung tissue is not ventilated. The gases in the bronchi and alveoli beyond the obstruction are rapidly absorbed, and the lung parenchyma then collapses, resulting in atelectasis. The signs and symptoms that follow depend upon the amount of lung tissue involved and vary from an asymptomatic shadow on an x-ray to acute respiratory distress. When a sufficient amount of lung is involved, there are signs of respiratory distress, and the mediastinal structures shift toward the affected lung because respiratory movements are diminished on that side. Unconsciousness, dehydration, and anesthesia predispose to atelectasis. The percussion note is dull; breath sounds disappear; and there is a loss of fremitus over the affected area.

Bronchiectasis—When a past infection or malformation of the bronchial walls results in dilatation of the bronchial structures, the condition is called *bronchiectasis*. The patient usually has had a history of recurrent episodes of pulmonary sepsis and sputum production, often accompanied by hemoptysis. Persistent râles are commonly heard over the diseased area of the lung.

Bronchopleural fistula—This is an abnormal connection between a bronchus and the pleural cavity. It usually occurs following infection, trauma, or surgery and results in empyema. When the patient is in certain positions, air passing into the pleural space produces the sound of air bubbling under water. Other findings are related to hydropneumothorax or to empyema.

Chronic obstructive lung disease—This is a generic term used to designate those diseases of which bronchial obstruction to airflow is a principal feature. It includes the following diseases:

Asthma—Asthma (now referred to as reversible airway obstructive disease) is acute, episodic, non-effort-related dyspnea which is brought on by narrowing of the airways of the lung. It may be due to inhalation of an extrinsic allergenic agent, or may be due to internal chemical disruptions which cause abnormal response of the smaller airways of the lung. Dyspnea and labored breathing occur. The chest becomes overinflated; exhalation is forced and prolonged. On auscultation, wheezes are heard throughout the lung fields, particularly during expiration.

Chronic bronchitis—The patient with chronic bronchitis should have a history of persistent coughing that cannot be explained by other causes and that occurs for at least three months in two successive years. Sputum production is persistent, and varies from glistening, white, tenacious, mucoid material to frank pus. Râles or wheezes may be heard over the lungs. Other findings depend upon the degree of airway obstruction.

Pulmonary emphysema—By definition "emphysema" refers to the presence of an abnormally large amount of air within the portions of the lung distal to the terminal bronchioles. It is commonly associated with degeneration of the alveolar walls, coalescence of the alveoli into larger air sacs, and the loss of bronchial supporting tissue. Expiration is prolonged in proportion to the degree of airway obstruction. Increased air in the alveoli and wasting of thoracic tissues results in hyperresonance of the chest on percussion; the areas of resonance extend beyond their usual boundaries. Breath sounds are distant. Wheezing may occur during forceful expiration. Bronchitis often accompanies emphysema and may give rise to additional findings.

Infarction of the lung—Pulmonary infarction follows embolization if the obstruction of the vascular bed is sufficient to cause necrosis of lung tissue. Classically, the findings are hemoptysis, fever, pleural pain, and a pleural friction rub that arises from the affected area.

Lung abscess—A lung abscess is a localized area of suppuration and cavity formation within the lung. Findings are varied and may include cough, fever, malaise, sputum production, râles, and pain over the affected lung. When the abscess drains by way of a bronchus, purulent sputum, often streaked with blood, is a principal finding.

Pleural effusion—A collection of fluid in the chest cavity between the parietal and visceral pleurae is called "pleural effusion." It may accompany heart failure, liver disease, or kidney disorders as well as primary disorders of the lungs and pleurae. Physical findings include dullness to percussion over the involved area, a shift of mediastinal structures to the side opposite the effusion, diminished fremitus, and poor transmission of breath sounds to the area of the chest wall that overlies the effusion.

Pleurisy—Acute inflammation of the pleura results in severe pain during respiration, a splinting of respiratory movements, and a friction rub. Later findings depend upon the amount of fluid that has accumulated in the chest cavity. Chronic inflammation and thickening of the pleura result in retraction of the chest wall, decreased respiratory movements, dullness to percussion, and diminished breath sounds. A friction rub may or may not occur.

Pneumonia—Any lung infection that involves the alveoli and causes them to fill with exudate or inflammatory secretions is called "pneumonia." Pneumonias usually involve a specific segment or lobe of the lung. Classically, lobar pneumonia is caused by *Diplococcus pneumoniae*. Pneumonia that does not involve complete anatomic segments of the lung is referred to as "bronchopneumonia." Physical findings vary according to the infectious agent and extent of infection. Cough, purulent sputum, and blood-streaked sputum may occur. If the infection extends to the pleural surface, pain is present during respiration; the patient splints his chest; and a pleural friction rub appears. When a sufficiently large area of lung is infected, bronchial breath sounds appear; râles are heard on inspiration and expiration; and the affected area is dull to percussion. When smaller areas of lung tissue are involved, only fever, malaise, and cough appear. X-ray study is then necessary to demonstrate the exudative changes in the alveoli.

Pneumothorax—An accumulation of air in the pleural space is called "pneumothorax." The patient may complain of shortness of breath or sudden pain in the chest. When there is sufficient air, mediastinal shift may cause displacement of the trachea and heart to the opposite side. Vocal fremitus and breath sounds disappear. The percussion note becomes hyperresonant or tympanitic.

Primary and secondary carcinoma of the lung—The clinical findings in cases of tumor of a lung or bronchus vary considerably. General symptoms include weight loss, fever, malaise. Clubbing of the fingers may be present in some patients; other patients present no symptoms and a few individuals develop bizarre metabolic or endocrine syndromes that mimic other diseases. The pulmonary signs and symptoms depend upon the location of the tumor. If the tumor is in a bronchus, cough, hemoptysis, and wheezing are the predominant findings. If the tumor obstructs the bronchus, atelectasis or persistent pneumonia gives rise to the principal physical findings. When the tumor involves a pleural surface, a friction rub may be heard, or if the lymphatic channels are blocked, a pleural effusion may develop.

Cancers in other organs of the body commonly metastasize to the lungs. Notably, carcinomas of the thyroid, kidney, breast, and gastrointestinal organs often spread to the lungs. The physical findings depend upon the site and upon the extent of involvement. Occasionally, tumors metastasize via lymphatic channels and result in considerable "stiffening" of the lung. When this occurs the patient is dyspneic and breathes rapidly and shallowly, but he may present few other findings to suggest the cause of his distress. An x-ray usually reveals a diffuse increase in markings throughout all lung fields.

Pulmonary edema—In pulmonary edema the lung capillaries are engorged with blood, and fluid accumulates in the alveoli and airways. The history should either reveal exposure to a noxious inhalant or provide clues to the presence of heart disease. When pulmonary edema is severe, the following signs are evident: rapid shallow breathing, cyanosis, copious perspiration, an appearance indicating extreme fear, and the production of frothy sputum, which may be bloody. Rales are heard throughout all lung fields during both inspiration and expiration. When the involved area is not extensive, the signs may be limited to percussion dullness over the lung bases and late inspiratory râles in dependent portions of the lungs.

Pulmonary embolus — When distal venous thrombi dislodge, they may reach the pulmonary capillary bed by embolization, and if infected, they give rise to areas of pneumonia or abscess. If the thrombi are sterile, signs and symptoms will result from alterations in the circulatory dynamics of the lesser circulation; i.e., sweating, tachycardia, cardiac arrhythmias, and tachypnea occur. If sufficiently large segments of the pulmonary circulation are blocked, changes are dramatic and include cyanosis and shock.

Pulmonary fibrosis — Fibrosis of the lungs may follow infections, irradiation injuries, certain systemic diseases such as scleroderma, or long-term inhalation and deposition of certain noxious fumes or particles that result in pneumoconiosis. Early changes may be detected only by functional measurements or x-ray changes. The findings are related to a loss of elasticity of the lungs and an impairment of gas transport across the pulmonary membrane. Thus the pattern of respiration may be shallow and rapid. Inspection of the thorax reveals wide changes in intrapleural pressure during ventilation with thoracic retraction and narrow interspaces. Resonance to percussion becomes impaired and breath sounds are usually diminished.

Pulmonary tuberculosis — The initial tuberculous infection of the lung is called the "primary" infection. This is a localized infection that spreads to regional lymph nodes. In children, lymph node involvement sometimes results in a cough or in atelectasis of a portion of a lung because of bronchial compression. Usually the lesion is self-limited and produces no symptoms. At other times the infection may disseminate to produce miliary tuberculosis. The principal physical findings in miliary tuberculosis may be limited to unexplained fever and weight loss.

Reinfection or progressive tuberculosis, so-called "secondary" disease, may occur in minimal, moderately advanced, or faradvanced states with cavitation of lung tissue occurring. Physical findings vary according to the stage of the disease and the amount of lung tissue involved. There may be no change other than that detected in the x-ray picture.

BIBLIOGRAPHY

Banoszah, E. F., Kory, R. C., and Snider, G. L.: Phonopneumography. Am. Rev. Resp. Dis., *107*:449, 1973.

Bates, D. V., Machlem, P. T., and Christie, R. V.: Respiratory Function in Disease. An introduction to the integrated study of the lung. 2nd ed. Philadelphia, W. B. Saunders Co., 1971.

Brock, R. C.: The Anatomy of the Bronchial Tree. New York, Oxford University Press, 1946.

Campbell, E. J. M., and Howell, J. B. L.: The sensation of breathlessness. Br. Med. Bull., *19*:36, 1963.

Cherniack, R. M., Cherniack, L., and Naimark, A.: Respiration in Health and Disease. 2nd ed. Philadelphia, W. B. Saunders Co., 1972.

Comroe, J. H., Jr., and Botelbo, S.: The unreliability of cyanosis in the recognition of arterial anoxemia. Am. J. Med. Sci., *214*:1, 1947.

Davis, H. L., Fowler, W. S., and Lambert, E. H.: Effect of volume and rate of inflation and deflation on transpulmonary pressure and response of pulmonary stretch receptors. Am. J. Physiol., *187*:558, 1956.

Dayman, H.: Mechanics of airflow in health and in emphysema. J. Clin. Invest., *30*:1175, 1951.

de Reuck, A. V. S., and O'Conner, M. (eds.): Ciba Foundation Symposium on Pulmonary Structure and Function. London, J. & A. Churchill, 1961.

Douglas, C. G., and Haldane, J. S.: The regulation of normal breathing. J. Physiol. (Lond.), *38*:420, 1909.

Ertel, P. Y., Lawrence, M., Brown, R. K., and Stern, A. M.: Stethoscope Acoustics. I. The doctor and his stethoscope. Circulation, *34*:889, 1967.

Fahr, G.: The acoustics of the bronchial breath sounds. Arch. Intern. Med., *39*:287, 1927.

Fenn, W. O.: Mechanics of respiration. Am. J. Med., *10*:77, 1951.

Finley, T. N., Swenson, E. W., and Comroe, J. H., Jr.: The cause of arterial hypoxemia at rest in patients with "alveolar-capillary block syndrome." J. Clin. Invest., *41*:618, 1962.

Fishman, A. P., Turino, G. M., and Bergofsky, E. H.: Editorial: The syndrome of alveolar hypoventilation. Am. J. Med., *23*:333, 1957.

Fletcher, C. M. (ed.): Ciba guest symposium report: Terminology, definitions, and classification of chronic pulmonary emphysema and related conditions. (Symposium, September 1958). Thorax, *14*:286, 1959.

Forgacs, P.: Crackles and wheezes. Lancet, *2*:203, 1967.

Forgacs, P.: Lung sounds. Br. J. Dis. Chest, *63*:1, 1969.

Fry, D. L., and Hyatt, R. E.: Pulmonary mechanics: A unified analysis of the relationship between pressure, volume, and gas flow in the lungs of normal and diseased human subjects. Am. J. Med., *29*:672, 1960.

Hunter, D.: The Diseases of Occupations. 3rd ed. Boston, Little, Brown & Co., 1962.

LeBlanc, P., MacKlem, P. T., and Ross, W. R. D.: Breath sounds and the distribution of pulmonary ventilation. Am. Rev. Resp. Dis., *102*:10, 1970.

Major, R. H.: Classic Descriptions of Disease. 3rd ed. Springfield, Illinois, Charles C Thomas, 1945.

McKusick, V. A., Jenkins, J. T., and Webb, G. N.: The acoustic basis of the chest examination. Studies by means of sound spectrography. Am. Rev. Tuberc., *72*:13, 1955.

Otis, A. B.: The work of breathing. Physiol. Rev., *34*:449, 1954.

Perry, M. A., and Sellors, T. H.: Chest Diseases. London, Butterworth & Co., 1963.

Sieker, H. O., and Hickam, J. B.: Carbon dioxide intoxication: The clinical syndrome, its etiology and management with particular reference to the use of mechanical respirators. Medicine (Baltimore), *35*:389, 1956.

9
THE CARDIOVASCULAR SYSTEM

THE HEART

The heart has always been an organ of extreme interest to man. The venerable Ebers Papyrus, compiled at least 16 centuries before the Christian era, states, "The beginning of the physician's secret: knowledge of the heart's movement and knowledge of the heart."

The modern era of cardiac diagnosis began with Auenbrugger, who pointed out in 1761 the method of determining by percussion the size and position of the heart, and with Laennec, who described in 1819 his invention, the stethoscope, with which he studied the heart sounds. The next advance was the invention of instruments for recording the pulse, such as Mackenzie's polygraph and the remarkable studies he made on cardiac irregularities.

Roentgen's discovery of the x-rays in 1895 made possible the accurate study of cardiac outlines and led to the later development of angiocardiography. The introduction of electrocardiography by Einthoven in 1901 was a revolutionary advance. The latest important development in the diagnosis of heart

358

disease was the introduction of cardiac catheterization in 1929 by Forssmann, who carried out his initial studies on himself. The spectacular triumphs of cardiac surgery in the last few years have been due in large measure to great advances in diagnostic and surgical techniques. The foundation stones of this success were—and remain—a meticulous history and a careful physical examination.

Inspection, Palpation, and Percussion of the Heart

Before beginning examination of the heart, remember that a single physiological event may produce many measurable phenomena. For example, a single cardiac cycle produces a measurable blood pressure, a palpable arterial pulse, a visible venous pulse, a visible and palpable precordial impulse, audible and palpable heart sounds, and, under certain circumstances, heart murmurs. All of these phenomena are manifestations of the same cardiac event and must be considered and assessed appropriately to ascertain the significance of a heart lesion. Figure 9–1 represents the temporal and hemodynamic relationships of the events that occur in a single cardiac cycle. For simplicity, only the left heart events are depicted. Refer to this diagram frequently as you attempt to understand the genesis of precordial movements, heart sounds, and murmurs.

It may be helpful at this point to review the topographical anatomy of the heart. Figure 9–2 is a diagram of the anatomy of the heart as projected against the anterior chest wall. Note that the right ventricle occupies the largest area, that the right atrium occupies a smaller area to the right of the ventricle, and that the left ventricle occupies a relatively thin strip along the left heart border. The aorta underlies the sternum. The main pulmonary artery is located at the second interspace to the left of the sternal border. In cardiac disease these relationships may be profoundly altered.

CARDIAC CYCLE

Systole (A-E)

1. Isometric contraction (B-C)
2. Maximum ejection (C-D)
3. Reduced ejection (D-E)
   Mitral valve open(G), close(B)
   Aortic valve open (C),close(F)

Diastole (E-A)

1. Protodiastole (E-F)
2. Isometric relaxation (F-G)
3. Rapid ventricular filling (G-H)
4. Diastasis (H-I)
5. Atrial contraction (I-A)

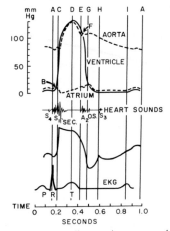

Figure 9-1. *The phases of the cardiac cycle as recorded by pressure tracings, phonocardiogram, apexcardiogram, and electrocardiogram.* **A₂** $= aortic$ *component of second heart sound;* **O.S.** $= opening snap;$ **P,R,T** $= waves of$ *atrial and ventricular depolarization and ventricular repolarization, respectively;* **S₁** $= first\ heard\ sound;$ **S₃** $= third\ heart\ sound;$ **S₄** $= fourth\ heart\ sound.$

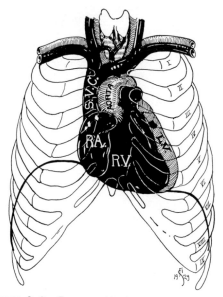

Figure 9–2. *Topographical anatomy of the heart.*

Inspection

Inspection of the heart is best carried out with the patient in the supine position or in the slight left lateral decubitus position. You should stand at the patient's right (Fig. 9–3).

On inspection look first for the point of maximal impulse (P.M.I.). This thrust of the heart was carefully studied by William Harvey, who wrote in his *De Motu Cordis:* "The heart is lifted, and rises to the apex, so that it strikes the chest at that moment and the beat may be felt on the outside." Although the apex itself may be 0.5 cm. to the left of the point of maximal impulse, for practical purposes the point of maximal impulse and the apex beat may be considered to be synonymous terms.

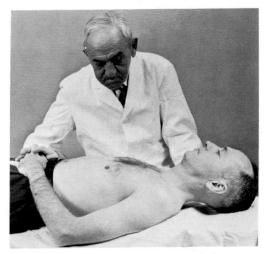

Figure 9-3. *Inspection of the heart.*

During systole the transverse diameter shortens more than the longitudinal diameter. As Hirschfelder has shown, the movements of the heart during systole push the apex of the heart against the chest wall, as the right and left ventricular free walls move toward the septum (Fig. 9-4).

The point of maximal impulse is most easily seen in patients who have a thin chest wall. In emaciated patients, the impulse may be so widespread and seem so forceful that cardiac disease may be suspected when none is present. When individuals have muscular or obese chest walls, the point of maximal impulse is less distinct; it may be absent in those with pulmonary emphysema. In dextrocardia the cardiac impulse is on the right instead of the left side.

Point of maximal impulse. When present, the point of maximal impulse is located in or about the fifth intercostal space inside the left midclavicular line. However, as Neehaus and Wright have pointed out, the "overall demonstrability of the

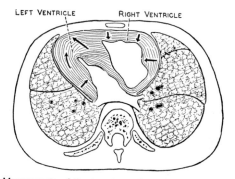

Figure 9–4. *Movements of the heart producing protrusions and retractions during systole. (Hirschfelder, A. D.: Diseases of the Heart and Aorta. Philadelphia, J. B. Lippincott Co., 1933.)*

apex for all ages and weights, and both sexes is only 24.6 per cent instead of the implied 100 per cent." Age, sex, and weight are important factors determining the presence of the apex beat.

The point of maximal impulse normally varies with deep inspiration and change of position. When the patient takes a deep inspiration and holds his breath, the point of maximal impulse moves downward from the fifth to the sixth interspace. When the patient lies on his right side, it moves slightly toward the right and when on his left side, it moves about 2 cm. toward the left. The absence of such mobility suggests an adherent pericardium. As Broadbent pointed out, deep inspiration may bring the lungs over the heart so that the impulse disappears altogether. This is especially true in patients who have emphysematous lungs. Therefore, disappearance of the impulse on inspiration does not necessarily mean that the heart is freely movable. Similarly, when the patient lies on his right side, the change in position of the point of maximal impulse may mean only that another part of the heart has been brought in contact with the chest wall, not that the apex has shifted.

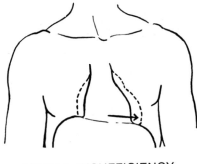

MITRAL INSUFFICIENCY

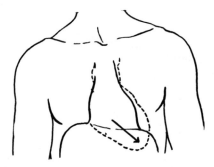

AORTIC INSUFFICIENCY

Figure 9–5. *Displacement of apex in mitral insufficiency and aortic insufficiency.*

Marked enlargement of the left ventricle displaces the point of maximal impulse to the left outside the midclavicular line and often to the anterior axillary line or even the posterior axillary line. With marked left ventricular enlargement, the apex is displaced downward as well as laterally (Fig. 9–5).

Any pathological process affecting the position of the heart may result in a displacement of the point of maximal impulse. A pleural effusion on the right side displaces the point of maximal impulse toward the left axilla, whereas a pleural effusion on the left displaces it toward the right. Pleural adhesions, mediastinal tumors, atelectasis, and pneumothorax may give rise to similar displacements.

The character of the impulse may give information of great value. The apex beat is composed primarily of an upward deflection due to left ventricular contraction. This large deflection is sometimes preceded by a smaller upward deflection that corresponds to the *a* wave of the venous pulse. This smaller presystolic deflection is a ventricular movement that results from left atrial contraction. An early diastolic deflection may also be identified, and is referred to as a rapid filling wave. This ventricular movement results from the rapid filling of the left ventricle immediately after the mitral valve opens (Fig. 9–6).[1] When left ventricular hypertrophy develops owing to systemic hypertension, aortic stenosis, aortic insufficiency, or coarctation of the aorta, a more forceful atrial contraction is required to complete ventricular filling. This produces a readily visible and palpable ventricular lift (Fig. 9–43).

---

[1]On the next several pages, a number of phonocardiographic tracings will be used as illustrations. In all of these, the upper line represents the sound vibrations, and the lower line is a reference tracing. The reference tracing may consist of an electrocardiogram, an indirect carotid pulse tracing, a venous tracing, or an apexcardiogram. The apexcardiogram records the chest wall vibrations at the point of maximal impulse. These vibrations are similar to those that can be seen by the naked eye during careful cardiovascular examination. The venous tracings are obtained from the external jugular vein, and the motions they record can be observed when the patient is properly positioned.

The recorded sound tracings are designated as either "stetho" or "log." The "stetho" tracing in effect records the low frequency vibrations to greatest advantage. This simulates listening with the bell of the stethoscope. The "log" tracing records the high frequency vibrations and is similar to listening with the diaphragm of the stethoscope. The position of the recording microphone is identified by the designation "aorta" for aortic area, "pulmonic" for pulmonary area, "LSB" for the lower left sternal border, and "apex" for the point of maximum impulse. These in essence conform to the aortic, pulmonary, tricuspid, and mitral auscultatory areas.

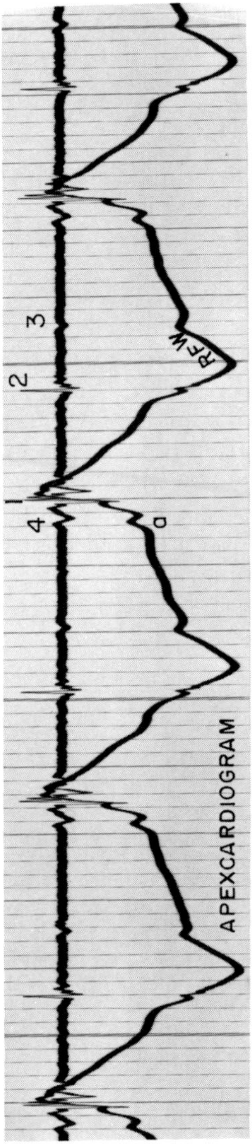

Figure 9–6. *Normal apexcardiogram.* **RFW** *indicates the rapid filling wave.*

The left ventricular systolic impulse is increased in amplitude and duration in these same pathological conditions. This slow, forcible lift of the interspace gives rise to the rounded or "dome-shaped" thrust that is characteristic of left ventricular hypertrophy. Mitral insufficiency and left heart failure are associated with a prominent rapid filling wave. Since mitral stenosis slows the passage of blood from left atrium to left ventricle, no rapid filling wave is present in this condition. In fact, moderate to severe mitral stenosis may be characterized by the absence of an apex beat.

The force of the impulse should be studied. The force and heart rate are often increased in persons with normal hearts who are nervous because of the examination. As the examination proceeds and the patient becomes more composed, the heart rate slows, the intensity of the cardiac contractions diminishes, and the force of the impulse lessens. The force of the impulse by no means corresponds to the force of the cardiac contractions. A soft, flabby, dilated heart may make greater excursions in systole than a smaller, more powerfully contracting heart and may not only show a larger area of pulsation, but may also appear to contract more powerfully.

The amplitude of the impulse depends in part upon the thickness of the chest wall, upon whether the point of maximal impulse lies under the rib or the interspace, and upon the character and thickness of the lung that covers the point. The extent of the area of the cardiac impulse depends largely upon the force and volume of the systole. In aortic insufficiency, when the heart beats forcefully, the area is extensive, but as previously mentioned, a dilated, flabby, weakly contracting heart may also show a large area of cardiac pulsation.

Systolic retraction. This phenomenon, also described as "negative cardiac impulse," was first studied by Skoda, who considered it to be a sign of adhesive pericarditis. It should be remembered, however, that during systole there is normally some retraction of the intercostal spaces near the point of maximal impulse. If the point of maximal impulse lies under a rib, you may see only the retraction of the intercostal spaces. According to some observers, however, this retraction of the precordium is caused by an unusually low intrathoracic pressure resulting from a hypertrophied right ventricle or an unusually forcible action of the heart.

Nonetheless, systolic retraction is a normal occurrence. Eden's advice is sound: that before we make a diagnosis of adhesive pericarditis, we should be sure "that not only the interspaces, but also the ribs themselves are retracted during systole."

Diastolic heart beat. Wood has described this phenomenon well: "The diastolic heart beat is an outward thrust that can be seen and felt during diastole, occurring in the absence of a normal apical systolic impulse, and accompanied by a protodiastolic sound." (See Fig. 9–7). This sign, first described by Skoda in 1852, is usually associated with systolic retraction of the precordium and sudden diastolic emptying of the cervical veins. A diastolic heart beat is a pathognomonic sign of constrictive pericarditis when the systolic apical impulse is absent and when accompanied by systolic retraction of the precordium and sudden diastolic emptying of the cervical veins.

Broadbent's sign. The sign, first observed by Sir William Broadbent and first reported in the literature by his son, Walter Broadbent, in 1895, is of value in the diagnosis of adherent pericardium. Walter Broadbent described four cases "in each of which there is a visible retraction synchronous with cardiac systole, of the left back in the region of the eleventh and twelfth ribs, and in three of which there is also systolic retraction of less degree in the same region of the right back." Sir William Broadbent later noted that "this indication is not infallible, as the tugging has been observed when the heart was hypertrophied without adhesions."

Rate and rhythm. The heart rate is increased in a variety of conditions, such as hyperthyroidism, anemia, and febrile illness. Paroxysmal supraventricular tachycardia is characterized by paroxysms of rapid heart action, the rate varying between 140 and 220 beats per minute. The episodes usually begin and end suddenly. The rapid heart action, obvious at the apex, is also ex-

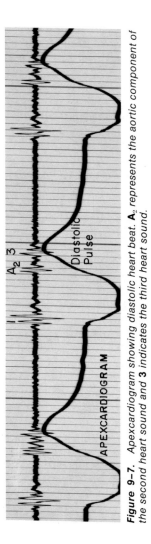

Figure 9–7. *Apexcardiogram showing diastolic heart beat.* **A**₂ *represents the aortic component of the second heart sound and* **3** *indicates the third heart sound.*

tremely forceful and is accompanied by forceful pulsations of the entire precordium. The heart rate is slowed in complete heart block; the slow rate of 20 to 40 may be readily recognized by observing the cardiac impulse.

Careful observation of the apex beat may be helpful in diagnosing other arrhythmias. Sinus arrhythmia, formerly called by Mackenzie "the youthful type of irregularity," is readily recognized. The heart beats more rapidly during inspiration than during expiration. Atrial and ventricular premature contractions are easily seen, but difficult to distinguish.

Atrial fibrillation is readily recognized by inspection of the point of maximal impulse. This condition was formerly called "delirium cordis" (cardiac delirium). Cardiac action is utterly irregular in both force and rhythm. Strong impulses alternate with weak impulses at times, then a series of strong beats and pauses of varying lengths alternate with runs of rapid beats in which the heart seems to be racing.

"Visible apical reduplication" has been described by King as an important diagnostic sign in bundle branch block, and Levine and Harvey note that "there is often a bifurcation of the apex impulse in many cases of bundle branch block especially if a gallop is present." A bifid apical pulse has been described in idiopathic hypertrophic subaortic stenosis.

The precordium. The precordium and the anterior surface of the chest should be carefully examined for the presence of abnormal pulsations. Marked pulsation in the first and second right interspaces outside the sternal border should make one suspicious of aneurysm of the ascending arch of the aorta. Similar pulsation occurs as a result of aortic insufficiency and poststenotic dilatation of the aorta. These conditions may also give rise to pulsations at the base of the heart. Aortic aneurysms may, in addition, cause a diffuse heaving of the sternum and pulsation in the sternal notch. Arteriosclerosis of the aorta may cause a similar pulsation in the sternal notch.

Some patients with atrial septal defects as well as patients with pulmonary valvular stenosis and poststenotic dilatation of the pulmonary artery have a pulsatile pulmonary artery that can be observed at the second interspace to the left of the sternal border. It is seen as a lift of the interspace during systole. Patients with right ventricular hypertrophy and dilatation due to atrial septal defect or mitral stenosis may demonstrate a systolic "precordial heave," which is a steady precordial lift seen at the left parasternal line.

In patients with marked pericardial effusion, a bulging in the epigastrium may be seen. This phenomenon is known as Auenbrugger's sign.

Palpation

The first aim of palpation should be to confirm the findings of inspection. You may be unable to see the impulse but can feel it, and thus gain information regarding the location and size of the heart. Observed disturbances in rate and rhythm can be confirmed by palpation.

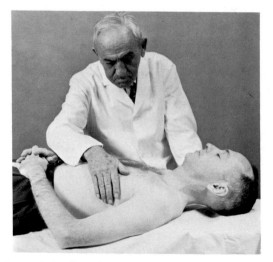

Figure 9–8. Palpation of the point of maximal impulse.

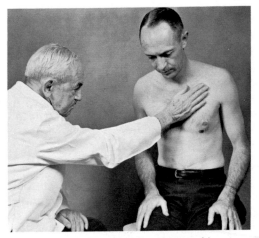

Figure 9–9. Palpation of base of heart.

Palpation gives a better impression of the force of the heart beat than does inspection. Often the impulse appears both forceful and extensive but on palpation proves to be weak, though present over a large area.

Method.   Although palpation can be carried out while the patient is standing or sitting, it is better done with your patient in the supine position. This position is advantageous since the patient is essentially immobile, and you will be in a more comfortable position. Sit at the patient's right side with the palm of your right hand over the precordium. Locate the apex beat exactly by palpation with the index finger. Palpable phenomena at the base of the heart can be examined in a similar fashion. In the presence of either a thick chest wall or pulmonary emphysema, the cardiac impulses may be palpable only when the patient is sitting upright or leaning forward.

The apex beat of the left ventricle is a forceful, prolonged heave when left ventricular hypertrophy is due to aortic stenosis or systemic hypertension. In aortic insufficiency and mitral insufficiency, when the ventricle is working against a low resistance, the apical impulse is also forceful but has greater amplitude and is more abrupt and lively. The apex beat of mitral insufficiency is shorter than that of aortic insufficiency. Both conditions are associated with increased systolic retraction over the right ventricle. Slight retraction in this region is normal.

When left ventricular hypertrophy is also accompanied by left atrial hypertrophy, the *a* wave of the apex beat may be palpable and is synchronous with the presystolic gallop sound (Fig. 9–1).

All of the heart sounds may be palpable. This includes the first sound, both components of the second sound, systolic ejection clicks, and the opening snap of mitral stenosis. Closure of the pulmonic valve is frequently palpable in normal individuals, but is more readily palpable when pulmonary hypertension is present. Systolic ejection clicks may be palpable over the aortic and pulmonic areas.

The dilatation of the pulmonary artery that occurs during systole may be distinctly palpable when there is increased pulmonary blood flow, as with atrial or ventricular septal defect. This is best felt at the second interspace to the left of the sternum with the patient in the supine position.

A steady heave of the right ventricle is palpable over the precordium to the left of the sternum when pulmonary hypertension is significant. In marked right ventricular hypertrophy, a strong right ventricular heave may be associated with apical retraction, resulting in a rocking motion that is the reverse of left ventricular rocking.

Pericardial friction rub. On palpation over the precordium, a friction fremitus may be felt in fibrinous pericarditis. This fremitus is synchronous with the heart beat and is not affected by respiration. It is produced by the roughened visceral and parietal pericardia rubbing upon each other. This sign was described by Hope as a "vibratory tremor generally perceptible to the hand." When a pericardial effusion follows fibrinous pericarditis, the friction rub often disappears.

Thrills. Corrigan showed that thrills could be produced by

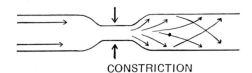

CONSTRICTION

Figure 9–10. *Production of a thrill in a tube by constriction.*

attaching a piece of rubber tubing to a water faucet, turning on the water, and constricting the tubing at a certain point. This constriction produces numerous eddies, twists, and turns in the part of the stream that is below the constriction, causing vibrations in the wall of the tubing. Such vibrations are felt as thrills and heard as murmurs (Fig. 9–10).

Palpation may thus be helpful in determining the presence of such thrills. They are best palpated when the chest is in the position of forced expiration, which brings the heart and great vessels closer to the anterior chest wall and retracts the lung from the position overlying the heart. This lessens the possibility of confusing the cardiac and respiratory phenomena. Almost all heart murmurs have associated palpable thrills.

PRESYSTOLIC THRILL. A presystolic thrill felt near the apex of the heart is pathognomonic of mitral stenosis. Corvisart, who first noted this sign, described it as a "thrill particularly difficult to describe, felt by the hand when applied to the pericardial region." Laennec, with more imagination, described it as similar to a cat's purring [frémissement cataire] and added that it "may be compared quite accurately to the vibration which accompanies the sound of satisfaction which a cat makes when one strokes it with the hand." Laennec remarked that a similar sensation may be produced by stroking the palm of a gloved hand with a rough brush.

The presystolic thrill of mitral stenosis is usually felt only over a small area at the point of maximal impulse. It is, as a rule, better felt if the heart is beating forcefully. It may not be felt when the patient is lying quietly in bed, but may be brought out by moving the patient up and down rapidly a few times and thus producing more active cardiac contractions. It may also be elicited by turning the patient on his left side.

The novice and, for that matter, the more experienced observer may have difficulty in timing the thrill. Careful examination, however, reveals that the thrill precedes the systolic shock or thrust by just a fraction of a second and is therefore presystolic in time. Simultaneous auscultation of the heart should convince you that the thrill is felt just before you hear the first heart sound.

SYSTOLIC THRILL. With aortic stenosis a rough purring systolic thrill may be felt over the precordium, with maximum intensity at the aortic area. It may also be felt in the carotid and brachial arteries as well.

The systolic thrill of pulmonary stenosis and atrial septal defect may be palpable at the second left interspace, the same area where the continuous thrill of a patent ductus arteriosus is palpable. The systolic thrill of a ventricular septal defect is best felt at the fourth or fifth interspace just to the left of the sternum, whereas the thrill of mitral insufficiency is best felt at the apex.

Percussion

Percussion of the heart was first performed by Auenbrugger, who observed on percussing the chest that "where the heart is located the sound obtained has a certain fullness showing clearly that the more solid portion of the heart, located there, dulls somewhat the ringing resonance." Corvisart used this method and discusses its value in his translation of Auenbrugger and in his treatise on heart disease. Laennec learned the procedure from his master, Corvisart. It was used and further developed by Piorry and Skoda.

Percussion of the cardiac outline has been the cause of more controversy than almost any other subject in the field of physical diagnosis. Some distinguished students of physical diagnosis have in recent years stated that percussion of the cardiac outlines is so notoriously unreliable that they no longer attempt it.

Instead, they rely solely upon the position of the point of maximal impulse as the only reliable index of the point to which the heart extends on the left. They also find that the only reliable guide to the size of the heart is the x-ray picture. Unfortunately, in many instances no cardiac impulse is visible, and in many instances the use of the x-ray is impossible. The physician always has his fingers and ears with him at the bedside of the patient.

The difference of opinion concerning the usefulness of percussion in determining the cardiac outline is explained in part by the remark of Friedrich Müller that "we must not explore the chest by percussing our ideas into it." Many of these ideas we obtain by studying the cardiac outlines in textbooks of anatomy rather than in roentgenograms. In one instance we see the inert heart hardened by formalin and distended to its maximum by embalming fluid injected under pressure, whereas the roentgenogram shows the heart as it is during life. A similar example occurs in comparing the pictures of the stomach as portrayed commonly in textbooks of anatomy with those obtained by studying the stomach under the fluoroscope.

Much of the distrust of percussion arises as a result of demanding more from the method than it will give. Percussion of the cardiac outlines is accurate only to a limited extent, but within these limitations it is a valuable method of examination. Differences of opinion between two examiners as to the extent of cardiac dullness are to be expected. One observer, on percussing the heart, may consider it enlarged, whereas a second observer disagrees. Similar differences of opinion may exist between two roentgenologists who examine the same plate of a patient's chest or between two pathologists who see the same heart at autopsy. Careful percussion will usually reveal whether the heart is approximately normal in size or whether it is definitely markedly enlarged. More than this we cannot expect of the most refined percussion.

Method of percussion. Many beginners, in attempting to outline the cardiac dullness, strike too forcibly and thus fail to hear the slight change in the percussion note caused by the thin layer of overlying lung. One should use the lightest percussion

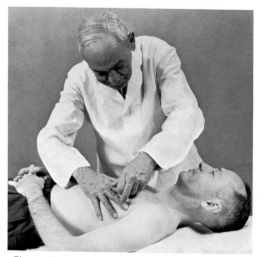

Figure 9–11. Percussion of the cardiac outline.

possible and, with experience, rely more and more upon the vibratory sense. In percussing, one should begin at the side and percuss toward the sternum, since it is easier for the ear to appreciate a change from resonance to dullness than vice versa (Fig. 9–11). Similarly, the plessimeter finger senses more readily a change from the vibration over a resonant area to the diminished vibration over a dull area.

Personally, we prefer to hold the plessimeter finger parallel to the outlines of the heart (Fig. 9–12) rather than at right angles to it, although good results may be obtained with the latter position. When the plessimeter finger is held parallel to the cardiac outlines, a larger number of vibrations cross the outlines than when the plessimeter finger is held at right angles to the cardiac outlines (Fig. 9–13).

AUSCULTATORY PERCUSSION. This method often gives satisfactory results when used to determine the cardiac outline. To

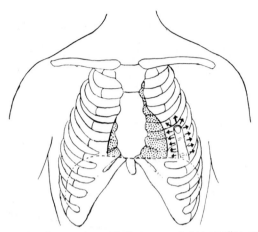

Figure 9–12. Percussion with finger parallel to cardiac outlines.

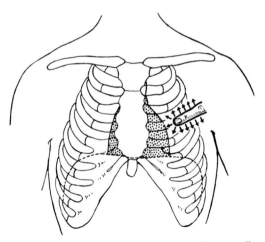

Figure 9–13. Percussion with finger at right angle to cardiac outline.

carry out auscultatory percussion, place your stethoscope over the lower part of the sternum, above the xiphoid, and rub or scratch lightly over the surface of the skin, beginning in the left anterior axillary line and gradually moving toward the sternum. Note first a soft rubbing or scratching sound; then, just as the border of relative cardiac dullness is reached, the sound abruptly becomes intense. The right border of the heart may also be outlined by this method.

Cardiac outlines. We have already noted that the left border of the normal heart and a part of both left and right ventricles are covered by lung tissue. Percussion over this part of the heart gives a note that is impaired, or diminished in resonance, but that retains a certain degree of resonance. This region is called the area of relative cardiac dullness (R.C.D.). Note, as you percuss toward the sternum, you presently encounter an area where the heart is no longer covered by the lung, there is no trace of resonance, and the percussion note is flat. This area is spoken of as the area of absolute cardiac dullness (A.C.D.). Most observers agree on these details. In an average normal man, the relative cardiac dullness extends 8 to 10 cm. to the left of the midsternal line in the fifth intercostal space, inside the midclavicular line.

The size of the heart should be expressed in terms of centimeters from the midsternal line (M.S.L.), and not in reference to the parasternal line, the mamillary line, or the midclavicular line. In women with large, pendulous breasts, it is often impossible to outline the left border of the heart by percussion. In most instances, however, if the breast is elevated you can determine the point to which relative cardiac dullness extends on the left. In some patients who are obese and who also have large breasts, it may be impossible to obtain by percussion any accurate knowledge regarding the size of the heart.

Cardiac dullness in abdominal distention. Just as the enlargement of the uterus during pregnancy causes a certain displacement of the abdominal organs and an elevation of the diaphragm, similarly a variety of pathological conditions such as ascites, an ovarian cyst, and peritonitis may cause an elevation of

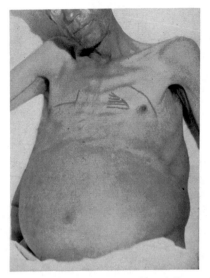

Figure 9–14. Increased width of the cardiac dullness due to ascites.

the diaphragm and an increase in the area of the cardiac dullness. This increase is, of course, due to the position of the heart and not to disease of the heart. The patient shown in Figure 9–14 had a marked upward displacement of the heart due to ascites and to a large abdominal cyst. The cardiac outlines shown here were verified at autopsy.

Changes in the position of cardiac dullness. Any condition that either pushes or pulls the heart to the right or the left will obviously alter the location of the cardiac dullness. A left-sided pleural effusion pushes the heart to the right and increases the cardiac dullness to the right of the sternum. The left border of the heart in such cases usually cannot be made out, since the cardiac dullness fuses with the dullness resulting from the effusion. A right-sided pleural effusion pushes the heart to the left, increasing the cardiac dullness on that side.

In the presence of a pleural effusion, the heart is displaced toward the normal side; but in massive collapse of the lung, the heart is displaced toward the affected side. This is a valuable diagnostic point.

Pleural adhesions may pull the heart to either side, giving rise to changes in the area of cardiac dullness that are similar to those that result from pleural effusions.

Decrease in the area of cardiac dullness. A decrease in the area of relative cardiac dullness may occur in pulmonary emphysema. The area of absolute cardiac dullness is usually decreased in emphysema, since the lung is increased in size and covers a greater area of the heart than normal. Indeed, in many cases of pulmonary emphysema, no absolute cardiac dullness can be found by percussion.

Increase in the area of cardiac dullness. An increase in the area of cardiac dullness is most strikingly seen in patients who have cardiac disease. This increase is usually more marked than the increase due to changes in the position of the heart. It should be emphasized, however, that we cannot detect by percussion an appreciable increase in the area of cardiac dullness in hypertrophy of the heart unless there is an accompanying dilatation. Hypertrophy of the heart in many cases of aortic stenosis cannot be detected by percussion; the hypertrophied and dilated heart in aortic insufficiency, however, is easily outlined. Enlargement of the left ventricle increases the area of relative cardiac dullness on the left, and often downward on the left. Enlargement of the left ventricle occurs in aortic insufficiency, mitral insufficiency, patent ductus arteriosus, ventricular septal defect, and long-standing hypertension.

Enlargement of the right ventricle and right atrium increases the area of cardiac dullness to the left and upward, often as high as the second rib, and on the right of the sternal margin. Gerhardt's dullness is described as a rectangular area of dullness in the second or third left intercostal space that is due to a dilated pulmonary artery.

Pericardial effusion. When there is a considerable effusion into the pericardial sac in exudative pericarditis, the cardiac

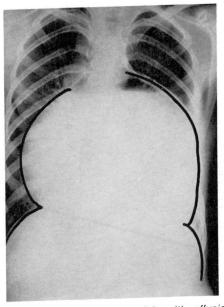

Figure 9–15. *Roentgenogram of pericarditis with effusion. Note large shadow and small area of air above fluid, the result of a small paracentesis.*

dullness increases in all directions and assumes a general globular enlargement (Fig. 9–15).

   Rotch's sign.   As Rotch pointed out in 1878, a large pericardial effusion causes dullness in the fifth right interspace and changes the cardiohepatic angle, which is normally a right angle, to an obtuse angle. Figure 9–63 shows a boy who has a large pericardial effusion and an obtuse cardiohepatic angle. The outlines shown in Figure 9–63 were obtained on percussion and verified shortly afterward at autopsy.

   Increased retrosternal dullness.   An increase in the area of retrosternal dullness occurs as a result either of tumors in the anterior mediastinum or of dilatation of the aorta in aortic aneurysms. Figure 9–16 shows a patient who has a marked increase in retrosternal dullness due to a mediastinal tumor. This tumor lay mainly on the right side and obstructed the venous outflow in the right arm with consequent enlargement of the arm. Figure 9–17 shows an area of increased retrosternal dullness in a patient suffering from mitral and aortic disease accompanied by marked widening of the aorta. Figure 9–78 shows an area of dullness to the right of the sternum in the second and third costal interspace that is due to an aneurysm of the ascending arch of the aorta. Over such an area of dullness an expansile pulsation is usually seen.

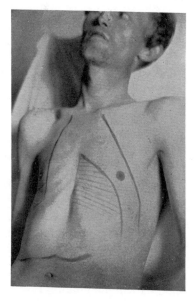

Figure 9–16. *Widened area of retrosternal dullness due to mediastinal tumor.*

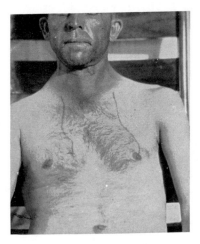

Figure 9–17. Increased retrosternal dullness due to dilatation of aorta.

BLOOD PRESSURE AND PULSE

Blood Pressure

In 1905 Korotkoff introduced the auscultatory method of estimating the blood pressure. This method has gained universal acceptance, for with it one can estimate both the systolic and diastolic pressures.

In order to carry out the auscultatory method, pump the arm cuff up until the pulse disappears. Place the stethoscope over the brachial artery at the bend of the elbow, and listen; nothing is heard—the period of silence. Slowly release the pressure and as the mercury falls in the manometer, note the point when beats become audible—the systolic pressure. As the mercury continues to fall, the sound of the beats becomes louder, then gradually diminishes until a point is reached at which there is a sudden marked diminution in intensity; the weakened beats are heard for a few moments and then disappear altogether—the diastolic blood pressure. This is the official recommendation of the American Heart Association.

Occasionally there is no disappearance of the sounds, and the beats are heard to zero pressure. This phenomenon has given rise to interesting but erroneous case reports of patients who "have no diastolic pressure." Obviously, every patient having a systolic pressure also has a diastolic pressure. The error arises from failing to estimate the diastolic pressure at the point where the sudden change in intensity occurs. We have encountered this phenomenon in patients who had aortic insufficiency or hyperthyroidism and, occasionally, in apparently normal persons.

The palpatory and auscultatory methods

COMPARISON.   Many observers use the auscultatory method to the exclusion of the palpatory. This we believe to be a mistake. For the estimation of the systolic blood pressure, the reading at which we can first palpate the pulse is obviously the systolic pressure, regardless of what we hear. Usually there is little difference between the systolic pressure as determined by the palpatory method and that obtained by using the auscultatory method,

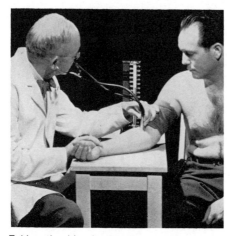

Figure 9–18. *Taking the blood pressure, employing both palpatory and auscultatory methods.*

although on the average the auscultatory method gives readings 10 to 15 mm. higher.

Occasionally, however, we can palpate the pulse when the manometer reading is 200 mm., but can hear nothing until the manometer falls to 170 or 160 mm. Obviously, in such conditions the systolic pressure is 200 mm., since the pulse appears at this level of pressure. Conversely, we occasionally hear the pulse sounds at 200 mm., but do not feel the pulse until 160 is reached. In this case we hear the column of blood beating against the compressed artery, which is somewhat relaxed but not patent, the pressure in the cuff not being sufficiently low to allow the pulse wave to pass through.

Since errors in determining the systolic blood pressure by auscultation are more likely to occur, the palpatory method is more reliable. However, it requires more practice to become adept in this method. A safe rule is to use both methods, but in case of difference to regard the palpatory findings as more reliable.

For the estimation of the diastolic pressure, the pressure is lowered slowly. Just before the diastolic pressure is reached, the pulse volume increases. At the diastolic pressure the pulse pressure diminishes abruptly. This technique is helpful when the pulse sounds can be heard to zero.

ACCURACY. The palpatory and auscultatory methods, like many methods used in clinical medicine, have only a relative accuracy. Estimations of the blood pressure by the direct method of introducing into an artery a needle connected with a sensitive recording apparatus show that the blood pressure taken by the Riva-Rocci sphygmomanometer often has an error of 10 to 20 mm. of mercury, sometimes too high, at other times too low. This holds for both the palpatory and auscultatory methods and for systolic as well as for diastolic pressure. However, we know what the average normal blood pressure is when estimated by the sphygmomanometer, so that it is the variations from this normal value that allow us to determine whether the blood pressure is normal, increased, or decreased.

The resistance of the tissues in the arm, which must be overcome by the arm band, is a factor of error. This probably accounts for the fact that the blood pressure as estimated with a sphygmomanometer is usually too high, since the pressure applied to the cuff must overcome the resistance of the tissues before compressing the brachial artery. For this reason patients with abnormally fat arms often show readings that are grossly inaccurate and far too high when a standard width cuff is used.

A more accurate systolic blood pressure determination can be obtained in obese individuals by placing the blood pressure cuff around the forearm and palpating the radial pulse, or by using a wider cuff. Errors in the auscultatory blood pressure reading also occur if the arm is dependent, if the cuff is inflated slowly, or if it is reinflated without allowing complete deflation. The "blood pressure" in the legs is always high because the large muscle masses strongly resist arterial compression.

Cardiac irregularities. Cardiac irregularities, caused by premature contractions and atrial fibrillation, are readily recognized when we use the auscultatory method of estimating the blood pressure. Mackenzie pointed out that the sphygmomanometer is of great value in determining the presence of a cardiac irregularity of force—pulsus alternans. This is usually a sign of heart failure or impending heart failure.

If you inflate the arm cuff well above the systolic pressure in a case of pulsus alternans and allow the pressure to fall slowly, you will presently hear the beats at the bend of the elbow coming through in a perfectly even and regular fashion, but at a rate one-half that of the pulse rate. As the pressure continues to fall, these beats become louder. Presently another set of softer beats appears, each soft beat following a loud beat, the rate now being exactly the pulse rate. This alternation in strength of the beats is clearly heard, and the condition can be distinguished from a bigeminal pulse by the regularity with which the beats are spaced.

The normal blood pressure. In the average normal adult from 20 to 40 years of age, the systolic pressure ranges from 90 to 120 and the diastolic pressure from 60 to 80 mm. of mercury. The pressure often goes higher as the age increases, not because an increase in pressure is normal with an increase in age, but because hypertension is a disease of middle age and not of youth. The "rule" that the systolic blood pressure should be the age plus 100 is not a rule but a superstition. Many persons seventy or eighty years of age have a systolic blood pressure of 120 to 140. It is a safe rule to consider a systolic blood pressure above 140 and a diastolic pressure above 90 as definitely elevated.

The blood pressure is not a constant factor. It changes from day to day, from hour to hour, and even from minute to minute. Although it shows these periodic changes, it does not rise above the normal limits in healthy individuals.

The range of blood pressure that can be considered normal varies with climate and race. The inhabitants of torrid and tropical zones have a lower blood pressure than do those living in temperate zones. Chinese, Japanese, and Malays have a lower blood pressure than Europeans. The blood pressure falls during sleep and may be strikingly elevated by fright or excitement.

Elevation of blood pressure: hypertension. The level of the blood pressure depends primarily on the peripheral resistance and the cardiac output. Significant increases in either of these factors may produce significant hypertension. An increase in stroke volume produces systolic hypertension. Anemia, hyperthyroidism, arteriovenous fistula, aortic insufficiency, and complete heart block are examples of this. A normal stroke volume pumped into a noncompliant arteriosclerotic aorta will also produce systolic hypertension.

Increased arteriolar resistance is the most common cause of hypertension. This increased resistance may occur secondarily to endocrine disease or renal disease, or the cause may be unknown, in which case it is called "essential hypertension."

ENDOCRINE CAUSES. The adrenal gland is intimately associated with the production of hypertension. Tumors of the adrenal medulla (pheochromocytomas) produce epinephrine and norepinephrine and may give rise to a paroxysmal form of hypertension. These paroxysms may last for minutes, hours, or days, during which the blood pressure is over 300 mm. of mercury.

Between paroxysms the blood pressure may be normal. Cushing's syndrome results from adrenal cortical hypersecretion of non-aldosterone steroids. It is characterized by truncal obesity, moon facies, muscle and skin atrophy, and hypertension. Aldosterone-secreting tumors of the adrenal gland, first described by Conn, give rise to hypertension without any of the clinical manifestations of Cushing's disease. Hyperthyroidism and hyperparathyroidism may also cause hypertension.

RENAL CAUSES. Renal hypertension may result from disease of the renal parenchyma or the renal vasculature. Parenchymal diseases include chronic glomerulonephritis, pyelonephritis, and polycystic disease of the kidney. Vascular lesions may be due to congenital or acquired malformation of the renal artery or to small vessel disease such as occurs in lupus erythematosus.

ESSENTIAL HYPERTENSION. This is the most common cause of a pathologically elevated blood pressure. The disease is quite prevalent; it shows a marked familial tendency, and it appears commonly in middle-aged people. Its victims usually die as a result of heart failure, cerebral hemorrhage, or uremia. It is one of the most common causes of left ventricular hypertrophy.

The blood pressure in essential hypertension may be quite labile, changing with emotions. The systolic blood pressure is more labile than the diastolic pressure. A marked elevation in the diastolic pressure is a bad prognostic sign. Blankenhorn showed that some patients with essential hypertension have a marked decrease in blood pressure, often to normal, during sleep, whereas others show no change. The prognosis is better in the first group.

The blood pressure in coarctation of the aorta. The systolic and diastolic blood pressure in cases of coarctation of the aorta is higher in the brachial arteries than in the femoral and tibial arteries, since the brachial arteries originate above the stenosis and the tibial arteries below. In this connection the well known physical law will be recalled that a partial obstruction to the flow of a fluid in a tube increases the pressure above the obstruction, but decreases it below. In coarctation of the aorta, the patient may show a brachial systolic pressure of 200 mm. or over, whereas the femoral systolic pressure is 100 mm. or less.

The demonstration of marked hypertension in a youthful person should always suggest the possibility of coarctation of the aorta, since the pressure is usually taken in the brachial artery.

Low blood pressure: hypotension. Hypotension results either from a decrease in cardiac output or from a decrease in peripheral resistance. Decreases in cardiac output occur in Addison's disease, myocarditis, myocardial infarction, pericarditis with effusion, and following hemorrhage. A marked decrease in blood pressure is a sign of serious prognostic import in pericardial effusion and is an indication for pericardiocentesis.

A sudden decrease in peripheral resistance (vasomotor collapse) may occur in pneumonia, septicemia, acute adrenal insufficiency (Waterhouse-Friderichsen syndrome), and drug intoxications. A sudden drop in blood pressure should be regarded as a grave sign.

The Pulse

Palpation of the pulse is one of the most ancient and time-honored practices of the medical profession.

Inequality of the pulses. The Chinese physician of old always felt both pulses of a patient simultaneously as the first procedure in the examination of his patient, and he laid great stress on the comparison of the two pulses. He diagnosed diseases of the heart, liver, kidney, and intestines from the left wrist and diseases of the lungs, stomach, spleen, and kidney from the right wrist. It would be wise for the physician of today to follow his example, but for a different reason. Inequality of the two pulses is readily determined and may be of diagnostic value. Retardation of the pulse is commonly present in arteries that are distal to an aneurysmal sac. An aneurysm of the transverse or descending arch of the aorta causes a retardation of the pulse wave at the left wrist. The artery feels smaller and is more easily compressed than usual. An aneurysm of the ascending aorta or innominate artery may result in similar changes in the pulse at the right wrist. Either a tumor pressing upon any of the large arterial trunks or an atherosclerotic plaque occluding a large artery may change the pulse in a manner similar to that of an aneurysm.

In coarctation of the aorta, the radial and carotid pulses are large and throbbing, whereas the femoral, popliteal, and dorsalis pedis pulses are scarcely palpable. The pulsations of the abdominal aorta may be difficult to feel and may be delayed. This lag is due to stenosis of the aorta, which also gives rise to collateral circulation between the upper and lower parts of the body, mainly through the internal mammary, intercostal, scapular, and deep epigastric arteries. These latter vessels are usually markedly dilated and show visible pulsations. The enlargement of the intercostal arteries may result in notching, or erosions, on the lower border of the ribs that are clearly seen in the x-ray photograph.

Palpation of the pulse. To examine the pulse, take the hand of your patient with the palm upward and place three fingers on the radial artery with your index finger nearest the heart (Fig. 9–19). With your fingers in this position, you should be able to feel the patient's pulse distinctly and to note its characteristics. Palpate the carotid, brachial, femoral, popliteal, posterior tibial, and dorsalis pedis arteries as well as the radial arteries.

Many misconceptions have arisen concerning the exact nature of the visible and palpable pulse. With each ventricular systole a volume of blood is suddenly ejected under pressure into the aorta. If the aorta were a rigid pipe, it would transmit this pressure immediately to the capillary bed. Since the aorta is elastic, a large part of the pressure of the ejection acts to distend the ascending aorta. The distention of the aorta accommodates the ejected volume of blood, and the pressure is transmitted as a wave through the entire aorta and its branches. This wave gives rise to several harmonic waves that may have a cumulative effect. The forward movement of blood follows this pressure wave. This pressure wave, along with its harmonics and with the

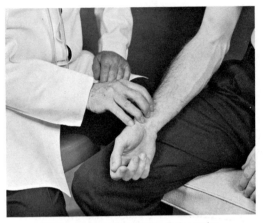

Figure 9–19. Palpation of the pulse.

expansion and elongation of the artery that it causes, constitutes the palpable and visible pulse.

The pulse is largely an index of the heart's action. In addition to the action of the heart, however, the elasticity of the larger vessels, the viscosity of the blood, and the resistance in the arterioles and capillaries play important roles in determining certain characteristics of the pulse.

Characteristics of the pulse. It is a common practice to speak of the force of the pulse, which depends in great measure upon the force of the systole, since the pulse obviously cannot be strong if ventricular systole is weak or if ventricular filling is incomplete. The pulse, however, may be feeble even though the cardiac contractions are very forcible. This is the case in aortic stenosis or in certain cardiac irregularities. The force of the pulse is not, therefore, an accurate index of the force of the cardiac contractions.

The use of the term "force" in relation to the pulse and the description of the pulse as "strong" or "weak" are open to serious objections. By the term "strong" one person means the volume of the pulse, whereas another may mean the pressure within the artery.

The terms "quick" and "slow" are often ambiguous, also, since they may refer to the pulse rate or to the character of each individual beat. The ancients were more accurate in their terminology. When referring to the pulse, they spoke of a pulsus frequens or pulsus rarus (frequent or infrequent), and when describing the character of the individual beat, they used the terms pulsus celer or pulsus tardus (quick or prolonged).

The pulse may be described most clearly in terms of the following characteristics:

1. Rate — pulsus frequens or rarus (rapid or slow).
2. Size — pulsus magnus or parvus (large or small).
3. Type of wave — pulsus celer or tardus (quick or prolonged).
4. Rhythm — pulsus regularis or irregularis (regular or irregular).
5. Tension — pulsus durus or mollis (hard or soft).

RATE. The average pulse rate in normal adults is 60 to 80 per minute; in children, 90 to 140; in the aged, 70 to 80.

Tachycardia. One hundred pulsations per minute may be considered the upper limit of normality. An acceleration of the pulse, tachycardia or pulsus frequens, is a normal occurrence during and after exercise. The pulse rate is decreased during sleep, increased after eating, and during coitus may rise to 140 per minute or more. It changes slightly during respiration, being faster during inspiration than during expiration. Excitement causes a temporary increase in the pulse rate, and the physician, in taking the patient's pulse, should wait two or three minutes before beginning to count the rate. In some patients the pulse may be rapid during the physical examination but fall to normal after the patient is completely relaxed.

In most diseases associated with fever, the pulse rate is elevated. The pulse rate usually bears a definite ratio to the height of the body temperature, the rate being increased on an average of five beats for every degree F. (eight beats per degree C.). An increased pulse rate is usually present in severe anemias, and after a severe hemorrhage the pulse is markedly increased in rate. Atropine increases the pulse rate.

One of the most common causes of persistent tachycardia is Graves' disease. This disease is also known as Basedow's disease, and more correctly as Parry's disease, since this syndrome was first observed by Caleb Hillier Parry 49 years before Basedow's publications. In Graves' disease the temperature is commonly elevated, but the increase in the pulse rate is out of proportion to the elevation in temperature. Basedow called attention to three outstanding findings in this disease: exophthalmos, tachycardia, and goiter. This combination of signs is often referred to as the "Merseburger triad," after Merseburg, the home of Basedow.

Persistent tachycardia is an important sign of myocardial disease and is almost invariably present in cardiac failure. Tachycardia may be the only pathological finding in acute and chronic myocardial disease. A fast pulse associated with indistinct heart sounds suggests myocardial disease.

Paroxysmal tachycardia. This condition was first described by William Stokes in 1854, but it was studied more extensively by Richard Cotton in 1867. Cotton's first case had a pulse rate of 230 per minute, and three weeks after the onset of the attack, "the patient entirely recovered; the action of the heart becoming suddenly in every respect natural, and the pulse eighty in the minute."

Léon Bouveret, in 1889, gave the disease the name of "essential paroxysmal tachycardia," and it is often referred to by the French as "Bouveret's disease." According to Bouveret, "each paroxysm begins and ends suddenly, in a few seconds. These sudden transitions from normal rhythm to a tachycardia rhythm, and vice versa, are accompanied sometimes by peculiar sensations in the head or in the precordial region."

A patient may have attacks of paroxysmal tachycardia for many years with no apparent impairment of health. The paroxysmal attacks vary in their duration from a few minutes or hours to days or weeks. Thyroid disease is a common cause of paroxysmal tachycardia, but this type of tachycardia usually occurs in otherwise normal individuals.

Pathognomonic of this disease is the abrupt onset and sudden termination, with a pulse rate between 140 and 220 per minute. The stimuli that give rise to these attacks may originate in the atrium or in the atrioventricular node. This differentiation can be made only with the electrocardiogram. Though the rate is rapid, the beats are regular.

Bradycardia. A slowing of the pulse, bradycardia or pulsus rarus, is noted during convalescence from certain infectious diseases, especially influenza and pneumonia. Myxedema, arteriosclerosis, and jaundice are common causes of bradycardia. Typhoid fever causes a relative bradycardia — the temperature is markedly elevated, whereas the pulse rate is only slightly increased. When increased intracranial pressure results in stimulation of the vagus nerve, the pulse rate is decreased.

The classic example of bradycardia occurs in heart block, first described by Morgagni as "epilepsy with a slow pulse," but better known as Stokes-Adams disease. Some patients with heart block may have epileptiform attacks when the pulse rate falls below 40 per minute. Almost all patients with heart block may have epileptiform attacks when the pulse rate falls below 16 per minute. In some cases this disease may exist for years with no apparent impairment of health. We once observed a patient who had a pulse of 40 for 50 years and died at the age of 84 from pneumonia.

The "sick sinus syndrome" may give rise to alternating periods of tachycardia and bradycardia. The modern use of implanted cardiac pacemakers provides an effective means of controlling severe bradycardias and preventing the deleterious consequences of sudden decrease in the pulse rate and fall in cardiac output.

Some persons can increase the pulse rate at will, and others can decrease the rate. This voluntary control of the pulse rate is rare, and its cause is not well understood. The alteration in rate is probably caused by sympathetic or vagus depression or stimulation.

SIZE. The size of the pulse is dependent upon the degree of filling of the artery during systole and of emptying during diastole. It is a measurement of the pulse pressure—the difference between systolic and diastolic pressure. A pulsus magnus has a high pulse pressure, a pulsus parvus a low pulse pressure. The collapsing pulse in aortic insufficiency is a good example of the pulsus magnus, whereas the pulse in aortic stenosis is the classic example of the pulsus parvus.

TYPE OF WAVE. The type of pulse wave that the palpating finger feels depends upon the rapidity with which the pulse pressure changes. The term pulsus celer does not refer to the pulse rate, inasmuch as it does not mean a rapid pulse, but refers to a quick pulse, one which rises quickly and falls quickly.

Since the size of the pulse and the type of the pulse wave are closely related, they are considered together in the following discussion, and some of the classic examples of disturbances in size and type are considered.

The pulse in aortic insufficiency. The pulse associated with aortic insufficiency is a pulsus magnus et celer (Fig. 9–20). It is a pulsus magnus because it has a high pulse pressure and a pulsus celer because it rises quickly and falls quickly.

The pulse in aortic insufficiency was first described in 1715 by Raymond Vieussens, who wrote that the "pulse, which appeared to be very full, very fast, very hard, unequal and so strong that the artery of first one then the other arm, struck the ends of my fingers just as a cord would have done which was very tightly drawn and violently shaken." James Hope, more

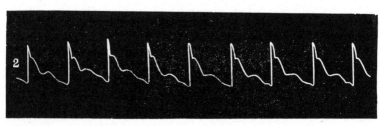

Figure 9–20. *Radial tracing of pulse in aortic insufficiency. (Marey, E. J.: La Méthode Graphique. Paris, G. Masson, 1878.)*

than a century later, described it as a jerking pulse, "the pulse of unfilled arteries." Corrigan wrote a classic paper on aortic insufficiency in which he called attention particularly to the throbbing carotids that are associated with this disease and in which he noted that the pulse was "invariably full." Corrigan's description of the pulse was so clear and vivid, his description of the clinical picture of aortic insufficiency so complete, that it has been customary since his day to speak of the "Corrigan pulse."

Other terms commonly used in designating this pulse are "collapsing pulse" and "water-hammer pulse." The term "collapsing" was applied since the extreme and marked change in pulse pressure imparts to the palpating finger the impression that the pulse has collapsed. The term "water-hammer" is more frequently used than understood. The water hammer was a toy or piece of physical apparatus widely used in the nineteenth century. A water hammer consisted of a thick glass tube about 1 ft. in length that was half filled with water, the air having been expelled by boiling the water just before sealing the end of the tube with a blowpipe. When such a tube is inverted, the water falls down through the vacuum like a solid body, and the hand feels a short hard knock. A similar sensation is often transmitted to the finger by the water-hammer pulse. The term "water-hammer pulse," according to Dock, was not used first by Corrigan, but by Sir Thomas Watson.

The water-hammer pulse has a high pulse pressure, the difference between the systolic and diastolic blood pressure often being 80 to 100 mm. of mercury as compared with 50 to 60 mm. in the normal person. This pulse is almost always associated with aortic insufficiency, but it may be seen occasionally in severe anemias, in arteriovenous fistula, in coarctation of the aorta, in patent ductus arteriosus, in ruptured sinus of Valsalva aneurysm, and rarely in Graves' disease.

Though this pulse is easily felt with the palpating fingers over the radial artery, it can best be felt by holding the patient's hand over his head.

The pulse in aortic stenosis. The pulse associated with aortic stenosis is the antithesis of that found in aortic insufficiency. The

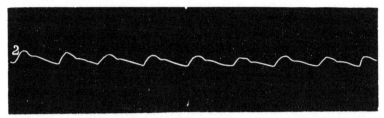

Figure 9-21. *Radial tracing of pulse in aortic stenosis. (Marey, E. J.: La Méthode Graphique. Paris, G. Masson, 1878.)*

pulse in aortic stenosis is small and hard, and it rises and falls slowly—a pulsus parvus et tardus (Fig. 9–21). The sphygmographic tracings clearly show this characteristic pulse.

Sphygmographic tracings in aortic stenosis frequently show two other types of pulse, the anacrotic pulse and the pulsus bisferiens. These two types of pulse will be considered later.

The pulse in mitral stenosis. The pulse in uncomplicated mitral stenosis is regular and small, but not feeble. It is the typical pulsus parvus. This small size is often of value in diagnosis.

Pulsus alternans. The classical pulsus alternans shows a regular alternation in the size of the beats. This pulse was first described by Ludwig Traube in 1872 as "a succession of high and low pulses, in such a manner that a low pulse follows regularly a high pulse, and this low pulse is separated from the following high pulse by a shorter pause than that between it and the preceding high pulse." Traube illustrated his article with the tracing shown in Figure 9–22. This alternation of the pulse is readily detected by the palpating finger, and occasionally is so

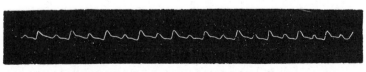

Figure 9-22. *Traube's tracing of pulsus alternans.*

striking that it can be seen on inspection, particularly on inspection of the brachial arteries in elderly arteriosclerotic patients.

Mackenzie regarded pulsus alternans as a grave prognostic sign. He states that he had noted this form of irregularity and had published some tracings in his book on the pulse that appeared in 1902. In 1905 Wenckebach called attention to these tracings and Mackenzie writes, "When I saw his account, I started to re-examine all my patients who had shown this condition (about a dozen), and I found they were all dead."

Pulsus alternans occurs chiefly in elderly patients suffering from myocardial disease, which is usually a result of arterial hypertension, coronary disease, or aortic lesions. This pulse is a cardinal sign of heart failure and is frequently accompanied by a gallop rhythm. When it occurs in the course of an attack of paroxysmal tachycardia or appears for only a few beats following an extrasystole, it has no sinister meaning.

Dicrotic pulse. A normal sphygmogram shows a second small wave on the declining limb of the wave produced by the radial pulse. In fever there is a marked relaxation of the arteries, and the dicrotic wave becomes exaggerated and can be felt as a small wave immediately following the pulse wave (Fig. 9–23). It is most marked when the diastolic pressure is low. The dicrotic

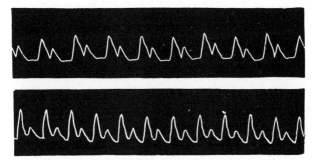

Figure 9–23. *Radial tracing of dicrotic pulse. (Broadbent, W. H.: The Pulse. London, Cassell & Co., 1890.)*

pulse is easily obliterated by slightly increasing the pressure of the examining finger.

Anacrotic pulse. The sphygmogram of the anacrotic pulse (Fig. 9–24) shows a small wave on the ascending limb of the pulse wave, analogous to the dicrotic wave on the descending limb. This pulse may be a result of aortic stenosis. Some observers consider it an artifact. It cannot be felt by the examining finger, and in diagnosis it is of no importance.

Pulsus bisferiens. The pulsus bisferiens is a pulse having two beats and showing two waves at the apex (Fig. 9–25). According to Broadbent, it differs from the dicrotic pulse in that the second wave of the dicrotic pulse is easily obliterated, whereas the pulsus bisferiens is brought out by firm pressure. Pulsus bisferiens occurs primarily in the presence of aortic stenosis and insufficiency. Its exact nature is unknown. Bramwell indicated that the second impulse is a tidal wave overlapping on the forcible, prolonged percussion wave. A combined aortic lesion may give rise to this phenomenon, since aortic insufficiency increases the force of the percussion wave, whereas aortic stenosis prolongs it.

Pulsus paradoxus. The pulsus paradoxus is characterized by a decrease in the size of the pulse, or even its momentary disappearance, during inspiration. This phenomenon is normally present during forced inspiration. When it occurs, not as the result of effort but during quiet respiration, it is pathological. The paradoxical pulse can be measured by placing a blood pressure cuff about the arm and measuring the drop in peak systolic pressure during inspiration. A drop of 5 mm. of mercury occurs normally. It is commonly found in patients who have constrictive pericarditis, but it has also been described in tumors of the mediastinum, heart failure, myocarditis, pericardial effusion, and pulmonary emphysema. This pulse is thought to result from the following mechanism: the downward movement of the diaphragm during inspiration stretches the pericardium over the heart, impeding venous return and subsequently reducing cardiac output. This mechanism gives rise to an increase in venous pressure during inspiration (Kussmaul's sign).

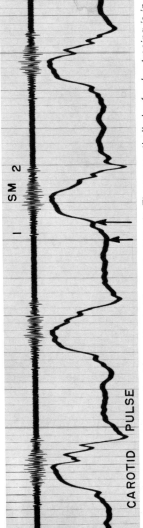

Figure 9-24. Anacrotic pulse in a patient with aortic stenosis. The anacrotic limb of pulse tracing is indicated by the arrows. **SM** indicates a systolic murmur.

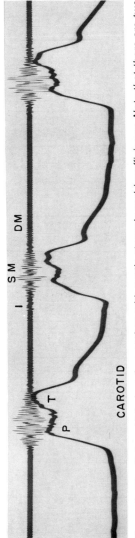

Figure 9-25. Pulsus bisferiens in a patient with aortic stenosis and insufficiency. Note that there are two distinct pulse waves, indicated as **P** and **T** (percussion wave and tidal wave). **DM** indicates a diastolic murmur.

RHYTHM.   The normal pulse is a series of rhythmic beats that follow each other at regular intervals—pulsus regularis.

The presence of an irregularity of the pulse, and therefore of the heart beat, is often the most significant feature of the entire physical examination. We should not forget, however, that a patient with a seriously damaged heart may have a regular pulse and that a patient with an excellent heart may have a definite irregularity.

This simple division of the pulse into pulsus regularis and irregularis was familiar to Rufus of Ephesus in the second century. Some of his descriptions of irregularities of the pulse almost allow us to make a diagnosis. "The pulsus caprisans is when a strong beat is followed by a weak one in such a manner that the artery appears ready for a new diastole without having entirely completed the systole" (extrasystole?). Until the early part of the twentieth century, however, the cause of cardiac irregularity was an unsolved mystery. The man who did the most to solve this mystery was James Mackenzie, a practitioner in the town of Burnley, England.

Mackenzie, at the beginning of his practice, saw many patients with irregular pulses. They were much disturbed and asked him what these irregularities meant. Unable to find out in any medical book or by consultation with colleagues, he determined to find out for himself and began taking radial tracings on all his cardiac patients, using a Dudgeon sphygmograph for this purpose. After several years' patient effort, he had collected a large number of such tracings but could make nothing out of them. He then devised an instrument of his own that took simultaneous tracings of the radial artery and of the jugular vein. His subsequent studies on cardiac irregularities were epochal and gave us a clear and entirely new insight into the origin of these irregularities.

Mackenzie's studies of the venous pulse showed that although the "movements in the neck seemed dancing, an analysis of a tracing refers each movement to a definite cause." He found the venous pulse to consist of three waves, one of which he labeled *a* because it resulted from the contraction of the atrium;

the second, v, from the contraction of the ventricle; and the third, c, from the carotid pulse. The v wave is actually caused by passive ventricular filling.

Mackenzie recognized three common varieties of irregularity. His classification has since been widely adopted.

Sinus irregularity. In this type of irregularity, the pulse rate is constantly changing, usually with respiration, and the palpating finger notes that the beats are equal in strength. Sinus irregularity is seen especially in youthful persons and, for this reason, was called by Mackenzie "the youthful type of irregularity." It is common in infants and can be induced in many persons by forced respiration, the pulse rate usually increasing during inspiration.

This type of irregularity is of vagal origin. The pulse slows on expiration owing to vagal stimulation and increases on inspiration. Sinus irregularity is not pathological. Mackenzie stated that "its presence indicates that the heart is healthy."

Premature contractions. These have been widely described as extrasystoles, which they usually are not, and also as "dropped beats." Mackenzie noted: "In many cases the finger fails to recognize the small pulse beat due to an early occurring systole." The finger receives the impression of a long pause, and then the normal rhythm is resumed. On listening at the apex of the heart, the premature contraction can usually be heard.

Tracings of such a pulse show the following sequence: a normal beat, a short pause, a small beat, a long pause, and a normal beat (Fig. 9–26). It should also be noted that the interval between the normal beat preceding the small beat and the next

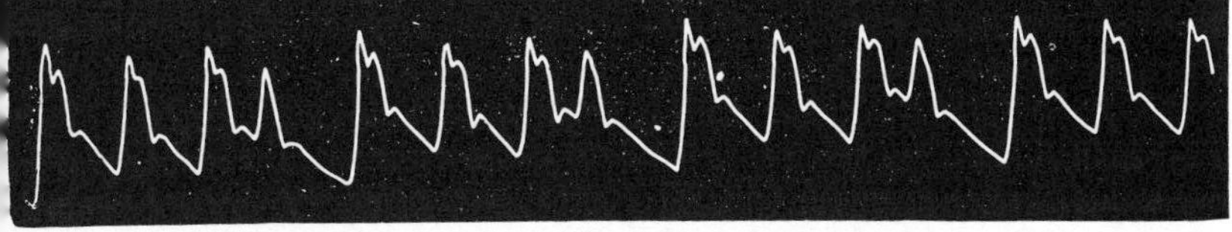

Figure 9–26. *Radial tracing of premature contractions (Mackenzie, J.: The Study of the Pulse. Edinburgh, Young J. Pentland, 1902.)*

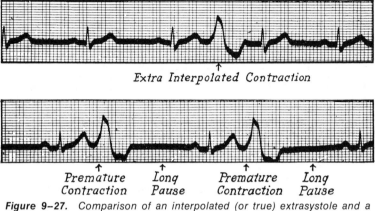

Figure 9–27. Comparison of an interpolated (or true) extrasystole and a premature (so-called) extrasystole.

normal is twice as long as the interval between normal beats. Mackenzie at first called this beat a "premature systole" but later spoke of it as an "extrasystole." Lewis and other observers have called it a "premature contraction." The term "premature contraction" is more accurate, since in most instances this systole is not a truly extra, interpolated contraction but is simply a contraction that has occurred prematurely (Fig. 9–27).

This premature contraction, as electrocardiograms and tracings of the venous pulse have shown, may have any one of three points of origin: it may be atrial, ventricular, or nodal (originating at the atrioventricular node).

In diagnosing premature contractions by palpation of the pulse, the important feature is the pause followed by a resumption of the normal rhythm. Premature contractions may appear in severe cardiac disease, but they may also be present for years without any apparent impairment of the heart. Mackenzie, after a lifetime spent in studying premature contractions, concluded that "when the extrasystole is the only abnormal sign, the prognosis is a favorable one, and where it is associated with other signs, the prognosis is to be based on the other signs."

Pulsus irregularis perpetuus. Irregularities in the pulse have been described for thousands of years, but in 1903 Hering drew attention to a particular type of irregularity that he called pulsus irregularis perpetuus — perpetually irregular pulse. Mackenzie encountered this irregularity early in his work on the pulse and described it as the "dangerous form of irregularity."

In this type of irregularity, there is a complete arrhythmia; beats follow each other at irregular intervals; and the strength of the individual beats shows great variation. This irregularity in both force and rhythm is readily detected by the finger and is graphically shown in a pulse tracing (Fig. 9–28). This type of irregularity differs from sinus arrhythmia and from extrasystoles in that these last two have a certain regular rhythm that is changed at times by the disturbing irregularity, whereas the pulsus irregularis perpetuus has no regularity at all.

The explanation of this irregularity began with the discovery by Mackenzie that tracings of the jugular veins of patients who suffered from this anomaly showed an absence of the normal *a* wave. In one of his old patients who had mitral stenosis with a loud presystolic murmur, Mackenzie saw that the appearance of this irregularity coincided with the disappearance of the presystolic murmur. Mackenzie came to the conclusion that this dangerous type of irregularity resulted from paralysis of the atrium. He reasoned that the *a* wave disappeared because the atrium did not beat, and for the same reason the heart was unable to pump the stream of blood through the narrowed mitral orifice with sufficient force to produce a presystolic rumble. He called the disease "paralysis of the auricle."

Later investigations showed the irregularity to be due to fibrillation of the atria. Atrial fibrillation was well known to physiologists and had been produced in the hearts of dogs by stimulating the atria with an electrode. As the electric current passes through them, the atria cease to beat regularly, and instead a series of twitchings or fibrillations occur at various points. Electrocardiographic studies carried out by one of Mackenzie's colleagues, Thomas Lewis, showed that the electrocardiogram in pulsus irregularis perpetuus was identical with that

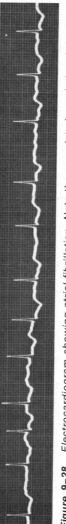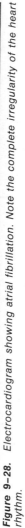

Figure 9-28. Electrocardiogram showing atrial fibrillation. Note the complete irregularity of the heart rhythm.

which resulted from electrically stimulating the dog's atria. Since this discovery that the cessation of atrial activity was due to fibrillation of the atria, the condition has been universally called "atrial fibrillation."

The extreme irregularity of the pulse in this condition is matched, of course, by the extreme irregularity of the heart. This led older writers to speak of "delirium cordis," a very descriptive term for the heart action.

Atrial fibrillation occurs most often as a complication of mitral stenosis, hyperthyroidism, arteriosclerotic heart disease, atrial septal defect, digitalis intoxication, or as an idiopathic paroxysmal arrhythmia. Mackenzie stated that 60 to 70 per cent of all cases of serious heart failure accompanied by dropsy owe the failure directly to atrial fibrillation or have had the failure aggravated by this condition. Embolism is a frequent occurrence in atrial fibrillation. Atrial fibrillation is not, however, incompatible with many years of relatively good health, particularly in the absence of a valvular lesion.

Pulse deficit. In atrial fibrillation many of the ventricular beats are so weak that, although they may be heard at the apex, they fail to come through at the wrist. If one counts the beats at the apex and at the wrist simultaneously, the apex rate is faster than the radial pulse. Upon cessation of fibrillation, this pulse deficit disappears. A pulse deficit also frequently accompanies premature contractions.

Heart block. Mackenzie's jugular pulse tracings showed conclusively that in heart block the sphygmograph often registers several atrial contractions before the *c* wave of ventricular contraction occurs (Fig. 9–29). This "epilepsy with a slow pulse" of Morgagni was due to the fact that some of the atrial contractions did not pass through the bundle of His and produce ventricular contractions, with the result that the radial pulse was markedly slowed.

Pulsus bigeminus. In pulsus bigeminus, the beats come in couples or twins, the second beat usually being somewhat weaker (Fig. 9–30). Pulsus bigeminus may be produced by the following two quite different mechanisms:

Premature contractions. When each normal systole is fol-

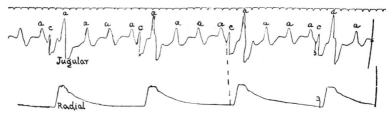

Figure 9–29. *Jugular wave in heart block. Four atrial beats to one ventricular—4:1 rhythm. (Mackenzie, J.: The Study of the Pulse. Edinburgh, Young J. Pentland, 1902.)*

lowed closely by a premature contraction, the premature contraction in turn is followed by a longer pause, and a coupling of the beats results. This coupling is readily perceived by the finger, and its mechanism is easily seen in an electrocardiogram (Fig. 9–31).

Partial heart block. When every third atrial contraction fails to pass through the bundle of His and cause ventricular contraction, a similar coupling of the beats occurs.

Premature contractions are a more common cause of the bigeminal pulse than is heart block. A bigeminal pulse frequently results from the administration of digitalis and disappears when use of the drug is discontinued.

Pulsus bigeminus is often confused with pulsus alternans.

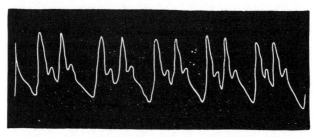

Figure 9–30. *Radial tracing of pulsus bigeminus. (Riegel.)*

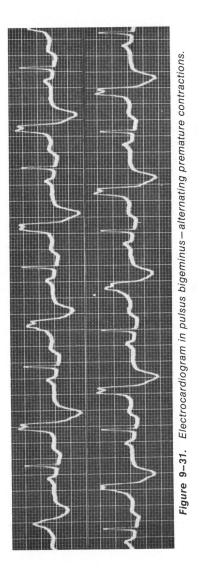

Figure 9–31. Electrocardiogram in pulsus bigeminus—alternating premature contractions.

In the latter condition, however, the rhythm is regular, whereas in pulsus bigeminus the weaker beat is followed by a pause. At times, however, differentiation may be so difficult that we must have recourse to a blood pressure apparatus, pulse tracings, or the electrocardiogram.

Pulsus trigeminus. In pulsus trigeminus every three beats are followed by a pause. This condition may result from premature contractions that replace each normal third beat, from heart block in which each fourth ventricular contraction is missing, and, according to Lewis, also from an extrasystole that replaces the fourth normal beat, this extrasystole failing to reach the wrist.

For convenience and completeness, Table 9–1 lists all of the recognizable arrhythmias, many of which may be recognized only with the help of the electrocardiogram.

TENSION. To estimate the tension of the pulse, it is necessary to use the fingers of both hands. Place the index finger of one hand distally over the radial artery, and exert firm pressure here to prevent the pulse from returning to the radial artery from the ulnar artery through the palmar arch. Then place the index finger and second finger of the other hand over the radial artery, exerting pressure with the index finger. The pulse is felt with the second finger. If the pressure necessary to obliterate the pulse is slight, we have a soft compressible pulse, a pulsus mollis, a pulse of low tension. If the pulse is obliterated with difficulty, we have a hard pulse, a pulsus durus, a pulse of high tension. The pulse tension corresponds to the diastolic blood pressure.

The normal radial artery is palpable only during systole and not during diastole. If the diastolic pressure is above 100 mm. of mercury, the artery may be palpable throughout the pulse cycle.

The older generation of physicians who estimated the tension of the pulse only with the palpating finger noted a low tension in fevers, in patients with failing hearts, and in nervous persons; high tension was associated with renal disease, gout, lead poisoning, and pregnancy.

TABLE 9-1. ARRHYTHMIAS OF CARDIAC MECHANISM

1. Atrial fibrillation
2. Atrial flutter
3. Atrioventricular block
   a. Incomplete A-V block (prolonged conduction time)
   b. Complete A-V block
4. Atrioventricular nodal rhythm
5. Escaped beats (ventricular escape)
6. Intraventricular block
7. Paroxysmal tachycardia
   a. Atrial
   b. Atrioventricular nodal
   c. Unknown supraventricular origin
   d. Ventricular
8. Premature contractions
   a. Atrial
   b. Atrioventricular
   c. Unknown supraventricular origin
   d. Ventricular
9. Electrical alternans
10. Sinus arrest (sinoatrial block)
11. Sinus arrhythmia
12. Sinus bradycardia
13. Sinus rhythm, normal
14. Sinus tachycardia
15. Ventricular fibrillation
16. Wandering pacemaker

A hard pulse or a soft pulse can be evaluated by palpation, but most attempts to estimate the blood pressure, in terms of millimeters of mercury, with the fingers, fail.

Vessel wall. The last procedure in palpating the pulse is to feel the vessel wall. In marked arteriosclerosis of the radial artery, the wall of the artery feels hard and irregular on light palpation; this is the so-called "pipe stem" or "goose neck" artery. In doubtful cases, the blood should be expressed from the artery by pressing the two second fingers firmly together over the radial pulse and then, keeping them on the artery, drawing them 2 or 3 inches apart. If the artery, after the blood has thus been forced out, can be distinctly felt by the two index fingers, it is definitely thickened.

The most common error made in palpation is to confuse the tension of the pulse with thickening of the vessel wall. In our experience, based on later pathological examination of radial arteries that had been palpated by competent clinicians, the diagnoses of "moderate" and "slight" arteriosclerosis are usually wrong. Palpation of the brachial artery may give a better appreciation of the degree of arteriosclerosis.

Capillary pulse. Capillary pulse is also known as Quincke's pulse, since the observations of Heinrich Quincke focused attention upon this phenomenon. It is best seen, as Quincke pointed out,

in the area between the whitish, blood-poor area and the red injected part of the capillary system of the nail-bed. In the majority of persons examined, there is, with each heart beat, a forward and backward movement of the margin between the red and white part, and he can convince himself that the increase of the redness follows a moment later than the apex beat and is still clearly systolic and rather rapid, while the backward movement of the edge of the redness seems to take place more slowly. That is, a lingering in the wave which can be seen by the eye, just as palpation and the sphygmograph show it in the pulse waves of the radial artery. . . . A large and rapidly falling pulse is seen especially in aortic insufficiency, and for this reason, the capillary pulse is especially clear in this condition. Even in a horizontal position of the hand, we see a very clear and rapid appearance and disappearance of the margin between the red and white zone and also a uniform coloration of the nail and lightning-like and evanescent reddening, so that the manner of the appearance and disappearance of the capillary pulse is, for the eye, a characteristic sign of active visibility of the capillary pulse in health, and in addition the transparency of the nails and the proper degree of elasticity of the arteries must be considered.

The pulse is often brought out especially well in white patients by rubbing the forehead until a red line is formed and then observing the change of color in this red line. Another excellent method consists of pressing a glass slide against the everted lower lip. The pulse may also be demonstrated by shining a light through the tip of the finger. The capillary pulse is most commonly seen in aortic insufficiency, but is also present at times in patients with hyperthyroidism or with severe anemia.

Venous pulse. The jugular venous pulse can be seen in most people. It is not palpable because of the very low pressure that produces it. The jugular venous pulse is best seen when the patient is in the supine position or has his head and shoulders slightly elevated. You should sit at the patient's right, with the patient's head turned away.

Since there are no venous valves between the right atrium and the external jugular vein, right atrial pressure is reflected in the external jugular vein. The sternal angle is 5 cm. above the right atrium when the patient is in either the supine or erect position. The vertical distance from the top of the venous column to the sternal angle is a measure of the venous pressure. Normally this distance should not be more than 5 cm. The venous pressure is elevated in right heart failure.

The venous pulse consists of an a wave due to atrial contraction, a c wave due to a transmitted carotid pulse and a pulse wave produced by an upward bulging of the tricuspid valve, and a v wave due to ventricular filling. The a-c waves are followed by an x descent that is due to atrial relaxation. The v wave is followed by a y descent which begins with the opening of the tricuspid valve and is due to ventricular filling (Fig. 9–32). The a wave is accentuated in pulmonary stenosis, pulmonary hypertension, tricuspid stenosis, tricuspid atresia, and Ebstein's anomaly. It disappears during atrial fibrillation. The v wave is prominent in tricuspid insufficiency, heart failure, and constrictive pericarditis. The x descent is absent in atrial fibrillation and tricuspid insufficiency. The y descent is accentuated in heart failure, constrictive pericarditis, and tricuspid insufficiency.

AUSCULTATION OF THE HEART

One of the first observations of the heart sounds was that of William Harvey. "It is easy," he wrote, "to see, when a horse

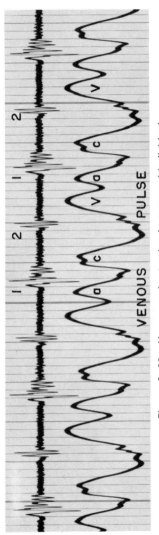

Figure 9–32. Venous pulse tracing in a normal individual.

drinks, that water is drawn in and passed to the stomach with each gulp, the movement making a sound, and the pulsation may be heard and felt. So it is with each movement of the heart, when a portion of the blood is transferred from the veins to the arteries, that a pulse is made which may be heard in the chest." Harvey's observations were not immediately accepted. Aemilius Parisanus wrote in 1647, "Nor we poor deafs, nor any other doctor in Venice can hear them, but happy is he who can hear them in London." This same sentiment might reflect the defeatist attitude of the novice as he first learns the art of cardiac auscultation.

Sound and Hearing

Sound consists of vibrations of the air that are audible because of their appropriate frequency and amplitude. There are three important characteristics of sound—*frequency, amplitude,* and *quality.* The frequency, or pitch, of a pure tone is the number of vibrations per second. Amplitude is the measured intensity of a given sound and is a reflection of the force that produced it. In addition to the fundamental vibration, which determines the pitch, most sounds have higher frequency components called "overtones." The combination of the fundamental vibration and the overtones determines the quality of a sound and permits the listener to determine the source of the sound. Two notes of identical pitch, one produced by a violin and the other by a clarinet, have different overtones that allow us to recognize the instrument that is producing the note. Musical sounds are composed of vibrations of regular frequency. Most cardiovascular sounds are composed of a mixture of vibrations of several frequencies.

Hearing may be defined as our ability to detect and analyze sound. The human ear can detect sound in the frequency range between 16 and 16,000 cycles per second (c.p.s.). We are most sensitive to sounds in the frequency range from 500 to 5000 c.p.s. Since the ear detects sound in a logarithmic fashion, a tone of 100 c.p.s. must be 100 times greater than a tone of 1000 c.p.s. in order to be heard with equal ease. Most cardiovascular sounds are near the lower end of the range of human audibility; 80 per cent of the frequencies that constitute the first and second sounds have frequencies of less than 70 c.p.s. The third and fourth sounds have frequencies of about 30 c.p.s.

When a low amplitude sound occurs immediately after a loud sound, it may not be detected. This hearing phenomenon, which is the inability to hear some sounds in the presence of others, is called "masking." This phenomenon makes it difficult to detect faint murmurs following loud sounds or faint sounds following loud murmurs.

Sound transmission is governed by the "inverse square law"; that is, the intensity of a sound diminishes in proportion to the square of the distance from the source. The quality of sound is altered as the sound passes from one medium to another. As sound passes through muscle, lung, and fat, the quality of the sound is altered so that the same murmur may have different quality when heard over two different areas of the chest. Other sensory stimuli may decrease auditory sensitivity. All of these auscultatory obstacles may be overcome by patience, training, and experience.

Listening to the Heart

The stethoscope is the instrument used to transmit sound from the patient's chest to the listener's ear. Appreciation of certain features of the stethoscope will be of considerable benefit in auscultation. The earpieces should fit snugly in the ears so that there is an airtight system from chest to tympanic membrane. If the earpieces fit properly, pressure on the diaphragm of the stethoscope will cause a painful sensation in the ear when the stethoscope is in place. The internal diameter of the tubing should be small, and the total length of the stethoscope should not exceed 16 inches.

There are two basic chest pieces, the bell and the diaphragm

(Fig. 8–24). The bell is best for transmitting low frequency sounds. It is important that the bell be placed very lightly on the skin. If the bell is placed firmly against the chest wall, the skin will be stretched taut and will act as a diaphragm. The diaphragm has a high natural frequency that tends to accentuate high frequency sounds but reduces the sensitivity to low frequency sounds. This gives the effect of a low frequency sound filter.

Valve areas. The areas over the heart where the sounds of the valves have the greatest intensity do not correspond to the anatomical location of the valves, as is seen in Figure 9–33. The mitral valve area is located in the fifth left intercostal space at the midclavicular line; the pulmonary valve area is in the second left intercostal space at the parasternal line; the aortic valve area is above the right second rib and in the right second intercostal

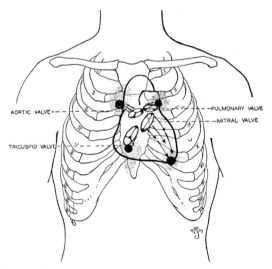

Figure 9–33. Anatomical location of heart valves and of the areas where sounds are best heard.

space at the parasternal line; the tricuspid area is over the sternum at the junction of the gladiolus, or corpus sterni, with the xiphoid process.

Abnormal sounds or murmurs arising from the various valves are usually heard at these valve areas, although their maximum intensity may be elsewhere, and their distribution may be quite different from that of normal sounds. These important features of abnormal valvular sounds will be discussed later.

TECHNIQUES OF AUSCULTATION. As with other techniques of physical diagnosis, the key to successful examination is the comfort of the patient and the examiner. The clothing should be removed from the area to be examined. The patient should be lying or sitting in a comfortable position with the examiner standing or sitting to the patient's right. All extraneous noise should be eliminated. The patient should be requested to breathe quietly and naturally.

Although most heart sounds and murmurs can be heard when the patient is in the supine position, the sounds and mur-

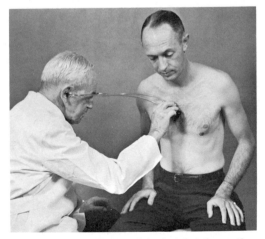

Figure 9–34. Auscultation of the heart at the aortic area.

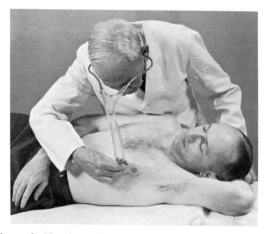

Figure 9–35. Auscultation of the heart at the mitral area.

murs originating from the base of the heart can be heard more easily when the patient is sitting and leaning forward slightly (Fig. 9–34). The faint murmur of aortic insufficiency may be heard only when the patient is in this position. The third heart sound, fourth heart sound, and diastolic murmur of mitral stenosis are often audible only when the patient is in the left lateral decubitus position. For these reasons the novice should always listen to the chest while the patient is in the supine, sitting, and left lateral decubitus positions (Fig. 9–35).

Since the carotid pulse rises shortly after the first heart sound, it is helpful in distinguishing systole from diastole. The apex beat may be used in a similar fashion, since it begins to rise shortly before the first sound. Palpation of the carotid pulse or the apex beat while listening to the heart is the best technique for timing murmurs (Figs. 9–6 and 9–7).

The human ear can distinguish sounds occurring 0.02 second apart. The human ear can also distinguish a single tone in the midst of many similar tones. This ability to discriminate is accomplished by directing attention to the specific sounds or tones we desire to hear. This well known phenomenon permits us to hear the violin in the midst of a symphonic rendition. It is important to concentrate on each heart sound, each murmur, each phase of the cardiac cycle in sequence so that you may properly appraise each auscultatory event. Certain combinations of heart sounds and murmurs develop a rhythmical quality. Duroziez suggested an onomatopoetic phrase (fout-ta-ta-rou) to describe the sounds associated with pure mitral stenosis. It is frequently helpful for the novice to think of this phrase as he listens for the murmur of mitral stenosis. An appreciation of other sounds may be obtained in a similar fashion by listening in the proper part of the cardiac cycle. By slowly inching the stethoscope from an area where the sounds are distinctly heard to an area in which the sounds are less clearly distinguished, one can perceive these rhythms and use them to identify the sounds characteristic of various disease states.

The Heart Sounds

Scientific study of the heart sounds began with Laennec's investigation of auscultation, and its application to the diagnosis of cardiac disease. Laennec wrote, "Normally this sound is double, and each beat of the pulse corresponds to two successive sounds: one clear, abrupt, like the clapping of the valve of a bellows, corresponds to systole of the auricles; the other duller, more prolonged coincides with the pulse beat as well as with the sensation of shock . . . and indicates the contraction of the ventricles." Laennec, as we see, believed that the first sound ("clear, abrupt") was due to atrial systole, whereas the second sound ("duller, more prolonged") was caused by ventricular contraction. James Hope, in 1835, after enumerating nine "erroneous or defective" theories, gave the explanation of the cause of the first and second heart sounds that is still widely accepted in the textbooks today. According to Hope, the first sound is caused by two actions: the closure of the atrioventricular valves and the muscular contraction of the heart. The second sound is produced by the closure of the semilunar valves. There has been unanimity of opinion that the second sound is valvular in origin, and many authorities still adhere to the view of Hope that the first sound has both muscular and valvular components.

William Dock, however, uncovered evidence that the first heart sound results from the sudden tension of the previously slack fibers of the atrioventricular valves. His experiments on dogs indicate that there is no muscular element in the first heart sound and that ventricular systole does not emit any sounds if tension of the atrioventricular valves is prevented. The weight of evidence now favors the view that both the first and second heart sounds are mainly valvular in origin. The first sound results mainly from tension or closure of the atrioventricular valves (mitral and tricuspid); the second sound results from tension or closure of the semilunar valves (pulmonary and aortic). Although the valve closure may not cause the sounds, the sounds occur synchronously with these events.

First heart sound. The first sound occurs with the onset of the apex impulse and corresponds to the beginning of ventricular systole (Fig. 9–1). The first sound is deeper and longer than the second and may usually be distinguished from the second by the rhythm. The time interval between the first sound and the second sound is usually shorter than the time interval between the second sound and the succeeding first sound (diastole is longer than systole). The first sound can be identified by placing a finger over the point of maximal impulse while listening to the heart. The rise of the finger will be synchronous with the first sound (Fig. 9–6). The carotid pulse is a reliable timing device, since it occurs immediately following the first sound (Fig. 9–36).

Since the first sound is a result of both mitral and tricuspid valve closure,.it has two valvular components. Normally, mitral valve closure precedes tricuspid valve closure. Ordinarily the time interval between mitral and tricuspid valve closure is short, and we are unable to distinguish between the two components. However, in some normal individuals and in patients with right bundle branch block, the duration of the interval is sufficiently

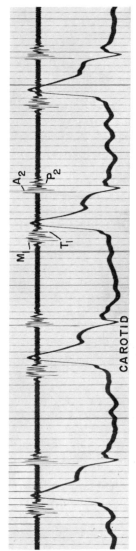

Figure 9–36. Phonocardiogram of split first and second heart sounds in a normal person. M_1 = mitral component of first sound; T_1 = tricuspid component of first sound; A_2 = aortic component of second sound; P_2 = pulmonic component of second sound.

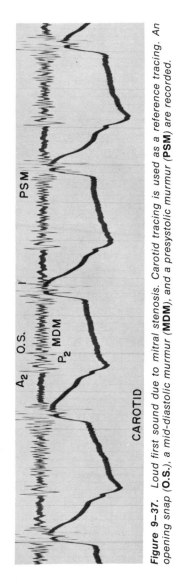

Figure 9–37. Loud first sound due to mitral stenosis. Carotid tracing is used as a reference tracing. An opening snap (O.S.), a mid-diastolic murmur (MDM), and a presystolic murmur (PSM) are recorded.

prolonged to allow both components of the first sound to be heard (Fig. 9–36). This splitting is usually best heard at the lower end of the sternum, probably because this site is nearest the softer tricuspid component, which is not well transmitted. The importance of the splitting of the first sound is in its differentiation from a fourth heart sound or a systolic ejection click. The term "splitting of the first sound" is preferred to "reduplication of the first sound," since the double sound results from the separation of the two major components of a "single" sound.

The intensity of the first heart sound depends upon the position of the valve leaflets at the onset of ventricular contraction, the pliability of the leaflets, and the force of ventricular contraction. If the valve leaflets are widely separated because of a prolonged flow of blood from atria to ventricles, they will swing through a greater arc in closing and will emit a louder sound (Fig. 9–37). This may occur when ventricular filling is prolonged as a result of obstruction of the atrioventricular valve or increased cardiac output. If the atrioventricular filling time is shortened as a result of tachycardia or a late surge of filling, such as occurs when atrial contraction immediately precedes ventricular contraction, the intensity of the first heart sound will be increased. In summary, the first heart sound will be accentuated in mitral or tricuspid stenosis, in conditions producing an increased cardiac output, in tachycardia, and in complete heart block when atrial contraction immediately precedes ventricular contraction.

The first sound is diminished in conditions in which sound transmission is impaired, such as obesity, pleural or pericardial effusion, and emphysema. If the mitral or tricuspid leaflets are calcified or immobile, the first sound will be reduced. When the heart muscle is weakened by myocardial infarction or myocarditis, the intensity of the first sound is reduced.

Second heart sound. The second sound has two components, one due to aortic valve closure and the other due to pulmonic valve closure (Fig. 9–1). Normally the aortic component precedes the pulmonic component. The aortic component of the second sound is transmitted over the entire precordium.

The pulmonic component is normally heard only over the pulmonic area. The second sound normally splits at the end of a normal inspiration (Fig. 9–38). This is due to a slight prolongation of right ventricular systole and a slight reduction in the duration of left ventricular systole. The split second sound can be heard by listening over the pulmonic area while the patient breathes quietly.

A great deal of information can be obtained by careful auscultation of the second sound at the pulmonic area. An unusually wide split of the second sound can result from a prolongation of right ventricular systole or a shortening of left ventricular systole. Delayed right ventricular depolarization, which occurs in right bundle branch block, results in a widely split second sound. In atrial septal defect there is an increase in the duration of right ventricular systole that is related to the increased diastolic volume of the right ventricle. This gives rise to the physical finding most characteristic of an atrial septal defect, the widely split second heart sound (Fig. 9–39). Right ventricular systole is also prolonged in pulmonary stenosis. The degree of prolongation is a measure of the severity of the pulmonary stenosis.

When pulmonary hypertension develops, right ventricular systole is shortened and either the second sound becomes single or "reverse splitting" occurs; that is, pulmonary valve closure may precede aortic valve closure. In aortic stenosis, also, the left ventricular systole may be so prolonged that pulmonary valve closure precedes aortic valve closure.

The intensity of the second heart sound is dependent upon the diastolic pressure in the aorta or pulmonary artery, the mobility of the valve leaflets, and the transmission of sound. The loudness of the aortic component of the second sound is increased in systemic hypertension and aortic insufficiency. It is decreased in aortic stenosis when the aortic valve is calcified and immobile (Fig. 9–40). Emphysema and obesity also decrease the loudness of the aortic component of the second sound. The pulmonary component of the second sound is increased when large left to right shunts exist, such as those that occur with atrial sep-

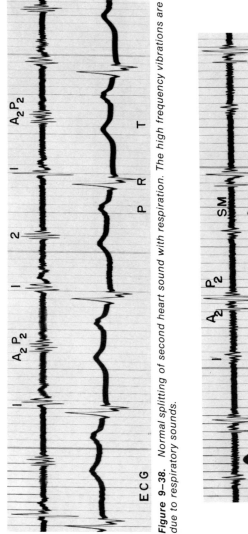

Figure 9–38. Normal splitting of second heart sound with respiration. The high frequency vibrations are due to respiratory sounds.

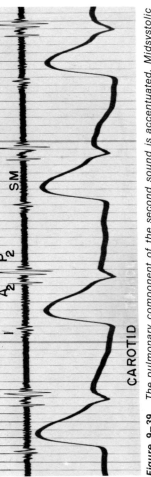

Figure 9–39. The pulmonary component of the second sound is accentuated. Midsystolic murmur is present (**SM**).

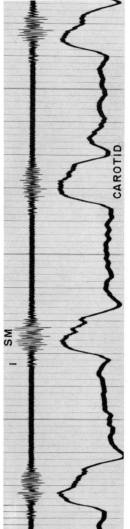

Figure 9–40. Midsystolic ejection murmur in aortic stenosis. The second heart sound is not recorded because of the calcified aortic valve.

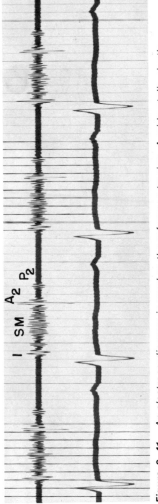

Figure 9–41. An electrocardiogram is used as the reference tracing. A midsystolic ejection murmur ending before pulmonary component of second heart sound is present. The A_2–P_2 interval is widely split.

tal defects, ventricular septal defects, and patent ductus arteriosus. Pulmonary hypertension also increases the intensity of the pulmonary component of the second sound. When the pulmonary component of the second sound is increased, it may be heard over a greater area of the precordium. If it is heard at the apex, pulmonary hypertension should be suspected. If the second sound is single, a comparison of its intensity at the aortic area with that at the pulmonic area will give some idea of the intensity of the pulmonic component, since this component does not ordinarily transmit to the aortic area.

The pulmonary component of the second sound is decreased in pulmonic stenosis (Fig. 9–41). When the stenosis is severe, the pulmonary component may be completely absent. It is usually absent in tetralogy of Fallot.

Opening snap. Sounds associated with the opening of the atrioventricular valves are normally inaudible (Fig. 9–1). However, in mitral stenosis these sounds become quite prominent. They have the same physical characteristics as the second sound. The mitral opening snap was first described in 1835 by Bouillaud, who referred to it as a "bruit de rappel." He described the rhythm of the first sound, second sound, and opening snap in mitral stenosis as that "of the hammer which after striking the iron, falls on the anvil, rebounds, and falls again motionless." The opening snap occurs shortly after the second heart sound and may be confused with a split second sound (Fig. 9–37). It is loudest at the lower left sternal border but may be transmitted to the base of the heart. The loudness of the opening snap is dependent upon the severity of the mitral stenosis and the pliability of the mitral valve. The sound is markedly diminished when the valve is moderately or seriously calcified. The time interval between the aortic component of the second sound and the opening snap is a reflection of left atrial pressure. In severe mitral stenosis the left atrial pressure is markedly elevated, and the time interval between the second sound and opening snap is correspondingly shorter. A tricuspid opening snap may also occur, but it is more difficult to hear and has less clinical significance.

Third heart sound. Thayer, in 1908, called attention to the third sound, the "early diastolic sound," when he wrote, "In certain young persons whose chest wall was not thick, palpation detected a slight shock, independent of and following the cardiac impulse. By means of auscultation, a third sound was audible, occurring shortly after the second heart sound during the phase of diastole and having the characteristic of a dull distant thud." This sound is a normal finding in most children and in adults. below the age of 40. It is heard most clearly when the patient is in the lateral position and is exhaling. The bell of the stethoscope should be held lightly against the skin over the apex of the heart. The third heart sound occurs about 0.13 to 0.18 second after the aortic component of the second sound.

The third sound is a very low frequency sound. The onomatopoetic phrase "lubb-tup-puh" may help to suggest the rhythmical relationship of this sound to the first and second sounds. The third sound is caused by the sudden distention of the ventricular wall when blood flows into the ventricle from the atrium during the period of rapid ventricular filling (Fig. 9–1).

The intensity of the third sound is dependent upon the cardiac output, the left atrial pressure, and the ventricular muscle tone. When cardiac output is increased owing to anemia, hyperthyroidism, ventricular septal defect, patent ductus arteriosus, or exercise, the third sound is loud. Mitral regurgitation gives rise to a distinctly palpable apical rapid filling wave and a very loud third sound; a similar situation exists in aortic insufficiency (Fig. 9–42). The flabby muscle of a failing heart is easily distended, giving rise to a very loud third sound that may be interpreted as a gallop rhythm. The loudest third sound occurs in constrictive pericarditis (Fig. 9–7).

A third sound may also emanate from the right ventricle; this sound is present in atrial septal defect and right heart failure. It is usually heard most clearly near the left sternal border.

Fourth heart sound. The normal fourth sound was first described by Clendinning in 1840. He stated that "the auricular systole is attended by an intrinsic sound resembling that of the ventricle, but more short, obtuse and feeble." The fourth sound results from distention of the ventricular wall due to left atrial

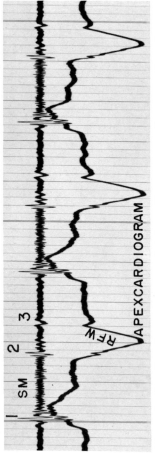

Figure 9-42. The phonocardiogram is taken with an apexcardiogram as the reference tracing. A pansystolic murmur is present. The third sound is synchronous with the rapid filling wave (**RFW**) of the apexcardiogram.

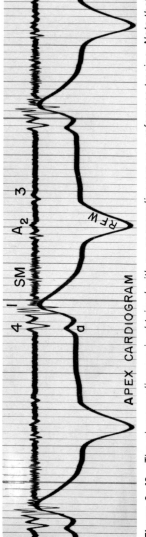

Figure 9-43. The phonocardiogram is obtained with an apexcardiogram as a reference tracing. Note that the fourth heart sound is synchronous with the a wave of the apexcardiogram. A third heart sound and systolic ejection murmur are also present.

contraction (Fig. 9–1). It precedes the first heart sound, is of very low frequency, and is heard most clearly at the apex, near the xiphoid or in the suprasternal notch (Fig. 9–43). A fourth heart sound is not always an abnormal finding, but it is usually associated with left ventricular hypertrophy due to systemic hypertension, aortic insufficiency, or aortic stenosis. It may also be heard when there is a prolonged P-R interval or atrioventricular dissociation. It is absent if atrial fibrillation is present.

A right atrial fourth sound may also occur. It is usually heard most clearly at the left sternal border, over the right precordium or over the right external jugular vein, and is usually associated with pulmonary stenosis, pulmonary hypertension, or atrial septal defect.

Ejection clicks. Early systolic ejection sounds were first described by Lian and Selti as "claquements protosystoliques." These high-pitched, early systolic sounds are caused by sudden dilation of the aorta and pulmonary artery (Figs. 9–1 and 9–44). The pulmonary systolic ejection click is heard most easily at the base of the heart and must be differentiated from a split first heart sound. It is usually associated with pulmonary hypertension, mild or moderate pulmonary valvular stenosis, or idiopathic dilatation of the pulmonary artery. The aortic systolic ejection click is transmitted over the entire precordium and is more difficult to differentiate from a split first sound than is the pulmonary click. It occurs accompanying aneurysm of the aorta, systemic hypertension, aortic stenosis, and aortic insufficiency.

Midsystolic click. Midsystolic clicks were initially thought to be due to pleuropericardial adhesions. However, most of these probably arise from the mitral valve owing to degeneration of the valve structure and elongation of the chordae tendineae. The sounds are due to the prolapse of the mitral leaflet into the atrium. They are pathognomonic of the so-called "floppy valve syndrome." They frequently are followed by a late systolic murmur. The click moves closer to the first sound when the patient moves from the supine to the erect position. This is due to the reduced ventricular volume (Fig. 9–45).

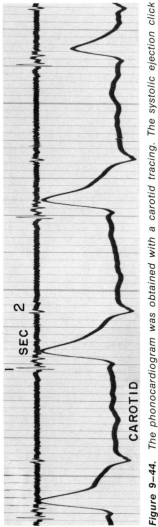

Figure 9–44. The phonocardiogram was obtained with a carotid tracing. The systolic ejection click (SEC) occurs on the ascending limb of the carotid trace.

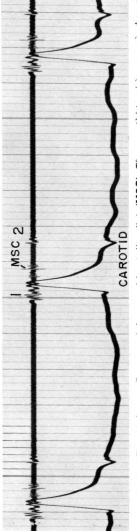

Figure 9–45. The phonocardiogram shows a midsystolic click (MSC). The carotid tracing was used as a reference tracing.

Gallop Rhythms

Gallop rhythm (bruit de galop) was so named by Bouillaud. The first published description of it was, however, by his pupil Potain. Potain recognized the concept that gallop sounds are an exaggeration of normal diastolic sounds. He stated, "If one auscultates a goodly number of healthy persons, one will not be long in discovering that diastole is not completely silent; that in the part of the cardiac cycle where the abnormal sound responsible for the gallop is located, there is sometimes already, in vestigial form, something which, when exaggerated, could become the sound in question." Potain's description of the presystolic or fourth sound gallop stated that

it precedes the first sound by a very short time but longer than that which separates the two parts of a reduplicated sound, much shorter than the short silence [between first and second sounds]. The sound is dull, much more so than the normal sound. It is a shock, a perceptible elevation, scarcely a sound. If one applies the ear to the chest, it affects the tactile sensation more perhaps than the auditory sense. If one attempts to hear it with a flexible stethoscope, it is barely audible. The place where one perceives it best is a little below the apex of the heart, somewhat toward the right, but sometimes one can distinguish it throughout the entire precordial region. The sound results from the abruptness with which the dilatation of the ventricle takes place during the presystolic period, a period which corresponds to the contraction of the auricle. It appears to be an indirect consequence of the excessive arterial tension which interstitial nephritis produces.

The only additions which can be made to these descriptions are that this gallop may also occur in aortic stenosis, aortic insufficiency, and coarctation of the aorta. This gallop is not necessarily a sign of heart failure. Since it is produced by atrial contraction, it cannot occur with atrial fibrillation.

The protodiastolic or third sound gallop is usually loudest at the apex. It is an accentuation of the third sound. The gallop cadence is a result of the increased intensity of the third sound and the shortened period of diastole that occurs with increased heart rate. The third sound or protodiastolic gallop is a sign of heart failure. It has been described as "the cry of the heart for help."

The mesodiastolic or summation gallop is produced by a fusion of the third and fourth sounds that occurs when the heart rate becomes so rapid that the atrium contracts immediately after the mitral valve opens. Since it is a combination of a third and fourth sound gallop, it is also a sign of heart failure. It may be caused by the failing hypertensive heart or by heart failure with prolonged P-R interval. Occasionally a quadruple rhythm may occur when both third and fourth sounds are present but not fused.

A systolic gallop may also occur. It is due to the presence of a midsystolic click and has no clinical significance.

Friction Sounds

Friction sounds heard over the heart and synchronous with the heart beat are pathognomonic of fibrinous pericarditis. Collin, who first called attention to this sign, described it as a "sound analogous to the creaking of new leather." He said that "this sound continued for the first six days of the disease, but disappeared as soon as the local symptoms indicated a slight liquid effusion into the pericardium."

The pericardial friction rub is synchronous with the heart beat and unaffected by respiration, which should distinguish it from a pleural friction rub or a pleuropericardial friction rub. There may be three components of the friction rub. They coincide with atrial systole, ventricular systole, and the rapid filling phase of early diastole. As the friction rub fades, the early diastolic component disappears first, the atrial systolic component next, and the systolic component last.

Pericardial friction rubs are not transmitted and nearly a century ago Stokes, one of the pioneers in the study of these sounds, noted that "in many instances we find that on removing the stethoscope but a single inch from the spot where the sound is best heard, it totally ceases, although we still hear the ordinary sounds of cardiac pulsation."

The pericardial friction rub changes in intensity with the position of the patient, increasing in intensity when the patient sits up. The sounds may also increase in the lateral decubitus position and in the supine position with the arms extended above the head during deep inspiration. Pressure on the bell of the stethoscope produces an increase in the loudness and distinctness of the friction sounds. This modification produced by pressure varies with the elasticity of the chest and is particularly evident in children and undernourished adults.

The character of the friction rub varies in different patients or at different times in the same patient. The sound has been compared in different instances to the rasping of wood, the grating of nutmeg, the rustling of silk, the crackling of parchment, and the creaking of new leather.

"It may strike the reader," Hope remarked, "as rather incredible that so many varieties of rubbing murmurs should be produced by a single affection; but his doubts will cease on finding that he may closely imitate the whole, even the creaking sound, by rubbing a damp finger with various degrees of force, and in various positions, against the back of his hand, while he listens with a stethoscope applied to the palm."

Cardiac Murmurs

Cardiac murmurs were first described in 1819 by Laennec, who mistakenly believed they were always produced by valvular lesions and added that "their situation, and the time at which they are heard, indicates obviously which orifice is affected." Later he denied any value to blowing murmurs in diagnosing valvular lesions, since he saw patients who had cardiac murmurs but showed no valvular lesions at autopsy. In this, Laennec fell into a second error greater than the first.

Bouillaud, Gendrin, Skoda, Hope, Forbes, and Stokes continued the studies begun by Laennec. James Hope's *Diseases of the Heart*, which first appeared in 1831, contained an account of all pathognomonic heart murmurs that are recognized today, each correctly described and its pathological significance correctly recognized. All these observers heard extracardiac as well as cardiac murmurs and speculated as to their causes. Potain systematically studied extracardiac murmurs, classified them, and advanced explanations as to their causes. The mistake made by earlier observers was largely a result of their attempt to determine from the character of the murmur alone whether or not it arose from organic disease of the heart. Potain showed that, with a few exceptions, there was no such single characteristic and that only a careful study of the individual murmur and associated physical findings would lead to a correct differential diagnosis.

Mechanisms of production of heart murmurs. Murmurs may be produced in a tube through which a fluid is flowing by four methods: (1), by increasing the rate of flow through the tube; (2), by producing a constriction in the tube; (3), by causing a dilatation of the tube; and (4), by inserting a taut string or membrane that vibrates as the fluid flows past. All four of these mechanisms are found to produce heart murmurs (Fig. 9–46).

The normal valves of the heart fulfill two functions: they prevent the backflow of the blood and they offer no impediment to the forward flow of the blood. Healthy heart valves fulfill these requirements perfectly. During ventricular systole, the mitral and tricuspid valves are closed and allow no blood to regurgitate; the aortic and pulmonary valves allow the blood to pass freely into the great vessels. During diastole the two sets of valves change their roles. The aortic and pulmonary valves are closed and prevent regurgitation from the great vessels; the mitral and tricuspid valves are open and allow free passage of blood from atria to ventricles (Fig. 9–47).

In a heart with a valve insufficiency, the valve does not close completely and an opening is left through which a portion of the blood regurgitates. This results in the murmur of valvular insufficiency. If a valve is stenotic or narrowed, the valve fails to open completely. The blood passing through this narrowed orifice en-

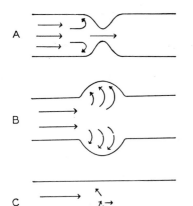

A

B

C

Figure 9–46. Methods of production of heart murmurs: A, constriction of elastic vessel; B, dilatation of vessel; C, vibrating flap in lumen.

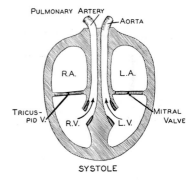

PULMONARY ARTERY — AORTA

R.A.   L.A.

TRICUS-PID V.   MITRAL VALVE

R.V.   L.V.

SYSTOLE

Figure 9–47. Diagram of positions of heart valves during systole and diastole.

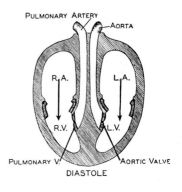

PULMONARY ARTERY — AORTA

R. A.   L. A.

R.V.   L.V.

PULMONARY V.   AORTIC VALVE

DIASTOLE

counters a resistance, turbulent flow results, and the murmur of stenosis appears.

Character of heart murmurs. Most heart murmurs are noises composed of vibrations of many discordant frequencies. Occasionally heart murmurs produced by vibrations of a single frequency have a musical quality. The pitch of a murmur depends primarily on the velocity of blood flow. When the velocity is great, the pitch of the murmur is high. This type of murmur is usually produced when there is a large pressure gradient across a small orifice. It occurs in pulmonic stenosis, in aortic stenosis, or with a small ventricular septal defect. Similarly, when the velocity is low, the pitch of the murmur is low. This type of murmur is produced when there is a small pressure gradient across an inadequate orifice and occurs in mitral stenosis. No murmur is produced by the large flow of blood across

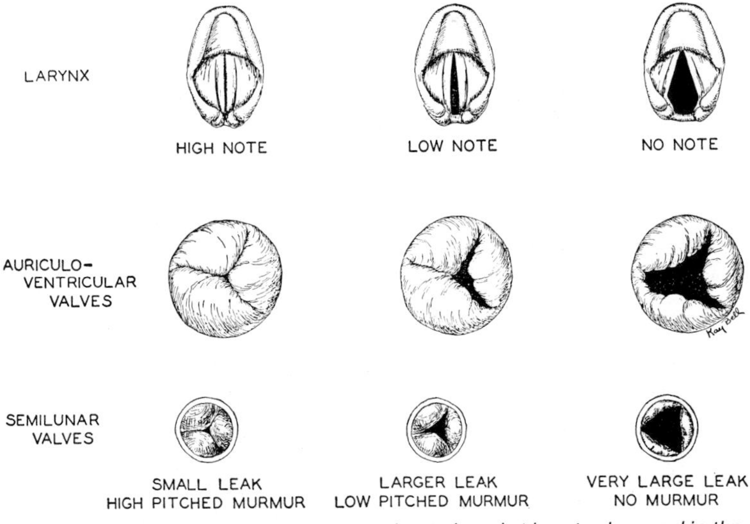

LARYNX

HIGH NOTE   LOW NOTE   NO NOTE

AURICULO-
VENTRICULAR
VALVES

SEMILUNAR
VALVES

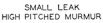

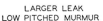

SMALL LEAK
HIGH PITCHED MURMUR

LARGER LEAK
LOW PITCHED MURMUR

VERY LARGE LEAK
NO MURMUR

Figure 9–48. *Similarity between sounds produced at heart valves and in the larynx. (Hirschfelder, A. D.: Diseases of the Heart and Aorta. Philadelphia, J. B. Lippincott Co., 1933.)*

an interatrial septal defect because of the low velocity of flow. The character of the orifice and the resonating properties of the surrounding structures also contribute to the character of a murmur. Hirschfelder has ingeniously compared a valvular orifice to the larynx with its vocal cords. When the cords are closely approximated, a high note is produced; when they are wider apart, the note is low; when they are lax and wide apart, the air moving over them produces no sound (Fig. 9–48).

Murmurs are either systolic or diastolic in time, occurring either with systole or diastole. They may also be characterized according to the valve area at which they are best heard.

Loudness of murmurs. Murmurs are occasionally so loud that they are heard by the patient himself and may be heard several feet away from the patient. This phenomenon was well known to Corvisart and Laennec and has been frequently observed. Loudness of murmurs, like loudness of heart sounds, is dependent on extracardiac factors, such as the thickness of the chest wall and the presence of emphysema. Levine graded the intensity of murmurs from I to VI. The numbers have the following connotation:

I	very faint
II	faint
III	moderately loud
IV	loud
V	very loud
VI	loudest possible

A Grade I murmur is the faintest murmur that is audible on the most careful auscultation. This murmur is not generally heard during the first few seconds of auscultation. Grade II murmurs are very faint murmurs which can be heard when the stethoscope is first applied to the chest. Grade VI murmurs can be heard without a stethoscope.

Transmission of murmurs. The point of maximum intensity of a murmur should be located. In general, this will correspond to the auscultatory valve area from which the murmur is originating. Murmurs are usually transmitted best in the direction of the blood flow. The murmur of aortic stenosis is heard best in the carotid arteries, whereas the murmur of aortic insufficiency is heard best along the left sternal border. The quality as well as the intensity of the murmur is altered as it is transmitted over the precordium. This alteration of the murmur is due to the distance from the source, the changes in conducting media, and the natural frequency of the chest wall.

Heart murmurs may be altered by respiration. Just as the normal heart sounds are increased during expiration when the lungs are contracted, cardiac murmurs may be more intense during expiration than during inspiration.

Systolic Murmurs

Leatham has proposed that systolic murmurs be classified in two major categories: midsystolic ejection murmurs and pansystolic regurgitant murmurs. Midsystolic ejection murmurs are produced by the forward flow of blood across the aortic or pulmonary valve.

Systolic ejection murmurs. Midsystolic murmurs may be produced under the following conditions: increased velocity of flow across a normal heart valve, stenosis of a valve or subvalvular area, deformity of a valve without hemodynamic stenosis, dilatation of a vessel beyond the valve, or a combination of these conditions. Midsystolic ejection murmurs of any cause have the following common characteristics: (1), there is an interval between the first heart sound and the onset of the murmur; (2), the murmur reaches peak intensity at some time during early, mid-, or late systole and diminishes during late systole, giving a crescendo-decrescendo quality; (3), the murmur ends before the appropriate component of the second heart sound (Figs. 9–1 and 9–40).

Aortic systolic murmurs. Aortic systolic murmurs are heard best over the aortic valve area. They are transmitted superiorly into the carotid arteries and inferiorly to the apex (Fig. 9–49). In some elderly individuals with emphysematous chests, the murmur is heard best at the apex and may be distinguished from mi-

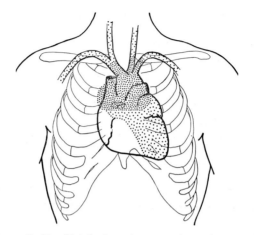

Figure 9–49. Distribution of murmur in aortic stenosis.

tral insufficiency because the murmur ends well before the second sound. The murmur produced by increased velocity of flow across a normal aortic valve occurs in patients with anemia, thyrotoxicosis, systemic hypertension, pregnancy, and in complete heart block. Since the rate of ejection and velocity of flow are greatest early in systole, all of these murmurs are characterized by early systolic accentuation.

The murmur of aortic stenosis was first clearly recognized by Hope who stated, "Its pitch, or key is usually that of a whispered *r*, from being superficial, and it accordingly conveys the idea of being near to the ear." In severe aortic stenosis, the murmur is harsh and reaches its peak intensity late in systole. Some elderly individuals with thickened and gnarled aortic valve cusps may have a similar murmur. This is presumably a result of the turbulent flow produced by the thickened valve leaflets. Similar murmurs also occur in the presence of an aortic aneurysm, dilated ascending aorta due to arteriosclerosis, luetic aortitis, and rheumatic aortic insufficiency. A dilated ascending aorta secondary to coarctation of the aorta may also give rise to a mid-systolic ejection murmur.

Pulmonary systolic murmurs. Pulmonary systolic murmurs are best heard over the pulmonic valve area (Fig. 9–41). When intense they may radiate over the precordium and into the neck. Pulmonary stenosis is usually a congenital defect and is frequently associated with other congenital heart lesions, such as ventricular septal defect or atrial septal defect. If there is a septal defect and the stenosis is severe, right to left shunting and cyanosis will occur.

Increased pulmonary blood flow is a frequent cause of a pulmonary systolic ejection murmur. A common cause of increased blood flow is a left to right intracardiac shunt due to an interatrial septal defect. Thyrotoxicosis, anemia, and pregnancy may also be associated with increased pulmonary flow and pulmonary systolic ejection murmurs.

Pansystolic regurgitant murmurs. Regurgitant murmurs are always pansystolic beginning with the first heart sound and continuing to the second heart sound. They are produced by the flow of blood from a chamber or vessel that is of higher pressure throughout systole than the receiving chamber or vessel (Fig. 9–1). This type of murmur occurs in mitral and tricuspid regurgitation, interventricular septal defect, and ductus arteriosus.

Mitral regurgitation. The murmur of mitral regurgitation or insufficiency is best heard at the apex of the heart, but is commonly heard over the greater part of the precordium. It is transmitted to the left axilla and may be heard in the back on the left side (Fig. 9–50). Laennec, who first heard and described it, compared it to the sound of a bellows—"bruit de soufflet." Stokes and other physicians of his time described the murmur as the "bellows murmur." It is usually soft and blowing, occasionally musical, and rarely harsh. The murmur is systolic in time because blood is flowing through a valve that should normally be closed during systole.

The lesion is usually due to rheumatic valvulitis, which causes shortening of the chordae tendineae as well as retraction of valve leaflets, preventing valve closure. Since the left ven-

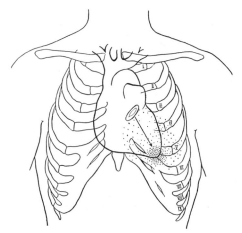

Figure 9–50. Location of murmur in mitral regurgitation.

tricular pressure exceeds left atrial pressure throughout systole, the murmur is pansystolic (Fig. 9–42).

Tricuspid regurgitation. Organic tricuspid regurgitation or insufficiency is rare, but functional tricuspid insufficiency due to dilatation of the right ventricle is not uncommon. It is usually associated with increased venous pressure, pulsating liver, and other signs of right heart failure (Fig. 9–51). The murmur is a pansystolic regurgitant murmur that has the same quality as the murmur of mitral insufficiency. It is located low along the left sternal border or at the xiphisternal angle. Frequently the intensity of the murmur increases with inspiration. This may help to distinguish this murmur from mitral regurgitation.

Interventricular septal defect. Perforation of the interventricular septum was first described by Henri Roger in 1879 and has since been known as Roger's disease. Roger described the murmur as follows: "A loud murmur, audible over a large area, and commencing with systole, is prolonged so as to cover the normal tic toc. It is maximum at the upper third of the precordial region. It is central like the septum, and from this central

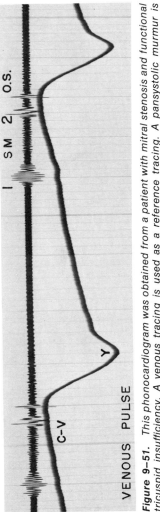

Figure 9–51. This phonocardiogram was obtained from a patient with mitral stenosis and functional tricuspid insufficiency. A venous tracing is used as a reference tracing. A pansystolic murmur is present. Note the diastolic collapse of the venous pulse.

point gradually diminishes in intensity in every direction. The murmur does not vary at any time, and it is not conducted into the vessels." The murmur is usually accompanied by a thrill. It is pansystolic because the left ventricular pressure exceeds right ventricular pressure throughout ventricular systole.

Continuous murmurs. Murmurs that continue through systole and diastole are caused by the continuous flow of blood from a higher to a lower pressure area (Fig. 9–52). This type of murmur is produced by patent ductus arteriosus, aortopulmonary septal defect, ruptured sinus of Valsalva aneurysms, coronary artery fistulas, and systemic or pulmonary arteriovenous fistula. These murmurs are characterized by patent ductus arteriosus, which is best heard at the second or third left intercostal space near the sternum and may be transmitted to the left clavicle, to the vessels of the neck, and backward to the interscapular area. It is described as a "machinery murmur" or, as described by Vaquez, "resembles the sound of a train in a tunnel." The murmur is usually accompanied by a thrill.

Diastolic Murmurs

Diastolic murmurs are produced by the flow of blood across the atrioventricular or semilunar valves during ventricular diastole. These murmurs may be divided into two major groups: ventricular filling murmurs and aortic or pulmonic regurgitant murmurs.

Ventricular filling murmurs. These murmurs are produced by obstruction of an atrioventricular valve, deformity of an atrioventricular valve without obstruction, and increased flow across a normal valve. Blood normally flows across the mitral and tricuspid valves during ventricular diastole in order to fill the ventricle in readiness for the next systole. Ventricular filling occurs in two phases: the first is a passive or rapid filling phase which may produce a mid-diastolic murmur; the second is due to atrial contraction and may produce a presystolic murmur (Figs. 9–1 and 9–53). A time interval is present between the sec-

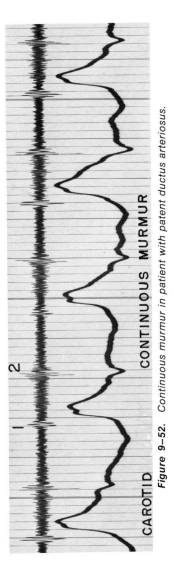

Figure 9–52. Continuous murmur in patient with patent ductus arteriosus.

DIASTOLE

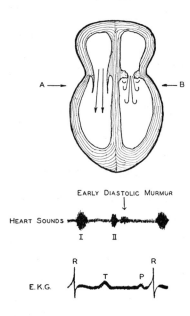

EARLY DIASTOLIC MURMUR

HEART SOUNDS

I   II

E.K.G.

Figure 9–53. A, *Blood flowing through normal valves in diastole produces no murmur. B, Blood flowing through stenosed valves in diastole produces early diastolic murmur. C, Blood flowing through normal valves during atrial systole produces no murmur. D, Blood flowing through stenosed valves in atrial systole produces late diastolic (presystolic) murmur.*

AURICULAR SYSTOLE

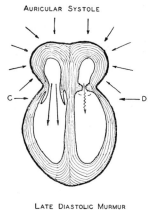

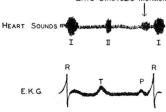

LATE DIASTOLIC MURMUR

HEART SOUNDS

I   II   I

E.K.G.

ond sound and the onset of the mid-diastolic murmur. This represents the time necessary for the ventricular pressure to fall below atrial pressure. The pressure gradient across the atrioventricular valves is small and the velocity of flow is correspondingly small, which accounts for the low frequency of these murmurs. Since very low frequency sounds are heard with great difficulty, these murmurs must have considerable amplitude to be heard and are poorly transmitted.

MITRAL STENOSIS. The murmur of mitral stenosis was first heard by Laennec, who described it as "bruit de scie ou de râpe" (noise of a saw or a grater) and compared it also to the noise produced by a wood file. Bertin pointed out its association with mitral stenosis, and Hope extended these observations. Duroziez invented the onomatopoetic phrase "fout-ta-ta-rou" and gave such a lucid description of "pure" mitral stenosis that the condition is frequently referred to as Duroziez's disease in the French literature.

The murmur is produced by obstruction to the flow of blood across the mitral valve during ventricular diastole. It is a harsh, low pitched, rumbling sound that is best heard at the apex (Fig. 9–54). It is not widely transmitted and frequently is heard only in an area as large as the bell of the stethoscope. The murmur is best heard with the patient in the left lateral position and the bell of the stethoscope pressed very lightly to the skin. It is sometimes necessary to have the patient exercise in order to bring out the murmur.

The murmur of mitral stenosis has two components, a mid-diastolic murmur and an atrial systolic or presystolic murmur. The mid-diastolic murmur is preceded by an opening snap which occurs about 0.05 to 0.10 second after the aortic component of the second sound. It corresponds to the passive filling phase of the ventricle and is produced by the flow of blood across the narrowed mitral lumen. This murmur is of longer duration than the presystolic murmur and is decrescendo in quality. The presystolic component of the murmur is produced by the powerfully contracting left atrium forcing blood through the constricted mitral orifice. This murmur corresponds with atrial

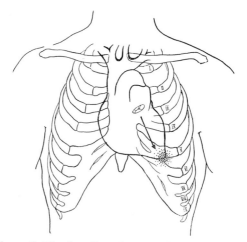

Figure 9–54. *Location of murmur in mitral stenosis.*

contraction, is presystolic in time and of short duration, and ends with a loud first heart sound (Fig. 9–37). The atrial contraction is absent in atrial fibrillation, resulting in the absence of the presystolic component of the diastolic murmur. This fact was known to Mackenzie (Fig. 9–55).

Mitral stenosis is usually produced by valvulitis occurring in acute rheumatic fever; however, the episode of rheumatic fever usually antedates the mitral stenosis by many years. Occasionally, a soft mid-diastolic rumble may occur with acute rheumatic valvulitis. This murmur is thought to be due to turbulence of flow produced by the diseased valve and is called Carey-Coombs murmur. This murmur has great value as a sign of acute rheumatic carditis.

Mitral mid-diastolic rumbles are also produced by increased flow across the valve. This type of murmur is heard in association with mitral insufficiency, ventricular septal defect, and patent ductus arteriosus. These conditions usually produce mid-diastolic rumbles associated with the rapid filling of the ven-

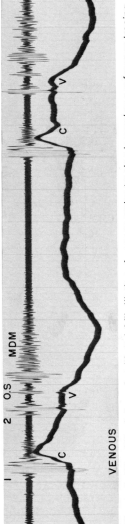

Figure 9-55. Mitral stenosis with atrial fibrillation. A venous pulse tracing is used as a reference tracing. The opening snap is synchronous with the peak of the v wave. There is no presystolic murmur.

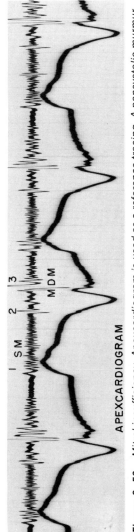

Figure 9-56. Mitral insufficiency. Apexcardiogram is used as a reference tracing. A pansystolic murmur and loud third heart sound are present. A mid-diastolic filling murmur is recorded.

tricle. The murmurs are usually short since there is no obstruction to produce a delay in ventricular filling. The diastolic filling murmur of mitral insufficiency is due to the rapid emptying of the dilated left atrium (increased flow across a valve) into the ventricle (Fig. 9–56). The frequent occurrence of this murmur with mitral insufficiency has led to the erroneous conclusion that mitral insufficiency is always accompanied by mitral stenosis.

The mitral valve may be obstructed in lupus erythematosus owing to verrucous endocarditis. Myxoma of the left atrium and large left atrial thrombi may also be responsible for mitral obstruction. All these conditions may produce mid-diastolic mitral murmurs, but the opening snap and loud first sound of mitral stenosis is usually not present in these conditions.

Austin flint murmur. This murmur was first described by Austin Flint, Sr., in 1862, in two patients who showed a diastolic aortic murmur, but who also had a marked presystolic murmur at the apex. At autopsy both patients showed aortic lesions, but normal mitral valves. Flint's observations have since been repeatedly confirmed and the importance of his observations has been generally appreciated. The Austin Flint murmur is frequently heard in aortic insufficiency.

Flint's explanation of the murmur is as follows:

In cases of considerable aortic insufficiency, the left ventricle is rapidly filled with blood flowing back from the aorta as well as from the auricle, before the auricular contraction takes place. The distention of the ventricle is such that the mitral curtains are brought into coaptation, and when auricular contraction takes place the mitral direct current passing between the curtains throws them into vibration and gives rise to the characteristic blubbering murmur. The physical condition is in effect analogous to contraction of the mitral orifice from an adhesion of the curtains at their sides.

This explanation accounts for the presystolic component of this murmur. The mid-diastolic component of the murmur is thought to be due to the impingement of the regurgitant stream from the aorta on the anterior leaflet of the mitral valve (Fig. 9–57). This displaces the leaflet into the stream of blood flowing from the mitral valve, producing a partial obstruction.

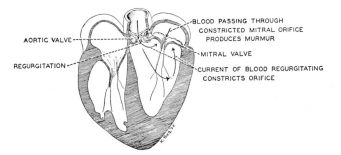

Figure 9–57. Diagram illustrating production of Austin Flint murmur. (Hirschfelder, A. D.: Diseases of the Heart and Aorta. Philadelphia, J. B. Lippincott Co., 1933.)

It is often extremely difficult to decide whether a patient suffering from aortic disease and showing a presystolic apical rumble has aortic insufficiency with an Austin Flint murmur or aortic insufficiency with mitral stenosis. On the basis of pathological findings the diagnosis of aortic insufficiency with an Austin Flint murmur is more often correct. A presystolic thrill is usually absent in an Austin Flint murmur and frequently present in mitral stenosis. If there is a small pulse instead of a bounding one, mitral stenosis is probably present.

TRICUSPID STENOSIS. This is a very uncommon lesion. The murmur is best heard at the lower part of the sternum at the left sternal border. The murmur is usually accentuated by inspiration because of the increased venous return. The murmur has the same quality and character as the murmur of mitral stenosis. The murmur may be produced by obstruction of the valve from rheumatic valvulitis, myxoma of the right auricle, or scarring secondary to a metastasized carcinoid tumor. A tricuspid middiastolic rumble is frequently heard when there is increased flow across the tricuspid valve because of a large atrial septal defect.

Aortic and pulmonic regurgitant murmurs. The aortic and pulmonic valves are normally closed during ventricular diastole. Aortic or pulmonic diastolic murmurs can occur only if there is incomplete closure of these valves, allowing the backward flow of blood into the ventricles. Since the diastolic pressure of the aorta exceeds left ventricular pressure at the time of aortic valve closure, backward flow across this valve will begin at this time and decrease as the ventricle fills. The pressure gradient across the aortic valve at the time of valve closure is great, giving rise to a high velocity flow and subsequently a high frequency murmur. Aortic and pulmonic regurgitant murmurs are high frequency decrescendo murmurs beginning with the second sound and ending in mid- or late diastole.

Aortic regurgitation or insufficiency. The murmur of aortic insufficiency was first clearly described by James Hope in 1831. Hope observed that "when there is regurgitation through the permanently open aortic valves, a murmur accompanies the second sound" and noted further that "it was louder and more superficial opposite to and above the aortic valves than at the apex," that it was "prolonged through the whole interval of repose," that it had "the softness of the bellows murmur, and inferior degree of loudness, and a lower key, like whispering the word awe during inspiration." It often becomes musical. The murmur is of high frequency, usually low amplitude, emanating from the aortic valve and radiating down the left sternal border (Figs. 9–58 and 9–59). It frequently is best heard at the third left interspace at the left sternal margin (Erb's area) with the patient sitting, leaning forward, and in forced expiration. The murmur is best heard with the diaphragm of the stethoscope. The murmur is so distinctive that it is rarely confused.

Aortic insufficiency usually results from rheumatic valvulitis, syphilis, hypertension, arteriosclerosis, and bacterial endocarditis. When the murmur has been caused by bacterial erosion of a valve cusp, it frequently has a musical quality (Fig. 9–60).

Pulmonary regurgitation or insufficiency. Pulmonary insufficiency is a rare congenital or rheumatic lesion. It is most frequently encountered in patients with pulmonary hypertension and is a murmur that is identical in quality and distribution to the murmur of aortic insufficiency. Although the murmur of pulmonary insufficiency begins with the pulmonic component of

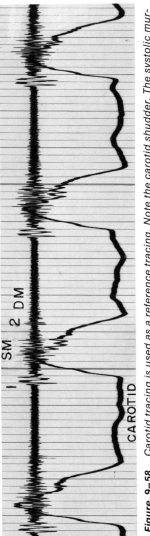

Figure 9–58. Carotid tracing is used as a reference tracing. Note the carotid shudder. The systolic murmur of aortic stenosis and the diastolic murmur of aortic insufficiency are both recorded.

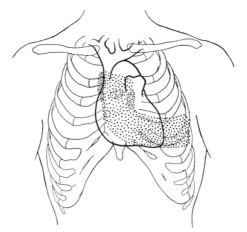

Figure 9-59. *Distribution of murmur in aortic insufficiency. Points at which dots are closer together indicate greater intensity.*

the second sound rather than with the aortic component, this feature does not usually permit clinical differentiation of these murmurs.

GRAHAM STEELL MURMUR.   In 1889 Graham Steell showed that in some patients with mitral stenosis an excessive pressure is produced in the pulmonary artery, causing dilatation of that artery with insufficiency of the pulmonary valve. This produces a soft diastolic murmur along the left border of the sternum. It is difficult to distinguish from aortic insufficiency and most murmurs that were initially thought to be Graham Steell murmurs have proved to be a result of aortic insufficiency. Physical findings of pulmonary hypertension should be present before considering a diagnosis of Graham Steell murmur.

The murmur of pulmonary insufficiency with normal pulmonary artery pressure is rare and distinctive. It begins a short interval after the pulmonary component of the second sound and has a crescendo-decrescendo quality. It is of short duration.

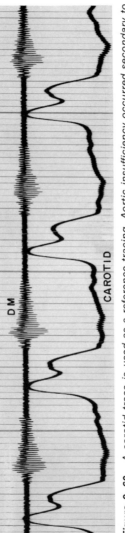

Figure 9–60. A carotid trace is used as a reference tracing. Aortic insufficiency occurred secondary to bacterial endocarditis. A loud musical murmur is recorded.

Functional Murmurs

In contrast to organic murmurs, which are produced by pathological changes in the heart valves, there is a group of murmurs that are not due to such changes, and the significance or importance of these is often difficult to determine. These murmurs are most commonly spoken of as functional, accidental, or hemic murmurs. They confused Laennec so much that he finally came to the erroneous conclusion that murmurs were of limited value in the diagnosis of cardiac disease. Potain made a most exhaustive study of functional murmurs. He found such murmurs present in one-eighth of all patients seen during his hospital service. They were present in practically all cases of Graves' disease, in 50 per cent of the cases of anemia, 5 per cent in measles and scarlet fever, and 10 per cent in pulmonary disease. He found the murmurs more common in young persons, the greatest frequency being between the ages of 20 and 30. There was a rapid decrease in frequency after the age of 30.

Functional murmurs may be classified as being of cardiac or cardiopulmonary (extracardiac) origin.

Cardiac functional murmurs. The most common functional murmur is the systolic murmur in the pulmonary valve area. White remarks: "It is the commonest of all heart murmurs, and if absent with the subject in the upright position, it can usually be brought out in the normal individual as well as in the cardiac patient by the assumption of the recumbent position, especially in full expiration. Therefore, the pulmonary systolic murmur may be considered to be a normal physiological event unless of considerable intensity in the upright position; even then it should be carefully analyzed before being called abnormal." Such murmurs are probably associated with slight displacement or distortion of the pulmonary artery.

Another common functional murmur is the mid- or late systolic musical or nonmusical murmur heard at the lower left sternal border or apex. These murmurs are frequently introduced by a midsystolic click. Although the exact cause of these murmurs is not known, it is thought to be of pericardial origin.

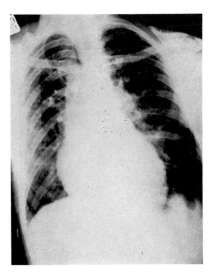

Figure 9–61. *Roentgenogram of of patient with severe anemia, showing marked cardiac dilatation.*

Murmurs associated with increased cardiac output or cardiac dilatation are also frequently classified as "functional" murmurs. These murmurs might be better described on an etiological basis, for example: a midsystolic aortic ejection murmur due to increased flow or a mitral pansystolic regurgitant murmur due to cardiac dilatation.

Extracardiac functional murmurs. These murmurs, better known as cardiorespiratory or cardiopulmonary murmurs, were first described by Laennec and later exhaustively by Potain.

Laennec, in 1826, noted that "in certain persons the pleura and the anterior borders of the lungs extend in front of the heart and cover it almost entirely. If one examines such a person at the moment when he notes the heart beats are rather forceful, the diastole of the heart compressing these portions of the lung and forcing the air out of them alters the breath sounds in such a manner that they imitate more or less closely the sound of a saw or that of a soft wood file. But with a little practice it is easy to

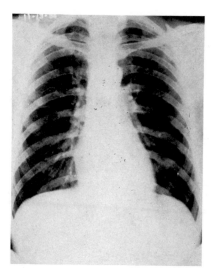

Figure 9-62. *Patient shown in Figure 9-61 after anemia was largely controlled.*

distinguish this sound from the bellows sound produced by the heart itself. It is more superficial. One hears below the normal sounds of the hearts; and on asking the patient to hold his breath, it diminishes markedly or ceases almost entirely."

Potain confirmed these findings and also showed that they are heard over areas where there is retraction of the heart, which produces a small area of increased negative pressure with a sudden expansion of the lung, causing air to rush in with the production of a murmur. This retraction is usually systolic and such murmurs are usually systolic, but occasionally the retraction is diastolic and the murmur is diastolic.

Hamman, in 1937, called attention to the presence of a "peculiar crunching, crackling, bubbling sound heard over the heart with each contraction." This sound may appear or disappear with a change in position. It occurs in mediastinal emphysema and is often heard without a stethoscope.

Auscultation of Blood Vessels

Arteries. In addition to the murmurs produced within the heart and transmitted to the arteries, murmurs may arise in the arteries themselves. A systolic murmur may be produced in a normal artery by compression.

The eddies in an aneurysmal sac may produce loud systolic murmurs which are transmitted for some distance along the arteries. A rough continuous murmur with systolic accentuation is heard over an arteriovenous fistula. Both types of murmurs are frequently accompanied by palpable thrills.

In coarctation of the aorta there is a soft systolic murmur over the innominate, carotid, and subclavian arteries and their branches. This is probably due to dilatation of the ascending aorta. A murmur is also heard at the angle of the left scapula. This may be early, mid-, or late systolic or continuous, depending on the severity of the coarctation.

In aortic insufficiency a loud first sound, or pistol shot sound, and Traube's double sound may be heard over the femoral arteries without exerting pressure.

Duroziez's sign is the "double intermittent crural murmur" in aortic insufficiency which, as Duroziez noted, "most commonly is not present and it is necessary to produce it by means of compression." On pressing the stethoscope firmly over the femoral artery in aortic insufficiency, one often hears this double murmur—"swish-swish." This murmur is usually not present unless the lesion is fairly severe.

Continuous arterial murmurs may be heard over the skull in the presence of arteriovenous fistulas, vascular brain tumors, and aneurysms; over bone in Paget's disease; over the thyroid in Graves' disease; over the pregnant uterus (uterine souffle); over the lactating breast (mammary souffle); and over a carotid artery partially occluded by an atherosclerotic plaque when collateral circulation is compromised. Bruits over the major vessels are usually due to atherosclerotic plaques which may represent sites of potential obstruction. The carotid arteries are accessible for auscultation in the anterior triangle of the neck, the vertebral arteries in the posterior triangle, and the subclavian arteries in the infraclavicular area. The renal vessels produce murmurs that may be heard in the flank or over the abdomen. The aortic and iliac vessels produce murmurs heard over the abdomen. The femoral vessels are easily accessible below the inguinal ligaments.

Veins.   A continuous humming or racing murmur is heard over the jugular vein in some cases of marked anemia and hyperthyroidism. It never ceases, occurs during systole and diastole, and has been called the "humming top murmur" and "bruit de diable." It is readily abolished by occluding the regular flow with a finger.

Loud murmurs are occasionally heard in cirrhosis of the liver over dilated veins connecting the portal and caval venous systems. This form of venous hum is called Cruveilhier-Baumgarten murmur.

PHYSICAL FINDINGS IN CARDIOVASCULAR DISEASE

Diseases of the heart and great vessels produce certain changes which can be recognized by inspection, palpation, percussion, and auscultation. The recognition of pericardial, myocardial, valvular, and congenital lesions is of fundamental importance to the physician. By physical examination he can establish a diagnosis, direct therapy, and determine the prognosis. In this chapter the outstanding physical findings in the most important cardiovascular diseases will be considered.

Pericarditis

Pericarditis may be due to infection, inflammation, neoplasm, trauma, certain metabolic disorders, and nonspecific or idiopathic causes. Pneumonia was the most common cause of pericarditis. Since the advent of antibiotic therapy, the incidence of bacterial pericarditis has markedly decreased, and nonspecific or idiopathic pericarditis is now the most common form of pericarditis. Infectious pericarditis is often the result of an extension of a pneumonic process from adjacent lung, pleura, or mediastinal lymph nodes. In this regard the staphylococcus and tubercle bacillus are still important etiological organisms. Infectious pericarditis may occasionally be due to a blood stream infection.

Inflammatory pericarditis may occur with acute myocardial infarction. The area of pericarditis is frequently localized to the area of infarction. Collagen diseases, such as rheumatic fever, rheumatoid arthritis, scleroderma, and disseminated lupus erythematosus, also produce an inflammatory pericarditis. Malignancies, particularly bronchogenic carcinoma, metastasize to the pericardium, producing pericarditis. Traumatic pericarditis may result from a stab wound, bullet wound, or a blow to the chest. Uremia is the most common metabolic disorder producing pericarditis. Pericarditis is often an unimportant but interesting complication of the disease and is frequently unassociated with symptoms.

Acute pericarditis may occur with or without effusion; this complication depends on the character of the exudate. If the exudate is fibrinous, no effusion occurs; if it is serous, an effusion appears. Three types of pericarditis are observed clinically: acute fibrinous pericarditis, pericarditis with effusion, and chronic constrictive pericarditis.

Acute fibrinous pericarditis. Acute fibrinous pericarditis is the most common and most benign form of pericarditis. The amount of exudate is usually small; the process may be localized to a small area or may be extensive. When the exudate is abundant, the fibrin may be in shreds, and the heart presents a shaggy or hairy appearance, the so-called cor villosum. The ancients considered such a heart a sign of great fortitude. According to Pliny, Aristomenes, the Greek hero who single-handedly put entire armies to flight, was found after death to have a heart "covered with hair."

Patients with acute fibrinous pericarditis may have fever.

The affection is usually painless unless the pleura or diaphragm is involved, in which case the pain is referred to the shoulder or chest.

Inspection. This is usually noncontributory.

Palpation. On palpation, fremitus due to the rubbing together of the pericardial surfaces is often felt.

Percussion. This reveals nothing abnormal.

Auscultation. The characteristic finding is the friction rub, which is triphasic but is not synchronous with the heart sounds. It may be an almost inaudible, soft, scratchy sound, or it may be loud and harsh, sounding like the creaking of new leather—bruit de cuir neuf. It may last only a few hours, then disappear and reappear a few hours later. This friction rub is most frequently heard over the right ventricle in the fourth and fifth left interspaces near the sternum, but it is often heard at the base. Its intensity may be increased by pressure over the bell of the stethoscope. It disappears when the pericardial exudate completely separates the visceral from the parietal pericardium, but it may persist in the presence of considerable effusion.

Pericarditis with effusion. Pericarditis with effusion is the direct sequel to acute fibrinous pericarditis and is usually regarded as its second stage. The physical findings are distinctive: they are due to stretching of the pericardium, pressure on the adjacent organs, or cardiac compression due to increased intrapericardial pressure.

Inspection. If the effusion is extensive, the patient may look anxious; the face is gray and cyanotic and covered with perspiration. Marked dyspnea may be present, the nostrils dilating with inspiration and the patient assuming a sitting posture for comfort. The superficial veins of the neck are engorged and distended. On inspiration the neck veins may become more distended (Kussmaul's sign). This is a reflection of the additional increase in intrapericardial pressure produced by the descent of the diaphragm. The venous pulse shows a rapid diastolic collapse or *y* descent (Friedreich's sign).

The cardiac impulse may not be visible. The disappearance of this impulse in a patient with acute fibrinous pericarditis is a sign that pericardial effusion is developing. The diaphragm and left lobe of the liver are pushed downward, causing a fullness in the epigastrium. This pressure on the diaphragm may produce hiccups. The stretching of the pericardium and adjacent pleura may also produce pain. Compression of the major bronchi produces cough.

Palpation. In large effusions the apex impulse is not felt. A pericardial friction rub may be felt in moderate effusions, but disappears in large effusions. In some patients the friction rub is felt when the patient is sitting, but disappears when he lies down.

Percussion. The area of cardiac dullness is definitely increased, particularly the absolute cardiac dullness. The outline of the cardiac dullness resembles that of a triangle with the base down (Fig. 9–63). The relative cardiac dullness extends further to the right and left in the fourth interspaces when the patient sits up than when he lies down.

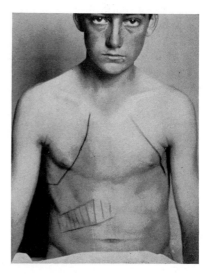

Figure 9–63. Outline of area of dullness in pericardial effusion.

Dressler has described a flat percussion note over the lower half of the sternum, on the left of the sternum in the third interspace, and to the right extending from the sternum between the third and sixth rib which he finds even more reliable than a single x-ray film in making the diagnosis of pericardial effusion.

Shifting dullness at the base of the heart is a valuable diagnostic sign. This dullness in the first and second interspaces, elicited best by direct or immediate percussion, shows a narrowing when the patient sits up. This change is the reverse of the findings in the fourth interspaces.

Rotch's sign, an obtuse cardiohepatic angle, may be present. The value of this sign is disputed by some observers.

Auscultation. The pericardial friction sound is usually audible with a moderate effusion, but disappears when the effusion is large. It may be heard in the erect but not in the recumbent position. When the pericardial effusion is absorbed, it may reappear.

As the amount of pericardial fluid increases, the heart sounds become distant and feeble.

Bamberger's or Ewart's sign is an area of dullness with bronchial breathing "at the left inner base, extending from the spine for varying distances outwards, usually not quite so far as the scapular angle line; commonly it does not extend higher than the level of the ninth or tenth rib" (Ewart). The area over which the sign is heard may be "no larger than the bell of the stethoscope or may occupy the entire left base of the lung below the tip of the scapula and extend from the midline in the back out to the posterior axillary line" (Christian).

The sign was first noted by Bamberger and later studied by Ewart. Pins, in 1889, described a similar sign found when the patient is lying down or seated leaning backwards; the sign disappears when he bends forward or assumes the knee-chest position. This has been described as Pins' sign.

Pulse. The pulse is rapid and small and may be irregular. A pulsus paradoxus may be present. This is a pulse which becomes weak or disappears on each inspiration. This pulsus paradoxus is, however, not always present, and is not pathognomonic of pericarditis with effusion.

The blood pressure is usually normal when the effusion is moderate, but falls as the amount of the effusion increases. A sudden fall in systolic pressure is a danger signal.

Chronic constrictive pericarditis. Constrictive pericarditis occurs when the fibrotic and thickened pericardium impedes the diastolic filling of the ventricles. The pericardium is frequently calcified. This condition is known as concretio cordis or hardening of the heart.

Inspection. The most important physical findings in chronic constrictive pericarditis are those of inspection. Although dyspnea is present, the patients are rarely orthopneic. There is moderate peripheral edema which is usually associated with ascites and hepatomegaly. The jugular venous pulse is elevated. Kussmaul's and Friedreich's signs may be present.

The area of the cardiac impulse may be broad and diffuse or totally absent. A systolic retraction of the rib and interspace in the region of the apex may replace the normal apex beat. The apex is fixed and does not change its position when the patient is turned first on the one side and then on the other.

Adhesions to the diaphragm may cause a marked systolic retraction of the eleventh and twelfth ribs in the back—the well known Broadbent sign.

Palpation. Palpation of the apex beat confirms the observation that it is fixed and does not alter its position as the patient's position is changed. The diastolic heart beat described by Skoda may be present. This consists of a systolic retraction followed by a diastolic lift of the apex beat (Fig. 9–7).

Percussion. Usually percussion of the heart is of very little diagnostic help.

Auscultation. On auscultation the most important finding is a loud third heart sound that is synchronous with the diastolic lift of the apex beat. This sound occurs earlier than a normal third heart sound and is considerably sharper. It is thought to be due to the early limitation of diastolic filling of the left ventricle produced by the rigid pericardium.

Pulse. About half of the patients with constrictive pericarditis have atrial fibrillation. In some patients a pulsus paradoxus may be present. The blood pressure is usually low.

Summary. In acute fibrinous pericarditis a fremitus is felt over the heart, which is synchronous with the to-and-fro friction rub heard on auscultation. There is no change in the area of cardiac dullness and no alteration in heart sounds.

In pericarditis with effusion, the precordium often bulges, and the cardiac impulse is usually neither visible nor palpable. A pericardial friction rub is felt in a moderate effusion, but disappears when the effusion is large. The area of cardiac dullness is increased. Shifting dullness at the base of the heart and an obtuse cardiohepatic angle are important findings. On auscultation, the pericardial friction sound may be audible in the early stages of effusion, but becomes fainter and disappears as the amount of effusion increases.

Chronic constrictive pericarditis is associated with hepatomegaly, ascites, peripheral edema, and engorgement of the jugular veins. A diastolic apical beat synchronous with a third heart sound is a helpful diagnostic sign. The apex beat is fixed and does not change its position when the patient turns from side to side.

Arteriosclerotic Heart Disease

Angina Pectoris. Angina pectoris has been recognized as a disease entity since the classic description by William Heberden in 1786. It is diagnosed from the history given by the patient. The disease may be readily feigned or simulated and you may find it difficult to determine whether a person is really suffering an attack of angina pectoris. Chest pain simulating angina pectoris may result from a number of neuromuscular disorders as well as from diseases of the thoracic and abdominal viscera. Heberden was familiar with this and observed that

the breast is often the seat of pains, which are distressing, sometimes even from their vehemence, oftener from their duration, as they continue to tease the patient for six, for eight, for nine, and for fourteen years. . . . There has appeared no reason to judge that they proceed from any cause of much importance to health, or that they lead to any dangerous consequences; and if the patient were not uneasy with what he feels, he needs never be so on account of anything which he has to fear. . . .

But there is a disorder of the breast marked with strong and peculiar symptoms, considerable for the kind of danger belonging to it, and not extremely rare, which deserves to be mentioned more at length. The seat of it, and sense of strangling and anxiety with which it is attended, may make it not improperly be called angina pectoris.

They who are affected with it, are seized while they are walking (more especially if it be uphill, and soon after eating) with a painful and most disagreeable sensation in the breast, which seems as if it would extinguish life, if it were to increase or continue; but the moment they stand still, all this uneasiness vanishes.

In all other respects, the patients are at the beginning of this disorder, perfectly well, and in particular have no shortness of breath, from which it is totally different. The pain is sometimes situated in the upper part, sometimes in the middle, sometimes at the bottom of the os sterni, and more often inclined to the left than to the right side. It likewise very frequently extends from the breast to the middle of the left arm. The pulse is, at least sometimes, not disturbed by this pain, as I have had opportunities of observing by feeling the pulse during the paroxysm. Males are most liable to that disease, especially such as have passed their fiftieth year.

After it has continued a year or more, it will not cease so instantaneously upon standing still; and it will come on not only when the persons are walking, but when they are lying down, especially if they lie on their left side.

Heberden notes further, and this point has been corroborated by numerous successors, that attacks could be brought on by "any disturbance of mind." John Hunter, who died during an attack of angina pectoris provoked by anger, had remarked for years that his "life was in the hands of any rascal who chose to worry him."

During a severe attack of angina pectoris the patient usually looks anxious. Drops of sweat appear on his face, and he stands or sits still and remains in this position awaiting the death which he thinks must surely come. The blood pressure may be high or low. A fourth heart sound may be heard during and immediately after an attack of angina in some patients. Paradoxical splitting of the second heart sound has also been reported during the acute anginal attack.

To many patients, the diagnosis of angina pectoris is terrifying. In spite of its serious import, it may not cause much impairment in the activities of some patients. John Hunter lived for 20 yeas after onset of his cardiac pains. Sir James Mackenzie and Sir Thomas Lewis lived 18 years after the onset of angina pectoris.

Heberden noted in one of his cases that "a very skillful anatomist could discover no fault in the heart, in the valves, in the arteries or neighboring veins," and successive generations of pathologists have reported the same lack of findings. On the other hand, the coronary arteries may, as in the case of John Hunter, be "in a state of bony tubes, which were with difficulty divided by the knife" or may show no more sclerosis than those of any other person of the same age. Although it is generally agreed that angina pectoris is associated with coronary atherosclerosis and reduced coronary blood flow, the exact mechanism of pain production is not known.

Acute coronary insufficiency. The term acute coronary insufficiency has been proposed to describe episodes of chest pain that last too long to be considered typical of angina pectoris but that do not produce clinical or electrocardiographic evidence of myocardial infarction. Except for the duration of pain, these episodes resemble angina pectoris. They are probably produced by more prolonged episodes of decreased coronary blood flow.

Acute myocardial infarction. Myocardial infarction occurs when a portion of the heart muscle is deprived of its blood supply for a period of time sufficient for cell death to occur and usually results from coronary occlusion. The first ante mortem diagnosis of coronary occlusion was reported by Adam Hammer in 1878. One of the first published reports on the clinical differentiation of angina pectoris and myocardial infarction was written by J. B. Herrick in 1912.

The appearance of a patient during an acute myocardial infarction may resemble that of a patient suffering from a severe attack of angina pectoris. The onset of pain in the precordium is usually accompanied by an appearance of profound shock. The patient's face has an ashen-gray color, and there is frequently a drenching perspiration, irregular pulse, and drop in blood pressure. The pain lasts longer than the pain of angina pectoris. As the pain subsides the patient's color becomes normal and the perspiration may disappear. The pain is frequently felt only in the abdomen and is associated with nausea and vomiting, simulating gallbladder disease.

Auscultation of the heart commonly shows some acceleration of the rate. Premature contractions are common and a third or fourth sound gallop rhythm is frequently heard. The first heart sound is soft. A pericardial friction rub is occasionally heard. Heart block or atrial fibrillation may immediately follow the attack of coronary occlusion and may persist after recovery from the acute attack.

The clinical picture of acute myocardial infarction is produced by practically no other disease, and the diagnosis can be made with a fair degree of accuracy. In addition, the patient usually has an elevation of temperature and a characteristic electrocardiogram. Occasionally there is no pain at all, and the only symptoms are fainting, dyspnea, syncope, and sweating.

The first myocardial infarction may prove fatal. However, the patient may recover completely and have no further attacks. More frequently he will recover from the initial attack but succumb to a subsequent attack after several years have passed. It is noteworthy that myocardial infarction often occurs when the patient is at rest or even asleep, whereas initial attacks of angina pectoris almost invariably occur during exercise.

Pathological studies have shown that occlusion of a coronary artery can be demonstrated in most patients dying from what had been previously diagnosed as angina pectoris. This does not, however, prove the identity of angina pectoris and coronary occlusion, since angina pectoris may occur in hyperthyroidism. The pain of angina pectoris, as Mackenzie pointed out, resembles the pains in the legs in intermittent claudication. Levine remarks, "Coronary thrombosis is related to angina pectoris in much the same way as an occlusion of a vessel of the leg with gangrene is related to intermittent claudication. The anginal state may be regarded as a transitory one leaving the heart in practically the same condition after an attack as before. . . . Sometime during the life of those suffering from angina a thrombosis of a coronary artery is apt to occur."

Hypertensive Heart Disease

The patient with essential hypertension does not have a unique physical appearance. The physical findings associated with hypertension are dependent on the severity of the disease. The effects of prolonged hypertension are reflected in the retina and may be observed on funduscopic examination. Changes in the retinal arterioles, such as increased tortuosity, segmentation, arteriovenous nicking, and thrombosis, are among the earliest signs. With progression of hypertension, the patient may experience hemorrhages, exudation, and papilledema. Papilledema is often accompanied by cerebral edema, in which case the patient may be somnolent and confused or may demonstrate focal neurological signs and have convulsions. This clinical state is called "hypertensive crisis."

Inspection. The apex beat is displaced to the left and downward. It may be in the sixth interspace at the anterior axillary line. A presystolic *a* wave may be noted in the apex beat, indicating left atrial hypertrophy.

Palpation. Palpation serves only to confirm the findings noted on inspection.

Percussion. Cardiac dullness is increased to the left.

Auscultation. Several auscultatory changes occur in hypertension. The intensity of the aortic component of the second sound is increased. An aortic systolic ejection click and a fourth heart sound may be present. If the heart rate is rapid and the fourth sound is loud, a fourth sound or presystolic gallop rhythm is heard. An aortic early systolic ejection murmur is often present. With severe hypertension an aortic diastolic regurgitant murmur may be heard along the left sternal border.

Pulse. The pulse is usually firm (pulsus durus), but the amplitude may vary considerably.

Cor Pulmonale

The term cor pulmonale has been used to categorize a group of cardiovascular disorders developing secondary to disease of the lung parenchyma. The most frequent causes are bronchiectasis, emphysema, tuberculosis, sarcoidosis, silicosis, and carcinomatosis. Multiple small pulmonary emboli may produce cor pulmonale (Castleman-Bland syndrome). The chief symptoms are dyspnea, chest pain, headache, and syncope.

Inspection. The patient appears dyspneic and is frequently cyanotic. Clubbing of the fingers and toes is present. The neck veins are distended and a prominent *a* wave is seen in the jugular pulse.

Palpation. A right ventricular heave as well as the shock of pulmonary valve closure is palpable.

Percussion. The cardiac dullness may be diminished by the overlying lung if pulmonary emphysema is present.

Auscultation. The auscultatory findings of cor pulmonale are similar to those of systemic hypertension except that the extra sounds and murmurs arise from the right heart. These findings are sometimes dampened by the over-distended lungs or are completely obliterated by respiratory sounds. The auscultatory findings include a fourth heart sound, a pulmonary systolic ejection click, an accentuated pulmonary component of the second heart sound, a pulmonary diastolic regurgitant murmur due to pulmonary valvular insufficiency, and a short pulmonary systolic ejection murmur. Tricuspid insufficiency is a common complication of cor pulmonale.

Similar findings occur in idiopathic pulmonary hypertension and in heart disease secondary to marked chest deformity (Fig. 9–64). Severe cor pulmonale with marked polycythemia and cyanosis is known as Ayerza's disease.

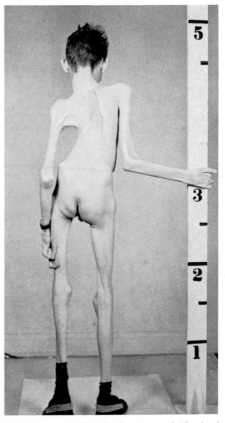

Figure 9-64. *Marked chest deformity in a boy of 15 who had an attack of poliomyelitis at the age of 9. Patient has cor pulmonale with myocardial insufficiency.*

Myocarditis and Myocardial Disease

Although there are many diseases that primarily affect the heart muscle, they comprise a very small percentage of patients with heart disease. This group of illnesses produces symptoms because the weakened myocardium is unable to maintain adequate cardiac output.

Myocarditis of infectious origin may be caused by viral infections such as influenza and infectious mononucleosis; by bacterial infections such as diphtheria, tuberculosis, and typhoid fever; by fungal infections such as histoplasmosis; and by parasitic infections such as toxoplasmosis. Fiedler's myocarditis is an idiopathic form of myocarditis.

Many of the collagen diseases cause inflammation and degeneration of the heart muscle. Systemic disorders, such as primary amyloidosis, hemochromatosis, progressive muscular dystrophy, thyrotoxicosis, and myxedema, produce myocardial degeneration. Myocardial degeneration may also result from the toxic effects of alcohol, emetine, potassium, and quinidine. Primary and secondary tumors of the myocardium produce a similar clinical picture.

Inspection. The patient frequently has a pale, waxy appearance. The skin may be cool and moist. The venous pressure is elevated and the neck veins are engorged. The point of maximal impulse is displaced to the left and inferiorly. The rapid filling wave may be the most prominent wave of the apex beat.

Palpation. Palpation serves to confirm the findings noted on inspection.

Percussion. The area of cardiac dullness is increased.

Auscultation. The first sound is diminished. A third sound, fourth sound, or summation gallop rhythm is usually present. There are no characteristic heart murmurs.

Pulse. The systolic pressure is low but the diastolic pressure is normal, resulting in a low pulse pressure and pulsus parvus. Atrial fibrillation and heart block are frequent complications. A pulsus alternans is frequently present.

Heart Failure

Heart failure occurs clinically when the heart is unable to maintain a cardiac output adequate for the patient's needs in spite of an adequate venous return.

Heart failure usually results from valvular lesions, chronic arterial hypertension, and myocardial infarction due to coronary occlusion. Less common causes are rheumatic carditis, thyrotoxicosis, congenital heart lesions, anemia, and uncontrolled tachycardia such as atrial fibrillation, atrial flutter, and paroxysmal atrial tachycardia. Several mechanisms are responsible for heart failure. Backward failure occurs when the ventricle cannot maintain a given work load. Forward failure occurs when the kidneys are unable to excrete salt and water load. Heart failure may be due to failure of the left ventricle, the right ventricle, or both. Failure of the left ventricle is more common and is the most common cause of right ventricular failure.

Left ventricular failure.   The earliest and chief symptom of left ventricular failure is dyspnea while at rest or when carrying out some physical activity which previously caused no discomfort. Dyspnea at rest is especially marked when the patient lies down (orthopnea) and may be relieved when he sits up. The onset of congestive heart failure in many patients coincides with the time they find it necessary to sleep sitting up in a chair instead of lying down in bed.

One striking type of dyspnea seen in left ventricular failure is acute paroxysmal nocturnal dyspnea, the patient being awakened with a sense of suffocating. This may be associated with signs of acute pulmonary edema. Acute paroxysmal nocturnal dyspnea, when associated with an asthmatic type of breathing, is called cardiac asthma. It resembles bronchial asthma so closely that a differential diagnosis may be difficult.

Inspection.   The patient is dyspneic and orthopneic. Cheyne-Stokes respiration is often present and cyanosis may appear. The point of maximal impulse is frequently displaced to the left and inferiorly as a result of the left ventricular dilatation and hypertrophy. A significant rapid filling wave may be noted in the apex beat.

Palpation and percussion. Palpation and percussion are helpful in confirming the left ventricular enlargement. If a pleural effusion is present, dullness and absent tactile fremitus will be noted.

Auscultation. The first sound is diminished. The pulmonary component of the second sound is frequently accentuated. A third sound or protodiastolic gallop is heard. Large moist râles and expiratory wheezes are heard in the lungs.

Pulse. The pulse rate is usually rapid. A pulsus alternans may be present.

Right ventricular failure. Right heart failure is characterized by systemic venous congestion and edema. Although left ventricular failure is the most common cause of right ventricular failure, right ventricular failure may occur in pure form with pulmonary hypertension, pulmonary embolus, pulmonary stenosis, and an atrial septal defect.

Inspection. The jugular venous pressure is elevated. Peripheral edema and ascites are present.

Palpation. Hepatosplenomegaly is present. The liver may be tender and pulsatile. The pitting characteristic of the edema can be fully appreciated by palpation. A hepatic jugular reflex may be noted by compressing the liver.

Chronic Valvular Heart Disease

Rheumatic fever is the most common cause of chronic valvular heart disease. Aneurysms of the ascending aorta may produce insufficiency. They are caused by lues, arteriosclerosis, Marfan's syndrome, or cystic medial necrosis. The mitral valve may be damaged in lupus erythematosus (Libman-Sacks disease), bacterial endocarditis, spontaneous degeneration (floppy valve syndrome), papillary muscle dysfunction, calcification of the mitral annulus, heart failure, and ventricular aneurysm. In older persons arteriosclerosis is a common cause of valvular disease.

Compiling statistics in more than 3000 cases, White found the mitral valve to be involved in 70 to 85 per cent of the cases, the aortic valve in 42 to 45 per cent, the tricuspid valve in 10 to 15 per cent, and the pulmonary valve in approximately 1 per cent. The mitral valve alone was diseased in 50 to 60 per cent, the aortic valve alone in 10 to 20 per cent.

Mitral stenosis.   Mitral stenosis demonstrates the serious aftereffects of acute rheumatic fever. It does not become clinically significant until many years after the initial injury. The lesion is more common in females than in males. The chief symptoms of mitral stenosis are dyspnea and hemoptysis.

Inspection.   Patients commonly have flushed cheeks. The point of maximal impulse is characteristically imperceptible in mitral stenosis.

Palpation.   The apex beat frequently cannot be located even by palpation. A presystolic thrill is often palpable and has been likened to a cat's purr. It is usually localized to a very small area near the apex. It has a very definite crescendo quality ending with the shock of mitral valve closure. The thrill may be present only after the patient has exercised. It is one of the most distinctive findings in physical diagnosis.

Percussion.   Percussion usually is of limited value since the primary cardiac enlargement occurs in the left atrium, which is posterior. When mitral stenosis is accompanied by severe pulmonary hypertension, the pulmonary artery may be enlarged. This can be percussed in the second interspace (Fig. 9–65).

Auscultation.   The characteristic auscultatory findings of mitral stenosis are a loud first sound, an opening snap, a mid-diastolic rumble, a presystolic rumble, and an accentuated pulmonary component of the second sound (Figs. 9–37 and 9–55). The presystolic murmur is associated with atrial contraction and disappears when atrial fibrillation occurs. The accentuated pulmonary component of the second sound is related to the degree of pulmonary hypertension. If the pulmonary hypertension attains sufficient severity, a diastolic regurgitant murmur can be heard at the left sternal border. This murmur of pulmonary insufficiency is the Graham Steell murmur. The loudness of the first sound and the opening snap are a clue to the pliability of the mitral valve. These sounds are diminished if the

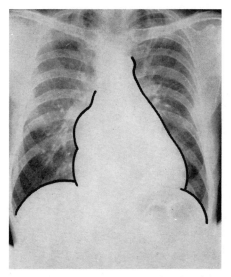

Figure 9-65. *X-ray of heart in mitral stenosis, showing convexity of left border and enlargement of the left atrium.*

mitral valve is fibrotic or calcified. The time interval between the aortic component of the second sound and the opening snap is a reflection of the severity of the mitral stenosis. The more severe the lesion, the closer the interval.

Pulse. The pulse of mitral stenosis is the pulsus parvus. Atrial fibrillation, a common complication of mitral stenosis, produces a characteristic totally irregular pulse.

Mitral insufficiency. Mitral insufficiency may be due to many different cardiovascular problems, including rheumatic carditis, bacterial endocarditis, Marfan's syndrome, spontaneous degeneration of the valve and its substructure, papillary muscle dysfunction, calcification of the mitral annulus, ventricular dilatation, and ventricular aneurysm. Palpitations and easy fatigability, the symptoms of mitral insufficiency, are much less striking than those of mitral stenosis.

Inspection. The apex beat is displaced to the left of the midclavicular line in the fifth or sixth interspace. It is hyperactive and a rapid filling wave is frequently seen.

Palpation. In addition to confirming the location of the point of maximal impulse, palpation helps to confirm the strong forceful character of the apex beat. The rapid filling impulse is often palpable. A systolic thrill may be felt at the apex. A left parasternal systolic lift is often present.

Percussion. Cardiac dullness is increased to the left, and may also be increased to the right.

Auscultation. The characteristic auscultatory findings of mitral insufficiency are a normal first sound, an apical pansystolic regurgitant murmur that encloses both the first and second sounds, and a loud third heart sound. The apical pansystolic murmur transmits to the axilla. A short mid-diastolic apical rumble is frequently present and is usually due to increased flow across the mitral valve rather than to organic obstruction (Figs. 9–42 and 9–56). The "floppy valve syndrome" produces a distinctive group of auscultatory findings. These are a midsystolic click followed by a late systolic murmur. When the patient assumes the sitting or standing position, the click moves closer to the first heart sound and the murmur becomes longer and louder. When mitral insufficiency results from rupture of the chordae tendineae of the anterior leaflet, the murmur may transmit to the top of the head.

Pulse. The peripheral pulse is small (pulsus parvus) and has an abrupt rise (pulsus celer).

Aortic insufficiency. Aortic insufficiency may result from rheumatic fever, syphilis, hypertension, aortic aneurysm, or arteriosclerosis. The condition usually does not produce symptoms until left heart failure occurs. The physical signs in aortic insufficiency are usually quite distinctive.

Inspection. On observing the head, it is often seen to jerk slightly with each heart beat—de Musset's sign. Inspection of the neck shows marked throbbing of both carotid arteries, one of the most distinctive signs of aortic insufficiency.

Inspection of the chest shows the cardiac impulse to be

displaced to the left and inferiorly. The apex beat is both hyper-dynamic and hyperkinetic, rising rapidly to a large volume which is momentarily sustained and then falling quickly. A rapid filling wave is frequently visible.

Palpation. The heaving apical pulse is readily palpable. A rapid filling impulse may be palpable.

Percussion. Percussion serves to confirm the cardiomegaly.

Auscultation. On auscultation, the characteristic aortic dias-tolic regurgitant murmur is heard over the aortic area and along the left sternal border. The murmur is usually soft and blowing and, as Hope noted, sounds "like whispering the word awe dur-ing inspiration." It is frequently heard best with the patient lean-ing forward in deep expiration (Figs. 9–58 and 9–59). An aortic systolic ejection murmur is also frequently heard. This is caused either by a concomitant aortic stenosis or by increased blood flow across the aortic valve. A third sound is frequently heard at the apex, as well as a fourth sound. Because of the dilatation of the left ventricle, a pansystolic mitral regurgitant murmur may be heard at the apex. A diastolic rumble is sometimes heard at the apex. This is the Austin Flint murmur. A to-and-fro mur-mur is heard over the femoral artery (Duroziez's sign), as well as the "pistol shot" sounds.

Pulse. The most striking feature on palpation is the char-acter of the pulse—the collapsing, water-hammer, or Corrigan pulse. This is a forceful pulse; it rises sharply and falls quickly (pulsus magnus et celer). Blood pressure determination shows a high pulse pressure due to an elevated systolic pressure and a lowered diastolic pressure.

The capillary pulse of Quincke is usually present. This al-ternate flush and pallor of the capillary bed may be elicited by gentle pressure on the tips of the fingernails. It may also be seen if an area of hyperemia is produced on the forehead or if a light is shined through the nail bed.

Aortic stenosis. Aortic stenosis may be congenital, rheu-matic, or arteriosclerotic in origin. Syncope, angina pectoris, and shortness of breath are the important symptoms of aortic ste-nosis and sudden death is not uncommon. Aortic stenosis may be supravalvular, valvular, discrete subvalvular, or hypertrophic subaortic stenosis.

Inspection. Patients with aortic stenosis experience concentric hypertrophy of the left ventricle. Although the thickness of the ventricle is significantly increased, the heart is not greatly enlarged. If the heart is enlarged, the point of maximal impulse will be displaced to the left and inferiorly. The apex beat is hyperdynamic (quietly heaving). An *a* wave may be visible in the apex beat (Fig. 9–43).

Palpation. Palpation serves to confirm the findings noted on inspection. A systolic thrill may be palpable over the precordium, maximum in the aortic area and at the apex, but frequently extending above the clavicles into the carotid arteries.

Percussion. Percussion may show nothing pathological, but in some patients an enlarged left ventricle can be demonstrated.

Auscultation. On auscultation a harsh systolic ejection murmur is heard in the second right interspace. This murmur radiates into the neck and down the left sternal border and is frequently heard at the apex. In some patients who have associated pulmonary emphysema, the murmur is best heard at the apex. A fourth sound is frequently heard at the apex when the lesion is hemodynamically severe. If the aortic valve is fibrotic or calcified, the aortic component of the second heart sound is diminished or absent. An aortic systolic ejection click is sometimes heard in mild to moderate lesions (Fig. 9–40).

Pulse. The pulse of aortic stenosis is often diagnostic. It is small, rises slowly, and falls away gradually — the classic pulsus parvus et tardus. If aortic stenosis is complicated by aortic insufficiency, a pulsus bisferiens may be present. The blood pressure in aortic stenosis is of some diagnostic value. In severe aortic stenosis the blood pressure is low and the pulse pressure is small. However, in mild or moderate aortic stenosis the blood pressure may be normal or elevated (Figs. 9–24 and 9–25).

Pulmonary stenosis and insufficiency. Pulmonary stenosis rarely occurs as a complication of rheumatic endocarditis. It is usually due to a congenital defect of the pulmonary valve. Acquired pulmonary stenosis has been described as a part of the "carcinoid syndrome." The findings of pulmonary stenosis will be discussed in the section on congenital heart lesions.

Pulmonary insufficiency rarely occurs as a result of an organic lesion of the pulmonary valve. Relative pulmonary insufficiency is seen in pulmonary hypertension and gives rise to the characteristic Graham Steell murmur. This is a soft pulmonary diastolic regurgitant murmur heard at the left sternal border which may be more intense immediately following a deep inspiration.

Tricuspid stenosis. Tricuspid stenosis is exceedingly rare and is usually complicated by mitral stenosis. The right atrium is markedly enlarged. The tricuspid component of the first heart sound is accentuated and a mid-diastolic rumble is heard that is loudest at the lower left sternal border rather than at the apex. A tricuspid opening snap may be present. Observation of the venous pulse may be diagnostic. The *a* wave is prominent and the *y* descent is prolonged.

Tricuspid insufficiency. Organic tricuspid insufficiency is also a relatively uncommon lesion, but functional tricuspid insufficiency is a common finding in right heart failure. The findings of tricuspid insufficiency are quite characteristic.

Inspection. The neck veins are engorged and the patient may have a plethoric cyanotic facies. Ascites and marked peripheral edema are commonly present. An enlarged liver with systolic pulsation may be noted. A precordial heave is noted along the left sternal border in systole, and a visible impulse may be present early in diastole associated with rapid filling of the right ventricle.

Palpation. Palpation of the abdomen confirms the presence of systolic pulsation of the liver. Pressure applied to the liver causes a distention of the jugular veins—the hepatic-jugular reflux. The right precordial systolic heave is palpable. A systolic thrill may be felt over the right ventricle.

Percussion. Percussion shows enlargement of the heart both to the right and to the left.

Auscultation. A pansystolic tricuspid regurgitant murmur may be heard over the right ventricle. The intensity of the murmur increases during inspiration when the lesion is mild or moderate and can occasionally be made to disappear by having the patient perform a Valsalva maneuver. When the lesion is severe it is unaffected by respiration. When the lesion is mild, the murmur may be present only on inspiration. A right ventricular third sound is often heard, and sometimes a short mid-diastolic tricuspid flow murmur can be heard at the lower left sternal border.

Pulse. The venous pulse of tricuspid insufficiency is quite characteristic. Since most patients with tricuspid insufficiency have atrial fibrillation, there is no *a* wave. The *c* and *v* waves fuse and the *y* descent is rapid. This produces the characteristic venous pulse — a systolic rise with a marked diastolic collapse (Fig. 9–51).

Endocarditis

Aside from acute rheumatic endocarditis, subacute bacterial endocarditis is the most common form of endocarditis. In this disease the patient may have a fever and show evidence of embolism before the findings in the heart become distinctive. Bacterial endocarditis has a predilection for hearts previously damaged by rheumatic fever or by congenital defects and usually develops on the surface of a valve. The first known illustration of valvular endocarditis, published by Sandifort in 1777, was in a patient with tetralogy of Fallot.

The signs of embolism are usually decisive in establishing the diagnosis. The most common locations of such emboli are the conjunctiva of the eyelid and in the fingers and toes, particularly under the nails where they have the appearance of "splinter hemorrhages" (Figs. 9–66 and 9–67). Hemorrhages may be seen in the retina on ophthalmoscopic examination. When the pulmonary or tricuspid valve is involved, the emboli are carried to the lungs and produce small pulmonary infarctions. Such infarctions cause pain in the chest, hemoptysis, and pleural friction rub.

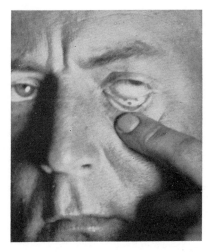

Figure 9–66. Conjunctival petechial hemorrhages in subacute infectious endocarditis.

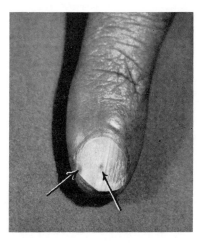

Figure 9–67. Splinter hemorrhage of left index finger. Two hemorrhages at tips of arrows.

Painful subcutaneous nodes, often slightly red in color, may appear early, especially in the pulp of the fingers and toes (Osler's nodes).

As the disease progresses, anemia and cachexia appear, petechiae become more numerous, and the heart gradually becomes enlarged. The spleen is often palpable in the early stages of the disease and later may show considerable enlargement. The previous heart murmur may show an increase in intensity or a change in quality. A changing heart murmur and fever always suggest bacterial endocarditis.

Congenital Heart Disease

Interest in congenital heart disease has increased greatly during the past few years because of the increased skill in diagnosis as well as the phenomenal advances in cardiac surgery. For years, many varieties of congenital heart lesions were diagnosed only by the pathologist after death. Today with the aid of x-ray, electrocardiogram, phonocardiogram, and cardiac catheterization studies, the physician can diagnose with accuracy most congenital heart lesions. These advances have not made physical diagnosis obsolete, but have proved that certain physical signs are pathognomonic of specific congenital heart lesions. By correlating the physical signs with the cardiac catheterization data, it is possible to estimate accurately the severity of many cardiac defects.

The commonest sign of a congenital heart defect is a heart murmur. However, many children have a heart murmur that is not associated with a heart defect. Cyanosis and clubbing of the fingers and toes are important signs of congenital heart defects. Cyanosis has been used as a basis for the classification of congenital heart defects as cyanotic or acyanotic. This group has been described under the term morbus caeruleus, the blue disease. Other signs and symptoms of congenital heart disease are growth retardation, ease of fatigue, tachypnea, and tachycardia.

Acyanotic Congenital Heart Disease

Atrial septal defect.   Embryonic atrial septal defects may be due to defects in the septum secundum or septum primum. Septum primum defects are frequently associated with insufficiency of the mitral and tricuspid valves. Patients with atrial septal defects may have an increased frequency of respiratory infections in childhood but are usually asymptomatic until late in adult life, at which time varying degrees of effort intolerance occur.

The most important physical findings of an uncomplicated atrial septal defect are a systolic ejection murmur and a widely split second sound that does not vary with respiration (Fig. 9–39). The systolic ejection murmur which is heard at the second left interspace is due to increased flow across the pulmonary valve. A soft mid-diastolic murmur is heard at the lower left sternal border in about 30 per cent of patients. It is caused by increased blood flow across the tricuspid valve.

Ventricular septal defect.   Patients with a ventricular septal defect may be completely asymptomatic or have severe growth retardation and heart failure. The severity of the symptoms is dependent to a large degree on the magnitude of the left to right shunt. The term "maladie de Roger" is reserved for mild cases.

A pansystolic regurgitant murmur that is maximal at the fourth or fifth interspace at the left sternal border is heard. This murmur is accompanied by a thrill and diminishes in intensity as the stethoscope is moved away from this area. A third sound and a mid-diastolic rumble are heard at the apex. The diastolic murmur is due to the increased flow across the mitral valve. The second sound is closely split. The third sound and diastolic rumble are present only when there is a significant left to right shunt. When these signs are absent and there is no evidence of pulmonary hypertension, the lesion is probably not clinically important.

Patent ductus arteriosus.   There are no symptoms in mild or

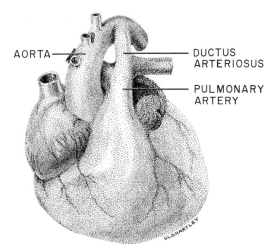

AORTA

DUCTUS ARTERIOSUS

PULMONARY ARTERY

Figure 9–68. *Patent ductus arteriosus.*

moderate cases. When a large left to right shunt is present, growth retardation and heart failure may occur (Fig. 9–68).

A continous thrill is palpable in the second interspace to the left of the sternum and on auscultation a continuous murmur is heard in this area (Fig. 9–52). Since the murmur increases in intensity late in systole, the second sound is usually masked. If the second sound can be heard, a paradoxically split second sound is a sign of a large left to right shunt. A third sound and mid-diastolic apical rumble reflect the increased flow across the mitral valve. The peripheral pulse characteristically has a water-hammer quality. The systolic blood pressure is normal but the diastolic pressure is low, resulting in a high pulse pressure.

These findings were once thought to be pathognomonic of patent ductus arteriosus, but the jugular venous hum, pulmonary atresia with bronchopulmonary anastomosis, pulmonary arteriovenous fistula, coronary artery–left atrial arteriovenous fistula, perforation of a sinus of Valsalva, and aortopulmonary septal defect all produce continuous murmurs that may be confused with patent ductus arteriosus.

Many of the acyanotic congenital heart defects are not associated wih intracardiac shunts. These include abnormalities of the individual heart valves and great vessels.

Coarctation of the aorta. Most patients with coarctation do not have symptoms when first seen. Headache, shoulder pain, and intermittent claudication are symptoms of coarctation. Other congenital anomalies such as bicuspid aortic valve, fibroelastosis, ventricular septal defect, and patent ductus arteriosus are present in about 20 per cent of patients with coarctation (Fig. 9–69).

The most striking physical finding in coarctation is absence of the femoral pulses. There is hypertension in the upper extremities and hypotension in the lower extremities. The carotid pulsations are vigorous, and intercostal pulsations may be visible and palpable.

The heart may be hypertrophied with displacement of the apex to the left. A systolic ejection murmur is frequently heard

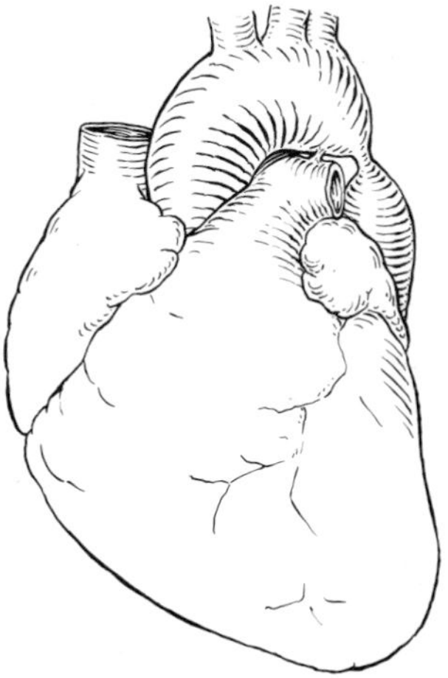

Figure 9–69. Coarctation of the aorta.

over the aortic area. A murmur is also heard between the scapulae. This murmur may be systolic, systolic and diastolic, or continuous. Notching of the lower margins of the ribs is a pathognomonic x-ray sign of coarctation of the aorta.

Aortic and subaortic stenosis. Aortic stenosis is the most common form of acyanotic congenital heart disease. It is often associated with hypoplasia of the left atrium, left ventricle, mitral valve, and aortic arch, comprising the hypoplastic left heart syndrome. The findings in congenital supravalvular and valvular stenosis are essentially the same as those in acquired valvular disease. Recently, considerable interest has been expressed in the investigation of a lesion that has been designated hypertrophic subaortic stenosis. This obstruction is produced by hypertrophied muscle mass in the left ventricular outflow tract. The characteristic physical findings include a bifid apical pulse, bifid carotid pulse, normal aortic component of the second sound, and absence of an aortic systolic ejection click. The murmur is characteristic in that it is usually maximal at the lower left sternal border, does not transmit into the neck, and sounds pansystolic. It is often confused with a ventricular septal defect or mitral insufficiency.

Dextrocardia. Complete dextrocardia is usually associated with situs inversus of the intestinal viscera. When dextrocardia is associated with situs inversus, bronchiectasis, and sinusitis it is known as Kartagener's syndrome. Dextrocardia with situs inversus is also associated with splenic agenesis and atrioventricular canal defects of the heart. This combination of defects is known as the splenic agenesis syndrome.

Pulmonary stenosis. Isolated pulmonary valvular stenosis is one of the more common congenital heart defects. The lesion usually does not produce symptoms unless it is severe, in which case dyspnea, syncope, and angina pectoris may occur.

The physical findings of pulmonary stenosis are related to the severity of the obstruction. The left ventricle may be rotated posteriorly so that the apex beat is neither visible nor palpable. A right ventricular heave is present. A harsh systolic ejection murmur is heard over the pulmonic area and is frequently accompanied by a palpable thrill. A fourth sound and a systolic ejection click may be heard. The second sound is widely split, but the pulmonary component of the second sound is diminished (Fig. 9–41). In severe pulmonary stenosis the pulmonary component of the second sound may be absent. The jugular venous pulse shows a very prominent *a* wave.

Cyanotic Congenital Heart Defects

Transposition of the great vessels. Transposition of the great vessels is the most common form of cyanotic congenital heart defect in newborn infants. Since most patients with this defect die in infancy or are modified by palliative or corrective surgery, it is not frequently encountered in the adult population. The clinical signs depend on the associated cardiac defects. X-ray and electrocardiographic findings are helpful.

Tetralogy of Fallot. This is probably the most common form of cyanotic congenital heart disease seen in the adolescent and adult population. Tetralogy of Fallot was first described by Nicholas Steno in an embryo in 1673. In 1777, Edward Sandifort reported a second case, describing not only the pathological findings but also the clinical course of the patient. His patient, a boy of 13, also showed endocarditis of the pulmonary valve at autopsy. Fallot, in 1888, published an analysis of 55 cases of cyanotic congenital heart disease and found that 74 per cent had a combination of four lesions: ventricular septal defect, pulmonary stenosis, dextroposition of the aorta, and hypertrophy of the right ventricle. This combination of four abnormalities has since been known as tetralogy of Fallot. These patients usually show marked cyanosis due to the pulmonary obstruction and the dextroposed overriding aorta, which allow unoxygenated right heart blood to get directly into the aorta and systemic circulation (Fig. 9–70).

Patients with tetralogy of Fallot complain of shortness of breath which is relieved by squatting. Syncope that occurs with exertion is a serious symptom which may precede a cerebral thrombosis. Physical examination reveals a plethoric, underde-

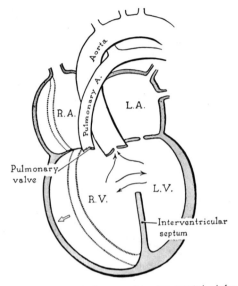

Figure 9–70. Tetralogy of Fallot: ventricular septal defect, pulmonary stenosis, dextroposition of the aorta, and hypertrophy of the right ventricle.

veloped, cyanotic individual with clubbing of the fingers and toes. The precordium is quiet and the apex beat is neither seen nor felt. A systolic thrill is usually palpable at the second and third interspace to the left of the sternum, and a systolic ejection murmur is heard in this area. The second sound, which is single and may be loud, results from closure of the aortic valve.

Pulmonary stenosis may occur with an atrial septal defect or with a ventricular septal defect without overriding of the aorta. The signs and symptoms of these disorders will depend on the severity of the pulmonary stenosis. If the pulmonary stenosis is severe, cyanosis will occur. If it is mild or moderate, there will be no cyanosis.

Eisenmenger's complex. This consists of an atrial septal defect, ventricular septal defect, or ductus arteriosus, pulmonary vascular hypertension, and right to left shunt. The markedly increased pulmonary vascular resistance is responsible for the right to left shunt, since the resistance to flow is less in the systemic circuit than in the pulmonary circuit. Patients with Eisenmenger's complex frequently have a late onset of cyanosis. They complain of shortness of breath, hemoptysis, and syncope.

The apex beat is neither visible nor palpable. A palpable pulsation over the pulmonary artery is frequently present and pulmonary valve closure is easily palpable. A systolic ejection murmur of varying intensity can be heard over the pulmonic area. The second heart sound is either single or very closely split, but if a pulmonic component of the second sound is heard, it is accentuated. A Graham Steell murmur of pulmonary insufficiency is often present.

Tricuspid atresia and truncus arteriosus. Tricuspid atresia and truncus arteriosus produce no characteristic physical findings.

The Electrocardiogram

In this book we have purposely omitted extensive discussion of the electrocardiogram. Electrocardiography is a science in itself. However, as an adjunct to physical diagnosis, the electrocardiogram has great diagnostic value.

The history of electrocardiography began with the discovery by Kölliker and Müller, in 1856, that each beat of the frog's heart was accompanied by the production of an electric current. In 1887 Waller showed that this current could be demonstrated in animals and in man by attaching electrodes to the front and back of the chest and connecting them with a capillary electrometer. Willem Einthoven, in 1903, substituted a string galvanometer of his own design for the capillary electrometer and introduced the electrocardiograph as a clinical instrument.

The electrocardiogram helps to determine whether premature contractions are atrial, nodal, or ventricular in origin. If tachycardia is present, the electrocardiogram can be used to differentiate sinus tachycardia, supraventricular tachycardia, atrial flutter, atrial fibrillation, and ventricular tachycardia. In congenital and rheumatic heart disease the electrocardiogram is helpful in distinguishing between left ventricular hypertrophy and right ventricular hypertrophy. It can also give information that allows one to determine whether the hypertrophy is due to the heart's pumping an increased volume of blood (diastolic overload) or the heart's pumping against an increased resistance (systolic overload).

In coronary occlusion with infarction, a characteristic electrocardiogram is seen, and usually it is possible to determine the area of the heart in which the infarction has occurred. The electrocardiogram may also show signs of myocardial ischemia without infarction, as well as evidence of pericarditis. Suggestive or confirmatory evidence of hyperthyroidism, myxedema, hyperpotassemia, hypopotassemia, hypercalcemia, hypocalcemia, dextrocardia, digitalis effect, and quinidine effect can be obtained from the electrocardiogram.

The X-Ray in the Diagnosis of Cardiac Disease

The chest x-ray and cardiac fluoroscopy are of great value to the clinician. First of all, the x-ray shows us the position, location, and size of the heart. Dextrocardia is obvious in an x-ray picture. An increase in the overall size of the heart or of individual heart chambers can be determined. Some changes are pathognomonic.

Patients with Addison's disease have very small hearts in contrast to patients with heart failure. Pericarditis with effusion presents a characteristic pear-shaped heart. The calcified pericardium of constrictive pericarditis can often be seen. In mitral stenosis the pulmonary artery and left atrial appendage are enlarged, producing a straight left heart border. The barium-filled esophagus is deviated posteriorly and to the right by the enlarged left atrium. Marked enlargement of the left ventricle is seen in hypertension and aortic insufficiency. The calcified aortic valve in aortic stenosis is best seen by fluoroscopic examination.

The chest x-ray of pulmonary stenosis is quite striking. The outline of the heart has been called the "sabot" heart from its resemblance to the sabot or wooden shoe worn by French peasants. This "sabot" heart is seen most frequently in tetralogy of Fallot. The egg-shaped heart occurring with transposition of the great vessels is also diagnostic.

In coarctation of the aorta erosion of the ribs is diagnostic. Aneurysms of the aorta are diagnosed with ease by x-ray examination.

PERIPHERAL VASCULAR DISEASE

Peripheral vascular disorders can result from abnormalities of the lymphatic vessels, capillaries, veins, and arteries. Disorders of the lymphatics, capillaries, and veins are usually due to organic lesions, but arterial disease may be either organic or functional (vasoconstrictive). Pain, paresthesia, edema, skin atrophy, ulceration, and gangrene are findings common to all forms of peripheral vascular disease.

History

Pain is the most frequent symptom that brings the patient with a peripheral vascular disorder to the physician. Patients with obstructive arterial disease complain of pain brought on by exertion (intermittent claudication). This pain is severe and causes the patient to stop his activity. Chronic venous insufficiency causes an aching or gnawing discomfort in the legs. It occurs while the patient is standing or when he reclines after having stood for a considerable time. Severe muscle cramps in the calves and feet, which awaken patients from sleep, also occur in patients with venous insufficiency. In Raynaud's disease pain occurs on exposure to a cold environment. Patients who have suffered frost bite, immersion foot, or chilblain (pernio) also experience pain on exposure to cold, but patients with erythromelalgia (Weir Mitchell disease) are uncomfortable in a warm environment, often plunging their extremities into ice water for relief. Pain may develop acutely with a peripheral embolus or acute arterial thrombosis, or slowly with a chronic arterial obstruction.

Coldness and paresthesias are frequent symptoms of peripheral vascular disease. The skin temperature is maintained by the superficial blood flow which is controlled by the autonomic nervous system. In general, unpleasant experiences cause vasoconstriction, whereas pleasurable experiences result in vasodilatation. The cold moist hands of the anxious patient are due to sympathetic overactivity, which causes both vasoconstriction and excessive perspiration.

In an arterial obstruction, the extremity is cold because of the inadequate blood supply. If there is a venous obstruction, the extremity may be cold not only because of associated arteriospasm but also because the blood remains in the extremity longer and loses more heat.

Paresthesias occur with both arterial and venous disease but are more common with arterial lesions. The paresthesias usually have a "stocking-glove" distribution and must be distinguished from primary neurological disorders.

Discoloration is a frequent complaint of patients with peripheral vascular lesions. Acute arterial obstruction produces pallor, but patients with chronic arterial insufficiency demonstrate cyanosis when the extremity is dependent. This is due to a combination of skin atrophy, capillary vasodilation, and reduced circulation. Patients with erythromelalgia have marked vasodilation; consequently their extremities are red and hot. Patients with Raynaud's phenomenon experience cyanosis as the arteriospasm and venospasm begin and marked pallor when the arteriospasm is severe. During the phase of vasodilation the extremities are red. Mottling is due to the uneven distribution of blood. This may occur because of vasoconstriction or organic obstruction with uneven distribution of collateral circulation. Acrocyanosis and livedo reticularis are vasospastic lesions associated with mottling of the skin.

Physical Examination

Peripheral vascular diagnoses are often made by inspection alone. A lesion previously seen is easily recognized. For this reason, inspection is the most important part of the physical examination.

Color.   In a warm room with the patient in a recumbent position, the foot has a pale pink color. The color increases if the room is warmed and blanches if the room is cooled. The skin color changes are a reflection of the cutaneous circulation and as such do not necessarily reflect disturbances of the deep circulation. When the foot is elevated 90 degrees, the veins empty and the skin has a cadaverous appearance if the arterial circulation is impaired. If the patient is then asked to sit with his legs in a dependent position, vascular filling of the feet can be observed. In patients with arterial impairment a cyanotic rubor occurs within two to three minutes (Buerger's test). When the patient performs this maneuver, one may also observe the veins on the dorsum of the foot which were collapsed with the legs elevated. In the dependent position these should fill in 10 to 15 seconds. If filling is delayed, this is a sign of compromised arterial circulation.

The anxiety of an interview may produce vasoconstriction and pallor. As the examination continues, the extremities will often assume a normal appearance. Mottling may disappear in a similar fashion as the patient relaxes.

Patients with chronic venous insufficiency have small, punctate purpuric lesions on the skin around their ankles. When these lesions are resolved, iron pigment remains in the skin, producing a brown punctate lesion. These lesions coalesce to produce the brownish discoloration about the ankles that is almost pathognomonic of chronic venous insufficiency.

Ulcers.   Skin ulceration is a common finding in most peripheral vascular disorders. The location of the ulcer is often a helpful clue to the correct diagnosis. Patients with Buerger's disease usually experience ulceration at the tips of the fingers and toes, whereas in patients with Raynaud's phenomenon the ulceration will frequently occur at the side of the finger, near the base of the nail. The ulcers of arteriosclerosis obliterans are usually locted at pressure points on the feet. Ulcerations from chronic venous insufficiency are located above the medial malleolus, whereas hypertensive ischemic ulcers occur more frequently on the lateral surface of the leg.

Atrophy. Skin atrophy is a common finding in all arterial lesions. The salient features of skin atrophy are loss of subcutaneous fat and secondary skin appendages (hair follicles, oil glands, and sweat glands). As a result, the fingers and toes are tapered, the hair is sparse, and there is no perspiration. This causes the skin to become dry and cracked. The toenails and fingernails develop longitudinal ridges, thicken, and curve over the tips of the fingers and toes.

Gangrene. The diagnosis of established gangrene is obvious; however, an attempt should be made to establish a cause. When gangrene is due to venous obstruction, infection, or superficial arterial lesions, the involved area may be purulent, moist, and edematous (wet gangrene). When the lesion is due to arterial obstruction, it is atrophic and mummified (dry gangrene). The unpleasant odor of putrefaction accompanies both types of lesions.

Skin temperature. Palpatory estimation of skin temperature is notoriously inaccurate, since the skin temperature is dependent on the ambient temperature as well as on the degree of vasoconstriction. Extremities are frequently cold in anxious patients who have no peripheral vascular disease. The extremities should warm if placed in a warm environment, particularly if the patient is given a potent vasodilator such as whiskey. Sympathetic nerve block removes vasoconstrictive stimuli, permitting maximum vasodilatation and increasing skin temperature. Maximum vasodilatation can be achieved by reactive hyperemia. This is achieved by occluding the circulation with a blood pressure cuff. The pressure is maintained until the extremity is painfully cyanotic. When the cuff pressure is released, blood rapidly fills the vessels which were maximally dilated by ischemic waste products. While estimating the skin temperature, it is convenient to note the skin texture. Edema can be detected by the persistence of a skin depression after digital compression.

Pulses. In the upper extemity the subclavian, axillary, brachial, radial, and ulnar arteries are readily palpated. The abdominal aorta and the femoral, popliteal, posterior tibial, anterior fibial, and dorsalis pedis arteries are palpable in the lower extremity. Arterial obstruction can be localized by careful palpation of the peripheral pulses. If the femoral artery is palpable and the popliteal artery is not, the obstruction must lie somewhere in between. Obstructions in other areas may be similarly located.

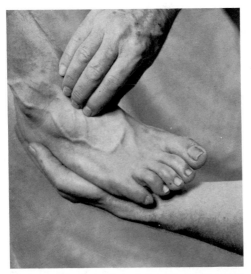

Figure 9–71. Palpation of dorsalis pedis artery.

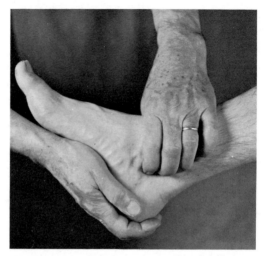

Figure 9–72. Palpation of posterior tibial artery.

Diseases of the Lymphatic System

Congenital or hereditary lymphedema was first described by Milroy in 1892. The term Milroy's disease should be reserved for those cases of lymphedema that are congenital and hereditary. Lymphedema may also occur idiopathically at puberty or may be secondary to tuberculosis, filariasis, phlebitis, lymphangitis, surgical removal of lymph nodes, and malignant invasion of the lymphatics.

The patient usually complains of a painless swelling of one or both lower extremities. As the edema becomes more severe, fatigue, tenderness, and paresthesia become prominent symptoms. Skin ulceration is not uncommon. Physical examination shows marked pitting edema of the involved extremities, which decreases when the patient is in the recumbent position. The skin of the edematous leg may have a rosy hue (Fig. 9–73).

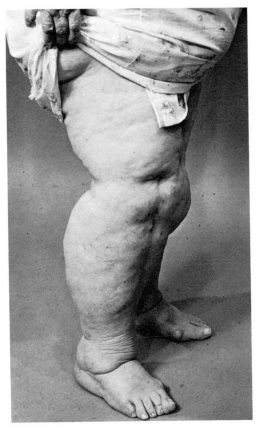

Figure 9–73. Milroy's disease.

Acute lymphangitis is the most common disorder of the lymphatic system and occurs in conjunction with acute infectious disorders of the extremities. It is characterized by the appearance of superficial red streaks along the course of lymphatic vessels. The streaks usually emanate from an area of cellulitis.

Diseases of the Veins

Varicose veins and thrombophlebitis are the two most common forms of venous disease. Phlebosclerosis, phlebofibrosis, and spontaneous rupture of veins are less common forms of venous disease.

Varicose veins. Varicose veins are dilated tortuous veins which may occur primarily or may be secondary to some other disease process. The primary form is often familial and is usually associated with congenital defects of the veins and their valves. Varicose veins can result from thrombophlebitis, trauma, increased venous pressure from abdominal tumors, pregnancy, portal hypertension, or heart failure. Varicose veins without venous insufficiency are asymptomatic. When venous insufficiency is present, patients complain of aching pain in the calves which is relieved by elevation of the extremities. These patients often ex-

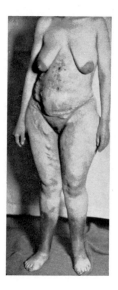

Figure 9-74. Varicose veins of the thighs and abdomen.

perience muscle cramps in the calves during sleep with excruciating pain from which the patient obtains relief by arising from bed and walking. Edema, pruritus, paresthesia, and skin ulceration are other common complaints of venous insufficiency.

Patients should be examined while they are standing so that the veins will be maximally distended. The varicose veins may be in the distribution of the greater saphenous or the lesser saphenous vein. In the familial form the lesions are usually bilateral, whereas unilateral lesions are more frequently encountered following acute phlebitis. If venous insufficiency has been present for a long time, the skin about the ankle develops a brown discoloration, becomes atrophic, and ulcerates. The brown discoloration is due to the deposition of iron pigment (Fig. 9–75).

Many tests have been devised to test the patency of the deep venous circulation when superficial varicosities are present. The simplest technique is to firmly apply an elastic bandage from the patient's toes to his thighs. If he is then able to walk rapidly for a considerable distance without experiencing pain, the deep veins are patent. If pain occurs and becomes increasingly more severe with exertion, deep vein obstruction may be present.

Thrombophlebitis. This is an obstructive disease of veins which usually occurs secondary to mechanical, chemical, or thermal injury; muscular strain; local inflammatory disease; and certain blood dyscrasias. Acute thrombophlebitis is associated with localized pain, tenderness, swelling, and fever. Arteriospasm may accompany the acute phlebitis, resulting in marked pallor of the extremity. The veins become firm and quite tender to palpation. When thrombophlebitis is present in the calf, dorsiflexion of the foot produces pain in the calf (Homans' sign). Another useful test is the cuff test, which is performed by gradually increasing the pressure in a blood pressure cuff that is wrapped around the calf. Each limb is tested, but pain occurs at a much lower pressure in the affected limb when phlebitis is present. Pulmonary embolism is a serious complication of thrombophlebitis. It may occur before the patient or physician is aware of the phlebitis.

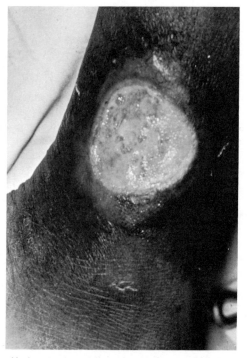

Figure 9–75. *Varicose ulcer. Note increased pigmentation around ulcer.*

Diseases of the Arteries

Arterial disease produces symptoms because of impaired circulation to the skin and muscle. Muscle weakness, atrophy, fatigue, and intermittent claudication occur when the blood supply to the muscle is impaired. Hair loss, skin atrophy, skin ulceration, and gangrene occur when the blood supply to the skin is restricted.

Arteriosclerosis obliterans. This is an obstructive degenerative disease that is characterized by the occlusion of large and small arteries by atheromata. The disease involves the legs to a greater extent than the arms. The onset may be sudden or gradual. The primary symptom of large vessel obstruction is intermittent claudication. The area in which intermittent claudication occurs is determined by the site of arterial obstruction. Obstruction at the bifurcation of the aorta produces bilateral intermittent claudication of the hips and impotence (Leriche syndrome). On physical examination, no pulses are felt in the

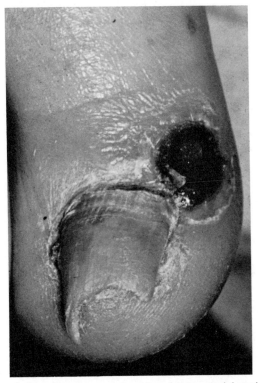

Figure 9–76. Gangrenous ulceration due to arterial occlusion.

lower extremities, although good pulsations are found in the upper extremities. If collateral circulation is adequate, hair loss and atrophy do not occur. When the common femoral artery is involved, symptoms are localized only to the side involved.

Sudden arterial occlusion as a result of embolism or thrombosis produces pain, pallor, paresthesia, paralysis, and coolness in the affected extremity. This is easily distinguished from a gradual occlusion in which collateral circulation has developed. When collateral circulation is inadequate, skin atrophy, hair loss, ulceration, and gangrene develop (Fig. 9–76).

Buerger's disease (thromboangiitis obliterans). This is an inflammatory disease that involves the arteries, veins, and nerves. It frequently produces obstruction of arteries, resulting in ulceration and gangrene. The disease occurs primarily in male smokers between the ages of 20 and 40 (Fig. 9–77).

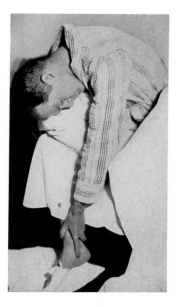

Figure 9–77. Posture in Buerger's disease.

Raynaud's disease. This is a vasoconstrictive disease of the arteries and arterioles of the hands and feet. The vasoconstriction is usually precipitated by nervousness or exposure to cold. The patient complains of color changes, pain, and paresthesias of the hands. At the onset of the vasoconstriction the fingers become blue because of partial arterial occlusion; as the vasoconstriction progresses, the fingers become white, and when vasodilatation occurs the hands become red. Ulceration and edema of the fingertips is not uncommon. Raynaud described this disorder as follows:

Without appreciable cause one or many fingers become pale and cold all at once; in many cases it is the same finger which is first attacked; the others become dead successively and in the same order. . . . The determining cause is often the impression of cold . . . sometimes even a simple mental emotion is enough [to bring on these changes]. . . . In the more pronounced cases, the pallor of the extremities is replaced by a cyanotic colour. . . . Finally a vermillion colour shows itself at the margin and little by little gains ground. . . . This patch gives place to the normal pink colour and then the skin is found to have entirely returned to the primitive condition.

This disease occurs frequently in nervous young women but may be secondary to lupus erythematosus or scleroderma. This phenomenon also occurs following traumatic injury to an extremity or in association with certain occupations, such as typists or pneumatic hammer operators, in which the extremities are exposed to constant vibration. Ergot and arsenic poisoning also produce severe vasoconstriction.

Cold exposure. Trench foot, immersion foot, and chilblain (pernio) are clinical disorders produced by exposure to cold. The clinical picture has three stages: prehyperemic, hyperemic, and posthyperemic. The prehyperemic stage occurs during cold exposure. Its primary symptom is hyperesthesia or anesthesia. When the exposed portion is warmed, the hyperemic stage occurs and is marked by pain, paresthesia, edema, and hemorrhagic bleb formation. The posthyperemic phase is marked by vasomotor instability. Coldness and sweating are primary symptoms.

Thoracic outlet syndromes. Since the subclavian artery exits from the thorax it is particularly vulnerable to compression by the anterior scalene muscle, the clavicle, and the insertion of the pectoralis minor muscle. This partial occlusion of the pulse gives rise to numbness, weakness, and paresthesia of the affected limb—a group of clinical entities known as thoracic outlet syndromes.

To test for obstruction by the anterior scalene muscle, ask the patient to turn his head to the affected side, extend the neck, and take a deep breath. Obliteration of the brachial pulse constitutes a positive test (Adson maneuver). Obstruction by the clavicle can be detected by having the patient hyperextend the shoulders while the physician palpates the brachial pulse. If the pulse disappears, the test is positive. Hyperabduction of the arms will obliterate the brachial pulse if the subclavian artery is obstructed by the insertion of the pectoralis minor muscle.

Aneurysm

Most of the aneurysms seen clinically are due to arteriosclerosis. Aneurysms may be congenital, traumatic, mycotic, or luetic in origin. Aneurysms also occur in Marfan's syndrome, pseudoxanthoma elasticum, and cystic medial necrosis.

Aneurysm of the thoracic aorta. Broadbent classified aneurysms as "aneurysms of signs" and "aneurysms of symptoms." Aneurysms of signs are those occurring in the ascending part of the arch of the aorta, whereas aneurysms of symptoms are located in the transverse and descending arch of the aorta. This second group may cause distressing symptoms but the diagnosis may be possible only by x-ray examination. Aneurysms of the arch and descending aorta are usually of arteriosclerotic origin.

Inspection. The pathognomonic sign of aneurysm of the ascending arch is a heaving, expansile pulsation in the upper part of the right chest at the level of the third rib to the right of the sternum. It sometimes extends over the manubrium, may involve the right sternoclavicular joint, or may be seen in the sec-

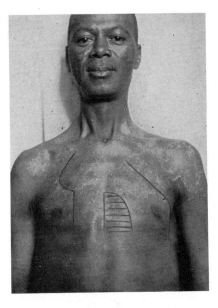

Figure 9-78. *Area of dullness to right of sternum in the second and third costal interspaces resulting from aneurysm of the ascending arch of the aorta.*

ond left interspace. A good light is helpful for the demonstration of such pulsation. The expansile character can often be brought out better by drawing a small notched area over the pulsation. As the aneurysm enlarges, it may extend forward and sometimes produces a swelling larger than a coconut. The pupil of the patient's eye may be dilated or contracted on one side.

Palpation. Palpation of the larynx may demonstrate a tracheal tug as noted first by Oliver. Palpation over the area of pulsation may disclose a diastolic shock, often intense, which is an important sign of aneurysm. A systolic thrill is sometimes felt.

Percussion. Dullness can usually be made out to the right of the sternum and may be extensive when pulsation is minimal. The percussion note over an aneurysm is flat (Fig. 9-78).

Auscultation. A systolic murmur is commonly present, and since the disease is frequently associated with aortic insufficiency, an aortic diastolic regurgitant murmur may also be heard. A continuous "humming-top" murmur is usually present when there is a communication between the aneurysm and the vena cava or the pulmonary artery.

Pulse. Palpation of the pulse may show marked difference between the pulse in the right and left radial arteries, one pulse being small and showing a definite lag in the time of its appearance as compared with the other.

Aneurysm of the abdominal aorta. On inspection of the epigastrium, there is a marked pulsation, sometimes a definite mass. A thrill is occasionally felt. The pulse is forceful and expansile. On auscultation a systolic murmur is usually audible.

Marked pulsation of the epigastrium is extremely common in thin, nervous patients, especially those with marked anemia. The diagnosis of an abdominal aneurysm should not be made by palpation alone unless the observer definitely feels a mass with expansile pulsation.

Dissecting aneurysm. Dissecting aneurysm of the aorta was noted by Morgagni as early as 1760. Pain is one of the most common findings, usually severe; it may, however, occasionally be slight or even absent altogether. The location of the pain depends upon the location of the part of the aorta undergoing dissection, whether in the chest, interscapular region, lumbar region, abdomen, sacral region, or hips. Weakness of the lower extremities, paresis of the legs, urinary retention, syncope, convulsions, coma, hypertension, and hemiplegia may occur. A diastolic aortic murmur, due to dilatation of the aorta, may appear. Logue and Sikes have pointed out the diagnostic significance of pulsation of the sternoclavicular joint in dissecting aneurysm of the aorta.

Arteriovenous aneurysm. An arteriovenous aneurysm (arteriovenous fistula or an abnormal communication between an artery or an adjacent vein) is usually the result of a wound, occasionally of an ulceration. Such aneurysms are found most commonly in the extremities and present a characteristic picture. The affected limb is larger and often has a definite cyanotic hue. The skin temperature is elevated in the neighborhood of the aneurysm. In young people the leg or arm, the seat of the aneurysm, may grow longer and develop more hair than the corresponding side. A systolic thrill can be felt over the aneurysm, and a continuous murmur with systolic accentuation is heard. Pressure over the aneurysm, closing the fistula, causes a sharp drop in the pulse rate (Branham's sign). The sign was first reported by Branham in 1890 in a case of arteriovenous aneurysm of the femoral vessels. He noted: "The most mysterious phenomenon connected with the case, one which I have not been able to explain to myself, or to obtain a satisfactory reason for from others, was slowing of the heart's beat, when compression of the common femoral was employed. . . . This symptom became more marked until pressure of the artery above the wound caused the heart's beat to fall from 80 to 35 or 40 per minute and so to remain until pressure was relieved. Compression of the artery of the sound limb would produce no such effect."

Accompanying the decrease in the pulse rate there is usually an elevation of both systolic and diastolic blood pressure. The decreased pulse rate, which is apparently of vagal origin, is corrected by the use of atropine. Holman believes that closure of the fistula increases the aortic pressure, causing a stimulation of the depressor fibers of the vagus in the arch of the aorta and a resultant slowing of the heart. An arteriovenous aneurysm in the extremities leads to cardiac hypertrophy and later to myocardial insufficiency.

Arteriovenous aneurysms of the vessels of the head or neck often cause great annoyance to the patient because of the constant whirring sound that is heard. A fistula between the thoracic aorta and the vena cava produces intense cyanosis of the upper part of the body.

Summary. Aneurysms of the ascending thoracic aorta, called "aneurysms of signs," show a heaving expansile pulsation, a diastolic shock over the pulsation, a flat percussion note, and a systolic murmur on auscultation. A tracheal tug is often present. The radial pulse often shows marked differences on the two sides.

Aneurysms of the descending arch of the aorta, "aneurysms

of symptoms," although producing distressing dyspnea and pain, are often recognized only after x-ray examination.

Aneurysms of the abdominal aorta produce a marked epigastric pulsation. The diagnosis, however, should not be made unless the examiner can definitely feel an expansile, pulsating tumor under his hand.

Arteriovenous aneurysms are commonly suspected from the patient's history. A systolic thrill is felt, and a systolic murmur is heard over the aneurysm. Pressure causes a sharp fall in pulse rate. The increase in temperature of the extremity involved is readily appreciated.

COMMON CLINICAL TERMS

Aneurysm—A dilated, thinned portion of a blood vessel or cardiac chamber.

Apex beat—Precordial movements produced by the impact of the contraction of the left ventricle.

Cyanosis—Blue appearance of tissues due to accumulation of excessive amounts of reduced hemoglobin.

Diastole—The portion of the cardiac cycle during which the ventricle fills.

Edema—Swelling produced by fluid collection in the interstitial spaces of body tissues.

Heart murmur—Noise made by the flow of blood across normal or diseased valves or through abnormal intra- or extracardiac communications.

Pericarditis—Inflammation of the pericardium.

Phlebitis—Acute inflammation of a vein.

Systole—The portion of the cardiac cycle when the ventricle contracts and expels blood.

Tachycardia—A rapid heart rate usually in excess of 120 beats per minute.

COMMON CLINICAL SYNDROMES

Angina pectoris—Precordial constricting chest pain precipitated by myocardial ischemia. The pain is precipitated by activity or emotion and relieved by rest.

Buerger's disease—A chronic, inflammatory, obliterative peripheral vascular disorder involving the artery, vein, and nerve resulting in gangrene.

Cor pulmonale — Right heart hypertrophy and/or failure resulting from some form of pulmonary disease.

Eisenmenger's syndrome — Cyanotic congenital heart disease due to pulmonary hypertension with right to left shunt at atrial, ventricular, or ductal level.

Fallot's tetralogy — A congenital heart defect with infundibular pulmonary stenosis, ventricular septal defect, dextroposition of the aorta, and right ventricular hypertrophy.

"Floppy valve syndrome" — Myxomatous or primary degeneration of the mitral valve causing mitral insufficiency. Clinically the syndrome is recognized by a systolic click and late systolic murmur.

Leriche syndrome — Thrombotic obliteration above or at the bifurcation of the aorta causing claudication and impotence.

Marfan's syndrome — A syndrome of arachnodactyly, ectopia lentis, and cardiovascular defects including aortic aneurysm.

Raynaud's disease — A peripheral vascular disease of unknown etiology in which spasm of digital arteries is produced by cold exposure or emotional distress. Pallor, cyanosis, and ulcers result. Rubor and paresthesia result from warming.

Stokes-Adams syndrome — Syncope with or without convulsions due to a cardiac arrhythmia, commonly heart block.

BIBLIOGRAPHY

Allbutt, C.: Diseases of the Arteries Including Angina Pectoris. New York, The Macmillan Co., 1915.

Allen, E. V., Barker, N. W., and Hines, E. A., Jr.: Peripheral Vascular Diseases. 3rd ed. Philadelphia, W. B. Saunders Co., 1962.

Bamberger, H.: Beitrage zur Physiologie und Pathologie des Herzens. Virchows Arch. Pathol. Anat., 9:328; 523, 1856.

Bean, W. B., and Schmidt, M. D.: Rupture of the aortic valve. J.A.M.A., 153:214, 1953.

Bishop, L. F.: A Key to the Electrocardiogram. New York, Wm. Wood & Co., 1923.

Blankenhorn, M. A.: The effect of sleep on normal and high blood pressure. Trans. Assoc. Am. Physicians, 40:87, 1925.

Blumgart, H. D., Schlesinger, M. J., and Zoll, P. M.: Angina pectoris, coronary failure and acute myocardial infarction. J.A.M.A., 116:91, 1941.

Boas, E. P., and Goldschmidt, E. F.: The Heart Rate. Springfield, Illinois, Charles C Thomas, 1932.

Bock, H.: Ueber die Verwendbarkeit des Differential-Stethoskopes nach Dr. Bock. Berlin, Klin. Wochenschr., 46:544, 1909.

Bock, K. D., and Collier, P. T.: Essential Hypertension. Berlin, Springer Verlag, 1960.

von Bondsdorff, B., and Wolf, H. J.: Weitere Erfahrungen mit der Registrierung absoluter Sphygmogramme der Arteria cubitalis. Z. Gesamte Exp. Med., 86:12, 1932.

Bramwell, C.: Gallop rhythm. J. Med., 4:149, 1935.

Bramwell, C.: Sounds and murmurs produced by auricular systole. Q. J. Med., 4:139, 1935.

Bramwell, C.: Arterial pulse in health and disease. Lancet, 2:239; 301; 366, 1937.

Branham, H. H.: Aneurysmal varix of the femoral artery and vein following a gunshot wound. Int. J. Surg., 3:250, 1890.

Broadbent, W.: The Pulse. London, Cassell & Co., 1890.

Broadbent, W.: Heart Disease. London, Baillière, Tindall & Cox, 1900.

Brown, J. W.: Congenital Heart Disease. New York, Staples Press, 1950.

Cabot, R. C.: Facts on the Heart. Philadelphia, W. B. Saunders Co., 1926.

Christian, H. A.: The Diagnosis and Treatment of Diseases of the Heart. New York, Oxford Book Company Inc., 1935, p. 67.

Coleman, W.: The vibration sense in percussion. Trans. Assoc. Am. Physicians, 50:278, 1935.

Corvisart, J. N.: Essaie sur les Maladies et les Lésions Organiques du Coeur. Paris, Migneret, 1806.

Corvisart, J. N.: Nouvelle Méthode pour Reconnaître les Maladies Internes de la Poitrine. Paris, Migneret, 1808.

Delp, M. H., and Maxwell, R.: Rupture of an aortic aneurysm into the pulmonary artery. J.A.M.A., 110:1647, 1938.

De Veer, J. A.: A mechanical explanation of sudden death in aortic stenosis. Am. Heart J., 15:243, 1938.

Dimond, E. G.: Electrocardiography. St. Louis, The C. V. Mosby Co., 1954.

Dock, G.: Dominic John Corrigan: His place in development of our knowledge of cardiac disease; water-hammer pulse. Ann. Med. Hist., 6:281, 1934.

Dock, W.: Mode of production of the first heart sounds. Arch. Intern. Med., 51:737, 1933.

Dressler, W.: Percussion of the sternum. Aid to differentiation of pericardial effusion and cardiac dilatation. J.A.M.A., 173:7, 1960.

Eggleston, C.: The persistence of a mitral stenotic murmur in the presence of auricular fibrillation. Trans. Assoc. Am. Physicians, 43:36, 1928.

Ewart, W.: Practical aids in the diagnosis of pericardial effusion. Br. Med. J., 1:717, 1896.

Fishberg, A. M.: Hypertension and Nephritis. Philadelphia, Lea & Febiger, 1930.

Floyer, J.: The Physician's Pulse-Watch. London, Smith & Walford, 1707.

Gasul, B. J., and Fell, E.: Salient points in the clinical diagnosis of congenital heart disease. J.A.M.A., 161:39, 1956.

Gevalt, F. C., Jr., and Levine, S. A.: The significance of Ewart's sign. Int. Clin., 4:1, 1940.

Gross, R. E., and Hubbard, J. P.: Surgical ligation of a patent ductus arteriosus: Report of first successful case. J.A.M.A., 112:729, 1939.

Gwyn, N. B.: On some venous murmurs found in hepatic cirrhosis and their confusion with murmurs of congenital heart disease. Trans. Assoc. Am. Physicians, 45:240, 1930.

Hamman, L.: Spontaneous interstitial emphysema of the lungs. Trans. Assoc. Am. Physicians, 52:311, 1937.

Harvey, W.: De Motu Cordis. Translated by Chauncey D. Leake. Springfield, Illinois, Charles C Thomas, 1931.

Harvey, W.: The Works of William Harvey, M.D. Translated by Robert Willis. London, Sydenham Society, 1847.

Hirschfelder, A. D.: Diseases of the Heart and Aorta. Philadelphia, J. B. Lippincott Co., 1933.

Holman, E.: The physiology of an arteriovenous fistula. Arch. Surg., 7:64, 1923.

Holman, E.: Arteriovenous aneurysm. Ann. Surg., 80:801, 1924.

Hope, J.: A Treatise on the Diseases of the Heart. London, J. & A. Churchill, 1839.

Horine, E. F.: An epitome of ancient pulse lore. Bull. Hist. Med., 10:209, 1941.

Janeway, T. C.: The Clinical Study of Blood pressure. New York, Appleton, 1910.

Joseph, G.: Geschichte der Physiologie der Herztone. Janus, 2:345, 1852.

King, J. T.: The clinical recognition and physical signs of bundle-branch block. Am. Heart J., 3:505, 1928.

Kölliker, A., and Müller, H.: Nachweis der negativen Schwankung des Muskelstroms am natürlich sich kontrahierenden Muskel. Verh. Phys.-Med. Ges. Würzb., 6:528, 1856.

Laubry, C., and Pezzi, C.: Les Rhythmes de Galop. Paris, Gaston Doin, 1926.

Leaman, W. G., Jr.: The history of electrocardiography. Ann. Med. Hist., 8:113, 1936.

Leatham, A.: Auscultation of the heart. Lancet, 2:703; 757, 1958.

Levine, S. A.: Clinical Heart Disease. 5th ed. Philadelphia, W. B. Saunders Co., 1958.

Levine, S. A., and Harvey, W. P.: Clinical Auscultation of the Heart. 2nd ed. Philadelphia, W. B. Saunders Co., 1959.

Lewis, J. K., and Dock, W.: The origin of heart sounds and their variations in myocardial disease. J.A.M.A., 110:271, 1938.

Lewis, T.: Notes upon the cardiorespiratory murmur and its relationship to other physical signs. Q. J. Med., 2:178, 1908.

Lewis, T.: Clinical Disorders of the Heart Beat. London, H. Frowde, 1921.

Lewis, T.: Clinical Electrocardiography. 3rd ed. London, Shaw & Sons, Ltd., 1924.

Lewis, T.: The Mechanism and Graphic Registration of the Heart Beat. 3rd. ed. London, Shaw & Sons, Ltd., 1925.

Lewis, T.: Pain in muscular ischemia. Arch. Intern. Med., 49:713, 1932.

Lewis, T.: Diseases of the Heart. New York, The Macmillan Co., 1933.

Logue, R. B., and Sikes, C.: A new sign in dissecting aneurysm of the aorta. J.A.M.A., *148*:1209, 1952.

Mackenzie, J.: The Study of the Pulse. Edinburgh, Young J. Pentland, 1902.

Mackenzie, J.: Principles of Diagnosis and Treatment in Heart Affections. London, Oxford University Press, 1918.

Mackenzie, J. Diseases of the Heart. London, H. Frowde, 1921.

Major, R. H.: The history of taking blood pressure. Ann. Med. Hist., *2*:47, 1930.

Major, R. H.: Raymond Vieussens and his treatise on the heart. Ann. Med. Hist., *4*:147, 1932.

Marey, E. J.: La Méthode Graphique. Paris, G. Masson, 1878.

Margin, S. J., and Gorham, L. W.: Cardiac pain. Arch. Intern. Med., *52*:840, 1938.

Matas, R.: On the systemic or cardiovascular effects of arteriovenous fistulae. Int. Clin. Ser. (35), *2*:58, 1925.

McKusick, V. A.: Cardiovascular Sound in Health and Disease. Baltimore, Williams & Wilkins Co., 1958.

McKusick, V. A.: The history of methods for the diagnosis of heart disease. Bull. Hist. Med., *34*:16, 1960.

McKusick, V. A., Murray, G. E., Peeler, R. G., and Webb, G. N.: Musical murmurs. Johns Hopkins Med. J., *97*:136, 1955.

Merrill, A. J.: Edema and decreased renal blood flow in patients with chronic congestive heart failure. J. Clin. Invest., *25*:389, 1946.

Mond, H., and Oppenheimer, E. T.: Gallop rhythm in hypertension. Arch. Intern. Med., *43*:166, 1929.

Mote, C. D., and Carr, J. L.: Dissecting aneurysm of the aorta. Am. Heart J., *24*:69, 1942.

Neuhof, S.: The Heart. Philadelphia, P. Blakiston's Sons & Co., 1923.

Pardee, H. E. B.: Clinical Aspects of the Electrocardiogram. 2nd ed. New York, Paul B. Hoeber, 1928.

Paulus Aegineta: Opus de re Medica, apud Andream Arrivabenum. Venice, 1542.

Paulus Aegineta: Seven Books. Vol. 1. Translated by Francis Adams. London, The Sydenham Society, 1844.

Pease, E. A.: Voluntary Control of the Heart. Boston Med. Surg. J., *120*:525, 1889.

Pins, E.: Ein neues Symptom der Pericarditis. Wien. Med. Wochenschr., *39*:210, 1889.

Potain, C.: Clinique Médicale de la Charité. Paris, G. Masson, 1894.

Prinzmetal, M., Corday, E., Brill, J. C., Oblath, R. W., and Kruger, W. E.: Auricular Arrhythmias. Springfield, Illinois, Charles C Thomas, 1952.

Pullen, R. L.: Medical Diagnosis, Applied Physical Diagnosis. 2nd ed. Philadelphia, W. B. Saunders Co., 1950.

Ravin, A.: Auscultation of the Heart. Chicago, The Year Book Publishers Inc., 1958.

Raynaud, A. G. M.: De l'asphyxie locale et de la gangrène symétrique des extrémités. Paris, Rignoux, 1862, p. 109.

Reich, N. E.: The Uncommon Heart Diseases. Springfield, Illinois, Charles C Thomas, 1954.

Reid, W. D.: The Heart in Modern Practice. Philadelphia, J. B. Lippincott Co., 1928.

Rosenbloom, J.: The history of pulse timing with some remarks on Sir John Floyer and his physician's pulse watch. Ann. Med. Hist., 4:97, 1922.

Rotch, T. M.: Absence of resonance in the fifth right intercostal space, diagnostic of pericardial effusion. Boston Med. Surg. J., 99:423, 1878.

Roth, I. R.: Cardiac Arrhythmias. New York, Paul B. Hoeber, 1927.

Routier, D., and van Heerswynghels, J.: À propos du bruit de galop, étude phonocardiographique. Arch. Mal. Coeur, 28:629, 1935.

Sancetta, S. M.: Clinical detection of "pulsating" liver. J.A.M.A., 158:922, 1955.

Sanctorii Sanctorii: Commentaria in Primam Fen. Primi Libri Canonis Avicennae. Venice, 1625.

Sandifort, E.: Observationes anatomicopathologicae. Leyden, Eyk and Vygh, 177–1781.

Scherf, D., and Boyd, L. J.: Cardiovascular Diseases, Their Diagnosis and Treatment. St. Louis, The C. V. Mosby Co., 1939.

Schnitker, M. A.: Congenital Anomalies of the Heart and Great Vessels. New York, Oxford University Press, 1952.

Seifert, O., and Müller, F.: Taschenbuch der medizinisch-klinischen Diagnostik. 15th ed. Wiesbaden, J. F. Bergmann, 1912.

Senac, J. B.: Traité de la Structure du Coeur. Paris, Jacques Vincent, 1749.

Smith, S. C.: Heart Records: Their Interpretation and Preparation. Philadelphia, F. A. Davis Co., 1923.

Sodeman, W. A., and Sodeman, W. A., Jr.: Pathologic Physiology. 5th ed. Philadelphia, W. B. Saunders Co., 1974.

Stewart, H. A.: Experimental and clinical investigation of the pulse and blood pressure changes in aortic insufficiency. Arch. Intern. Med., 1:102, 1908.

Stieglitz, E. J.: Arterial Hypertension. New York, Paul B. Hoeber, 1930.

Stokes, W.: The Diseases of the Heart and the Aorta. Dublin, Hodges and Smith, 1854.

Thayer, W. S.: On the early diastolic heart sound (the so-called third heart sound). Boston Med. Surg. J., 48:173, 1908.

Thayer, W. S.: Further observations on the third heart sound. Arch. Intern. Med., 4:297, 1909.

Tice, G. M.: Radiographic evidence of cardiovascular disease. Bull. Univ. Kansas School Med., 5:8, 1934.

Traube, L.: Gesammelte Beitrage zur Pathologie und Physiologie. Berlin, Hirschwald, 1878.

Vaquez, H.: Diseases of the Heart. Philadelphia, W. B. Saunders Co., 1924.

Vaquez, H., and Bordet, E.: The Heart and the Aorta. Translated by James A. Heneij and John Macy. New Haven, Yale University Press, 1920.

Vierordt, H.: Die Messung der Intensitat der Herztone. Tübingen, H. Laupp'sche Buchhandlung, 1885.

Vierordt, K.: Die Lehre vom Arterienpuls in gesunden und kranken Zustanden. Brunswick, Friedrich Vieweg, 1855.

Vieussens, R.: Traité nouveau de la structure et des causes du mouvement naturel du coeur. Toulouse, Jean Guillemette, 1715.

Waller, A. D.: A demonstration on man of electromotive changes accompanying the heart's beat. J. Physiol. (London), 8:229, 1887.

Warren, J. V., and Stead, E. A., Jr.: Fluid dynamics in chronic congestive heart failure. Arch. Intern. Med., 73:138, 1944.

Weiss, O., and Joachim, G.: Registerung und Reproduktion menschlicher Herztone und Herzgerausche. Arch. Gesamte Physiol., 123:341, 1908.

West, H. F., and Savage, W. E.: Voluntary acceleration of the heart beat. Arch. Intern. Med., 22:290, 1918.

White, P. D.: Heart Disease. 4th ed. New York, The Macmillan Co., 1951.

Wiggers, C. J.: Principles and Practice of Electrocardiography. St. Louis, The C. V. Mosby Co., 1929.

Wiggers, C. J.: Circulatory Dynamics. New York, Grune & Stratton, 1952.

Willius, F. A.: Clinical Electrocardiography. Philadelphia, W. B. Saunders Co., 1922.

Wilson, R. M.: The Beloved Physician, Sir James Mackenzie. New York, The Macmillan Co., 1927.

Winsor, T.: Peripheral Vascular Diseases. Springfield, Illinois, Charles C Thomas, 1959.

Wolf, H. F., and von Bonsdorff, B.: Blutige Messung des absoluten Sphygmogramms beim Menschen. Z. Gesamte Exp. Med., 79:567, 1931.

Wong, K. C., and Wu, L.: History of Chinese Medicine. Tientsin, Shanghai, China, National Quarantine Service, 1932.

Wood, F. C., Johnson, J., Schnabel, T. G., Jr., Kuo, P. T., and Zinsser, H. F.: The diastolic heart beat. Trans. Assoc. Am. Physicians, 64:95, 1951.

Wood, P.: Diseases of the Heart and Circulation. Philadelphia, J. B. Lippincott Co., 1956.

10
EXAMINATION OF THE BREAST

The physical signs of breast disease are of greater significance for diagnosis than are the symptoms that the patient may relate. Self-discovered nodules or such symptoms as pain, tenderness, and nipple discharge may prompt the patient to seek medical consultation specifically for breast examination. When the physician is so alerted, discovery of breast disease, while requiring diligence, demands no great astuteness or refinement of skills. Discovery of an asymptomatic breast lesion during a routine periodic health examination, however, requires persistence and thoroughness in the application of practiced skills. Such a discovery is particularly rewarding if the lesion is malignant, since early discovery markedly enhances the chance for cure.

A major impediment to thorough routine breast examination is a degree of sensitivity and embarrassment surrounding breast examination on the part of most women and, all too frequently, of the physician. The pursuit of accurate diagnostic information leading to prompt adequate treatment can ill afford such subjectivity in the examination of any female patient.

The primary concern regarding any breast lesion is the detection of malignant change at the earliest possible time. Astute and thorough clinical examination of the breasts provides the

517

clues to proper management. In most instances, however, specific diagnosis requires microscopic examination of excised tissue by a pathologist.

Should there be any questionable findings of a breast mass or if the breast is difficult to examine by virtue of its large size or firm consistency, mammography should supplement the physical examination.

HISTORY OF THE PATIENT

If the patient presents with complaints referable to the breast, questioning should be immediately directed to this area. If the consultation is for a routine health survey or an unrelated complaint, during the system review inquire regarding pain, nipple discharge, changes in appearance of the breast, and the presence of any abnormal masses.

Breast pain (mastodynia) is common in teenage girls and young women in the several days preceding the onset of menses. This is due to normal physiological stimulation of the breast and accompanies a sensation of breast enlargement, often noted by the patient by the observation that her brassiere fits more tightly than usual. This type of mastodynia is characterized by its cyclic nature and by its alleviation or disappearance with the onset of menses. The discomfort is more common in the axillary tail of the breast than elsewhere. Pain that is not cyclic or that is well localized may indicate a benign tumor, such as fibroadenoma or localized cystic disease. Pain is not a common presenting complaint of patients with breast carcinoma, but a history of intermittent, sharp, or jabbing pain in a breast without obvious cause should increase suspicion of breast carcinoma.

Query should be made regarding any spontaneous discharge from the breast. This may be clear and watery, bloody, gray-green, or milky, and is often seen only as a stain on the brassiere. Its frequency, amount, and character should be carefully noted. Occasionally in a middle-aged woman, squeezing the nipple area may produce a drop of thick gray material. This is a normal discharge from ectatic ducts and differs significantly from conditions producing a spontaneous discharge.

Several breast lesions (e.g., carcinoma, traumatic fat necrosis) may cause retraction signs, such as "dimpling" of the skin due to fibrosis involving Cooper's ligaments. This may be the patient's first recognition of breast disease. Carcinomas located near the nipple cause retraction or inversion of the nipple. Whenever nipple inversion exists, ask the patient about its duration, since it may occur as a normal variation.

Increase in the size of one breast (or both) may be described by the patient. The giant fibroadenoma (cystosarcoma phyllodes) involving one breast and juvenile hypertrophy involving one or both breasts are obvious to patient and examiner alike. Redness of the breast indicative of cellulitis may occur as a primary inflammation, generally in the postpartum period or as a companion to carcinoma (inflammatory carcinoma).

Has the patient noted a mass? Many breast masses are discovered by the patient as she bathes herself, as she examines her breasts during self-examination, or when she rolls over in the bed and notes an unusual sensation.

An important part of the history is previous breast disease, an earlier breast operation, or aspiration of a breast tumor. Since breast disease is related to a patient's reproductive and menstrual history, such data should be carefully recorded. Notation of current medications, particularly hormones, should be made.

EXAMINATION OF THE PATIENT

The requirements for examination of the breast are good lighting, warm hands, and a sympathetic manner.

After a thorough history has been taken, inspect the breasts first with the patient sitting upright, then leaning forward, and finally in the supine position. When the patient is sitting, ask her to extend the arms straight out in front and then directly overhead (Figs. 10–1 to 10–3). Attention should be directed to sym-

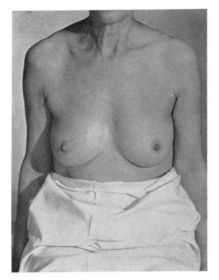

Figure 10-1. Inspection of the breasts with the arms at the sides. (Hopkins, H. U.: Leopold's Principles and Methods of Physical Diagnosis. 3rd ed. Philadelphia, W. B. Saunders Co., 1965.)

Figure 10-2. Inspection of the breasts with the arms raised. (Hopkins, H. U.: Leopold's Principles and Methods of Physical Diagnosis. 3rd ed. Philadelphia, W. B. Saunders Co., 1965.)

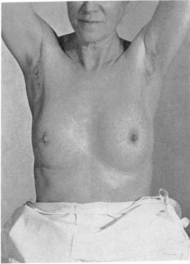

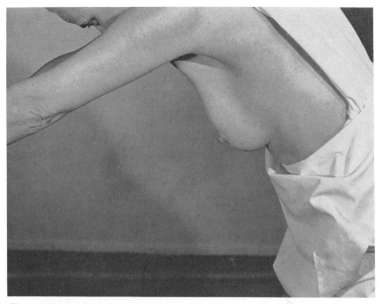

Figure 10–3. *Inspection of the breasts with the patient leaning forward.*
(Hopkins, H. U.: Leopold's Principles and Methods of Physical Diagnosis, 3rd
ed. Philadelphia, W. B. Saunders Co., 1965.)

metry of form and mass (Fig. 10–4), whether there is any retraction of the skin (Fig. 10–5), and whether there is retraction or inversion of one or both nipples (Fig. 10–6).

Note the appearance of the skin. Is it edematous, reddened,
or discolored? Is it warmer than normal to touch? Is an obvious
mass present? Occasionally the skin overlying an infiltrating
tumor takes on the appearance of an orange peel (peau
d'orange) (Fig. 10–7). An eczematoid appearance of the nipple,
e.g., dry, scaling crusts that are papular with or without erythema, most generally indicates Paget's disease (Fig. 10–8).

Palpation should then be done with the patient sitting and
supine. Stand beside the seated patient and palpate the breasts

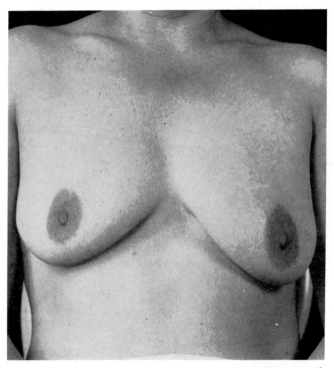

Figure 10–4. *Asymmetric elevation of the right breast due to carcinoma. (Haagensen, C. D.: Diseases of the Breast. 2nd ed. Philadelphia, W. B. Saunders Co., 1971.)*

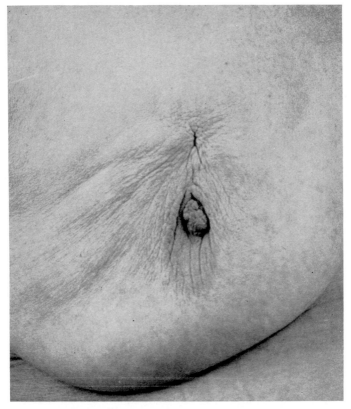

Figure 10–5. *Marked retraction resulting from carcinoma of the upper central portion of the breast. (Haagensen, C. D.: Diseases of the Breast. 2nd ed. Philadelphia, W. B. Saunders Co., 1971.)*

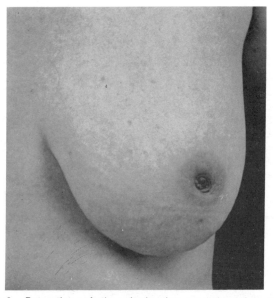

Figure 10-6. *Retraction of the nipple due to subareolar carcinoma. (Haagensen, C. D.: Diseases of the Breast. 2nd ed. Philadelphia, W. B. Saunders Co., 1971.)*

with the flat part of the hand. Learn to recognize the feel of normal breast tissue. If an abnormal mass is felt, outline it with your fingers. Then with the patient lying down, elevate the shoulder with a pillow on the side being examined and repeat the palpation (Fig. 10–9). Masses that are not apparent in one position may be evident in the other.

If a mass is found, note whether it is painful, what its contour is, what its consistency is (firm and rubbery, or unyielding), whether there is adjacent inflammation, and whether it is attached to the underlying pectoral muscle. The latter is best determined by having the patient place her hands on her hips and

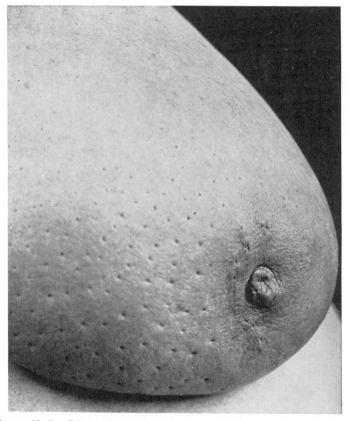

Figure 10–7. *Edema of the skin of the breast due to underlying carcinoma. (Haagensen, C. D.: Diseases of the Breast. 2nd ed. Philadelphia, W. B. Saunders Co., 1971.)*

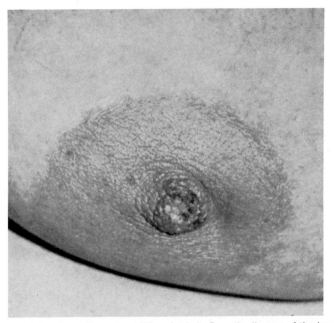

Figure 10–8. *A small erosion of the nipple in Paget's disease of the breast. (Haagensen, C. D.: Diseases of the Breast. 2nd ed. Philadelphia, W. B. Saunders Co., 1971.)*

adduct her arms as forcibly as possible, thus tensing the pectoral muscle (Fig. 10–10*A*). If the tumor becomes elevated or otherwise moves and becomes fixed with this motion, then first degree fixation is present. Second degree fixation is present if, when the patient is supine, pectoral contraction causes sharp fixation and immobility of the tumor mass (Fig. 10–10*B*), and third degree fixation is evident when the mass is clearly fixed with the pectoralis relaxed. Pay particular attention to the sharpness of separation of the mass from the surrounding tissue. Is it well

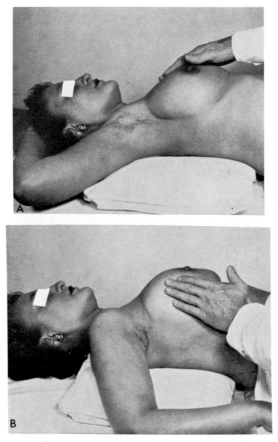

Figure 10-9. A, *Palpation of the inner half of the breast with the arm above the head;* B, *palpation of the lateral half of the breast with the arm at the side. (Haagensen, C. D.: Diseases of the Breast. 2nd ed. Philadelphia, W. B. Saunders Co., 1971.)*

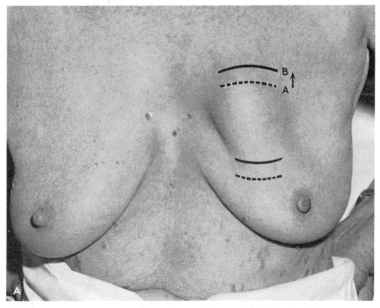

Figure 10–10. A, *A marked example of first degree fixation of a tumor to the pectoral fascia. Contraction of the pectoral muscle elevated the carcinoma 2 cm. and accentuated the skin retraction.*

Illustration continued on opposite page.

delimited or does it blend into the surrounding tissue with only an obscure line of demarcation?

Fluctuation should be determined by isolating the mass between two fingers of one hand and gently palpating with the other hand. A yielding sensation suggests a cyst filled with fluid. This lesion may then be examined for transillumination by darkening the room and holding a flashlight against the suspected cyst.

Finally, examine the adjacent axillary and supraclavicular spaces for lymph node enlargement (Figs. 10–11 and 10–12).

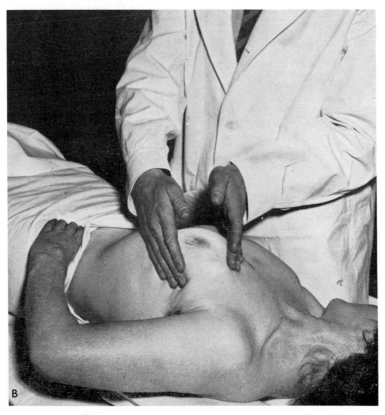

Figure 10–10 (Continued). B, *Testing the mobility of a tumor for second degree fixation. (Haagensen, C. D.: Diseases of the Breast. 2nd ed. Philadelphia, W. B. Saunders Co., 1971.)*

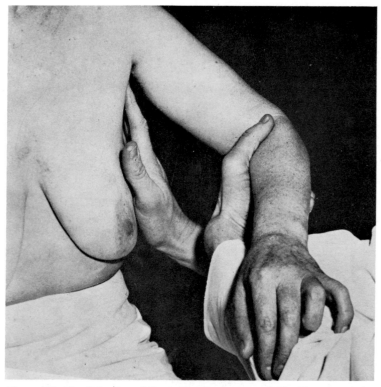

Figure 10–11. *Palpation of the axilla. (Haagensen, C. D.: Diseases of the Breast. 2nd ed. Philadelphia, W. B. Saunders Co., 1971.)*

A description as well as a line sketch of any breast findings should be a part of the record. Specifically, notation should be made about asymmetry of the breast, retraction signs, the presence and size of any mass, its consistency, its mobility, the skin of the breast and nipple, and lymph nodes in the axilla and supraclavicular regions.

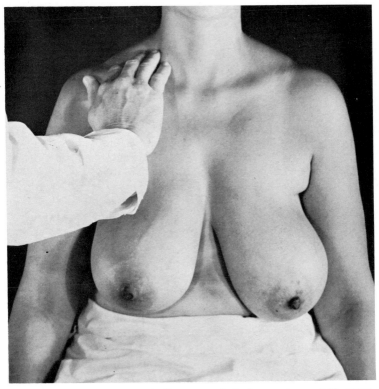

Figure 10–12. Palpation of the supraclavicular and cervical areas. (Haagensen, C. D.: Diseases of the Breast. 2nd ed. Philadelphia, W. B. Saunders Co., 1971.)

BREAST CANCER

Breast carcinoma is the most common cancer in women and, according to the most recent statistics, is the most common cause of death in women between the ages of 35 and 50. Any breast tumor in a woman past the menopause is very likely to be a carcinoma, since its frequency increases with age and other breast tumors decrease in frequency in later life.

Most patients with breast cancer present with the complaint that they have discovered a tumor mass. Nipple discharge, pain, and retraction signs may also cause them to seek medical advice. Between 5 and 10 per cent of breast carcinomas are discovered during a routine periodic examination or "check-up"—the patient having experienced no symptoms.

Carcinoma of the breast is most frequently found in the upper outer breast quadrant and in the subareolar area. The mass is hard, usually not tender, and obviously different in consistency from the surrounding breast tissue. In spite of this latter characteristic, the mass is not well delineated. The physician should look carefully for retraction signs (Fig. 10–13) as well as for mobility or fixation of the mass to the pectoral fascia. Retraction signs may also occur with traumatic fat necrosis and in Mondor's disease (Fig. 10–14).

Observe the nipples for discharge, inversion, edema, or redness. Inspect the supraclavicular and axillary areas for lymph node involvement. Gentle but firm palpation is essential. Too vigorous prodding is not only painful but potentially capable of dislodging tumor cells into the blood.

Haagensen lists the following reasons that breast cancers are missed:

1. Failure to carry out adequate breast examination while treating the patient for another disease.

2. Failure to find a tumor discovered by the patient and thus dismissing her.

3. Mistaking a cancer for an infection.

4. Mistaking a cancer for a benign lesion without benefit of biopsy.

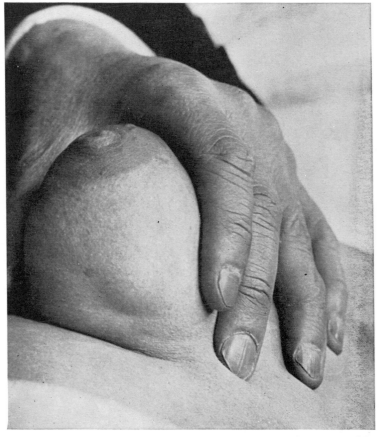

Figure 10–13. Dimpling in the lower half of the breast demonstrated by gentle compression of breast tissue and tumor. (Haagensen, C. D.: Diseases of the Breast. 2nd ed. Philadelphia, W. B. Saunders Co., 1971.)

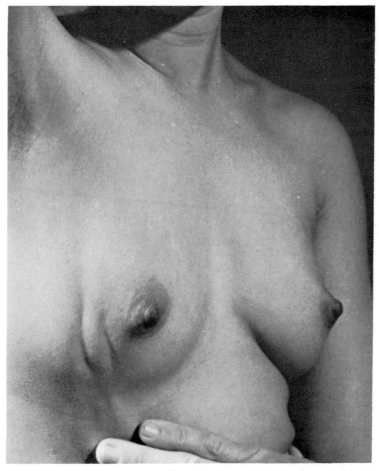

Figure 10–14. Grooves across the lateral aspect of the breast, due to thrombophlebitis of branches of the thoracoepigastric vein, accentuated by caudad traction. (Haagensen, C. D.: Diseases of the Breast. 2nd ed. Philadelphia, W. B. Saunders Co., 1971.)

5. Disregarding a history of acute, sharp pain in the breast.
6. Disregarding retraction signs.
7. Failure to determine the cause of nipple discharge.
8. Reliance on unreliable methods of diagnosis.

The alert physician, by conducting a thorough breast examination in all female patients, will discover nonsymptomatic breast cancers. Such discoveries, usually made early in the course of the disease, provide a markedly improved chance of survival and cure—they depend predominantly upon the skill and perseverance of the examining physician. Finally, it must be noted that breast cancer occurs in men but is, fortunately, rare.

INTRADUCTAL PAPILLOMA

Usually small (2 to 4 mm. average size), these neoplasms may produce no palpable tumor. Characteristically, they cause a serous, faintly yellow or a bloody discharge. They rarely cause pain and seldom cause retraction signs. Gentle palpation may cause nipple discharge and localize an otherwise nonpalpable tumor (Fig. 10–15).

Intraductal papillomas are usually located in the central subareolar breast region. A clinical pattern of breast or tumor enlargement followed by appearance of a nipple discharge and regression of the tumor intermittently suggests an intraductal papilloma.

Definite diagnosis requires a surgical biopsy because the tumors may be malignant and because the same signs and symptoms may be produced by a carcinoma.

PAGET'S DISEASE OF THE BREAST

Paget's disease, a carcinomatous disease of the breast, is readily apparent early in its course but proper treatment is frequently delayed because of the innocuous appearance of the lesion (see Fig. 10–8).

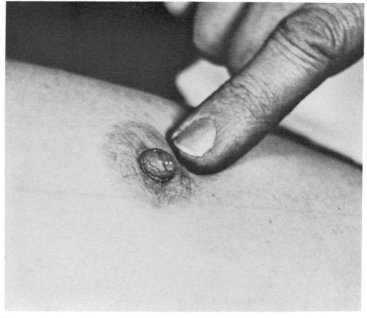

Figure 10-15. The expression of a drop of discharge from the nipple in a patient with intraductal papilloma, by gentle pressure over the site of the papilloma in the subareolar region. (Haagensen, C. D.: Diseases of the Breast. 2nd ed. Philadelphia, W. B. Saunders Co., 1971.)

The earliest symptom is usually itching or burning of the nipple followed by erythema, erosion with exudation, and crust formation. The eczematoid appearance may lead the physician to treat a case of Paget's disease as a dermatitis, but it does not respond to such management. As a rule an erosion that involves only the nipple is due to Paget's disease, whereas eczema involving the skin of the breast but sparing the nipple is not.

A tumor may or may not be palpable in the underlying tissue. A biopsy is mandatory in all such lesions involving the nipple and areola, whether a mass is present or not.

FIBROADENOMA

Fibroadenomas occur predominantly in young women as one or more discrete, smooth, round to ovoid masses of rubbery consistency, usually 1 to 5 cm. in diameter. Sharply delimited and lacking any fixation to the surrounding breast tissue, they are usually "accidentally" discovered because they seldom cause pain, tenderness, or discharge.

A small percentage of fibroadenomas are classified as cystosarcoma phyllodes. This type occurs more commonly in older women and is characterized by rapid growth to great size (Fig. 10–16). They are well delimited, rounded, lobulated masses that

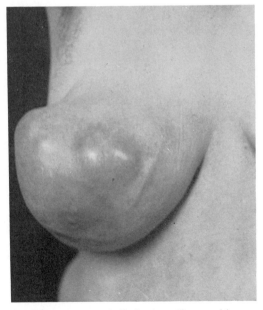

Figure 10–16. *Cystosarcoma phyllodes in a 48 year old woman. (Haagensen, C. D.: Diseases of the Breast. 2nd ed. Philadelphia, W. B. Saunders Co., 1971.)*

are relatively mobile. Retraction signs are rare despite the size of the tumor mass. Though generally benign, 10 to 15 per cent metastasize.

CYSTIC DISEASE OF THE BREAST

This disease, the most common disorder affecting the breast, occurs most frequently in the third and fourth decades; it is infrequently seen following the menopause. The cysts are usually multiple and involve predominantly one breast. The tumor masses are frequently discovered during a routine examination because they may produce no symptoms, although some patients note pain and tenderness. When such symptoms are present, they are often exaggerated during the premenstrual period. Pain is more common with cystic disease than with either carcinoma or fibroadenoma.

The cysts are frequently quite variable in both appearance and behavior. Disappearance and changes in size are common. Nipple discharge occurs but rarely, and retraction signs do not occur although distortion of breast contour may be apparent if the cysts are large. They are usually mobile like fibroadenomas and are round and well delimited; but if they are deep in the substance of the breast, these characteristics may be obscured. If many cysts are present in close proximity, the mass thus formed may suggest carcinoma. A biopsy is essential for definitive diagnosis, particularly since malignant changes do develop in cystic lesions.

Two variants are noted: sclerosing adenosis in which the fibrous stroma predominates and the cystic changes (epithelial proliferation) are minimal, and the solitary "blue-domed" cyst. The latter is a large (several centimeters), thin-walled cyst, often solitary, that appears blue through its capsule after excision.

BREAST HYPERTROPHY

True breast hypertrophy most commonly follows a normal pubescence and normal subsequent menarche. Though usually

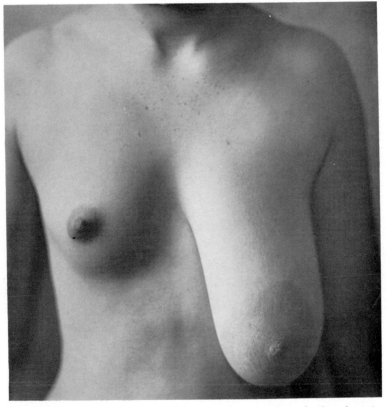

Figure 10–17. *Asymmetrical adolescent hypertrophy of the breast. (Haagensen, C. D.: Diseases of the Breast. 2nd ed. Philadelphia, W. B. Saunders Co., 1971.)*

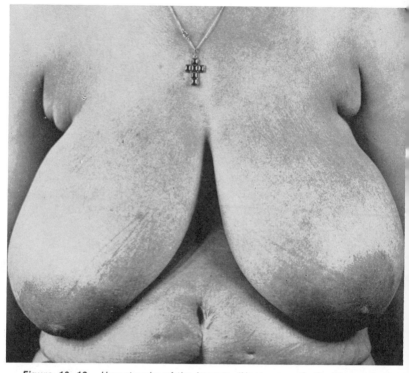

Figure 10–18. Hypertrophy of the breasts. (Haagensen, C. D.: Diseases of the Breast. 2nd ed. Philadelphia, W. B. Saunders Co., 1971.)

bilateral, it may involve one breast (Fig. 10–17) more than the other. Sufficiently large breasts may cause pain because of traction from their excessive weight (Fig. 10–18) and may be so pronounced that the patient is comfortable only when lying down. Enlargement does not regress with age. Microscopic examination reveals normal architecture.

Gynecomastia (hypertrophy of breast tissue in the male)

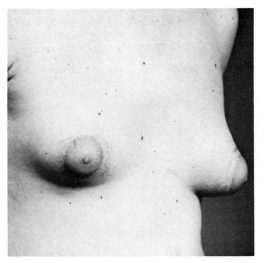

Figure 10–19. Gynecomastia in a man taking spironolactone for Laennec's cirrhosis.

occurs in a variety of illnesses. Eunuchs and men with Klinefelter's syndrome frequently have breast enlargement. Liver cirrhosis, particularly that related to alcoholism, is also associated with gynecomastia (Fig. 10–19). Hyperthyroidism, Addison's disease, some testicular and adrenocortical tumors, and malnutrition have all been associated with gynecomastia. Some medications, notably estrogenic substances, spironolactone, and digitalis preparations, may cause breast enlargement in men.

BREAST INFECTIONS

Breast abscesses occur most commonly during lactation and may be subcutaneous, intramammary, or retromammary. In the

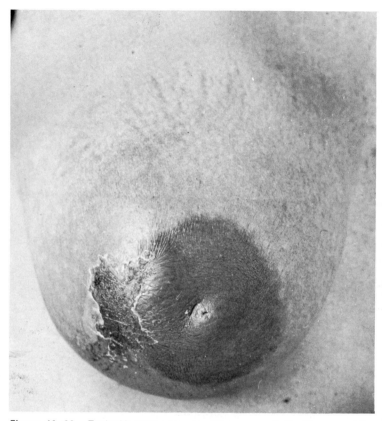

Figure 10–20. *Typical lactation abscess. (Haagensen, C. D.: Diseases of the Breast. 2nd ed. Philadelphia, W. B. Saunders Co., 1971.)*

first two locations, the abscess produces the classic signs of pain, erythema, heat, tenderness, tumor, and fluctuation. If, however, the abscess develops beneath the gland, these signs, particularly tumor and fluctuation, may be less obvious (Fig. 10–20).

TRAUMATIC FAT NECROSIS

Trauma to the breast may lead to abscess formation if the patient is lactating or to fat necrosis if she is not. In more than half of the patients no history of trauma is obtained.

The affected area is tender, edematous, and usually superfi-

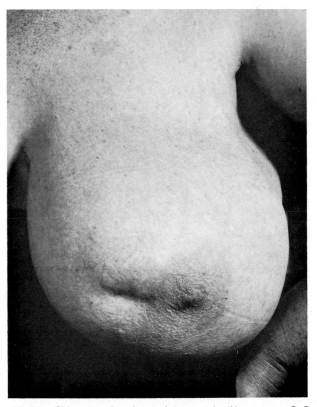

Figure 10–21.   Skin retraction due to fat necrosis. (Haagensen, C. D.: Diseases of the Breast. 2nd ed. Philadelphia, W. B. Saunders Co., 1971.)

cial. Ecchymosis overlying the area is common. A mass is usually palpable, firm, fixed, and well delimited. Retraction signs may be evident, making the differential diagnosis from carcinoma difficult if physical findings alone are considered (Fig. 10–21).

COMMON CLINICAL TERMS

Accessory breast — A fairly common anomaly in which supernumerary breasts or nipples occur. It is often hereditary. The accessory breasts are usually in the embryologic milk line between the axilla and the groin. The most common site is the axilla, followed by the area below the normal breast, but they may occur (rarely) in the inguinal region and the vulva.

Carcinoma en cuirasse — A far advanced stage of breast carcinoma in which the adjacent and overlying skin and breast are thickened, hard, dark red, fibrotic, and edematous. There may be plaques of rough skin resembling leather. This is due to invasion of the skin and subcutaneous tissues by carcinoma cells and lymphocytes. Named by Velpeau after the piece of armor worn about the chest by knights.

Cooper's ligament — Fibrous ligaments between the breast tissue and the superficial fascia. When fibrosis occurs (e.g., in carcinoma or traumatic fat necrosis) these ligaments contract and cause dimpling of the skin.

Mammography — Soft-tissue roentgenography of the breast. More recently this has been superseded by xeroradiography, which requires less irradiation and gives better soft tissue detail.

Peau d'orange — "Orange peel" appearance of the skin due to obstruction of the subdermal lymphatics. The skin is thickened and the orifices of the cutaneous glands are separated and deepened (see Fig. 10–7). It may be due to malignant or inflammatory disease.

Polythelia — The presence of more than one nipple for a breast, a rare anomaly.

Retraction signs — Signs produced by the fibrosis generally secondary to malignancy, but not always (e.g., traumatic fat necrosis, abscess). These signs are skin dimpling, fixation of the breast to the pectoral muscles, retraction, inversion or flattening of the nipple, and a change in the axis in which the nipple points.

COMMON CLINICAL SYNDROMES

Adenosis (or sclerosing adenosis)—A variant of cystic disease in which there is epithelial proliferation and excessive fibrosis, more than that usually seen in ordinary cystic disease. It may occur microscopically or be large enough to form a palpable tumor. Clinically it is firm, rubbery, and poorly delineated from adjacent breast tissue. Retraction signs are rarely present, but otherwise it simulates carcinoma. Some believe it occurs chiefly in young or middle-aged females taking estrogen preparations.

Adolescent (juvenile) hypertrophy of the breast—Excessive growth of one or both breasts after puberty. It is usually bilateral, but may be unilateral (see Fig. 10–17 and 10–18).

Cystosarcoma phyllodes (Mueller)—A large, bulky, and irregularly nodular tumor of the breast often preceded by a fibroadenoma of many years' duration. The diagnosis is made by microscopic examination of tissue although the gross irregular nodular appearance of the breast suggests the diagnosis (Fig. 10–16). Most cystosarcomas grow rapidly and, although they may appear malignant microscopically, only a few (10 to 15 per cent) metastasize.

Fibrocystic disease of the breast (called also chronic cystic mastitis; in France, Reclus' disease; in Germany, Schimmelbusch's disease; and cystic disease)—A disease of the breast characterized by cysts, varying in size, accompanied by (microscopic) epithelial proliferation and fibrosis. Probably 10 per cent of all women have cystic disease of the breast. Most common between the ages of 25 and 50 years. Sclerosing adenosis and the blue-domed cyst are variants of this disease.

Galactocele—A cyst containing thick inspissated milk. It occurs in lactating women when nursing has been terminated abruptly. Usually located at the central part of the breast, it mimics a benign tumor since it is freely movable and well demarcated. The milky fluid on aspiration is pathognomonic.

Gynecomastia—Hypertrophy of one or both breasts in the male. Primary gynecomastia may occur at puberty or in old age. In other instances it is secondary to endocrine abnormalities (diseases of the testis, adrenal cortex, pituitary, thyroid, and liver and ACTH-producing tumors of the lung), malnutrition, and the ingestion of various drugs (including androgens, estrogens, digitalis, diuretics) (see Fig. 10–19).

Inflammatory carcinoma of the breast—The worst type of breast carcinoma. It is characterized by generalized breast tenderness and pain. The breast is enlarged and firm; the overlying skin is red or dusky. Often there is generalized edema of the skin and induration of the breast. The erythema is not uniform, and an underlying tumor mass may be palpable. It is an extremely virulent type of carcinoma and is generally considered to be inoperable.

Lactation mastitis and abscess—A localized area of inflammation with pain, induration, and tenderness to palpation with fever developing in the breast of a female who is nursing a baby (mastitis). This initial mastitis may progress to obvious erythema and edema of the skin with fluctuation (abscess). Almost all postpartum abscesses are caused by coagulase-positive *Staphylococcus aureus,* often resistant to penicillin (see Fig. 10–20). Any abscess in a nonlactating breast should be suspected to be carcinoma.

Mondor's disease (thrombophlebitis of the superficial veins of the breast)—A rare disease, but important because of its differential diagnosis, this lesion is characterized by pain in the lateral aspect of the breast followed by a shallow groove extending upward across the outer breast towards the axilla. Palpation reveals a cord-like thickening beneath the groove. This represents phlebitis and fibrosis of the thoracoepigastric vein (see Fig. 10–14).

Paget's disease of the breast (James Paget, 1874)—An eczematoid eruption of the nipple and areola, generally accompanied by itching or a burning sensation, progressing to erosion of the nipple and a discharge secondary to an underlying breast carcinoma. Histologically, specific cells called Paget cells are seen invading the epithelium.

Papillary tumors of the breast—May be benign intraductal papillomas, which are the most frequent, or malignant papillary carcinomas, which are rare. These are the most common cause of serous or bloody discharge from the nipple. Nipple discharge in females is due to benign intraductal papilloma in 70 per cent of cases and to malignant papillary carcinoma in 12 per cent. The nipple discharge is serous in 45 per cent of cases and bloody in 55 per cent. The benign papillomas are usually small and often (about 60 per cent of cases) no tumor is palpable—but the nipple discharge can be provoked by examination (see Fig. 10–15).

Traumatic fat necrosis of the breast—A palpable tumor in the subcutaneous tissue of the breast due to necrosis of the fat. The initial necrosis, which may be secondary to trauma (but is in less than half of the patients) is followed by fibrosis and signs of retraction. Because of the retraction signs (skin dimpling, nipple retraction or deviation) this lesion mimics carcinoma. It can also simulate a breast abscess. Traumatic fat necrosis generally occurs in females with large breasts with a generous amount of subcutaneous fat (see Fig. 10–21).

BIBLIOGRAPHY

Haagensen, C. D.: Diseases of the Breast. 2nd ed. Philadelphia, W. B. Saunders Co., 1971.

Hopkins, H. U.: Leopold's Principles and Methods of Physical Diagnosis. Philadelphia, W. B. Saunders Co., 1965.

11
EXAMINATION OF THE ABDOMEN

Careful examination of the abdomen may yield signs of disease or injury not detected by history, radiologic examination, endoscopy, or laboratory tests. Moreover, any physical finding increases in significance when coupled with these other means of collecting information. Radiologic procedures in particular have added to the accuracy of diagnosis largely through use of contrast media, such as air, iodized solutions, barium, and radioisotopes. The ordinary upright and flat abdominal roentgenogram yields important adjunctive information to physical examination.

Examination of the abdomen for abnormalities in the intra- and extraperitoneal spaces should routinely include palpation of the left supraclavicular space and digital rectal palpation of the pelvic peritoneal area. These maneuvers should be as much a part of routine abdominal examination as inspection, palpation, percussion, and auscultation of the abdomen proper. Palpation of the left supraclavicular space (the upper terminus of the thoracic lymphatic duct) may reveal an enlarged lymph node as an important sign of a silent intra-abdominal malignancy; rectal examination of the caudad extremity of the peritoneal cavity may elicit points of tenderness, pelvic peritoneal masses, or a "rectal shelf" that otherwise would have been hidden during "anterior" abdominal examination.

548

The most satisfactory placement of the patient for examination of the abdomen is a completely relaxed supine position, arms to the side and head flat on a pillow (see Fig. 11–13*A*). The knees should be flexed only slightly, if at all. If the head or shoulders are elevated there is a tendency for the patient to watch the examination, which has the effect of tightening the abdominal musculature. Another hindrance to examination is flexion of the hips and knees, which is frequently employed but which causes the knees to interfere with palpation of the lower abdomen. The supine position is satisfactory for all parts of the examination except when examining for shifting dullness or for demonstrating the psoas sign or, more commonly, for showing bulges of the abdominal wall or hernias, which are best revealed in the standing position. The proper position for examination of the rectum and the pelvic peritoneum is the lateral Sims position with marked flexion of the hips and knees.

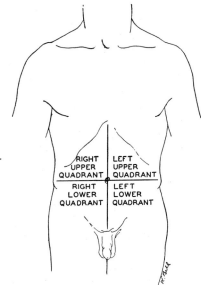

Figure 11–1. *Division of the abdomen into quadrants.*

Although one cannot say that any one aspect in the examination of the abdomen is of greater importance than another, palpation more often elucidates signs of disease or injury than do inspection, percussion, or auscultation; and even though all are important, auscultation, often neglected or omitted, commonly supplies the crucial information leading to a correct diagnosis.

Topographical anatomy of the abdomen is useful for describing areas in which findings are made; the most practical is into four quadrants, drawing a horizontal and vertical line through the umbilicus (Fig. 11–1). More specific terms, such as the epigastrium, flank, suprapubic areas, hypochondrium, or periumbilical, are used when appropriate.

INSPECTION

William Osler emphasized to medical students the importance of inspection when he said, "The whole art of medicine is in observation. Don't touch the patient—state first what you see.

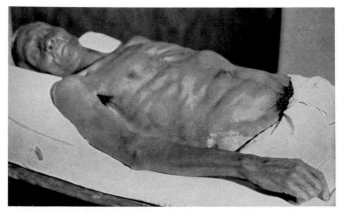

Figure 11–2. Emaciation with intestinal pattern evident on inspection of the abdomen, typical of chronic partial small bowel obstruction.

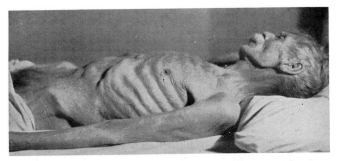

Figure 11–3. *Extreme emaciation with mass in epigastrium. Carcinoma of stomach.*

See—then reason and compare. Medicine is learned at the bedside, not in the classroom. Live in the ward. Don't waste the hours of daylight in listening to that which you may read at night."

A few moments of inspection, too often omitted, may give important clues as to which part of the remaining examination should be particularly emphasized. Presence or absence of distention, symmetry or asymmetry, and midline protuberances are best seen when the examiner stands or sits to one side looking across the surface of the abdomen.

Asking the patient to inspire deeply during inspection may bring out useful information. For example, "catching his breath" at the maximal point of inspiration may indicate infection of the pleura or involvement of the diaphragm by an infection such as a subdiaphragmatic abscess or acute cholecystitis. Deep inspiration may also reveal enlargement of the liver and spleen, distention of the gallbladder, and the prominence of pancreatic cysts. The liver, spleen, and gallbladder move with respiration because of the action of the diaphragm. An enlarged liver can be seen to pulsate in tricuspid insufficiency of the heart. Asking the patient to cough may bring out the "bulge" in hernias of the abdominal wall. A cough may also help to localize pain; particularly with acute appendicitis the patient, on coughing, will point to the area of pain in the right lower quadrant. Coughing may also elicit a point of pain in the exact midline between the umbilicus and the xiphoid process when an otherwise elusive epigastric herniation of properitoneal fat is present.

Inspection of abdominal skin for pigmentation, dehydration, or malnutrition is no more revealing than observation of the skin elsewhere. Dilation of abdominal veins, however, is indicative of an obstruction in either the portal vein or the inferior vena cava (Fig. 11–4). Caput medusae, a cluster of dilated veins radiating from the umbilicus, may occur in cases of obstruction of the portal vein but, as Cabot has stated, the caput medusae is "commonly found in text books, but rarely seen in cirrhosis of the liver." The umbilicus, however, should be carefully inspected for telltale signs of intra-abdominal abnormalities. Blue or yellowish blue discoloration around the umbilicus suggests that hemorrhage has occurred either intraperitoneally or retroperitoneally, such as in acute pancreatitis, exacerbation of chronic pancreatitis, duodenal injury with retroperitoneal hem-

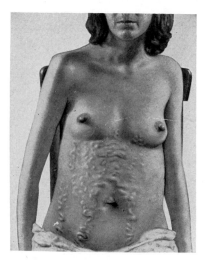

Figure 11–4. Dilated abdominal veins in obstruction of the vena cava.

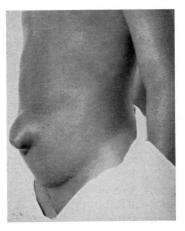

Figure 11-5. *Umbilical hernia.*

orrhage, or rupture of a tubal pregnancy. Nodules of the umbilicus may be the only sign of metastasizing intra-abdominal malignancy. Herniation at the umbilicus is usually just cephalad to the umbilicus proper (Fig. 11-5) and is made more prominent by abdominal ascites or tumors.

Striae of the skin of the abdominal wall are commonly seen in pregnant women and in women who have borne children. In pregnant women they are pinkish or slightly bluish depressed lines over the lower abdomen, parallel to the long axis of the body. In women who have borne children they are a glistening, silvery white color. They are produced by rupture of the elastic fibers of the skin and can be observed also in nonpregnant women and in men when there has been a rapid increase in size of the abdomen, as in the case of abdominal tumors, obesity, or Cushing's syndrome (see Fig. 15-8).

The abdomen may be grossly enlarged as a result of obesity, ascites, tumor, or gastrointestinal distention. A presumptive impression as to which of these is the cause can often be made upon inspection. Obesity of the abdomen often appears as folds or aprons of fat in the suprapubic or flank areas. When obesity is associated with hypopituitarism, the fat is centrally and not peripherally distributed. Ascites (from askos, a bag), the presence of free fluid in the peritoneal cavity, when moderate in amount, produces an enlarged abdomen that is flattened anteriorly with bulging in the flanks when the patient is in the supine position. It is distinguishable from a large ovarian cyst, which usually causes a domed, protuberant abdomen without bulging flanks. When ascites is severe, however, the contour of the abdomen is likewise rounded but can be differentiated from a tumor by demonstration of shifting dullness and a fluid wave (see Fig. 11–19). Ascites may occur with cardiac failure, as shown in Figure 11–6. This patient shows, in addition to a tense, shiny abdomen, marked cyanosis of the lips and nose and is dyspneic. Diagnosis in such patients is aided by the presence of an enlarged, tender liver and of cardiac enlargement with murmurs. Chronic adhesive pericarditis may likewise cause ascites but is associated with a normal-sized heart, distant heart sounds, and venous engorgement of veins in the neck and trunk. Cirrhosis of the liver is the

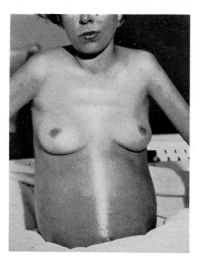

Figure 11–6. Ascites with cardiac failure. Note dark shade of the lips resulting from cyanosis.

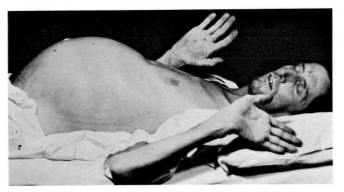

Figure 11–7. Wasting in cirrhosis of the liver.

classic cause of ascites. Atrophy of the chest and arms, gyneco-mastia, dilated veins of the abdomen, edema of the legs, an enlarged spleen, and spider nevi of the skin may be seen with hepatic cirrhosis (Figs. 11–7 to 11–10). Ascites is rarely seen with serum hepatitis or prolonged calculary obstruction of the com-mon bile duct, the latter circumstance probably being attributa-

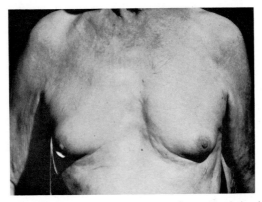

Figure 11–8. Gynecomastia in a patient with cirrhosis.

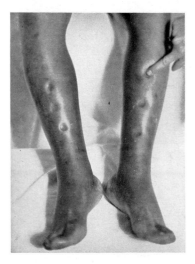

Figure 11-9. Edema of legs in cirrhosis of the liver.

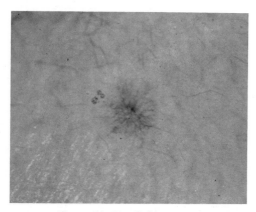

Figure 11-10. Spider nevus.

ble to lymphatic obstruction. Ascites may occur in vascular occlusions of the mesentery, strangulating obstructions of the intestine, polyserositis, tuberculosis of the peritoneum, nephritis, nephrosis, and abdominal carcinomatosis. In the last instance, a search for metastases to Virchow's node (left supraclavicular), umbilical nodularity, and Blumer's (rectal) shelf should be made.

When gastrointestinal distention occurs, careful inspection is imperative in order to determine the cause of distention. Most of the diagnostic features associated with gastrointestinal distention at any age are included in Table 11–1. When inspecting a distended abdomen, note carefully whether the distention is diffuse over the entire abdomen or limited to a portion of it, such as the upper or epigastric region. The detection of a mass or the visible outline of the intestine, such as the colon in congenital aganglionic megacolon (Hirschsprung's disease, Fig. 11–11), is also important. Intestinal movement or activity is rarely seen in the distended abdomen, but when "churning" of the intestine is apparent it is most certainly diagnostic of chronic partial small bowel obstruction. Acute small intestinal obstruction always results in distention of varying degrees, and is usually part of a triad of symptoms and signs: vomiting, abdominal distention, and abdominal cramping pains associated simultaneously with intestinal hyperperistalsis (borborygmi). When all three features are present in a patient, mechanical small bowel obstruction is present and upright abdominal x-rays usually will confirm its presence. If any one part of the triad is absent, the findings are not diagnostic of mechanical obstruction. In peritonitis, for instance, when paralytic ileus mimics the vomiting and distention, exaggerated bowel sounds will be absent even though pain may be present. Mechanical small bowel obstruction may be due to extrinsic, intrinsic, or obturator mechanisms, which often can be differentiated upon inspection by associated physical findings. For example, small bowel obstruction due to adhesions usually is associated with a skin scar that has healed in an ugly fashion. (See Table 11–1 for additional examples.)

Text continued on page 566.

TABLE 11-1. DIFFERENTIAL DIAGNOSIS

| Typical Age | Typical Sex | Triad[1] | | | |
		Abdominal Distention	Vomiting	Colic	Borborygmi
0–6 wks.	Either	Epigastric	+	0	0
1–7 days	Either	Epigastric only	+	0	0
1–7 days	Either	Epigastric only	+	0	0
1–7 days	Either	Diffuse	+	0	0
1 wk.	Either	Diffuse	+	0	+
1 wk.	Either	Diffuse	+	+	+
1 wk.	Either	Diffuse	+	±	±
1–3 wks.	Male	Epigastric	+	0	0
0–5 yrs.	Either	Diffuse	±	0	0

[1]*Triad* refers to a combination of symptoms and signs that are pathognomonic of a mechanical small bowel obstruction: distention, vomiting, and cramping abdominal pains simultaneous with borborygmi.

OF GASTROINTESTINAL DISTENTION

Associated Signs	Additional Clues	Confirmatory Tests	Probable Diagnosis
Bile-stained vomitus	Minimal air in intestine	Cecum in RUQ or LUQ	Duodenal band obstruction due to malrotation
Bile-stained vomitus	Minimal air in intestine	Double-bubble sign[2] Cecum in RLQ[3]	Duodenal stenosis or annular pancreas
Bile-stained vomitus	No air in intestine	Double-bubble sign Cecum in RLQ	Duodenal atresia
Shock	Dehydration	Fluid levels in localized loops	Volvulus due to malrotation
Bile-stained vomitus	No stools	No air in colon	Obstructing atresia of ileum
Several sausage-like masses	Positive sweat test	Fluid levels Occasional intra-peritoneal calcification	Obstructing inspissated meconium in ileum
Anal dimple	No stools May have fistula	Upside-down x-ray[4]	Obstructing anal atresia (imperforate anus)
Pyloric "tumor"	Delayed onset of vomiting No bile in vomitus	Minimal air in intestine Narrow pyloric opening	Congenital pyloric stenosis
Full rectum	Onset of constipation later than time of birth	Dilatation down to anus	Psychogenic megacolon

[2]Double-bubble sign is seen in an upright x-ray of the abdomen when there are two air-luid levels at different heights: one in the stomach, the other in the abdomen.

[3]Position of the cecum is best determined by a barium enema.

[4]"Upside-down x-ray" is a radiologic test taken with infant held up by the legs to determine e distance of an air bubble from the anal dimple (described by Wangensteen and Rice).

Table continued on following page.

TABLE 11-1. DIFFERENTIAL DIAGNOSIS

Typical Age	Typical Sex	Triad[1]			
		Abdominal Distention	Vomiting	Colic	Borborygmi
0–15 yrs.	Either	Diffuse	±	+	±
1 yr.	Male	Diffuse	+	+ (Severe)	+
5–15 yrs.	Either	Diffuse	+	+	+
6 yrs.	Either	Diffuse	+	+	+
15–25 yrs.	Female	Diffuse	+	+	+
Young adult	Either	Upper	+	+	+
Any age	Either	Diffuse	+	+	+
Any age	Either	Diffuse	+	+	+

OF GASTROINTESTINAL DISTENTION *(Continued)*

Associated Signs	Additional Clues	Confirmatory Tests	Probable Diagnosis
Visible colon "Pot" belly Empty rectum	Constipation since birth	Barium enema Narrow rectosigmoid Rectal biopsy, aganglionic	Congenital aganglionic megacolon (Hirschsprung's disease)
A sausage-like mass, upper or left abdomen	Currant-jelly[5] stool on rectal glove	Barium enema Spring sign[6]	Intussuception
Pigmentation of oral mucosa	Familial	X-ray signs of intussusception	Obstructing intussusception due to small bowel polyp (Peutz-Jeghers syndrome)
Anemia	Occult blood in stool	Fluid levels	Obstructing Meckel's diverticulitis
Mass RLQ (?)	Intermittent, alternating with diarrhea	String sign[7]	Obstructing regional ileitis
Recurrent peptic ulcer	Obstruction alternating with steatorrhea	Marked gastric hypersecretion Hypertrophic rugae of stomach	Obstructing jejunal ulcer with stricture (Zollinger-Ellison syndrome)
Incisional scar, usually "ugly"	History of prior perforated appendicitis or operation	Fluid levels	Small bowel obstruction due to adhesions
Inguinal bulge	Nonreducible hernia	Fluid levels	Obstructing incarcerated inguinal hernia

[5]"Currant-jelly stool" is the characteristic appearance of blood slightly altered in color and ᵏed with mucus.
[6]Spring sign is seen by a barium enema when there is telescoping of the small intestine into colon.
[7]The string sign refers to a narrow, irregular lumen of the terminal ileum and is best demon-ᵃted by a barium enema.

Table continued on following page.

TABLE 11-1. DIFFERENTIAL DIAGNOSIS

Typical Age	Typical Sex	Triad[1]			
		Abdominal Distention	Vomiting	Colic	Borborygmi
Any age	Female	Diffuse	+	+	+
45 yrs.	Female	Diffuse	+	+	+
45+ yrs.	Female	Diffuse	+	+	+
50 yrs.	Either	Upper	+	+	+
Adult	Either	Diffuse	+	+	+
Adult	Either	Diffuse	+	+	+
Adult	Either	Diffuse	+	+	+

OF GASTROINTESTINAL DISTENTION *(Continued)*

Associated Signs	Additional Clues	Confirmatory Tests	Probable Diagnosis
Femoral tenderness (?)	Institutionalized patient[8]	Fluid levels	Obstructing incarcerated femoral hernia or Richter's hernia[9]
Fat Flatulent	Intermittent bouts	Air in biliary tract[10]	Obstructing gallstone in ileum (gallstone ileus)
Rectangular area of telangiectatic discoloration of skin, inferior abdomen (radiodermatitis)	Intermittent Chronic Visible peristalsis History of carcinoma of cervix, treated by x-ray	Fluid levels	Obstructing irradiation stricture of ileum
History of edema, hypertension, or cardiovascular disease	Ingestion of potassium-coated pills	High jejunal obstruction	Obstructing potassium-induced stricture of jejunum
Intermittent Acute onset	Occasional relief by knee-chest position Commonly diagnosed as neurotic	Fluid levels	Obstructing internal hernia
Pallor Anemia	Occult blood in stool	Positive bone marrow	Obstructing lymphosarcoma of small bowel with ulceration
Movable mass, midabdomen (±)	Feeble-minded patient	Fluid levels	Bezoar in ileum[11]

[8]Feeble-minded patients commonly do not call the examiner's attention to pain or tenderness associated with occult femoral hernias.

[9]Richter's hernia is one in which only a portion of the circumference of the small intestine ncarcerated in the hernial ring.

[10]Air in the biliary tract is seen in an upright x-ray of the right upper quadrant when there is a ula between the gallbladder and duodenum. It is caused by the perforating passage of a ge gallstone into the duodenum; obstruction occurs later when the stone reaches the ileum.

[11]The bezoar may be composed of hair, persimmon peel, or other foreign objects such as shcloths.

TABLE 11–1. DIFFERENTIAL DIAGNOSIS

Typical Age	Typical Sex	Triad[1]			
		Abdominal Distention	Vomiting	Colic	Borborygmi
Adult	Either	Diffuse	+	+	+
Adult	Either	Diffuse	0	±	0
Adult	Either	Diffuse	0	±	0
60+ yrs.	Male	Diffuse	±	0	0
Adult	Either	Diffuse	+	0	0
Any age	Either	Diffuse	+	0	Silent
Any age	Either	Minimal	±	+	±
Adult	Either	Diffuse	+	0	Silent

OF GASTROINTESTINAL DISTENTION *(Continued)*

Associated Signs	Additional Clues	Confirmatory Tests	Probable Diagnosis
Mass RLQ	Anemic	Defect in cecum	Obstructing carcinoma of cecum at ileocecal valve
Mass on rectal examination	Blood in stool	Annular lesion	Obstructing carcinoma rectosigmoid
Tender LLQ	Blood in stool	Barium enema Long lesion with diverticulae of colon	Obstructing sigmoid diverticulitis
Sudden onset	History of prior attack	Large, air-filled viscus	Obstructing volvulus of sigmoid colon or cecum
Tender Rigid	Shock Tetany	Elevated serum amylase	Acute pancreatitis
Boardlike rigidity	History of ulcer[12]	Air under diaphragm as seen in upright chest x-ray	Peritonitis due to perforated peptic ulcer
Diarrhea	Borborygmi not simultaneous with abdominal pains	Air in colon	Acute gastroenteritis
Shock	Presystolic mitral murmur	Air in both small bowel and colon	Embolic occlusion of mesentery vessels

[12]Occasionally a duodenal ulcer will perforate in a patient who denies any prior history of ulcer disease.

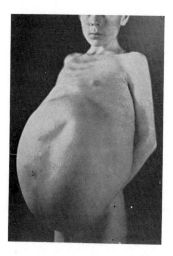

Figure 11-11. *Hirschsprung's disease. (Courtesy of Frederic M. Hanes.)*

There is a marked enlargement of the abdomen in women with pseudocyesis, or pseudopregnancy. In this interesting condition the patient imagines or wishes herself pregnant and the abdomen enlarges accordingly. She may almost convince her physician that she is pregnant even if her menstruation has not ceased. Under anesthesia this abdominal "tumor" disappears. The cause of pseudocyesis has never been fully explained, but it apparently is a psychoneurotic condition, probably best classified as hysteria.

PALPATION

Palpation is, in many respects, the most important procedure in the physical examination of the abdomen. It requires concentration, patience, practice, and experience. One important feature of palpation is to confirm and amplify the findings of inspection. A mass, for instance, that is just visible on inspection, may be firm or soft, smooth or irregular, fixed or movable, tender, fluctuant, or cystic. Frequently a mass that is not visible is easily felt on palpation.

The proper position of the patient for palpation of the abdomen is the supine, flat position, except for palpation of herniations, in which case an upright posture is more informative. Every effort should be made to secure complete relaxation of the patient to eliminate guarding by the abdominal muscles; to aid this satisfactory state, the patient should be assured by a confident attitude and gentle, unhurried movements. He should be asked to breathe easily through his mouth, with his head at rest and his arms loosely at his sides. Needless to say, the patient's undergarments constitute bothersome impediments to a thorough examination and should be removed, maintaining a sense of modesty for the patient with an appropriately placed sheet or towel.

As suggested earlier in this chapter, the examination of the abdomen includes palpation of the pelvic area by rectal examination and (in the female) vaginal examination. Parenthetically, abdominal palpation for abdominal aortic pulsation is a necessary initial part of the examination of the blood supply of the lower extremities.

When palpating the abdomen your hands should be warm and placed flat and held parallel to the surface of the abdomen. The tips of the fingers or the edges of the hands, when held at right angles, cause muscular resistance, which blocks successful palpation. Palpation should be at first soft, gentle, and superficial; then as the tenseness of the muscles relaxes, deeper palpation may be attempted. When palpating a mass in the abdomen, make every effort to note as many as possible of the following characteristics of the mass: location, size, consistency, tenderness (dolor), temperature (calor), color (rubor), fixation or mobility or attachments, fluctuation, ballottement, and transillumination. Obviously not all of these features may be discernible.

Palpation is of special value in determining the outlines of the liver, spleen, kidneys, uterus, and bladder when these organs are enlarged; determining the presence and characteristics of

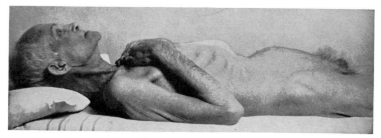

Figure 11–12. *Retention of urine with distention of the bladder.*

abdominal masses; determining the presence of tenderness or rigidity; and confirming the presence of herniations.

When palpating for enlargement of the liver, you may find it advantageous to place your left hand under the patient's right flank, lifting gently upward to elevate the bulk of the liver into a more easily accessible location. A folded towel may be used for the same purpose (Fig. 11–13). The positioned right hand is then moved downward and slightly upward just as the patient takes a deep breath. The descent of the diaphragm during deep inspiration carries the liver down, and its margin as well as an enlarged gallbladder may be palpated by the fingers of the examining hand. The liver may be enlarged because of chronic passive congestion, hepatic cirrhosis, primary or secondary malignancy, abscess, or hepatitis. The nodularity of metastatic disease or portal cirrhosis is easily felt. In tricuspid insufficiency a pulsating liver may be felt. An enlarged gallbladder may be palpated and in the absence of jaundice usually signifies acute cholecystitis due to a calculous obstruction of the cystic duct with hydrops or empyema of the gallbladder or even a pericholecystic abscess. On the other hand, a palpably enlarged gallbladder in the presence of jaundice usually indicates an obstruction of the distal bile duct as a result of malignancy of the head of the pancreas or the sphincter of Oddi (see Table 11–2). Courvoisier's law, it should be emphasized, applies only to the jaundiced patient, in whom the distention of the gallbladder secondary to

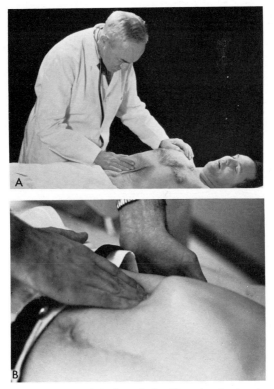

Figure 11–13. *Palpation of the liver.* A, *Position of patient and examiner;* B, *position of examiner's hand.*

TABLE 11–2. DIFFERENTIAL DIAGNOSIS

Typical Age	Typical Sex	Palpable Gall-Bladder	Associated Findings	Occult Blood in Stool	Serum Bilirubin
Infant	Either	0	Enlarged liver, onset at birth	0	Direct
Young	Either	0	Intermittent familial anemia	0	Indirect
Adult	Either	+	Anemia	+	Direct
Adult	Either	+	Anemia	+	Direct
Adult	Either	+	Silent	0	Direct
Adult	Either	0	Silent	0	Direct
Adult	Either	±	Discomfort RUQ	0	Direct
Adult	Either	0	Recent scar of cholecystectomy	0	Direct
Adult	Either	0	History of chlor-promazine medica-tion	0	Direct
Adult	Either	0	Nodular liver	0	Direct
Adult	Female	0	Colic ± fever ± tender RUQ	0	Direct

OF JAUNDICE

Alkaline Phosphatase	Other Tests	X-Ray Findings	Probable Diagnosis
+		Nonconfirmatory	Biliary atresia
0	Spherocytosis Erythrocyte fragility Hyperplastic bone marrow Reticulocytes Coombs' test Urine urobilinogen	Slightly enlarged spleen	Hemolytic anemia
+	Minimal urine urobilinogen	Duodenal defect	Carcinoma of ampulla of Vater
+	Absent urine urobilinogen	Widened duo- denum "E" sign	Carcinoma of head of pancreas
+	Low urine uro- bilinogen	Normal duo- denum	Carcinoma of distal common bile duct
+	Low urine urobilinogen	Normal duodenum	Carcinoma of common hepatic duct
.±	Normal	Normal duo- denum	Carcinoma of gall- bladder
+	Elevated SGOT (±)	Biliary fistula	Stricture of common bile duct
+	Elevated SGOT	Reduced rose bengal I-131 Hepatic scan	Chlorpromazine jaundice
Slight elevation		Defects in hepa- tic scan	Hepatic metastases
+	Elevated serum amylase	Normal duo- denum	Impacted stone in distal common bile duct

Table continued on following page.

TABLE 11–2. DIFFERENTIAL DIAGNOSIS

Typical Age	Typical Sex	Palpable Gall-Bladder	Associated Findings	Occult Blood in Stool	Serum Bilirubin
Adult	Male	0	Nodular liver Ascites Spider nevi Dilated veins Alcoholic	+	Direct Indirect
Any age	Either	0	History of contact or transfusion Tender liver	0	Direct

pancreatic obstruction is possible only if the gallbladder has not been previously contracted and fibrotic with calculary disease.

In jaundiced patients gallbladder enlargement due to carcinoma of the head of the pancreas or ampulla of Vater is usually associated with anemia because of ulceration of the duodenal mucosa, which leads to the associated finding of occult blood in the stool. On the other hand, in carcinoma of the distal common bile duct, occult blood in the stool is unusual and the duodenum is normal on radiologic examination. Carcinoma of the common hepatic duct with jaundice is rarely associated with palpable gallbladder or anemia. A stone impacted in the distal common bile duct will not usually cause distention of the gallbladder, since it is nondistensible because of the scarring of chronic disease. Elevation of the serum amylase is occasionally present and signifies that the impacted stone also is obstructing the pancreatic duct. Tenderness of a palpably enlarged gallbladder on inspiration (Murphy's sign) is an important indication of cholecystitis; the sign may also be present in patients with hepatitis. "The most characteristic and constant sign of gallbladder hypersensitiveness," wrote John B. Murphy, "is the inability of the patient to take a full, deep inspiration when the physician's fingers are backed up deep beneath the right costal arch below

OF JAUNDICE *(Continued)*

Alkaline Phosphatase	Other Tests	X-Ray Findings	Probable Diagnosis
+	Reduced serum albumin Thrombo- cytopenia ($\pm$)	Esophageal var- ices Splenomegaly	Hepatic cirrhosis
+	Very high SGOT	Reduced rose bengal I-131 Hepatic scan	Viral hepatitis

the hepatic margin. The diaphragm forces the liver down until the sensitive gallbladder reaches the examining fingers, when the inspiration suddenly ceases as though it has been shut off. I have never found this sign absent in a calculous or infectious case of gallbladder or duct disease."

Palpation of the spleen should be carried out by the following method: With the patient lying on his back, stand at the patient's right side and place your right hand flat against the abdominal wall, just at the costal margin in the anterior mammillary line. The procedure is assisted by placing your left hand under the splenic area and gently lifting upwards (Fig. 11–14). Ask your patient to inspire deeply, which causes the spleen to descend with the diaphragm and, when enlarged, to touch the tips of the fingers of your right hand. At times the spleen, although not felt when the patient lies on his back, is readily palpable if the patient lies on his right side. A normal-sized spleen will not be felt, as is often the case in congenital hemolytic anemia and thrombocytopenic purpura; however, the huge spleens found in the leukemias, Hodgkin's disease, malaria, and typhoid fever are easily felt (Fig. 11–15). The consistency of the enlarged spleen is often important. In typhoid fever it feels soft; in malaria, hard and firm. In Vaquez' disease the spleen is enlarged, hard, smooth, and painless. Pulsation of the spleen is a rare phenomenon, although it had been noted as far back as 1652 by Nicholas Tulp. It has been described in patients with aortic insufficiency who had splenic enlargement, usually due to malaria or typhoid fever. It occasionally occurs in combined mitral and tricuspid diseases. (See Chapter 16, Examination of the Hemic and Lymphatic Systems.)

The procedure for palpating the kidneys is similar to that used in palpating the liver. With deep inspiration the kidneys may descend, but mobility of the kidneys is not clinically significant. The kidneys are best examined by bimanual palpation of the flank, with one hand behind and one anterior to the organ;

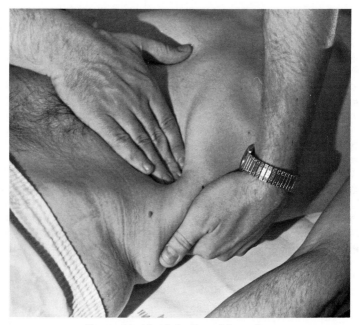

Figure 11–14. Palpation of the spleen.

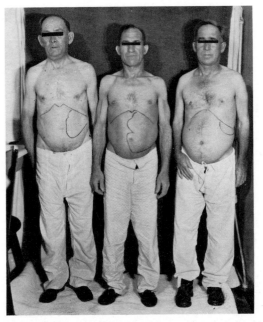

Figure 11–15. *Enlarged spleen in leukemia. Patient on right with smallest spleen has lymphatic leukemia. Two patients with larger spleens have myelogenous leukemia. Note splenic notch.*

if a mass in the flank is felt by both hands in this fashion, it is probable that it is a renal mass, i.e., hydronephrosis or renal tumor (Figs. 11–16 and 11–17). If the mass is palpable only anteriorly, it more likely is intraperitoneal, i.e., cecal carcinoma, appendiceal abscess, or regional ileitis.

Pulsation in the epigastrium of thin patients is apparent almost routinely on palpation and usually results from the normal pulsation of the aorta lying over the vertebral bodies. If a mass is associated with the pulsation, it most likely is a transmitted pulsation through a pancreatic tumor or cyst or a gastric tumor. If,

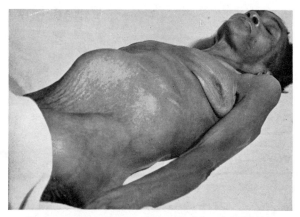

Figure 11–16. *Hypernephroma of the right kidney.*

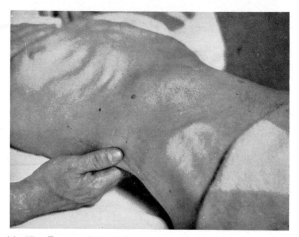

Figure 11–17. *Tumor of the right kidney made visible by pressure under the right back.*

on the other hand, the pulsation is expansile and associated with a mass, it quite possibly is an abdominal aortic aneurysm. Back pain usually is associated with aneurysms, and a lateral x-ray may show calcification of the aorta at that level with possible erosion of the vertebral bodies. It is important to keep in mind that the bifurcation of the aorta is more cephalad than is usually suspected, usually lying at the level of the umbilicus, or 2 or 3 inches superior to the sacral promontory. An expansile epigastric mass may therefore actually be an aneurysm located between the renal vessels and the bifurcation.

Uterine masses are best felt with one hand on the lower abdomen and the other with fingers inserted in the vagina. Vaginal examination in the pregnant woman should be done under sterile conditions. A distended bladder may be felt in the suprapubic region.

The detection and perception of abdominal rigidity and tenderness is of utmost importance in judging the severity of intraperitoneal disease. Voluntary muscle guarding should be recognized and eliminated by reassuring the patient, by using firm (nontickling) motions, and by warming your hands. When confidence and relaxation are obtained, involuntary guarding and various degrees of muscle rigidity can be detected in the area where disease may be present. When abdominal rigidity is diffuse, it signifies that the peritoneal cavity is generally involved (not localized). Rigidity is present in acute pancreatitis, acute mesenteric vascular occlusion, and generalized peritonitis. The most severe degree of abdominal rigidity, the "boardlike" abdomen, is felt in acute perforation when free spillage of air or gastrointestinal contents into the peritoneal cavity from perforation of a peptic ulcer of the anterior duodenum, stomach, or jejunum or from perforated ulcerative colitis or regional ileitis occurs. Remember that when these perforations occur in patients receiving corticosteroid therapy, the intensity of the pain and the rigidity and tenderness are ameliorated so much that detection of these findings may be very difficult. Boardlike rigidity is also felt in patients with rupture of tubo-ovarian abscesses or bursting of other collections of pus secondary to ruptured appendicitis or colonic diverticulitis. The rapid development of abdominal rigidity after some diagnostic procedures, such as gastroscopy, sigmoidoscopy, barium enema, or dilation with curettage of the uterus, should warn the physician that perforation and soilage of the peritoneal cavity has occurred. Moderate rigidity of the abdominal muscles after thoracic operations is sometimes noted but has no apparent clinical significance, and its cause is not understood.

Occasionally moderate localized rigidity is felt in the right lower quadrant associated with occult pneumonia of the right lung. On more than one occasion this finding has suggested a diagnosis of acute appendicitis, resulting in the removal of a normal appendix. A higher than usual leukocyte count and temperature elevation should alert the physician to the possibility of pneumonia, and a chest x-ray should be obtained in such instances. A lateral chest x-ray is especially important here, because pneumonia in the superior segment of the right lower lobe, through pleural involvement, can mimic acute appendicitis and will not be discernible on an ordinary posterior-anterior chest film because the pneumonic process will be hidden behind the right pulmonary hilus. A diagnosis of acute appendicitis is also erroneously suggested in cases in which there is really a stone high in the right ureter or renal pelvis without radiation of pain down the right thigh. When such a differentiation is considered, urinalysis and an intravenous pyelogram usually demonstrate the presence of the stone. A classic difficulty is encountered in women, in differentiating between acute appendicitis and an acute inflammation of the right uterine tube and ovary (acute salpingitis or pelvic inflammatory disease). In the latter, the point of maximal rigidity and tenderness will be more inferior in the right lower quadrant, movement of the cervix will cause exquisite pain, and a smear of the cervical discharge may reveal gonococcal organisms; a history of sexual contact may or may not be admitted by the patient. Rupture of a right tubal pregnancy also may produce physical findings suggestive of acute appendicitis. In such instances, the rigidity and tenderness

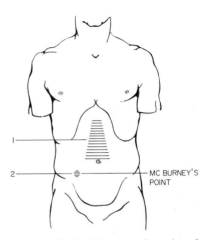

Figure 11–18. *The pain in appendicitis is commonly first felt in the epigastrium (1) and later localized over the appendix, near McBurney's point.*

are not as well localized and there usually is a history of a missed menstrual period.

·The physical findings in acute appendicitis are not always the typical finding of "fingerpoint pain" at McBurney's point on coughing, with direct tenderness and moderate rigidity (Fig. 11–18). Tenderness on the right upon rectal examination is frequently present, and accentuation of the pain when the psoas muscle is stretched suggests a retroceal appendicitis. The psoas sign is elicited by asking the patient to lie on his left side, then hyperextending the patient's right thigh on the hip. Of utmost importance in the history of the patient with acute appendicitis are the presence of nausea with localization of the pain in the right lower quadrant and the sensation of wanting to have a bowel movement but being unable to do so, often prompting the use of a laxative or enema. It is interesting that the diagnosis is still missed occasionally long after the early description of the clinical features of appendicitis in 1886 by Reginald Fitz. Physical findings are often obscure, particularly in infants, the elderly, and patients taking antibiotics. The presence of a surgical scar in the right lower quadrant does not always mean that the patient has had an appendectomy.

When local or general rigidity of the abdomen is palpated, the detection of the degree, extent, and type of tenderness is mandatory. The mechanisms of the various types of tenderness must be understood by the examiner for accurate evaluation of his findings. It is generally accepted that pain resulting from the pressure of palpation is due to the stretching of the visceral peritoneum over the abdominal organ (*direct tenderness*). Tenderness on pressure may be localized if the area of visceral peritoneal or chemical irritation is localized, such as with early acute appendicitis, acute cholecystitis, a penetrating (but not perforating) duodenal ulcer, Meckel's diverticulitis, sigmoid diverticulitis, or any situation in which there is local involvement of the visceral peritoneum. *Rebound tenderness*, elicited by suddenly lifting the hand off the abdomen, releases the direct pressure of palpation and provokes sharp abdominal pain. The presence of rebound tenderness is highly significant because it means that the parietal peritoneum is involved in the progressive disease process. The sudden stretching of the involved parietal peritoneum upon release of the hand produces exquisite pain. Both direct and rebound tenderness may be localized or diffuse over the abdomen; when there is diffuse tenderness there is usually, but not always, a diffuse rebound tenderness, signifying that not only the visceral peritoneum is involved but also the parietal portion of the peritoneal sac. Tenderness and rigidity are more difficult to evaluate in infants because the examiner must also watch for responses that suggest pain on palpation.

The *abdominal reflex* has very little clinical significance. The reflex may be obtained by stroking the skin of the abdomen on either side parallel to the costal margin or to Poupart's ligament. This stroking causes an obvious contraction of the rectus muscles. The abdominal reflex does not appear until several months after birth. Often it is absent in acute intraperitoneal inflammatory processes, such as acute appendicitis or perforated peptic ulcer, simply because of involuntary splinting. The absence of the abdominal reflex in a young person, when it is associated with other appropriate signs, may suggest multiple sclerosis.

A *fluid wave* is pathognomonic of fluid in the abdominal cav-

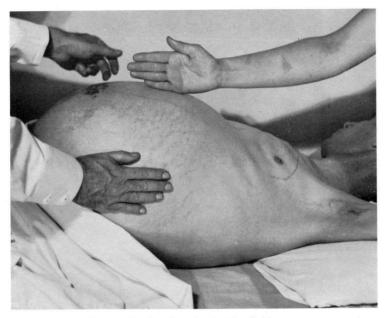

Figure 11–19. *Examination for fluid wave.*

ity and, when associated with shifting dullness, confirms the presence of free fluid. In eliciting a fluid wave it is important to exclude waves produced in the subcutaneous tissue. For this reason it is necessary to have an assistant hold his hand on the midline, with the ulnar margin pressed gently but firmly against the surface of the abdomen (Fig. 11–19). Place the fingers of one hand against the lateral wall of the abdomen and tap firmly with the other hand. This produces a fluid wave transmitted to the hand on the other side of the abdomen and felt as a bump. The wave is sometimes more readily detected with the patient standing, rather than when lying down. A fluid wave is sometimes visible. Celsus, more than 900 years ago, observed that "the fluid often collects within the abdomen so that if it be shaken by any movement of the body the fluctuation of the fluid can be seen."

PERCUSSION

Percussion of the abdomen is of prime importance in determining whether the abdomen contains predominantly fluid or air. Normally percussion over the abdomen produces a hollow sound because of air within the gastrointestinal tract. An exception to this occurs over the liver, where there normally is dullness. Complete absence of liver dullness indicates the presence of air in the peritoneal cavity and most commonly results from a perforated peptic ulcer. When there is free fluid in the abdomen, the fluid gravitates to the flanks, and the intestines float upward when the patient lies on his back. Under such conditions the percussion note is tympanitic over the anterior surface of the abdomen and dull in the flanks. The crucial test, however, is to turn the patient on one side; if there is free fluid in the abdomen the dullness shifts, the percussion note on the side that is uppermost becomes tympanitic, and the note on the lower side is dull. Shifting dullness is pathognomonic of free fluid and is more reliable than the test for a fluid wave. Percussion of the abdomen and flanks is of utmost importance in the examination of the patient suspected of having an injury to an intraperitoneal organ with resulting hemorrhage. An area of increasing dullness in the left flank is perhaps the most useful confirmation sign of a suspected traumatic rupture of the spleen.

Lawson and Weissbein have described a method that may indicate the presence of as little as 120 ml. of free fluid in the peritoneal space. Have your patient lie on his abdomen a few minutes and then position himself on hands and knees (Fig. 11–20). Place the head of a Bowles stethoscope over the lowest part of the suspended abdomen where puddling would occur, then repeatedly flick the near flank with your finger, while the stethoscope head is progressively repositioned toward the opposite flank. A positive sign consists of a marked change in the

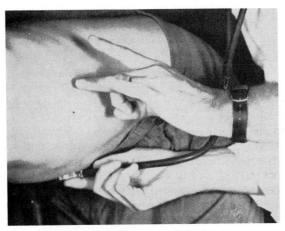

Figure 11–20. Puddle sign. (Lawson, J. D., and Weissbein, A. S.: The puddle sign—an aid in the diagnosis of minimal ascites. N. Engl. J. Med., 260:652, 1959.)

intensity and character of the percussion note as the stethoscope is moved toward the opposite flank. To the ear the intensity of the note seems to increase, and a point of demarcation is noted that correlates well with the amount of fluid present. To complete the method have the patient sit up while you hold the stethoscope on what was the dependent area. Now the percussion note becomes loud and clear, if the initial impression is correct.

In acute perforations of the gastrointestinal tract, the percussion note is hypertympanitic. Riverius, in the quaint translation of Nicholas Culpepper, stated, "The Dropsie called Tympanites hath its name from *tympanum*, a drum, because the abdomen is stretched out like a Drum, and if you strike it with your hand, it sounds like it. This stretching comes from wind shut up in the Cavity of the Abdomen. But sometimes this wind is in the Cavity of the Guts." In obstructions of the gastrointestinal tract there is an accumulation of swallowed air which produces only a resonant sound on percussion.

AUSCULTATION

Listening to the sounds of the abdomen can be rewarding if you wish to clinch a diagnosis in certain patients with grave abdominal pain. Interpretation of bowel sounds requires practice and a fundamental knowledge of the causes of the sounds. First, it must be realized that any intestinal sound requires that both fluid and air are in interphase in the lumen of the intestine, that neither alone is productive of sound. Second, movement of the air and fluid in the intestine produces normal sounds that range from low feeble rumbles to higher pitched tinkling sounds (the tighter the intestine is stretched, the higher the tinkle). Third, a normal peristaltic wave produces audible sounds of air and fluid moving along a tube. Significant abnormalities of the bowel sounds present themselves at two extremes: a virtual lack of normal sounds when motility of the bowel is inhibited by inflammation, gangrene, or reflex ileus; and a marked "rush" of peristaltic activity producing sounds called borborygmi, consisting of waves of loud gurgling and tinkling sounds as if exaggerated peristalsis were attempting to push fluid and air against an obstruction. An increase in intestinal activity is heard in gastroenteritis with diarrhea, but the intensity of the sounds is greater in mechanical obstruction in which the borborygmi are associated simultaneously with colicky pain. The borborygmi associated with cramping pains are part of the diagnostic triad (with vomiting and distention) that is pathognomonic of small intestinal obstruction (see Table 11–1).

The paramount importance of auscultation of the abdomen is emphasized in making a distinction between peritonitis and mechanical small bowel obstruction. In generalized peritonitis, there is an ileus or paralysis of intestinal movement with consequent lack of bowel sounds. In small intestinal obstruction, on the other hand, there are audible peristaltic rushes (borborygmi) that are heard simultaneously with abdominal cramping pain every 10 to 20 minutes. To be certain that an episode of borborygmi is not missed by the examiner, it is important that a sufficient period of time (20 minutes) be monitored. So that this time does not seem wasted, it is expedient to remove one of the stethoscope's ear pieces from your ear so that you can continue taking the patient's history and at the same time listen to the sounds of the abdomen. Ask the patient to tell you when intestinal cramping occurs so that particular attention can be paid to auscultation at the time of colic.

Auscultation of the abdomen for sounds other than intestinal activity has limited usefulness, although a systolic bruit over aneurysms of the abdominal aorta or constricted aortic branches is a significant finding. Soft murmurs over tortuous splenic arteries are heard normally in thin patients. A peritoneal friction rub is occasionally heard over the liver in cases of malignant deposits in the liver; such metastases usually have central necrosis with fine fibrinous peritoneal adhesions. A low grade fever also may be present.

PHYSICAL FINDINGS AND DIAGNOSTIC PROBABILITIES

Physical examination of the abdomen may yield an extraordinary amount of information leading to diagnoses that can be confirmed by laboratory determinations, by endoscopic and radiologic examinations, and, in appropriate instances, by surgical operations. The data gained by the techniques of observation by the eyes, ears, and hands are merely a collation of clues, each insignificant by itself, but which when put together point finally to an "obvious" diagnosis. Sherlock Holmes spoke to his doctor friend of this when he said, "You see, my dear Watson, it is not really difficult to construct a series of inferences, each dependent upon its predecessor and each simple in itself. If, after doing so, one simply knocks out all the central inferences and presents one's audience with the starting point and the conclusion, one may produce a startling, though possibly meretricious, effect."

In the preceding tables, observational clues obtained by examination are placed with confirmatory findings leading to highly probable diagnoses. Of course, many patients will present findings that do not fit in with those in the tables. As has often been said, exceptions to the rule make medicine all the more interesting and stimulating.

COMMON CLINICAL TERMS

Ascites—Excessive fluid within the peritoneal cavity which is usually associated with hepatic cirrhosis, congestive heart failure, or intra-abdominal malignancy.

Borborygmi—The audible sounds of hyperactive intestinal peristalsis; a diagnostic sign only when coupled simultaneously with cramping abdominal pain and associated with distention and vomiting.

Courvoisier's sign—A palpably enlarged gallbladder in a jaundiced patient usually indicative of obstruction of the common bile duct due to neoplasm; the sign does not apply to the non-jaundiced patient in whom a palpably enlarged hydropic gallbladder is usually indicative of calculous obstruction of the cystic duct.

Hematemesis—The vomiting of blood.

Ileus—A paresis of intestinal motor activity causing a reduction in audible bowel sounds and usually associated with intestinal distention due to the accumulation of swallowed air in postoperative patients or in patients with peritonitis.

Melena—The passage of black stool darkened by altered blood; if tarry in color and consistency, it usually connotes origin from the foregut (acid alteration); if dark maroon in color, the origin is usually from the midgut.

Murphy's sign—The inability of the patient to take a deep breath because of pain on inspiration when the examiner's fingers are pressed under the right hepatic and costal margin, indicative of gallbladder disease.

Rectal shelf (Blumer's shelf)—A nodular mass(es), palpable by rectal examination, located anterior to the rectum; indicative of implantation of malignant cells from a carcinoma of the gastrointestinal tract to the inferior most dependent portion of the peritoneal cavity.

Shifting dullness—Dullness on percussion of an area which shifts its location on the abdomen when the position of the patient is changed; indicative of free fluid in the peritoneal cavity.

Virchow's node—A hard, palpably enlarged lymph node situated in the left supraclavicular region; usually diagnostic of a carcinoma of the gastrointestinal tract which has metastasized via the thoracic lymphatic duct.

COMMON CLINICAL SYNDROMES

Boerhaave syndrome—"Spontaneous" rupture of the esophagus; in 1724, H. Boerhaave of Leyden published the case history of the Count of Wassenaer, who developed a sudden onset of severe vomiting (probably instigated by emetics) followed by difficulty in swallowing, substernal pain, cough, difficulty in breathing, fever, suffocation, and death.

Budd-Chiari syndrome—Hepatomegaly, ascites, and cirrhosis due to the occlusion of the hepatic veins and often associated with edema, thrombophlebitis of the inferior vena cava, and portal hypertension.

Carcinoid syndrome (Cassidy syndrome)—Episodic flushing of the skin after eating, dyspepsia, dyspnea, and hypertension in adults with hepatic metastases from carcinoid tumors of the small intestine, usually associated with an elevation of plasma serotonin and the appearance of urinary hydroxy-indole-acetic acid. Right-sided cardiac insufficiency may occur. Carcinoid tumors also occur in the bronchus, stomach, duodenum, appendix and rectum, but the syndrome depends upon serotonin by-pass of the liver.

Cholangitis syndrome—Fever, chills, and jaundice in patients with partial biliary duct obstruction due to stones or surgical biliary-enteric strictures. An elevated alkaline phosphatase is usually present.

Hirschsprung's disease—Congenital aganglionic megacolon which is usually present in infants and children who have constipation from the time of birth, abdominal distention progressing to a "pot-belly" appearance, episodes of intestinal obstruction, an empty rectum, radiologic findings of megacolon proximal to a narrow rectosigmoid, and histologic evidence of absent ganglion cells, but numerous nerve fibers in the intermuscular layer of the rectum.

Mallory-Weiss syndrome—Massive, painless gastric hemorrhage with hematemesis from erosive lacerations of the esophagogastric mucosa due to vomiting, usually after severe alcoholic intoxication.

Pancreatic cholera syndrome (diarrheogenic tumor syndrome; watery diarrhea, hypokalemia, and achlorhydria [WDHA] syndrome)—Symptoms of severe diarrhea producing hypokalemia with gastric achlorhydria in patients, often debilitated, having islet cell tumor(s) of the pancreas. The involved polypeptide hormone has not been isolated but is thought to be the gastric-inhibitory-polypeptide (GIP) and not secretin, gastrin, glucagon, or insulin.

Peutz-Jeghers syndrome—Familial intestinal polyposis–cutaneous pigmentation syndrome in which young patients usually develop an acute onset of intussusception (triad of mechanical small intestinal obstruction: distention, vomiting, and abdominal cramping pain associated with simultaneous borborygmi) due to intussuscepting polyps of the small intestine, and who have pigmentation of the buccal mucosa and/or skin and a dominant family history.

Whipple's triad (organic hypoglycemia syndrome)—In 1938 Whipple described a diagnostic triad of "attacks of nervous or gastrointestinal disturbances coming on in the fasting state, associated with hypoglycemia with blood sugar values below 50 mg. per 100 ml., and immediate relief of symptoms following the ingestion of glucose." The symptoms and signs can be imitated by a prolonged fast which unmasks the hyperinsulinism from a beta islet cell tumor of the pancreas or fibrous mesothelioma. However, the early symptoms of tremor, sweating, palpitation, and nervousness are due to compensatory hyperadrenalinism while the late symptoms of mental confusion, "black-out spells," and coma are due to cerebral hypoglycemia.

Zollinger-Ellison syndrome—Ulcerogenic tumor syndrome. Symptoms of severe ulcer pain, perforation or hemorrhage, often fulminating, and diarrhea in relatively young adults with a longstanding history of duodenal ulcer who have an association of marked gastric acid hypersecretion, recurrent duodenal or jejunal ulceration, and gastrin-secreting islet cell tumor(s) of the pancreas. Radiologic findings of gastric hyperrugation and intestinal hypermobility as well as immunochemical assays of the serum for increased gastrin levels are confirmatory. When this syndrome is in combination with pituitary acromegaly and hyperparathyroidism, in families, it is sometimes called **Wermer's syndrome or multiple endocrine adenomatosis syndrome, type 1.**

BIBLIOGRAPHY

Boerhaave, H.: Atrocis, nec descripti prius, morbi historia. Boutesteniana, 1724.

Dunphy, J. E., and Botsford, T. W.: Physical Examination of the Surgical Patient. 4th ed. Philadelphia, W. B. Saunders Co., 1975.

Hirschsprung, H.: Stuhltragheit Keugeboreuer infolge von dilatation und hypertrophie des colons. Jahrb. Kinderh., 27:1, 1888.

Jegher, H., McKusick, V. A., and Katz, K. H.: Generalized intestinal polyposis and melanin spots on the oral mucosa, lips and digits. A syndrome of diagnostic significance. N. Engl. J. Med., 241:993, 1949.

Lawson, J. D., and Weissbein, A. S.: The puddle sign – an aid in the diagnosis of minimal ascites. N. Engl. J. Med., *260*:652, 1959.

Major, R. H., and Black, D. R.: A huge hemangioma of the liver associated with hemangiomata of the skull and bilateral cystic adrenals. Am. J. Med. Sci., *156*:469, 1938.

Mallory, G. K., and Weiss, S.: Hemorrhages from lacerations of the cardiac orifice of the stomach due to vomiting. Am. J. Med. Sci., *178*:506, 1929.

Moore, S. W.: Physiological basis for diagnostic signs of an acute abdomen. Surg. Clin. North Am., *38*:371, 1958.

Murphy, J. B.: The diagnosis of gallstones. Med. News (N.Y.), *82*:825, 1903.

Osler, W.: Lectures on the diagnosis of abdominal tumors. N.Y. Med. J., *49*:129, 161, 193, 260, 385, 417, 477, 481, and 545; *50*:65 and 97, 1894.

Sailer, J.: Pulsating spleen in aortic insufficiency. Am. Heart J., *3*:447, 1928.

Sircus, W., Brunt, P. W., Walker, R. J., Small, W. P., Falconer, C. W. A., and Thomson, C. G.: Two cases of "pancreatic cholera" with features of peptide-secreting adenomatosis of the pancreas. Gut, *11*:197, 1970.

Stucky, D.: A physical sign of patent ductus arteriosus in infancy. Med. J. Aust., *2*:681, 1957.

Sutton, D. C., and Rawson, V.: A case of pulsating spleen in mitral and tricuspid disease. Am. Heart J., *10*:1096, 1935.

Weiss, S.: Diseases of the Liver, Gall Bladder, Ducts and Pancreas: Their Diagnosis and Treatment. New York, Paul B. Hoeber, 1935.

Wermer, F.: Genetic aspects of adenomatosis of endocrine glands. Am. J. Med., *16*:363, 1954.

Whipple, A. O.: Surgical therapy of hyperinsulinism. J. Internat. Chir., *3*:237, 1938.

Zollinger, R. M., and Ellison, E. H.: Primary peptic ulceration of the jejunum associated with islet cell tumors of the pancreas. Ann. Surg., *142*:709, 1955.

12
EXAMINATION OF THE MALE GENITALIA AND RECTUM

Exhaustive examination of the genitourinary organs is a science in itself, but no thorough physical examination is complete without at least inspection and palpation of the external genitalia and a careful rectal examination. Such evaluation may engender more patient concern than examination of other areas of the body because of the personal and emotional significance of the sexual organs. Brief, candid explanation of the purpose and procedure beforehand will help allay patient apprehension.

INGUINAL AREA

Examination of the inguinal area naturally follows the examination of the abdomen. Observation and palpation of the external genitalia should begin in the inguinal area, since lymph from the skin and superficial structures of these organs and the lower extremities passes to the regional inguinal nodes. Enlargement of these nodes may indicate inflammatory or neoplastic disease of the drainage area. Lymph from the urethra, testes, and associated structures passes to the iliac and periaortic lymph nodes.

Inguinal hernias. Inguinal hernias may be seen and palpated as masses presenting medial to the inferior epigastric vessels when direct inguinal herniation occurs, or they may occur as masses in the inguinal canal or scrotum when the hernia is indirect. If an indirect hernia is in the canal, it may be felt by gently unfolding the loose skin of the scrotum with the small or index finger and then gently passing the finger along the spermatic cord through the external inguinal ring (Fig. 12–1). When the patient responds to your request to cough, the impulse can be felt as the peritoneal sac is pushed farther down the canal by the increased intra-abdominal pressure. Although normally this is a sensitive area for examination, the patient may be hypersensitive, usually because of heightened anxiety resulting from lack of understanding of what is to transpire. Such increased anxiety frequently intensifies sensory perception and may lead the patient to overinterpret sensitivity as pain. This is more common in younger patients.

GENITALIA

Penis. Deviations from normal size of the genitalia are immediately evident. *Infantilism,* usually due to hypopituitarism, is characterized by extremely small genitalia. The patient shown in Figure 12–2 is 17 years old, but his genitalia are the size of those of a small child. This boy, suffering from Fröhlich's syndrome, is fat and lacks pubic hair and sexual desire.

Virilism is the opposite of infantilism. The genitalia shown in Figure 12–3 belong not to a man, but to a boy of five. This condition, due to excessive androgen formation, is usually associated with an adrenocortical tumor but may occur with precocious puberty of a benign type. The boy shown in Figure 12–3, when examined at 14 years of age, was quite normal, and his penis was not abnormally large for his age.

The psychological ramifications of deviation in penile size are too extensive to consider here, but it should be pointed out that the patient's concern about unusually large or small penis

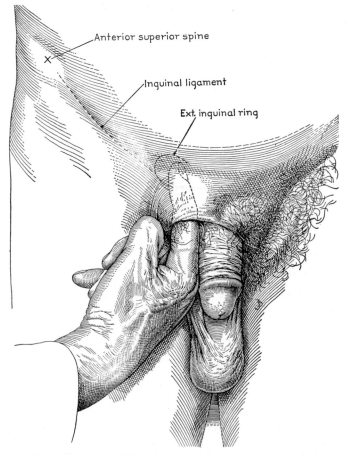

Figure 12–1. *Technique of invagination of the scrotum to permit thorough palpation of the inguinal canal. (Dunphy, J. E., and Botsford, T. W.: Physical Examination of the Surgical Patient. 4th ed. Philadelphia, W. B. Saunders Co., 1975.)*

Figure 12–2. *Genitalia in boy of 17 suffering from infantilism.*

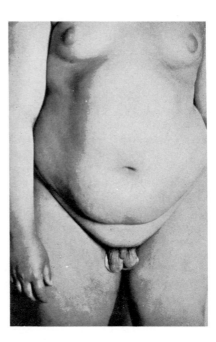

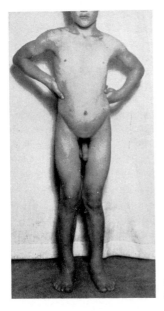

Figure 12–3. *Genitalia in boy of five suffering from virilism.*

size is real, regardless of its validity according to scientific data. Suffice it to say that during examination of such patients, an objective attitude which conveys a professional and personal respect for the patient's overt or covert concern is essential. Recognition of these psychological factors should be an essential part of the development of overall treatment plans for such patients.

Elephantiasis of the penis and scrotum, a relatively common condition in the tropics and occasionally seen in temperate zones, is due to inflammation and obstruction of the lymphatics with resultant hypertrophy of the skin and subcutaneous tissues. In the tropics, lymphatic obstruction is commonly produced by the Filaria sanguinis-hominis (*Wuchereria bancrofti*). In temperate zones the cause of such obstruction is usually not apparent.

Hermaphrodism, a rare condition, is characterized by the presence of both male and female sex organs.

Phimosis, a disorder in which the prepuce cannot be retracted over the glans penis, though sometimes congenital, is more commonly due to nonspecific infection of the glans and foreskin; it may be a complication of chancroid or gonorrhea. An attempt to retract the prepuce in phimosis may lead to paraphimosis, in which the prepuce is caught behind the glans and cannot be drawn forward to its normal position. Paraphimosis produces marked edema and discomfort in the glans penis.

Balanitis, inflammation of the glans penis, may be caused by filth or lack of cleanliness and sometimes results from gonorrhea. Balanitis rarely occurs in men who have been circumcised or who maintain good personal hygiene. In balanitis, the mucosa of the glans is swollen and reddened, the surface shows irregular areas of desquamation, and often a purulent secretion forms at the corona.

The penis and scrotum may show marked *edema* in ascites secondary to cardiac disease with cardiac failure, nephritis, or cirrhosis with ascitic decompensation. In such cases the penis may be swollen to twice its normal size, and urination may be difficult.

Examination of the urethral meatus may reveal a purulent

discharge indicative of either nonspecific or gonorrheal *urethritis*. A Gram stain of the exudate is usually sufficient for diagnosis. Examination of the voided urine under the microscope will also show the presence of pus when infection is present. If urethritis is suspected, it may be necessary to milk the urethra in order to obtain pus. Mild urethritis is occasionally seen as the result of injecting irritating antiseptic solutions to prevent venereal infection. The urethral meatus may be congenitally small, or previous infection may have produced stricture. When this occurs, the meatus may be of only pinpoint size and cause severe urinary obstruction. If possible, male patients should be observed during urination so that the character of the urinary stream can be seen. A normal urinary stream should have an adequate caliber and arc and be uninterrupted.

Scabies sometimes attacks the penis. The lesions consist of minute multiple elevations with burrows in the center; they itch intensely and are associated with similar lesions elsewhere, especially between the fingers.

Herpes of the penis is common and occasionally confused with a chancre. The lesions consist of small vesicles, usually on the glans but also on the prepuce, causing some pain and itching which usually disappear in a few days, leaving no scars.

Penile warts, condylomata acuminata, verrucae, and *venereal warts* (Fig. 12–4) are sometimes mistaken by the layman for chancres. They have nothing in common with chancres except that penile warts, like other warts, are of viral origin, are mildly contagious, and are possibly transmitted by sexual intercourse. The most important factor in their production is not venereal exposure, but irritation, uncleanliness, and phimosis with poor hygiene.

Chancroid, gonorrhea, and syphilis are the three most common venereal diseases. *Chancroid* is commonly referred to as a soft chancre, in contrast to the hard chancre of syphilis. It is produced by the Ducrey bacillus.

The simple chancroid appears as a number of small, superficial punched-out ulcers located about the corona. If this lesion does not heal, because of lack of cleanliness or continued irrita-

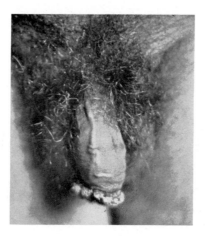

Figure 12–4. Venereal warts.

tion, the ulcers become larger. Edema of the prepuce appears and, with it, phimosis. A bubo or inguinal lymphadenitis appears so commonly in chancroid that it is classed as part of the disease picture. These enlarged inguinal lymph nodes break down and frequently become suppurant.

Chancre, the primary lesion of syphilis, is almost always located on the penis, just behind the glans, or on the prepuce (Fig. 12–5). John Hunter, it may be recalled, inoculated himself on the penis with some pus from the urethra of a gonorrheal patient; unfortunately, the patient had syphilis as well and a chancre developed. Since this memorable experiment in 1767, the chancre of syphilis has been spoken of as a hunterian sore or hunterian chancre.

As a rule, within a month after exposure, the chancre appears as a small red papule which slowly enlarges and then breaks, forming a small ulcer. The small ulcer is often partially covered by a grayish membrane and the tissue around it becomes indurated and soon has a hard, cartilaginous consistency. This cartilaginous thickening is characteristic of a true syphilitic chancre. It is also noteworthy that it is practically painless.

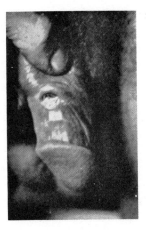

Figure 12-5. *Chancre.*

Chancres are usually single and are not autoinoculable, so that a chancre of the penis in contact with the scrotum will not cause a chancre on the scrotum. Chancroids are usually multiple, are autoinoculable, and are commonly associated with suppurating inguinal buboes. In spite of these clinical differences, chancres and chancroids are frequently indistinguishable; and before the physician makes a positive diagnosis, a smear from the lesion should be examined by the darkfield technique and a serological test for syphilis obtained.

Granuloma inguinale is found more frequently in black than in white patients. The lesion begins as a small papule, which later ulcerates and persists as an indolent, eroding ulcer with a shallow crater, the base of which is covered by granulation tissue. The edges of the ulcer are often redundant and seem to overlap the healthy skin margins. The lesions are not painful or sensitive, are commonly extensive and usually multiple, and are most often seen in the groin and on the prepuce, glans, vulva, perineum, buttocks, and anus.

Patients with apparent venereal lesions need careful examination, not only to prevent physician contamination, but to establish the trustworthy relationship essential for treatment planning and identification of sexual partners. A scientific, understanding, nonjudgmental attitude assists measurably in examination and postexamination follow-up. Overconfidence in penicillin and drug therapy, more casual attitudes about sexual relations, and use of "the pill," are some of the factors to which the marked increase in venereal lesions has been attributed.

Carcinoma of the penis is usually located on the glans, and less commonly on the prepuce. It is always a squamous epithelioma and is the second most common of all skin cancers. Two types of carcinomas are observed—one a papillary, cauliflower type (Fig. 12–6) and the other an indurated ulcer. The lesion, at first appearing as either a small ulcer or wart, grows slowly and causes no pain or untoward symptoms. Later, after attaining some size, it causes pain, for which the patient seeks medical at-

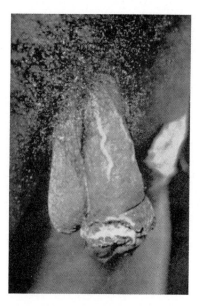

Figure 12–6. Carcinoma of penis.

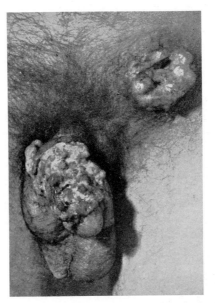

Figure 12–7. *Carcinoma of penis. Note metastasis in inguinal lymph glands.*

tention. It sometimes grows to considerable proportions, becomes a large bleeding mass, and even metastasizes to the inguinal and femoral lymph nodes (Fig. 12–7) before the patient consults a physician. Circumcision in early infancy is thought to be an almost absolute prophylactic against this form of cancer.

The scrotum and testicles. The scrotum normally contains two testes exquisitely tender to physical pressure of any sort, including that occurring during examination or resulting from disease. Hence examination should be thorough and gentle. Careful palpation and transillumination allow accurate identification of both normal and abnormal structures in the scrotum.

Varicocele consists of a dilation and engorgement of the veins of the pampiniform plexus of the spermatic cord. It usually occurs in a mild form, is present generally on the left side, and causes no serious physical inconvenience. Surgery is seldom indicated for this condition and it has no relationship to impotence. Varicocele is a common complaint of the neurotic or psychotic patient who exaggerates the significance of this condition.

A marked collection of fluid in the tunica vaginalis of the testis produces *hydrocele* (Fig. 12–8). Acute hydrocele is always secondary to inflammation of the testis or epididymis. Chronic hydrocele is most common between the ages of 40 and 60. It usually develops slowly and insidiously and may attain considerable size before causing any discomfort. Although most examples have been described as chronic idiopathic hydrocele, further examination usually discloses disease of the epididymis. In hydrocele the swelling is painless and fluctuates. The skin, tense, shiny, and somewhat reddened, has a translucent appearance. A

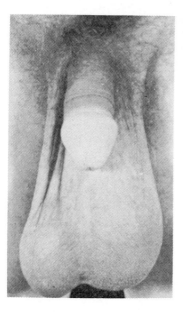

Figure 12–8. Hydrocele. (Boyce, W. H., and Politano, V. A.: Infections and diseases of the scrotum. In Campbell, M. F., and Harrison, J. H.: Urology. Vol. 1. 3rd ed. Philadelphia, W. B. Saunders Co., 1970.)

light held behind and against the scrotum will transilluminate the hydrocele sac. Upon aspiration of the fluid in a hydrocele sac, occasionally one will find many sperm; the structure is then called a *spermatocele.*

Hematocele, a collection of blood in the tunica vaginalis, is generally caused by trauma. Transillumination is impossible in this condition.

Acute painful *enlargement of the testis* may occur in viral orchitis. Diagnosis is not difficult as the condition is always secondary to viral parotitis and enlargement is confined entirely to the testicle. Painful *enlargement of the epididymis* can always be differentiated from a primary testicular condition and is generally associated with urinary tract infection. Sometimes the epididymis will reach the size of a lemon.

Torsion of the testicle, most common in a preadolescent boy, is associated with a history of sudden severe pain in the testicle. The finding of a twisted spermatic cord with the testicle in a higher than normal position is diagnostic of this condition. Unless the testicle and spermatic cord are untwisted immediately, the testis is rapidly destroyed.

Undescended testis or *cryptorchidism* is a common anomaly. Normally the testes descend into the scrotum before birth. If both testicles are undescended, the condition may be associated with infantilism and pituitary deficiency. Both testes should be present in the scrotum before the onset of puberty because sterility will occur if they are left in the abdomen. The incidence of malignant tumors of the testis is also many times greater in the undescended testicle.

Tumors of the testis are uncommon, but are among the most malignant neoplasms that occur. The majority of such tumors occur in patients between the ages of 20 and 40 and are easily identified as a painless, hard enlargement of the testicle proper.

RECTAL EXAMINATION

Examination of the genitalia is usually followed by a careful rectal examination. Once again, the patient's sensitivity, both physical and emotional, must be considered when performing a rectal examination. A brief explanation of the purpose and procedure helps allay anxiety and failure to provide it may make the examination more difficult.

This examination can be done either with the patient supine with thighs flexed on the pelvis or with the patient standing and bending well forward, his hands placed on a bed or chair. External hemorrhoids, which are dilated and prolapsed hemorrhoidal veins, are commonly seen around the anus. After the gloved index finger is well lubricated, it is inserted into the anal canal by exerting gentle but firm pressure on the anterior margin of the anal ring. As your finger passes through the anal canal note the tone of the anal sphincter muscle. If the muscle of the anorectal canal is flaccid, serious neurological disease is present or the anal sphincter has been injured by disease or trauma. Once your finger is inside the anal canal, gently feel the prostate anteriorly as a bilobate structure with a groove between the two lobes. The normal postpubertal prostate generally weighs 12 to 15 grams and has the consistency of one's nose. If the prostate is hard and irregular, a neoplasm should be suspected. Occasionally the seminal vesicles can be palpated above the prostate in the region of the floor of the bladder. After the prostate has been examined, turn your finger to examine the entire circumference of the rectum noting any masses, induration, or other abnormalities. Internal hemorrhoids may often be felt just inside the anal sphincter.

No rectal examination is completed until you have removed the external lubricant from the examined area with tissue and invited the patient to assume a more comfortable position.

COMMON CLINICAL TERMS

Anuria—Complete lack of urinary output.
Bacteriuria—Bacteria in the urine.
Chordee—Distortion and deformity of penis during erection resulting from fibrotic changes in the corpora cavernosa.
Cystitis—Urinary bladder inflammatory reaction.
Dysuria—Painful urination.

Enuresis—Involuntary urination during sleep.
Oliguria—Decrease of urinary output to less than 400 ml. per 24 hours.
Priapism—Sustained nonerotic and painful erection.
Proteinuria—Presence of protein in the urine.
Stress incontinence—Spontaneous and involuntary loss of urine during increased intra-abdominal and intravesical pressure likely to occur during lifting, coughing, or straining.

COMMON CLINICAL SYNDROMES

Adrenogenital syndrome—Congenital adrenal hyperplasia in females, resulting in faulty synthesis of adrenal cortical steroids with progressive secondary virilization, precocious puberty, pseudohermaphroditism, hirsutism, growth disorders, acne, and muscular hypertrophy.

Genital tuberculosis—Often asymptomatic, but patients may have irritative urinary symptoms, or complain of a painless purulent discharge from the scrotum. Examination reveals a hard and irregular prostate suggestive of neoplasm. The seminal vesicles can be palpated as ropy, indurated, and obliquely directed masses above the prostate. The globus minor or tail of the epididymis (at the lower pole of the testis) will commonly develop nonpainful cold abscesses which may develop spontaneous fistulas to the scrotal skin.

Klinefelter's syndrome—Gonadal dysgenesis resulting from an XXY chromosomal pattern. These males have small testes, and gynecomastia, furcap hairline, lack of beard, and female pubic hair distribution are also common. Azoospermia and resultant infertility is invariably present, and testicular biopsy reveals hyalinization of the seminiferous tubules.

Leriche's syndrome—Pain or coldness in legs, intermittent claudication, impotence, and absence of pulses in common iliac secondary to occlusion of the abdominal aorta at the bifurcation.

Münchausen's syndrome—A person will feign illness in order to be admitted to a hospital and receive treatment, usually with narcotic drugs. One frequently seen pattern is the patient who claims severe colicky flank pain as from a ureteral stone. Hematuria will be produced by self-inflicted urethral trauma. These patients are invariably from "elsewhere" and are "allergic" to diagnostic iodide contrast media.

Peyronie's syndrome—Plastic induration of the penis.

Posterior urethral syndrome—Usually seen in a young man who complains of perineal discomfort variously referred to the low back, the rectum, the suprapubic area, the testes, the glans penis, and the inner aspect of the thighs. Irritative urinary symptoms are usually present and the patient may complain of a scanty urethral discharge especially on arising. The prostate may be boggy or tender on examination, and after gentle prostatic massage, many white blood cells, and proteinaceous casts may be identified on microscopic examination of the prostatic fluid. The urinalysis is usually normal.

Reiter's syndrome—Triad of arthritis, conjunctivitis, and urethritis.

Uremic syndrome—Azotemia from renal failure with resulting manifestations of fatigability, headache, anorexia, vomiting, depression, epitaxis, dyspnea, Cheyne-Stokes respiration, fetid breath, dehydration, coma, anemia, elevated blood urea nitrogen, and low specific gravity of the urine.

Yo-Yo testis syndrome—Physiological retractile testis is a common finding in adolescent boys. In this condition, a hyperactive cremaster muscle periodically pulls the testis out of the scrotum and into the inguinal area. This condition must be carefully differentiated from a true cryptorchid, since no surgery or treatment is needed for the Yo-Yo testis.

13
EXAMINATION OF THE FEMALE GENITALIA

PATIENT'S HISTORY

The following items should be evaluated in taking the history of all women:

Menstrual history. The age at which menses began, the duration of each period of menstrual flow, the interval between periods, their regularity, and the age of cessation of flow in menopausal women are all of importance. Ask, in addition, for an estimate of the quantity of menstrual flow in terms of the number of pads or tampons used. Always question regarding any occasions when menstrual flow ceased or changed in character, because severe illness and some metabolic disorders, such as thyroid disease and adrenal disorders, are associated with abnormal menstruation. Are the menstrual periods associated with excessive cramping, nausea, or excessive weight gain? Has any bleeding or spotting occurred in the interval between menses? The date of the last menstrual period must always be recorded.

Pregnancy. Record the number of pregnancies the patient has had and their outcome. Were they all full-term? Did miscarriages or abortions occur and, if so, when and under what conditions? Note any complications that occurred with any of the pregnancies, such as excessive weight gain or hypertension and whether any problems were associated with delivery. The birth weights of infants and the presence of any anomalies should be listed. Diabetic women frequently bear infants weighing over 10 lbs.

Finally, in married women who have not borne children, inquire regarding fertility problems and whether she is using any contraceptive medications or devices.

Sexual intercourse. This part of the history is frequently avoided even by experienced physicians. Most women, however, are quite willing to relate this part of their history when asked in a straightforward manner. Indeed, many welcome the opportunity to discuss with a physician real or imagined problems regarding sexual function and activities. So much has been written regarding psychosexual development and conflict that the fundamental human desire for this aspect of the relationship between man and wife has been obscured and subjected to innuendo and folklore. Thoughtful, tactful inquiry regarding your patient's sexual experience is a pertinent and essential part of each woman's medical history.

Begin by asking how she gets along with her husband and if their marital relations are satisfactory. Note any problems she has experienced for discussion after the initial interview, when you have established a clear, understanding physician-patient relationship. Probably in no other area of history taking is tact so essential, nor can the door to knowledge of the patient be closed more quickly by the attitude of the physician.

General information. Record any history of vaginal discharge, perineal itching, or pain. Diabetes occasionally presents as severe pruritus involving the perineum. Inquire further regarding any disturbance of urinary frequency, burning, urgency, or pain on urination. In older women who have borne children, a history of uncontrollable loss of urine upon sneezing or coughing suggests a detached urethra with or without cystocele, frequently termed stress incontinence. In addition, obstipation or difficulty in evacuating the rectum may occur when a rectocele has developed. In young women, cystitis may appear following intercourse, giving rise to the term "honeymoon cystitis." Finally, inquire regarding any history of kidney infection or nephritis and the accompanying signs of discolored urine, fever, chills, and flank pain.

PELVIC EXAMINATION

In the evaluation of pelvic structures it is useful to recall the homology between the male and female genitalia, since many anomalies and variations occur that otherwise would be difficult to explain. Since there are distinct differences between the pelvic findings in infants, prepubertal girls, adults, and postmenopausal women, the examination outline relates to the adult with subsequent reference made to other age groups.

Prior to examination the patient should empty her bladder and rectum. The table should be firm, well padded, and comfortable to promote relaxation. Position the patient on her back with buttocks extending just beyond the edge of the table. Then place her feet in the stirrups with the knees flexed and separated. A sheet should be draped across the abdomen and folded over both legs. This arrangement, the most commonly used, is called the dorsolithotomy position (Fig. 13–1). Other positions may be used when required, notably the lateral or Sims position. Remember that the patient will be unable to see you during the examination, so speak so that she can hear you and inform her of each step in the examination. A good light source completes the arrangements for the examination.

Observe the distribution of the pubic hair as well as its color and texture. Normal pubic hair in the female is distributed in an inverted triangle with the base centered over the mons pubis. It is darker and coarser than the remainder of the body hair. In some women with familial hirsutism the hair may extend onto the abdominal wall toward the umbilicus, similar to the male escutcheon. However, extensive distribution of hair onto the abdomen, if associated with abnormal hair on the face, chest, and other body surfaces, suggests the possibility of disturbed ovarian or adrenal function or both.

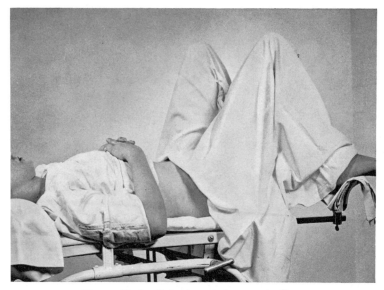

Figure 13–1. Patient ready for examination.

Next inspect the labia majora (homologous to the scrotum of the male) for ulcerations, discoloration, furuncles, or papillomatous growths. Lying internally and between the labia majora in the midline is the clitoris and its associated labia minora (homologous to the penile skin of the male) (Fig. 13–2). The clitoris is usually 1.5 cm. in length and somewhat blue-gray in color. The labia minora begin in the midline superior to the clitoris and extend posteriorly, terminating in the midline at the entrance of the vagina. This area should be inspected for ulcerations, leukoplakia, and any wartlike condylomas. Below the juncture of the labia minora in the area of the fourchette is the median raphe of the perineal body which terminates at the anus. Note any scars in the area (Fig. 13–3).

Inguinal hernias may be evident as swellings in one or both labia majora and occasionally a degenerative, cystic peritoneal

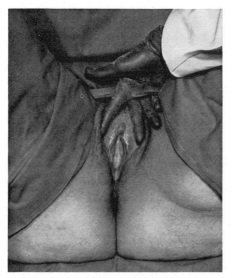

Figure 13–2. Examination of the external genitalia.

sac lying along the round ligament may be evident—a *hydrocele* of the canal of Nuck (Fig. 13–4). *Lipomas* are also found in the labia majora, as are small sebaceous cysts. *Edema* of the vulva may occur with renal or cardiac disease and also when lymphatic obstruction occurs with carcinomas in the pelvic region. *Melanomas* occur on the vulva and should be noted, particularly in pubertal girls. *Herpes* of the vulva is characterized by numerous small blisters or vesicles that are exquisitely painful when touched. *Erysipelas* of the vulva is a rapidly spreading inflammation accompanied by fever and chills; the external genitalia are swollen and reddened, and the patient experiences throbbing and burning in the area.

Pruritus vulvae accompanied by marked reddening and excoriation may occur with monilial vaginitis, trichomonas vaginitis, leukoplakia, and lichen sclerosis atrophicans. Monilial vaginitis is frequently seen in diabetic women, in pregnant women, and in patients using the oral progestin–estrogen contraceptive drugs. The vaginitis due to *Trichomonas vaginalis,* a flagellated protozoan, often macerates the skin. The whitish plaques and tissue thickening of leukoplakia are difficult to distinguish from lichen sclerosis atrophicans, a progressive disorder producing atrophy and loss of normal pigmentation of the vulva. Specific diagnosis of the cause of vulvar pruritus may require examina-

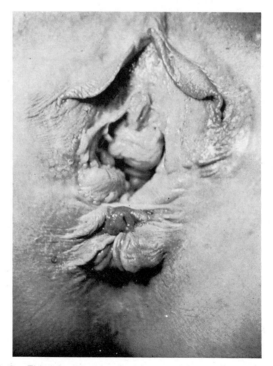

Figure 13–3. *Third degree tear of perineum with eversion of rectal mucosa. (Huffman, J. W.: Gynecology and Obstetrics. Philadelphia, W. B. Saunders Co., 1962.)*

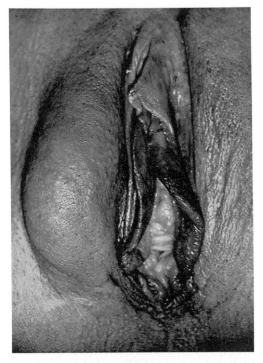

Figure 13-4. *Vulvar hydrocele, or cyst of the canal of Nuck, lying within the labium majus. (Huffman, J. W.: Gynecology and Obstetrics. Philadelphia, W. B. Saunders Co., 1962.)*

tion of a "hanging-drop" preparation, cultures, or a biopsy. Proper treatment based on accurate diagnosis brings great relief from the intense itching.

Pediculosis pubis or *scabies* may involve the vulva causing characteristic small red papules with lice seen on the hair follicles. Allergic reactions to poison ivy and other sensitizing agents are also seen occasionally.

Ulcerations involving the vulva may be caused by a number

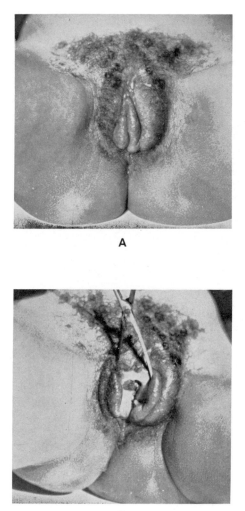

Figure 13–5. A, *Edema of vulva in patient with chancre;* B, *exposure of chancre upon separating labia.*

of factors. *Lipschütz ulcers*, small superficial ulcerations of the labia and vagina, are probably due to Döderlein's bacillus and related to poor hygiene. *Chancroid* causes an irregular ulceration with a punched-out appearance and a purulent granulating surface that is painful to touch (Fig. 13–5). *Granuloma inguinale* causes a papular lesion that may ulcerate and extend toward the groin. More often seen in warm climates, it is caused by a protozoan and produces progressive and extensive destruction of the genitalia. Diagnosis rests upon discovery of the characteristic Donovan bodies. *Lymphogranuloma venereum* is viral in origin and begins as a small papule with subsequent ulceration involving the entire vulva, groin, and rectal areas. A distinguishing lymphedema called esthiomene accompanies this ulcerative lesion. A Frei skin test may be useful in establishing the diagnosis.

Syphilis, caused by *Treponema pallidum,* produces a hard, raised, circular lesion with a pinkish surface and serous discharge. So-called "kissing lesions" on the apposing surfaces of the labia may be present. Darkfield examination of a properly prepared specimen should reveal the causative organism. Sec-

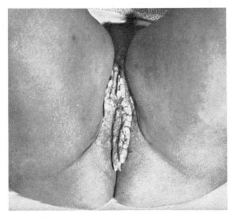

Figure 13–6. Condylomata lata.

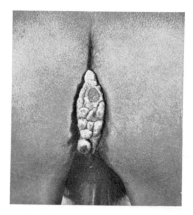

Figure 13–7. Condylomata acuminata.

ondary lesions of syphilis or condylomata lata occur as slightly elevated, plateau-like growths that are gray and moist and frequently join together to form aggregates (Fig. 13–6). These must not be confused with condylomata acuminata, which are papillomatous cauliflower lesions of the vulva and are viral in origin (Fig. 13–7). The latter are tender to touch and are often seen during pregnancy. Tuberculous vulvitis is a rare finding marked by small, discrete, punched-out ulcerations.

Carcinoma of the vulva is predominantly a disease of older women. In the early stages it may present as a small raised area of skin with some scaling that ultimately breaks down with ulceration. "Kissing lesions" are not uncommon and are frequently associated with considerable inflammation. All vulvar lesions should be studied until a specific diagnosis is achieved; frequently this requires a biopsy.

Following inspection of the labia and associated structures, observe the fossa navicularis just superior to the fourchette. It is usually quite obvious in young women but may be obscured in older persons. Superior to the fossa note the hymen surrounding or covering the entrance to the vagina, the introitus. In the nulliparous woman this membrane has a papillomatous appearance, with a crescentic or cribriform opening. In rare instances it may be imperforate, in which case it bulges forward with a blue-gray appearance because of retained menses. After childbirth and frequent coitus the hymenal remnants appear as small tags or carunculae. Following childbirth relaxation of the bulbocavernous muscles may leave the introitus gaping and the vagina exposed.

Proceeding superiorly, note the urethral meatus at the superior end of the rima pudendi. In young nulliparous women the urethral opening may be well concealed by many small folds of tissue. Along either side of the urethra are a series of small paraurethral glands, which are homologous to the prostate in the male. When acute infectious processes such as gonorrhea in-

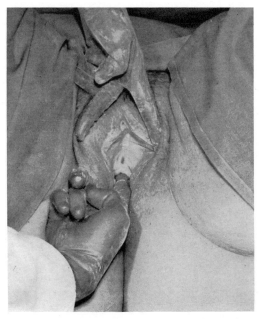

Figure 13–8. *Procedure of "milking" the urethra.*

volve the urethra, gentle massage along the urethra under the anterior vaginal wall may produce a small amount of pus for bacteriological study (Fig. 13–8). When chronic urethritis occurs, particularly in postmenopausal women, a small polypoid lesion, termed a "urethral caruncle," may be observed on the posterior surface of the urethral opening. *Carcinoma of the urethra* is an uncommon lesion but should be suspected if a papillary, firm growth involves the urethra, particularly in older women. A biopsy should be taken of suspicious lesions.

On either side of the hymen and external to it at approximately four and eight o'clock are two small depressions where the ducts of the two Bartholin or greater vestibular glands enter.

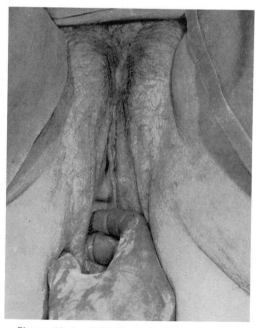

Figure 13–9. *Palpation of Bartholin's gland.*

These glands lie deep to the bulbocavernous muscles and secrete, under sexual stimulation, a mucoid lubricant. With age they gradually lose their ability to secrete. As a result of trauma or infection with coliform organisms or gonorrhea the glands may become distended, producing swelling of the lower perineum and severe pain. Following resolution of infection or trauma, obstruction of the duct may occur, resulting in distention of the gland with secretions producing a *Bartholin duct cyst*. These may be detected by placing the thumb and index fingers on either side of the labia and vagina and palpating the cyst (Fig. 13–9).

SPECULUM EXAMINATION

The vaginal speculum allows direct observation of the vaginal walls and cervix. However, before introducing the speculum, place two fingers in the introitus just beyond the hymen and press gently downward. At the same time ask the patient to strain downward. Note the extent to which the urethra and anterior and posterior vaginal walls bulge and whether the cervix appears in view. Prolapse of the urethra downward and outward is commonly termed a *urethrocele*. A more proper term is *detached urethra*. When such detachment is present and the patient is asked to cough, urine may spurt from the urethra verifying the presence of *stress incontinence*. If the anterior vaginal wall bulges downward, it is termed a *cystocele* (Fig. 13–10); and similarly, if the posterior wall bulges upward into the vagina, a *rectocele* is present (Fig. 13–11). The latter must be differentiated from a hernia between the rectum and vagina that occurs as a result of a congenitally deep cul-de-sac between the uterus and rectum, allowing descent of the small intestine into a cul-de-sac hernia, commonly called an *enterocele*. If, when the patient strains downward, the cervix appears at the introitus, a *prolapse* or *procidentia* of the uterus is present. Prolapse is graded as follows: first degree, the cervix appears at the introitus; second degree, the cervix or part of the uterus and vagina extend beyond the in-

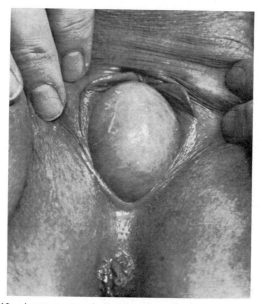

Figure 13–10. Large cystocele bulging from the introitus. (Huffman, J. W.: Gynecology and Obstetrics. Philadelphia, W. B. Saunders Co., 1962.)

troitus; and third degree, the entire uterus with vagina extends beyond the introitus (Fig. 13–12).

Inspect the vagina, noting the normal circular folds of tissue, termed rugae. Longitudinal breaks as a result of childbearing may frequently be seen.

Prior to removal of the fingers from the introitus, ask the patient to tighten the pelvic muscles and evaluate the tone of the levator ani and bulbocavernous muscles.

Following this general inspection, moisten the speculum with warm water. Water is the preferred lubricant since a Papanicolaou smear cannot be made when any other lubricant is employed. Spread the labia apart with the fingers, and holding the speculum with the blades closed, introduce it at an angle a

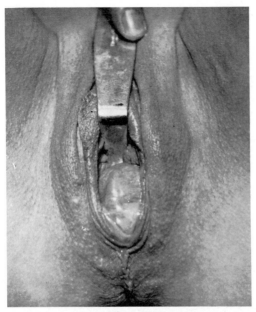

Figure 13-11. *Rectocele. (Huffman, J. W.: Gynecology and Obstetrics. Philadelphia, W. B. Saunders Co., 1962.)*

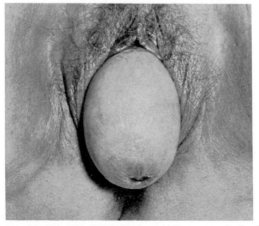

Figure 13-12. *Procidentia. (Parsons, L., and Sommers, S. C.: Gynecology. Philadelphia, W. B. Saunders Co., 1962.)*

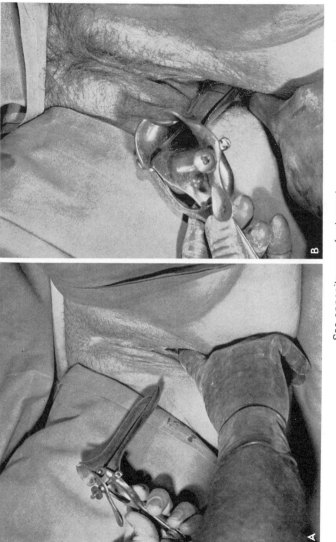

See opposite page for legend.

Illustration continued on opposite page.

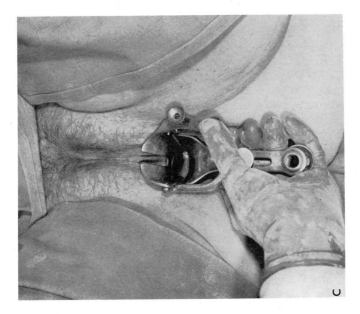

Figure 13–13. A and B, Introduction of vaginal speculum, blades closed; C, vaginal speculum in position.

little above the horizontal. Then, with gentle rotation, bring the blades to a horizontal position. While inserting the instrument, direct the blades posteriorly as far as the posterior blade will enter. Then open the blades gently and observe the cervix and vaginal wall (Fig. 13–13).

The Vagina

The color of normal vaginal epithelium varies with the phase of the menstrual cycle during which the examination is made. In the first or estrogenic phase, the epithelium appears pinkish with a white coating of desquamated cells covering the surface. During the second portion of the cycle the mucosa appears somewhat thinner and more vascular. Just prior to menstruation it may take on a bluish haze. Look in the posterior fornix of the vagina for a pool of cervical secretions containing exfoliated vaginal, cervical, and endometrial epithelium. Along the lateral walls of the vagina you may see small, thin-walled cystic masses of varying size called mesonephric duct cysts. They contain a mucoid secretion and represent vestiges of the male reproductive system.

Lesions of the vaginal mucosa. Numerous disorders may affect the vaginal mucosa. An erythematous appearance with a thick, white, cheesy exudate is characteristic of *monilial vaginitis* caused by *Candida albicans.* The exudate is easily scraped away and, if examined under a microscope, shows the typical branching mycelia of the fungus. In contrast, *trichomonas vaginitis* caused by *Trichomonas vaginalis*, causes a profuse discharge that is yellow in color. The epithelium may have a strawberry appearance because of many small punctate hemorrhages in the mucosa. Diagnosis may be made by preparing a hanging-drop slide. Trichomonas and monilial infections may be coexistent. *Atropic* or *senile vaginitis* is characterized by an epithelium that appears thin with an absence of prominent rugae. The discharge is yellow and frequently contains flecks of blood arising from punctate hemorrhagic areas. The discharge is usually malodorous.

Endometriosis, or ectopic endometrium, may involve the vagina. When it does, it is most evident in the posterior fornix as a direct extension through the cul-de-sac. The lesions are papular with a dark, reddish blue appearance and, if traumatized, reveal the presence of old, dark blood.

Primary carcinoma of the vagina, usually squamous in type, is a papillary growth with associated ulceration. Induration is usually present and the tumor mass bleeds easily if touched. *Secondary malignancy* (metastases) involving the vagina may result from extension of carcinoma of the cervix to the vagina or from endometrial carcinoma from the body of the uterus. Direct invasion of carcinoma from the bladder and rectum are far less common. *Choriocarcinoma* may also involve the vagina, producing red-blue lesions that bleed quite easily. *Primary sarcoma*, seen predominantly in children, has a characteristic papillary or grapelike appearance, giving rise to the term *sarcoma botryoides* (Fig. 13–14). This tumor is of embryonal origin and is of mixed mesodermal type.

The Cervix

Next inspect the cervix, noting its shape, the type of secretion in the external os, the configuration of the external os, and the color of the epithelium. The normal nulliparous cervix may be round to conical with an external os measuring 3 to 5 mm. (Fig. 13–15*A*). The surface is pale pink. Secretions from the cervix vary according to the time in the menstrual cycle. During the postmenstrual and premenstrual periods, the mucus is scant, tenacious, and opaque. During the preovulatory and ovulatory periods, because of high estrogen activity, the endocervical cells secrete large amounts of clear, mucoid fluid which can be drawn out in large bandlike threads, or spinnbarkeit. Following menopause, there is little or no cervical secretion.

Lesions of the cervix. The most common cervical lesion is often, but improperly, termed a *cervical erosion*. In the nulliparous woman, this lesion is usually the result of an outgrowth of columnar epithelium from the cervical canal onto the vaginal

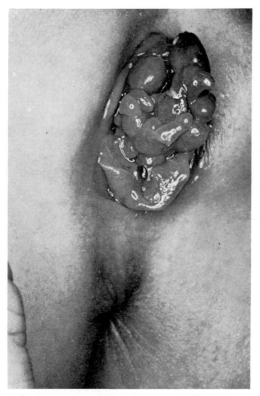

Figure 13–14. *Sarcoma botryoides. (Huffman, J. W.: Gynecology and Obstetrics. Philadelphia, W. B. Saunders Co., 1962.)*

Figure 13–15. *Types of cervicitis: A, grossly normal nulliparous cervix; B, lacerated, everted cervix; C, markedly lacerated and cystic cervix; D, lacerated, everted multiparous cervix; E, leukoplakia, metaplasia, and erosion of cervix. (Huffman, J. W.: Gynecology and Obstetrics. Philadelphia, W. B. Saunders Co., 1962.)*

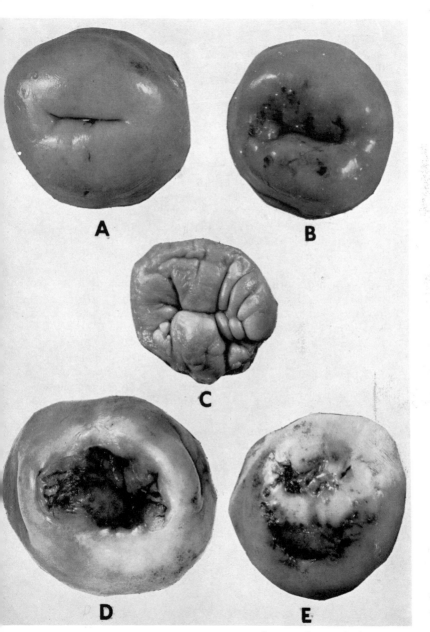

See opposite page for legend.

portion of the cervix, displacing the normal squamous epithelium and causing a characteristic cherry-colored lesion. In the parous woman, this may be an *ectropion,* that is, a patulous external cervical os that allows easy visualization of the endocervix and secondary outgrowth of cervical canal epithelium onto the vaginal portion (Fig. 13–15*B* to *E*). When this occurs and secondary infection is superimposed, the term *endocervicitis* is employed. If the squamous epithelium of the vaginal portion overgrows the columnar epithelium of the cervical canal, the secretions may be trapped in the submucous layers, producing nabothian cysts.

Gonorrheal cervicitis produces marked inflammation with a thick, purulent, yellow discharge coming from the cervix. True erosion of the cervix (ulceration) of benign origin is rare. When present, it is usually due to trauma or the presence of a foreign body within the cervical canal, such as a stem pessary. *Cervical polyps,* which are bright red in color, appear as tonguelike protrusions through the external os. They are attached in the endocervical canal or endometrial cavity, may be multiple or single, and bleed easily when subjected to trauma. Removal by curettement is required for the detection of any malignant change. *Condylomata acuminata* occur and appear as previously described (see p. 614).

Tuberculosis or *sarcoidosis* of the cervix, although uncommon, produce no specific clinical features other than erythema. *Endometriosis* involving the cervix appears as described (see p. 623). *Leukoplakia* of the cervix is characterized by white plaques of varying size that bleed easily and do not stain purple if Lugol's solution (dilute iodine) is applied to the cervix.

Squamous cell carcinoma of the cervix is the most common gynecological cancer encountered. Early lesions may be entirely asymptomatic and the cervix may appear quite normal. The most suggestive initial finding is the presence of a lesion on the cervix that bleeds with the slightest trauma and a watery vaginal discharge in the posterior fornix that is frequently purulent and malodorous. The lesion may be ulcerative or papilliform, producing a cauliflower-like growth.

Cervical carcinomas are classified in five stages as follows: *Stage 0*, intraepithelial lesions or carcinoma in situ; *Stage I*, invasive carcinoma confined to the cervix regardless of size or character; *Stage II*, extension of the tumor into the paracervical and parametrial tissues, sometimes involving the upper two-thirds of the vagina, but without the cervix being fixed; *Stage III*, involvement of the paracervical and parametrial tissues as far as the lateral pelvic wall, fixing the cervix on one or both sides and sometimes involving the lower third of the vagina; *Stage IV*, involvement of other organs, such as the bladder or rectum, and extension of the tumor beyond the pelvis.

Adenocarcinoma of the cervix originates in the endocervix primarily or as a result of extension from the endometrium. The cervix may be enlarged with blood exuding from the os. Frequently a hard mass can be palpated within the endocervical canal. Other cancers such as sarcoma botryoides may involve the cervix, as may metastatic lesions from the ovary and large intestine.

Papanicolaou smear.   A major advance in achieving early diagnosis of malignant lesions of the cervix is the study of exfoliative cytology of the cervix and posterior fornix vaginal pool after the method of Papanicolaou. No patient, regardless of age, should have a pelvic examination without a Papanicolaou study. To obtain material for cytologic study with the speculum in place, introduce a disposable spatula or tongue blade into the cervical canal, twisting it firmly through 360 degrees. The material obtained is then spread on a slide marked "cervix." Then remove the speculum and smear the material in the posterior blade upon a slide marked "vagina." The slides should not be allowed to dry in air but should be immediately fixed in 3 per cent acetic acid, 50 per cent ethyl alcohol solution. Submitted with the slides should be information regarding the date of the patient's last menstrual period, the age of the patient, whether she is pregnant, and the number of pregnancies. This information is essential to proper interpretation of the results of the cytology by the pathologist. Similar material for examination may be obtained if desired from the endocervix by aspiration with a small glass tube fitted with a suction bulb. If a speculum examination is impossible, material for study may be obtained by inserting a cotton applicator stick or cotton pledget grasped in uterine forceps into the vagina to the depth of the posterior fornix.

Squamous carcinoma of the cervix is usually associated with an abnormal Papanicolaou smear. However, the absence of a positive study does not preclude the presence of endometrial, tubal, or ovarian neoplasm. If in doubt, a punch or cone biopsy should be performed. The level of estrogen effect as estimated by a count of mature and immature cells of the vagina is invaluable in determining ovarian activity, especially at the menopause.

BIMANUAL EXAMINATION

The objectives of this procedure are to palpate the uterus and the adnexa between the vaginal and abdominal hand and to combine vaginal and rectal with abdominal palpation to outline the organs of the pelvis. The choice of which hand to use vaginally is a matter of personal preference. Most physicians use the left hand if naturally right-handed and vice versa. One or two fingers of the vaginal hand are moistened with lubricant and gently inserted into the introitus. Whether one or both fingers are used depends upon the age of the patient and the size of the introitus.

Following insertion of the fingers into the vagina, the examiner should place his foot (the right foot if the right hand is being used and vice versa) on a small stool and rest the elbow of the examining hand on the knee. This avoids placing undue pressure on the pelvic structures and offers a more controlled examination. Palpate the walls of the vagina as the fingers are inserted and, upon striking the cervix, note its consistency and the presence of any lesions previously seen. In addition, the presence of pain on movement of the cervix with reference to its severity and referral to other areas should be noted. Then place

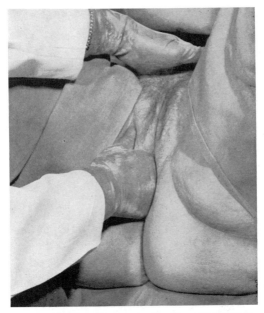

Figure 13–16. *Bimanual palpation of the uterus.*

the fingers into the posterior fornix and, with the other hand, gently but firmly palpate the midline of the abdomen approximately one third of the way to the umbilicus. Then, with the vaginal fingers lift the cervix and uterus upward in order that they can be felt between your two hands (Fig. 13–16). Note the position, size, shape, consistency, tenderness, and mobility of the uterus.

Determine if the uterus is anterior, lying upon the bladder with the cervix facing downward and backward. If the cervix is in its normal position but the body of the uterus is angulated sharply forward, anteflexion is said to be present. In contrast, if the body of the uterus is angulated backward, making it difficult to outline its posterior surface, retroflexion is present. When the cervix and fundus are in a normal relationship to each other but the cervix appears to be facing the anterior vaginal wall and the body of the uterus is located in the hollow of the sacrum, retroversion is said to exist. Similarly, if the normal cervix-fundus orientation is present but they are shifted downward and backward, then retrocession is present.

The normal uterus is approximately 7.5 cm. long, although its length varies with individuals. Note the firmness and contour of the fundus, particularly the presence of nodular areas. Observe and record the following findings if present:

Is any softening present between the body and cervix? Can arterial pulsations be felt by the vaginal fingers as the uterus is gently brought forward by the examining hand? Is the uterus of normal configuration (pear-shaped) or is it irregular? Are there any masses attached to it? Does pressure cause pain or does manipulation produce discomfort? If pain is produced by manipulation, is it referred? Can the uterus be moved up and down or does it seem to be attached to other organs or to the abdominal wall? Do not forget that one of the most common "tumors" palpated within the abdomen is a full bladder.

Pregnancy produces the most common abdominal "tumor" in women during the childbearing years. The pelvic signs of pregnancy include the following: A violaceous hue seen in the vulva, vaginal mucosa, and cervix is termed *Chadwick's sign.* A palpable softening of the cervix is called *Goodell's sign.* At approximately the sixth week of gestation *Hegar's sign* is present, manifested by a movable cervix felt by the vaginal fingers and a uterus of rubbery consistency palpated by the abdominal hand. The mobility results from enlargement and softening of the uterus. The uterus rises out of the pelvis at about 12 weeks of gestation, extends halfway to the umbilicus at 16 weeks, and is just below the umbilicus at 20 to 22 weeks. It reaches the xiphoid process at 36 weeks and then recedes below the xiphoid at approximately 40 weeks.

Congenital uterine anomalies vary from partial to complete duplications. The most common intrinsic tumor involving the corpus of the uterus is a *leiomyoma.* These are smooth muscle tumors that vary from 5 mm. in diameter to the size of a baseball or larger. They may be within the body of the uterus (intramural), under the peritoneal surface (subserous), or pedunculated. Malignant degeneration does occur within "fibroids" but fortunately is not common.

Endometrial carcinoma may cause no palpatory abnormalities or the uterus may be asymmetrically enlarged and feel soft. When the tumor spreads beyond the confines of the body of the uterus, its position becomes fixed and immovable.

Next, turn your attention to the tubo-ovarian areas or adnexa. Place the abdominal hand over the lateral border of the rectus muscle on the side to be examined and gently flex the fingers. At the same time bring the vaginal fingers anteriorly to meet the abdominal hand. A cord, felt anteriorly close to the symphysis, is the round ligament. The uterine tube is difficult to outline because of its consistency and mobility. When pelvic inflammatory disease has been present, cystic masses may be felt in the adnexa. The degree of tenderness and induration surrounding these masses gives a clue to the activity of the process.

The ovary may be detected as a firm, tender mass approximately 2 by 3 cm. in size. Ovarian masses may be cystic or firm and benign or malignant. All of the benign cystic tumors of the ovary have a malignant variant except the normal, functional follicular or lutein cyst. If in association with an ovarian mass there is evidence of precocious puberty, an estrogen-producing tumor should be suspected, whereas if progressive hirsutism has appeared, an androgen-secreting tumor or arrhenoblastoma is likely. The benign solid tumors of the ovary, such as fibromas, fibroadenomas, thecomas, and Brenner cell tumors, may occur during any period of life. Malignant solid tumors may be adenocarcinomas or hormone-producing tumors, such as granulosa cell tumors, arrhenoblastomas, dysgerminomas, and sarcomas. Teratomas or dermoids involve the ovary and may frequently be differentiated from other tumors because they appear to float on palpation, and an x-ray examination may reveal calcification or a fluid level in the tumor mass.

If a tumor is detected on one side, careful inspection of the opposite adnexa is imperative, since many ovarian tumors appear bilaterally. Notably, serous and mucinous cystadenomas and cystadenocarcinomas develop on both sides in 25 to 50 per cent of the cases. Teratomas appear bilaterally less often.

Endometriosis in the abdominal cavity may cause a progressive increase in ovarian size but cannot be differentiated except by history from other ovarian tumors.

In young women, ovarian cysts may appear on a functional basis and may be safely re-evaluated at intervals over one or two months if the patient is otherwise asymptomatic. However, in women over 35 any ovarian mass larger than 5 cm. requires immediate definitive evaluation. In menopausal and postmenopausal women no ovarian mass should be discounted. The presence of ascites should raise suspicion of ovarian malignancy, particularly if an ovarian mass is present. Metastatic lesions from the cervix, endometrium, gastrointestinal tract, and breast must all be considered when ovarian masses are felt in conjunction with the presence of a malignancy discovered at another site.

Following completion of the adnexal examination, move the examining fingers to the posterior fornix and palpate the uterosacral ligaments and the cul-de-sac of Douglas. Undue tenderness in the uterosacral ligaments as well as nodularity suggests the presence of endometriosis. Occasionally a prolapsed ovary in the cul-de-sac may be detected, and if a cul-de-sac hernia is present, the small intestine may be palpable.

In the differential diagnosis of masses in the pelvis, the possibility of ectopic pregnancy, either within the confines of the tube or ruptured into the peritoneal cavity, must be included. When rupture into the peritoneal space occurs, blood and the products of conception may be felt in the cul-de-sac.

Following bimanual examination, combined rectovaginal examination is done to evaluate the tone of the anal sphincter muscle and its competency and to detect hemorrhoids or other rectal disease (Figs. 13–17 and 13–18). Place the vaginal finger beneath the cervix then lift upward gently, placing strain on the uterosacral ligaments. The rectal finger is then moved upward and lateralward to meet the abdominal hand to further evaluate

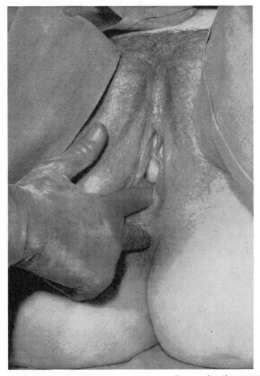

Figure 13–17. *Bidigital palpation with one finger in the vagina and the other in the rectum.*

the adnexa, the cul-de-sac, and the shape and position of the uterosacral ligaments. Following this examination, check the rectal finger for the presence of blood and the color of the stool.

It should be pointed out that use of the left hand allows more accurate examination of the left adnexa and conversely for the right side. If examination is not felt to be adequate the hands should be reversed and the procedure repeated.

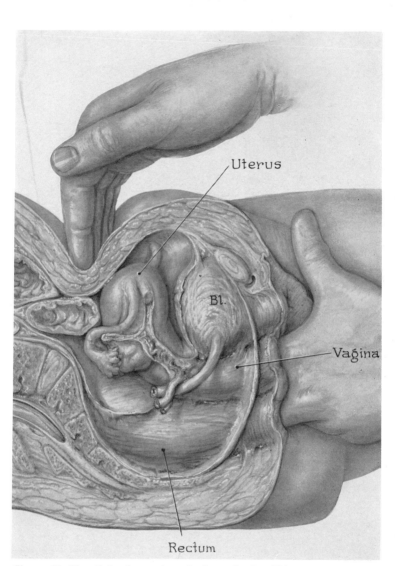

Figure 13–18. *Abdomino-rectovaginal examination. This maneuver permits palpation of lesions in the bases of the broad ligaments, which cannot be defined by vaginal examination. (Huffman, J. W.: Gynecology and Obstetrics. Philadelphia, W. B. Saunders Co., 1962.)*

To complete bimanual examination palpate the bony ligamentous structures of the pelvis for the presence of tenderness, tumors, or abnormal fixation.

PREVENTIVE MEDICINE

Pelvic examination must be a routine part of any physical examination of a female. In the premenarchal years a rectal examination may suffice. Many disorders, such as congenital anomalies, apparent in adult life escape early detection because a methodical, thorough pelvic examination has not been performed.

At the menarche, a Papanicolaou smear should be done at least once a year until the childbearing years when a six-month interval becomes proper practice if the "Pap" smear is not consecutively Class I. Class II requires six-month follow-ups. Classes III, IV, and V necessitate immediate repetition and further steps to rule out the presence of malignant disease. Do not neglect the Papanicolaou study and pelvic examination in pregnant women as well as at the six-weeks' postpartum visit. Additional, more specialized procedures such as endometrial biopsy and culdocentesis have proved of great value in detection of pelvic disease. It is your responsibility as a physician to educate your patients of the necessary preventive practices in order to help them to live fruitful reproductive lives and to aid in correction of any detectable abnormalities.

COMMON CLINICAL TERMS

Abortion—Termination of pregnancy before the fetus has become viable.

Amenorrhea—Absence of menses.

Dysmenorrhea—Painful menstruation.

Dyspareunia—Painful coitus in women.

Menorrhagia—Excessive menstrual flow.

Menopause—Cessation of menses in a normal manner at the end of the reproductive years.

Miscarriage—A lay term for loss of a fetus before it is viable.

Multipara—A woman who has borne more than one child.
Nullipara—A woman who has not produced a viable offspring.
Primigravida—A woman pregnant for the first time.

COMMON CLINICAL SYNDROMES

Abruptio placentae—Premature separation of the normally implanted placenta, often of unknown cause.
Chiari-Frommel syndrome—Persistent amenorrhea and galactorrhea after delivery, perhaps secondary to excessive prolactin secretion.
Endometriosis—Disseminated endometrial tissue implants outside the uterus that produce abdominal pain, backache, dysmenorrhea, and sterility.
Meigs' syndrome—Pleural effusion and ascites due to a benign fibroma of the ovary.
Preeclampsia—A syndrome of hypertension and proteinuria, with or without edema, occurring near the end of pregnancy; if convulsions occur, the condition is known as eclampsia.
Placenta previa—Implantation of the placenta on the lower uterine segment, low enough that expansion of the cervix causes tearing of placenta tissue and bleeding.
Sheehan's syndrome—Pituitary failure secondary to necrosis because of hemorrhage and shock complicating delivery.

BIBLIOGRAPHY

Huffman, J. W.: Gynecology and Obstetrics. Philadelphia, W. B. Saunders Co., 1962.
Parsons, L., and Sommers, S. C.: Gynecology. Philadelphia, W. B. Saunders Co., 1962.

14
EXAMINATION OF THE BACK AND EXTREMITIES

Examination of the back and extremities relies mainly on inspection and palpation, with percussion and auscultation playing minor roles for obvious physical reasons. Percussion, dependent upon variations in the air space in underlying tissues, has little value in the solidly constructed extremities. Likewise, auscultation is seldom applicable save for detection of crepitation upon joint motion, for detecting flow murmurs over blood vessels, or for the diagnosis of fractures of the hip. We shall consider inspection and palpation together since the two methods are intimately related, each serving to confirm and augment the findings of the other.

Palpation of the back and extremities requires finer discrimination than palpation of the intra-abdominal organs. The distance between the spinous processes of the vertebrae and the paraspinal muscles, between the joint line and the origin and insertion of the medial collateral ligament of the knee, and so forth, may be only a fingerbreadth.

Locomotion and support are the functions of the musculoskeletal system; therefore, observe the patient as he walks to and from the examining room, as he carries out the coordinated activities required in undressing, and as he climbs on and off the examining table. Much specific information can be gathered by

637

requesting the patient to do special tasks or assume various positions. These maneuvers are essential, specialized features of the examination of the musculoskeletal system and are detailed in subsequent sections of this chapter.

GENERAL INSPECTION

For proper examination, clothing must be removed to reveal the habitus, or physical characteristics, of the patient. Body symmetry and proportion may be disturbed by deformity or disproportion. Total height and the relationship of trunk length to extremity lengths vary with dwarfism, giantism, dyschondroplasia, and other disturbances of growth and development. Right and left halves of the body may be asymmetrical. Obesity, distribution of fat, muscular development, and muscle wasting must all be noted.

Careful inspection of the skin is important (see Chapter 3, Examination of the Skin). It may reveal the café au lait spots of neurofibromatosis or of fibrous dysplasia of bone, the increased pigmentation associated with prolonged and excessive use of local heat, or the psoriasis associated with psoriatic arthritis (see Fig. 3–25). Inspection may also reveal the lesions of herpes zoster (see Fig. 3–21), which can mimic nerve root compression syndromes; or boils and furuncles (see Fig. 3–24), which may be the primary site of infection in patients with hematogenous osteomyelitis and arthritis. In patients with acute injuries and multiple fractures, the appearance of petechial hemorrhages in the axillae, across the anterior chest wall and in the subconjunctival sacs, establishes the clinical diagnosis of fat embolism. Atrophy of skin appendages, e.g., nails and hair, should be carefully noted. Likewise, clubbing of the nails or cyanosis of the nail bed may be the first clue to cardiopulmonary disease. Transverse ridging of the nails may accompany nutritional disturbances, and the nails and hair may be brittle in patients with myxedema.

Are there telltale calluses, pressure sores, abrasions, even tire marks or other evidence of external violence? Old scars may be the result of previous injuries or operations. The absence of a breast, removed for cancer, in a patient with bone pain may be significant. In such a patient, edema of the arm on the side of breast removal may be the result of extensive surgery involving the lymphatic drainage of the arm. Is the skin temperature above or below normal? Is the skin dry or moist? Shake hands with the patient and note the strength and character of the grip. Patients with cirrhosis have a characteristic soft, feminine skin and a flaccid grip. Is the palm moist and warm, as in the thyrotoxic individual, or moist and cool, as in the patient with an anxiety reaction? Does the patient withdraw from a firm grip because of pain due to rheumatoid arthritis? A child seen in the emergency room with a fresh injury may exhibit bruises and burn scars of various ages suggesting the battered-child syndrome.

GAIT AND STANCE

Gait is the manner in which a person walks; it varies widely in normal persons, being quite distinctive in particular individuals. We can all identify certain persons at a distance by the way they walk, as may a blind man by the sound of their footsteps. For purposes of analysis, gait is divided into a high energy, stance phase (heel strike, mid stance, push off), when the leg supports the weight of the body, and a low energy phase (acceleration, swing through, deceleration), when the leg is not bearing weight. The arms should be moving rhythmically and symmetrically in a coordinated manner.

A normal gait propels the body with the greatest efficiency, i.e., with the least expenditure of energy. The center of gravity of the body, located at or just in front of the second sacral segment, moves approximately 2 in. up and down and from side to side with normal gait. Gaits that displace the center of gravity more than this consume more energy and are inefficient. Thus, the increased energy consumption required by a limp or abnormal gait contributes significantly to physical disability. A normal gait requires an intact neuromuscular mechanism, a normal skeleton, and normal joints. Injury to, or disease of, any of these systems will result in a gait disturbance. There are ataxic gaits, staggering gaits, steppage gaits, antalgic gaits, spastic gaits, waddling gaits, and many others that are characteristic of a wide spectrum of disease processes. Some of these are discussed in Chapter 4, Examination of the Nervous System.

The stance or posture that the patient assumes may indicate fatigue, dejection, tension, relaxation, and many attitudes of either physical or emotional background. The position of the head alone can suggest a myopic individual peering through his bifocals, a deaf person straining to hear, or a patient with wryneck. Gaits and postures are the stock in trade of the actor and mimic because they add so much to the reality of a portrayal. In a similar way, the patient reveals himself to you.

JOINT MOTION

One of the better systems for recording range of motion at a joint is that adopted by the American Medical Association and published in its *Guide to the Evaluation of Permanent Impairment of the Extremities and Back.* While the practiced eye alone may suffice for estimating range of motion, more accurate measurements can be made with a device that incorporates a protractor, e.g., a goniometer (Fig. 14–1). Children may have very flexible joints, whereas the elderly are likely to have a limited range of joint motion. Motion at a joint in one extremity should have the same range of motion as the corresponding joint in its counterpart. By careful comparison of an affected joint and its normal partner, small differences can be appreciated.

Range of motion at a joint may be limited because of disease within or outside the joint. If joint motion is uniformly restricted in all directions, the disease process is almost always within the joint, whereas limitation of motion in only one direction is usually the result of a bony or soft tissue block outside the joint.

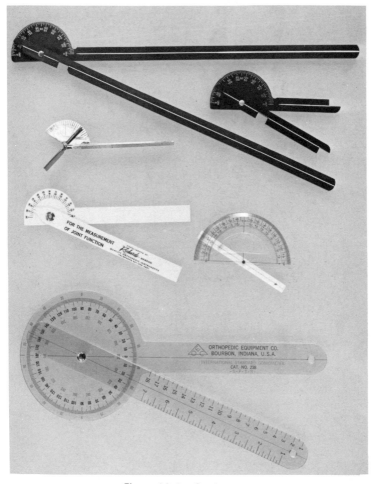

Figure 14–1. Goniometers.

When motion can be carried through a range greater than normal, the joint is unstable. Excessive motion ordinarily occurs in only one direction and results from injury to a specific ligament or ligaments, as in a sprain. Careful palpation of a joint at the points of attachment of the various ligaments will allow exact anatomical identification of the ligament injured, since the point of maximum tenderness indicates the site of injury. Sprains are classified as first, second, or third degree injuries, depending upon the extent of damage and the amount of instability. Gross instability of a joint, permitting grotesque motion, is characteristic of neuropathic disease. This type of condition is readily seen in the Charcot joints associated with tabes dorsalis in syphilis (Fig. 14–2). Generalized hyperflexibility of joints is a hereditary trait. An individual exhibiting this trait may say he is "loose jointed" or "doubled jointed." Rarely, generalized hyperflexibility is accompanied by excessive elasticity, friability of the

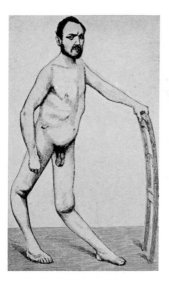

Figure 14–2. Charcot's knee. (Westphal.)

skin, and fragility of the subcutaneous blood vessels as in the Ehlers-Danlos syndrome.

Swelling of a joint may be caused by fluid within the joint space or within an overlying bursa. When fluid exists within a joint, palpation with the examining finger reveals this over the entire joint area, but when the fluid is in a bursa, the area of swelling is smaller and is sharply localized. Diffuse thickening of the synovial lining of a joint is a chronic slow change, the joint being firm to palpation and of a boggy consistency. A rise in the local skin temperature about a joint suggests inflammation. Determining whether a joint or bursa contains fluid, blood, or pus may require aspiration. If the swelling is due largely to a thickened synovium, very little fluid will be obtained.

Snapping, grinding, or crepitation that is apparent on motion may be caused by the friction of sliding tendons or of fibrous bands about the joint or by the actual binding of the cartilaginous joint surfaces as they glide upon one another. This latter phenomenon is related to chondromalacia, i.e., softening of the cartilage, and is most commonly encountered on the under surface of the patella. A clicking or locking during motion may indicate the presence of a loose body or a torn meniscus within the joint. A loose body may result from an osteochondral fracture, osteochondritis dissecans (Fig. 14–3), or osteochondromatosis. Such "joint mice" are cartilaginous in nature and usually cannot be seen on x-ray photographs of the joint, although the roentgenogram may demonstrate the spot from which the loose body arose. Fortunately, loose bodies can often be palpated through the joint capsule, and the diagnosis established in this way. Fibrocartilaginous menisci are found in the temporomandibular joints, in joints at either end of the clavicle, and in the knee; therefore, these are the only joints in which cysts of the menisci are found. Injuries of the menisci occur almost exclusively in the knee and are characterized by tenderness localized to the joint line, with clicking or snapping on controlled motion at the joint.

Small tumors commonly found on the extensor, and to a lesser degree the flexor, surfaces adjacent to the joints of the

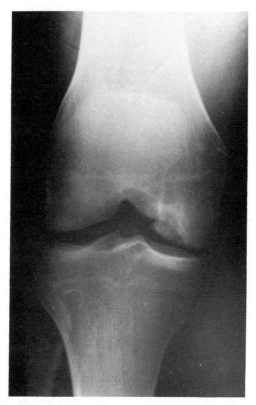

Figure 14–3. *Osteochondritis dissecans of medial femoral condyle. (Gartland, J. J.: Fundamentals of Orthopaedics. 2nd ed. Philadelphia, W. B. Saunders Co., 1975.)*

arms and legs are called ganglia. They are cysts arising from the synovial tendon sheaths and are filled with synovial fluid. A large synovial cyst associated with the hamstring tendons in the popliteal area is called Baker's cyst. Malignant soft tissue tumors occur adjacent to joints, particularly in the lower extremities.

These are firm, fleshy tumors adherent to the underlying tendons and fascia. Bony tumors palpable about the joints are usually osteochondromas arising in the adjacent metaphyses.

EXAMINATION OF MUSCLES

Congenital anomalies of muscles occur most frequently in the sternocleidomastoid muscles and in the pectoralis major. Portions of these muscles may be absent. Enlargement of muscles or muscle groups is found in congenital hypertrophy (Fig. 14–4) and in pseudohypertrophic muscular dystrophy. The calf muscles of a child with pseudohypertrophic muscular dystrophy have a firm, doughy consistency that is characteristic. Diminution of muscle mass can be associated with disuse or can be the result of neuromuscular disease—as in poliomyelitis, diseases of the brain or spinal cord, peripheral neuropathy, or peripheral nerve injury. Atrophy of muscles may also, of course, be the result of primary muscle disease, e.g., muscular dystrophies and myotonia. Palpation of the muscles gives a good idea of muscle tone and degree of atrophy. Measurement of the circumference of a calf, thigh, forearm, and arm, when compared with similar measurements on the opposite, uninvolved side, will give a rough indication of any loss of muscle mass. The small tender nodules often palpated in the periscapular, back, and gluteal muscles are called fibrocytic nodules. Tumors of the muscle are very rare.

Muscle testing, the evaluation of the strength and function of individual muscles, is a sophisticated and highly technical procedure requiring a thorough knowledge of anatomy and kinesiology. Muscle strength is commonly graded on a sacle of 0 to 5, zero indicating complete absence of contraction and five indicating normal strength. Additional diagnostic information regarding the muscles may be obtained by electromyography.

When an injured muscle has been torn from either its origin or its insertion, contraction of the muscle produces an abnormal muscle mass, since the muscle is no longer restrained by attach-

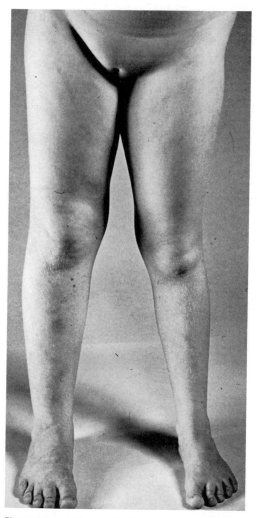

Figure 14–4. *Congenital hypertrophy of right leg.*

ment at both ends. In the biceps brachii, for example, this phenomenon results from a tear of the long head of the biceps in the bicipital groove or from avulsion of its insertion into the radius. Ossification of an intramuscular hematoma (myositis ossificans) results in a palpable mass. This is seen most frequently in the quadriceps muscles of the thigh and in the upper, outer portion of the arm.

Among football players, myositis ossificans is found in the quadriceps muscles in backs, and in linemen myositis ossificans of the arm muscles is so typical it is called "blocker's node."

EXAMINATION OF THE CERVICAL SPINE

Ask the patient to hold his head erect and level. Note that the cervical spine normally has a forward, or lordotic, curve. A flattening of this curve is indicative of disease or injury. Next, stand behind the patient and observe as he moves his head and neck through forward flexion, bending to the side, ear to shoulder, and turning right to left. Motion of the head on the neck is either "yes," forward and backward, or "no," from side to side. In the former, motion occurs between the occiput and first cervical vertebrae; in the latter, motion occurs between the first and second cervical vertebrae. Disease at a specific joint will result in limitation of the corresponding motion. Limitation of motion is rarely symmetrical. Muscle strength is tested by requesting the patient to hold his head firmly in the neutral position while the examiner pushes the head forward, backward, and from side to side. As the patient resists, the various muscle groups contract, allowing weakness and pain to be localized. Tenderness of the anterior neck muscles accompanied by pain on swallowing is found frequently in patients with hyperextension injuries of the neck. Generalized atrophy of the cervical muscles is associated with prolonged use of cervical collars and braces as well as with arthrosis of the cervical spine.

Other findings relating to the cervical area are detailed in Chapter 5, Examination of the Head and Neck.

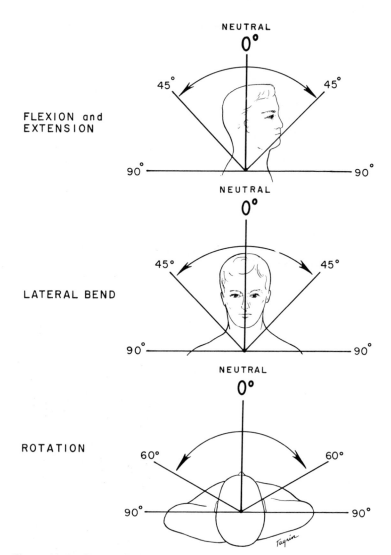

Figure 14-5. Range of motion of the cervical spine. (American Academy of Orthopaedic Surgeons: Measuring and Recording of Joint Motion. Everett, Massachusetts, Glenwood Press, 1963.)

EXAMINATION OF THE BACK

The thoracic spine normally has a slight backward rounding, kyphosis, whereas the lumbar spine has a forward, or lordotic, curve. Excessive rounding of the back, the most frequent deformity associated with osteoporosis, also occurs with Marie-Strümpell ankylosing spondylitis (Fig. 14–6). When kyphosis is long-standing and severe it is accompanied by a compensatory lordosis of the cervical spine with hyperextension of the head. The senile kyphosis of osteoporosis is caused by the collapse and anterior wedging of thoracic vertebrae. Rounding of the back in teenagers just prior to cessation of growth of the spine is called "juvenile kyphosis" or "adolescent round back." This is caused by epiphysitis of the lower thoracic vertebrae, or Scheuermann's disease.

Sharp forward angulation of the spine, presenting a more localized deformity, or gibbus, results from destruction or deformity of a vertebral body. In infants it is seen in lipochondrodystrophy and dyschondroplasia. A gibbus is the classic de-

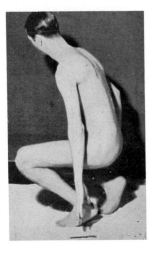

Figure 14–6. Characteristic attitude assumed by patient with poker spine (Marie-Strümpell disease) when picking a pencil from the floor.

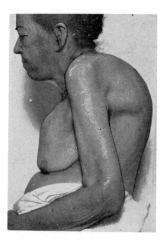

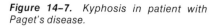

Figure 14–7. Kyphosis in patient with Paget's disease.

Figure 14–8. Gibbus due to tuberculosis of spine.

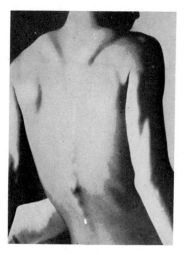

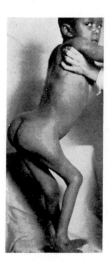

Figure 14–9. Lordosis in patient with tuberculosis of the hip.

formity of Pott's disease, or tuberculosis of the spine (Fig. 14–8), and is occasionally found after severe compression fractures of vertebral bodies.

Increased lordosis is found in patients with spondylolisthesis and spondylolysis, and particularly in individuals with very tight hamstring muscles. It is also seen in association with hip disease, especially in patients with congenital dislocation of the hips and in persons with flexion contractures of the hips who hyperextend the lumbar spine in order to stand erect.

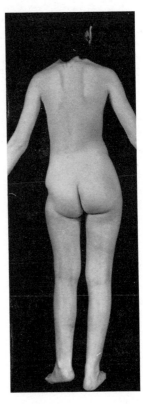

Figure 14–10. *Listing stance in patient with slipped capital epiphyses in childhood. Note the equinovarus foot position. (Howorth, M. B.: A Textbook of Orthopedics. Philadelphia, W. B. Saunders Co., 1952.)*

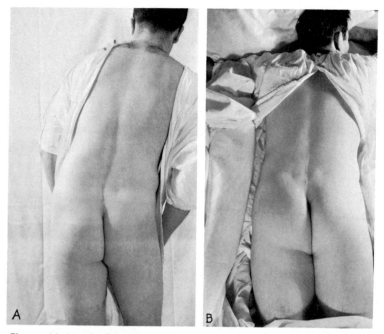

Figure 14–11. A, *Paravertebral muscle spasm with obliteration of lumbar lordosis, elevation of left side of pelvis, and list of spine to the right;* B, *the postural deformity disappears once the patient is relaxed in the prone position.* (Gartland, J. J.: Fundamentals of Orthopaedics. 2nd ed. Philadelphia, W. B. Saunders Co., 1975.)

A deviation of the spine to one side is called a "list" (Figs. 14–10 and 14–11). This is easily observed in patients whose legs are of unequal length. Lists may result from muscle spasms caused by herniation of an intervertebral disc or by acute fibromyositis of the paraspinal muscles. The trunk may list toward or away from the affected side in patients with sciatic pain. Occasionally the patient will list first to one side and then the other. Such lists disappear when the patient sits, or after the

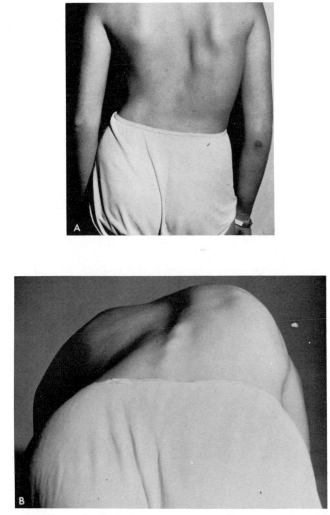

Figure 14–12. A, *Scoliosis in a young woman;* B, *exaggeration of abnormality with bending.*

pain disappears. This is in contrast to the permanent list produced when scarring and fibrosis of the back muscles follows a fracture of a transverse vertebral process.

Scoliosis is a more complicated deformity than kyphosis, lordosis, or a list, because not only does the spine bend in one direction or the other, but the vertebral bodies rotate one upon the other. Since most of the rotating vertebrae are thoracic and have ribs attached to them, the ribs are also displaced — forward on one side and backward on the other. Those that are displaced backward develop a sharp angulation. It is this displacement and angulation of the ribs that results in the more obvious part of the deformity. Bending forward accentuates this deformity (Fig. 14–12). Examination of the patient with scoliosis should include a search for congenital anomalies (particularly congenital heart disease), the stigmata of neurofibromatosis, and any residual muscle weakness or paralysis. Most commonly, scoliosis is idiopathic. It occurs most frequently in adolescent girls.

Inspection may reveal a congenital deformity of the scapula, Sprengel's deformity, in which the scapula is elevated and possibly attached to the lower cervical vertebrae by a palpable band of fibrous tissue or bone (the omovertebral bone).

Spina bifida cystica, with a cystic or fungating mass in the midline, usually occurs in the lumbar or sacral region (Fig. 14–13). Patients with this disorder usually have paralysis and loss of sensation in the lower limbs and perineum. Lesser skin stigmata, e.g., excess hair, a dimple, or a blind sinus tract, may occur in the midline at the lumbosacral junction in association with a spina bifida occulta. Still lower, a pilonidal sinus may be found.

Motion of the spine is best evaluated by observing the patient from behind as he bends forward, backward, from side to side, and rotates from side to side (Fig. 14–14). Measurement of chest expansion is an indirect measurement of thoracic spine motion, since rotation of the ribs takes place at the costovertebral joints, very near the facet joints. In rheumatoid arthritis of the spine (Marie-Strümpell ankylosing spondylitis), chest expansion is severely restricted. This may be the first clinical finding of this disease, which occurs primarily in young men.

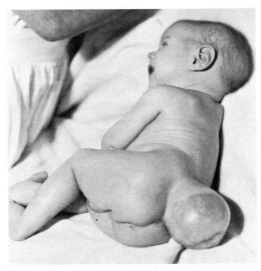

Figure 14–13. *Spina bifida cystica.*

Palpation of the back should reveal the spinous processes, the interspinous ligaments, and the paraspinal muscles. Muscle spasm and pain on palpation of the muscles is often associated with fibrocytic nodules, a condition which may extend into the gluteal muscles. Pain over the spinous processes and interspinous ligaments is more indicative of disease of the spine. Percussion of the spine will produce pain in patients with osteoporosis, carcinomatosis, and infections of the bodies of the vertebrae. Percussion over the costovertebral angles may cause pain in patients with kidney disease. Tenderness to pressure in the midline at the lumbosacral junction is present in patients with herniated intervertebral discs and in patients with spondylolysis or spondylolisthesis. A palpable step, or shelf, may be present in patients with spondylolisthesis in whom the body of the fifth vertebra slips forward on the body of the sacrum. Tender, fatty

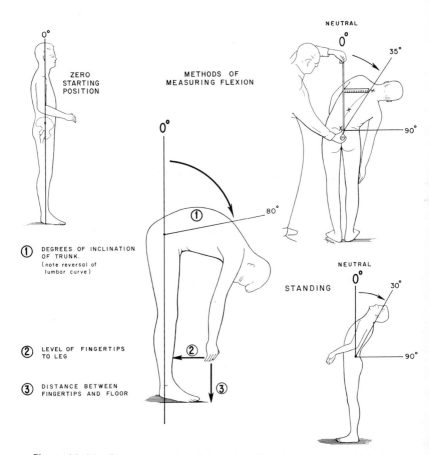

Figure 14–14. Range of motion of the spine. (American Academy of Orthopaedic Surgeons: Measuring and Recording of Joint Motion. Everett, Massachusetts, Glenwood Press, 1963.)

nodules are commonly palpable adjacent to the sacroiliac joints just below the edge of the ilium.

Localizing pain to joints requires examination for that purpose. Patrick's sign, positive in patients with sacroiliac disease, is elicited by placing the patient supine and asking him to place his heel on his thigh just above the opposite patella. The leg is then fully abducted, producing pain posteriorly over the joint if sacroiliac disease is present.

Rectal examination is essential in a patient with low back pain, since chronic prostatitis is a common cause of backache. Also, this is the only way deformities and injuries of the coccyx can be evaluated. A pelvic examination should be done in all women with back complaints.

EXAMINATION OF THE SHOULDER

All joints participating in shoulder motion – the sternoclavicular, acromioclavicular, scapulothoracic, and glenohumeral – can be easily observed and palpated as they move in concert in normal scapulohumeral action. Limitation of motion resulting from injury or disease of any of these joints distorts scapulohumeral motion, most often restricting abduction and internal rotation. If motion of the shoulder becomes progressively limited, a "frozen shoulder" may result.

Scapulohumeral rhythm and range of motion is best observed from behind the patient as he raises his arms above his head. The extent of rotation, seen as the patient puts his hands first behind his head and then behind his back, may be measured by placing the patient's arm at his side, elbow bent to a right angle, whence the patient is requested to move his hand away from his body, keeping his elbow at his side.

Inspection of the shoulders from behind may reveal a horizontal displacement of one shoulder. Such asymmetry may be due to Sprengel's deformity (congenital upward displacement of the scapula), scoliosis, or weakness of the muscles supporting one of the scapulae. If the patient is then asked to push his

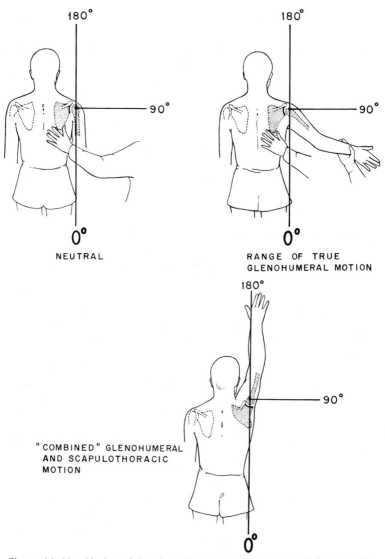

Figure 14–15. Motion of the shoulder. (American Academy of Orthopaedic Surgeons: Measuring and Recording of Joint Motion. Everett, Massachusetts, Glenwood Press, 1963.)

hands firmly together, either or both of the scapulae may project backward. Here the medial border of the scapula swings out away from the chest wall, producing "winging of the scapula," a deformity resulting from poliomyelitis, muscular dystrophy or atrophy, or isolated injury to the long thoracic nerve of Bell. Atrophy of the supraspinatus and infraspinatus muscles may be visible, and tender fibrocytic nodules can frequently be palpated at the medial superior border of the scapulae.

Observation of the patient from the front may reveal congenital absence of the clavicles with abnormal hypermobility of the scapulae, i.e., cleidocranial dysostosis as well as partial or complete absence of the pectoralis major. The sternoclavicular joint may be the site of acute arthritis, usually due to a gonorrheal infection. Instability or deformity of this joint is caused by subluxation or dislocation due to recent or old injuries. Rarely, cystic degeneration of the fibrocartilaginous meniscus may produce a visible and palpable mass at the joint.

Fractures of the clavicle can be easily appreciated by palpation, since it is subcutaneous throughout its length. The acromioclavicular joint at the outer end of the clavicle is a common site of injury in athletes. The joint may suffer partial or complete separation resulting in a "knocked down" or "dropped" shoulder, the deformity of which can be increased by pulling down on the arm. Injury commonly leads to arthritis of this joint. Swelling accompanied by tenderness on the anterior chest wall at a costochondral junction of one of the upper ribs is indicative of a chondritis, e.g., Tietze's syndrome.

Inspection and palpation of the upper arm at the shoulder will reveal the bicipital groove on the anterior aspect of the head of the humerus. Pain localized to this area is associated with acute or chronic tendinitis of the long head of the biceps brachii. The diagnosis can be confirmed by eliciting pain that is localized to the bicipital groove as the patient, with his arm at his side and the elbow flexed to a right angle, supinates his forearm against resistance. Additionally, if the long tendon of the biceps is ruptured, usually as a result of attrition from chronic tendinitis, this maneuver causes the biceps muscle to ball up into an abnormally

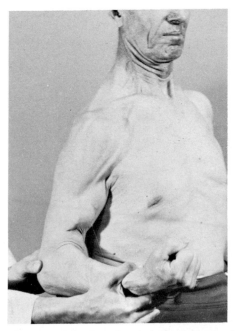

Figure 14–16. *Rupture of the long head of the biceps tendon. (Bateman, J. E.: The Shoulder and Neck. Philadelphia, W. B. Saunders Co., 1972.)*

rounded mass rather than to assume its usual fusiform shape, since one end of the muscle is no longer firmly anchored (Fig. 14–16). This finding also occurs in the rare disorder of avulsion of the insertion of the biceps tendon into the radius.

Pain in the shoulder due to subacromial bursitis or to a rotator cuff tear is commonly referred distally to the level of the insertion of the deltoid muscle. Careful palpation of the lateral aspect of the shoulder is necessary to differentiate between a rotator cuff tear at the insertion of the cuff into the tuberosities of the humerus and a tender subacromial bursa, which is only slightly more superior. Ask the patient to abduct his arm to 90 degrees and maintain it in this position while you push downward. Contraction of the rotator cuff muscles, to maintain the position of the humerus, causes pain at the point of a rotator cuff tear.

Bony masses palpable about the upper end of the humerus are usually osteochondromas, or they may be bony masses of myositis ossificans (blocker's node), frequently the result of blocking with the upper arms in football.

Dislocation of the shoulder is a common injury. In the young it is rarely accompanied by a fracture of the humerus, whereas in the middle-aged patient, associated fractures of the tuberosity of the humerus are the rule. When dislocation occurs, the head of the humerus is not in its normal relationship with the glenoid and cannot be palpated under the tip of the acromion. In the more common anterior dislocation, the arm is held in external rotation, the elbow away from the side of the body; the head of the humerus can be felt in a position inferior or medial to the coracoid process. The patient cannot touch his opposite ear with the affected hand. Posterior dislocations of the shoulder are rare and are almost always associated with uncontrolled muscular violence, e.g., a convulsion. With posterior dislocation, the arm is characteristically held in marked internal rotation and cannot be externally rotated, and the head of the humerus is more difficult to palpate posteriorly.

Brachial plexus injury may occur with difficult obstetrical deliveries and may affect the upper portion of the plexus (Erb's palsy), the lower portion of the plexus (Klumpke's palsy), or the entire plexus. If such an injury has occurred, the infant holds the arm in internal rotation and will not actively move it. In children or adults, marked limitation of external rotation of the humerus is evident along with muscular weakness or paralysis corresponding to the level and extent of injury to the plexus.

Complete evaluation of the patient who complains of pain and disability of the shoulder must include thorough examination of the neck and axilla and a thorough neurological examination.

EXAMINATION OF THE ELBOW

Although it is an oversimplification to call the elbow a hinge joint, for the purpose of measurement its motion is considered in only one plane. The normal range of motion at the elbow is flexion to 60 to 70 degrees and extension to 180 to 190 degrees. Hyperextension at the elbow is frequently seen in children, especially in those with generalized hyperflexibility. When the forearm is extended to 180 degrees, it becomes apparent that the arm and forearm do not make a straight line, but have a slight lateral angulation. This normal "carrying angle" is greater in women than in men. Injuries about the elbow may result in an increase (cubitus valgus) or decrease (cubitus varus) in the carry-

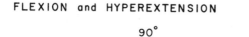

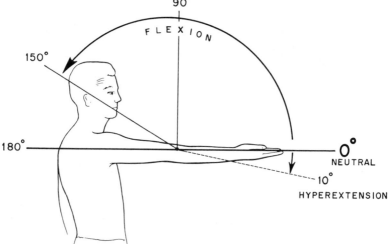

Figure 14–17. Joint motion as measured in degrees of a circle. (American Academy of Orthopaedic Surgeons: Measuring and Recording of Joint Motion. Everett, Massachusetts, Glenwood Press, 1963.)

ing angle. Severe cubitus varus, following a malunited supracondylar fracture, is referred to as a "gunstock deformity." Deformities of this type are not conspicuous when the elbow is partially flexed but become obvious when the forearm is extended as the arm hangs at the side. Cubitus valgus is often associated with a tardy ulnar palsy caused by chronic stretch injury of the nerve as it is angulated and stretched in its groove at the medial side of the elbow. When this occurs the nerve may be tender to palpation and thickened as it is felt posteriorly and medially in the ulnar groove, commonly called the "crazy bone." The symptoms of a tardy ulnar palsy are confined to the hand and consist of numbness, tingling, loss of epicritic sensation of the fifth and the medial half of the fourth fingers, and weakness and atrophy of the intrinsic muscles of the hand.

The lateral epicondyle of the humerus is the point of origin for the extensor muscle mass of the forearm. When these muscles are repeatedly stressed, this area of origin becomes quite painful, giving rise to a lateral epicondylitis, or "tennis elbow." The pain can be accurately localized and reproduced by asking the patient to maintain his hand and wrist in dorsiflexion against a resistance provided by the examiner. Similarly, the flexor muscle mass of the forearm originates from the medial epicondyle of the humerus, and a medial epicondylitis may result from repeated stress on these flexor muscles. This is such a frequent problem with adolescent ball players that it is referred to as "Little League elbow."

Pronation and supination of the forearm require full motion of the head of the radius on the capitellum and at the proximal radioulnar joint, as well as full motion at the distal radioulnar joint. Injuries of the head of the radius, which limit this motion, can be diagnosed by grasping the patient's hand as in shaking hands and, with the opposite hand, grasping the back of the forearm. With the elbow bent at 90 degrees, pronate and supinate the forearm with the thumb on the head of the radius. As the head of the radius resolves under the thumb, any irregularities can be felt, and pain may result from the pressure. A displacement of the radial head that has resulted from dislocation may also be detected. Occasionally, congenital or post-traumatic synostosis of the radius and ulna occurs, producing inability to pronate and supinate the arm. In such cases, however, flexion and extension of the forearm are unimpaired. Limitation of motion at the elbow may follow an injury that results in myositis ossificans. In such a case, a well defined bony mass may be palpated in the brachialis muscle in the antecubital space.

A previous injury to the bursa over the tip of the olecranon may cause it to rapidly fill with blood after subsequent slight injuries, or it may become chronically irritated and swollen, a condition often called "miner's elbow."

EXAMINATION OF THE WRIST

The distal radioulnar joint is not a part of the wrist joint, being separated from it by a triangular fibrocartilage. Occasionally, it is partially or completely dislocated as a result of injury, and the head of the ulna can be easily slipped in and out of joint by the examiner. Injuries or degeneration of the triangular fibrocartilage give rise to clicking sounds and pain during pronation and supination.

Motion at the wrist joint itself consists of dorsal and palmar flexion and radial and ulnar deviation. Fractures about the wrist are frequent injuries and result in classical deformities such as Colles' fracture, a transverse fracture of the distal end of the radius in which the radius is shortened. The styloid processes of the radius and of the ulna are then at the same level, instead of exhibiting the normal extension of the radial styloid — approximately a fingerbreadth beyond that of the ulnar styloid. In addition, the articular surface of the radius is tilted dorsally or backward, producing the "silver fork deformity," with local swelling and tenderness. The same deformity can result from a separation of the distal radial epiphysis in a child. The major deformity of a malunited Colles' fracture is prominence of the head of the ulna, which results from shortening of the radius and from radial deviation of the hand. In some fractures of the lower end of the radius, the distal fragment is displaced toward the palm. This occurs in Smith's fracture, in which again there is shortening of the radial styloid process; but since the radial fragment is displaced forward away from the head of the ulna, the head of the ulna becomes very prominent on the back of the wrist.

Fractures and dislocations of the carpal bones are difficult to diagnose either by examination or by x-ray. Pain and limitation of motion at the wrist always occur with dislocation of the lunate forward into the carpal tunnel, and the patient may be unable to actively or passively extend the third and fourth fingers without experiencing pain referred to the wrist. Fractures of the navicular can be diagnosed by palpation of the anatomical snuff box on the radial side of the wrist. The wrist should be in ulnar deviation, which rotates the navicular from behind the radial styloid process. Pain on pressure in this area indicates a fracture. This is an important finding, since x-rays do not always demonstrate such a fracture for several weeks after injury.

De Quervain's disease, a form of stenosing tenosynovitis that involves the tendons of the abductor pollicis longus and the extensor pollicis brevis as they pass through a tunnel on the radial styloid process, is most commonly found in women, often during the postpartum period. Pain and slight swelling of the dorsum of the wrist extend distally along the tendons to their attachment to the thumb. When the patient grasps his thumb with the other fingers of the hand and the fist is forced firmly into ulnar deviation, there may be acute pain at the radial styloid process, a positive Finklestein's test, which is diagnostic of de Quervain's disease. Other forms of acute or chronic tenosynovitis are seen on either the dorsal or palmar surfaces of the wrist and may be suppurative, associated with rheumatoid arthritis, or due to tuberculosis (Fig. 14–18). Frequently, small, firm, slightly movable tumors called "ganglia" are found about the wrist and are associated with the tendon sheaths or the wrist joint. Xanthomas of tendon sheaths may present as soft tissue tumors that move with the tendons as they glide to and fro.

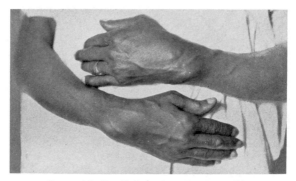

Figure 14–18. Tuberculous tenosynovitis.

EXAMINATION OF THE HAND

The hand, the most interesting area in the physical diagnosis of the extremities, is not only affected by intrinsic diseases and injuries, but it also participates in a wide spectrum of distant and systemic disease processes.

There are a wide variety of congenital malformations of the hand, such as polydactyly, syndactyly, and lobster-claw hand; typical configurations of the hand occur in many genetic abnormalities, such as achondroplasia and lipochondrodystrophy.

Fractures of the metacarpals can be diagnosed by eliciting pain when pushing on the fully extended fingers and by palpating the fracture-deformity on the dorsum of the hand. Fractures of the base of the first metacarpal and of the neck of the fifth metacarpal are usually incurred in fighting. Fracture of the neck of the fifth metacarpal results in a "dropped knuckle" when the fist is clenched, and dislocations of the metacarpophalangeal and interphalangeal joints produce easily interpreted deformities. Avulsion of the long extensor tendon from the base of a distal phalanx results in a "baseball finger" deformity. A "boutonnière deformity" results from a splitting of the extensor hood over the proximal interphalangeal joint.

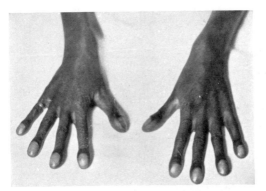

Figure 14–19. *Clubbing of fingers with congenital heart disease.*

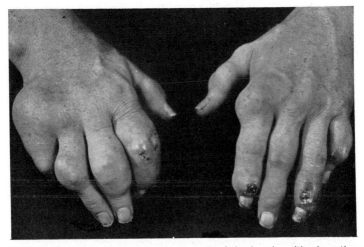

Figure 14–20. *Advanced tophaceous gout of the hands, with ulcerations. (Smith, L. H., Jr.: Disorders of purine metabolism. In Beeson, P. B., and McDermott, W. (eds.): Cecil-Loeb Textbook of Medicine. 13th ed. Philadelphia, W. B. Saunders Co., 1971.)*

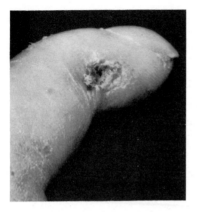

Figure 14–21. *Scleroderma: tightness of the skin, limitation of motion, and ulceration. (Shelley, W. B.: Consultations in Dermatology I. Philadelphia, W. B. Saunders Co., 1972.)*

The intrinsic muscles of the hand are supplied by the ulnar nerve, which also supplies sensation to the medial side of the fourth finger, to all of the fifth finger, and to the medial border of the hand. Atrophy of the intrinsic muscles of the hand can be most easily seen in the space between the thumb and index finger at the first dorsal interosseous muscle. Intrinsic muscle atrophy combined with loss of sensation in the area supplied by the ulnar nerve indicates a peripheral lesion of the ulnar nerve, such as a tardy ulnar palsy. Intrinsic muscle atrophy without sensory loss indicates disease of the central nervous system, such as amyotrophic lateral sclerosis, Charcot-Marie-Tooth progressive peroneal dystrophy, or disuse, as in the later stages of rheumatoid arthritis.

The median nerve supplies the muscles of the thenar eminence of the palm and supplies sensation to the palmar surface of the first, second, third, and the lateral half of the fourth fingers, and to the major portion of the palm. Tingling, numbness, and decreased epicritic sensation in these areas coupled with atrophy of the thenar and hypothenar eminences is usually due to the carpal tunnel syndrome, which results from local pressure on the median nerve at the wrist by the transverse carpal ligament. Fine sensory loss, i.e., light touch or two point discrimination, without corresponding motor loss, may be the earliest sign of nerve compression following injury. This may be caused by chronic synovitis of the flexor tendons, malunited fractures of the wrist, or unreduced dislocations of the wrist. Atrophy of the thenar eminence together with normal sensation is usually the result of poliomyelitis.

None of the muscles that originate in the hand are innervated by the radial nerve. The radial nerve, however, provides sensory fibers to a limited area on the back of the hand at the base of the thumb and second finger.

Fibrosis of the palmar fascia occurs frequently and is usually found at the base of the fourth finger. It may be associated with an increased incidence of stiff or frozen shoulders and chronic myofibrositis. When fibrosis of the palmar fascia is more extensive, it extends across the palm and out into the fourth and occasionally the fifth finger, producing Dupuytren's contracture (Fig. 14–22).

Although stenosing tenosynovitis can occur in any of the flexor tendon sheaths, the thumb is usually involved, being flexed at the interphalangeal joint, and cannot be extended at all or only with a click or snap, i.e., "trigger thumb." A small palpable mass can usually be felt in the flexor tendon at the base of the thumb. It is more common in infants than in children and adults. Stenosing tenosynovitis of the fourth finger is a common ailment of female typists and is associated with wearing a ring on this finger. The finger clicks and locks on extension and flexion, and again a small palpable nodule is usually felt in the superficial flexor in the palm at the base of the finger.

Rheumatoid arthritis results in fusiform swelling of the interphalangeal joints during the acute phase of the disease (Fig. 14–23). Later, as joint destruction occurs in the hand and wrist, a characteristic "flipper" deformity occurs, the hand in ulnar deviation and fingers flexed at the metacarpophalangeal joints (Fig. 14–24). This deformity can be prevented by proper management of the disease.

Heberden's nodes, which are hard, bony nodules at the dis-

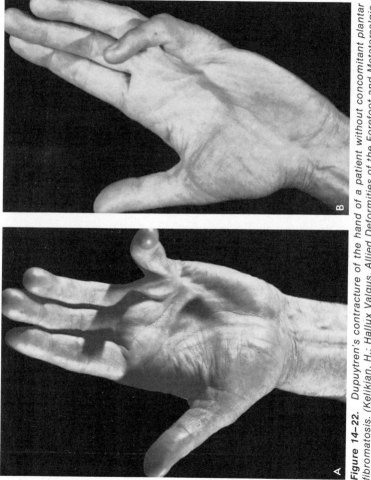

Figure 14–22. Dupuytren's contracture of the hand of a patient without concomitant plantar fibromatosis. (Kelikian, H.: Hallux Valgus, Allied Deformities of the Forefoot and Metatarsalgia. Philadelphia, W. B. Saunders Co., 1965.)

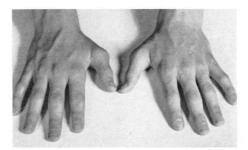

Figure 14-23. *Fusiform swelling of fingers in rheumatoid arthritis, sometimes called Haygarth's nodosities.*

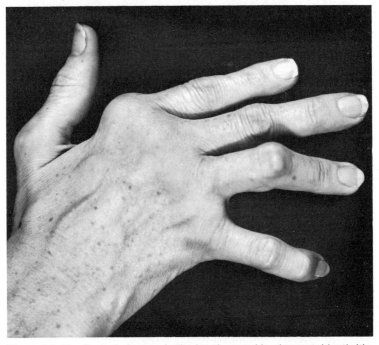

Figure 14-24. *Typical changes in the hand caused by rheumatoid arthritis. (Gartland, J. J.: Fundamentals of Orthopaedics. 2nd ed. Philadelphia, W. B. Saunders Co., 1975.)*

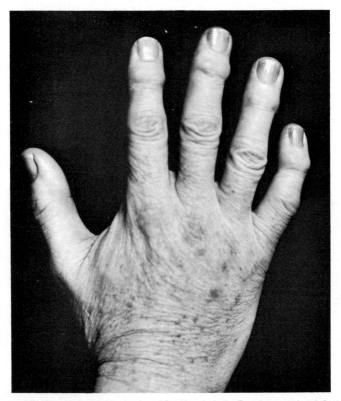

Figure 14–25. Heberden's nodes. (Gartland, J. J.: Fundamentals of Orthopaedics. 2nd ed. Philadelphia, W. B. Saunders Co., 1975.)

tal ends of the middle phalanges, are seen frequently in women and are probably hereditary (Fig. 14–25). Care must be taken when inspecting the hands to look for Osler's nodes, which are tender, reddish bumps that are a sign of embolic lesions in subacute bacterial endocarditis. Splinter hemorrhages at the tip of the nail bed are likewise a sign of this disease (see Fig. 9–67).

Spider nevi occur commonly on the backs of the hands in cirrhosis of the liver, and other telangiectatic lesions frequently are evident on the hands (see Fig. 11–7).

EXAMINATION OF THE HIP AND LOWER EXTREMITIES

Measurement of leg length, a basic procedure in examination of the lower extremities, should be made from the anterior superior spine of the ilium to the tip of the medial malleolus with the patient supine on an examining table. Differences in leg length of 1/4 in. or less are considered normal. If the legs differ by more than 1/4 in., the examiner must decide which leg is normal and which abnormal. Note that the primary concern is with relative length, not absolute length. Shortening may be related to residual paralysis from poliomyelitis, to spastic hemiplegia of cerebral palsy, to malunited fractures and epiphysial injuries, or to any of a number of other factors. Lengthening may result from congenital arteriovenous fistuls, congenital lymphangiomatosis, or simple congenital hypertrophy. Occasionally, it is difficult to determine which leg, the long or short, is abnormal, and why.

THE HIP

Hip motion involves flexion-extension, abduction-adduction, and internal-external rotation (Fig. 14–26). For measurement of the first two, examine the patient while he is supine on a firm examining table. Ask the patient to pull one knee against his abdomen and chest so as to fix his pelvis. With the patient in this position, the thigh of the other leg should lie flat on the table. If a flexion contracture is present, the thigh will not lie flat but will pull up into flexion as the opposite knee and hip are fully flexed and pulled onto the chest and abdomen (Thomas

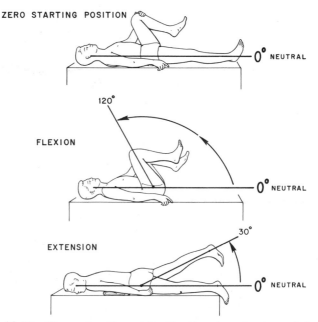

Figure 14–26. *Range of motion of the hip. (American Academy of Orthopaedic Surgeons: Measuring and Recording of Joint Motion. Everett, Massachusetts, Glenwood Press, 1963.)*

Illustration continued on opposite page.

test, Fig. 14–27). Measure the range of hip motion while the patient is in position with his pelvis firmly fixed (Fig. 14–28). Note also that in such a patient, when he is supine with both thighs flat on the table, you can pass your hand easily under his back, indicating an abnormal degree of lordosis.

Rotation of the hip is measured most accurately when the patient is prone, with knees flexed at a right angle. The feet are then separated (internal rotation) and brought together and crossed (external rotation). With the legs acting as a pointer on

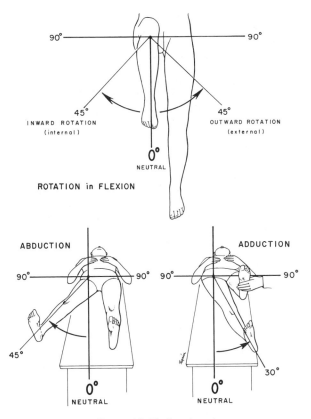

Figure 14–26. *Continued*

an imaginary protractor, the range of rotation can be easily estimated. When the patient's condition will not permit this maneuver, rotation can be estimated with the patient supine. The hip and knee are flexed to a right angle, and the leg is used to internally and externally rotate the hip.

In a few children, examination demonstrates a normal total range of rotation, but it is made up of excess internal rotation

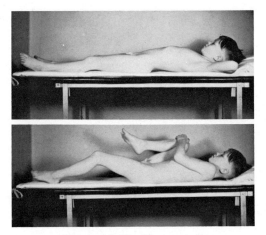

Figure 14–27. Thomas test.

LIMITED MOTION in FLEXION

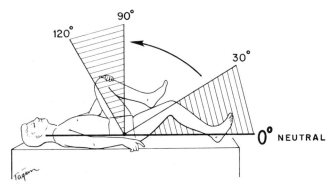

Figure 14–28. Test for hip flexion contracture. (American Academy of Orthopaedic Surgeons: Measuring and Recording of Joint Motion. Everett, Massachusetts, Glenwood Press, 1963.)

and decreased external rotation. Such children "toe in" when walking and may have had congenital dislocations of the hip, in which the femoral neck joins the shaft at a greater than normal angle of rotation and is said to be "anteverted." Similar findings may result from malunited fractures of the femur that heal with rotary displacement.

Congenital dislocation of the hip on one or both sides occurs most commonly in girls and may be associated with other congenital deformities. To examine for this deformity, place the child supine and observe the skin wrinkles in the groin and on the medial aspect of the thighs. Then, holding the legs together, flex the hips to a right angle and observe the skin wrinkles on the buttocks and thighs. Asymmetry of the skin wrinkles usually accompanies unilateral dislocation of the hip. In bilateral dislocations, the skin wrinkles are asymmetrical on both sides, and the perineum is widened. Next, flex the hips and knees to a right angle and press downward against the examining table. In unilateral dislocation, the dislocated hip lies further posteriorly, the thigh appears shorter, and the knees are not quite at the same level. When the leg is pulled forward against the counter pressure of the examiner's hand on the ilium, a click may be noticed as the head of the femur clears the posterior rim of the acetabulum (Ortolani's sign). Finally, separate the thighs while pressing downward and outward into abduction. Limitation of abduction is one of the most constant findings in congenital dislocation of the hip. X-rays of the pelvis should be made in any patient in whom the physical findings suggest congenital dislocation of a hip.

Hip disease in childhood usually becomes evident because of a limp. Pain arising in the hip is commonly referred to the knee; therefore, any child complaining of knee pain must have a careful examination of the knee and the hip. Measurable atrophy of the thigh muscles is a constant accompaniment of chronic hip disease. Flexion contracture and limitation of rotation are the most frequent findings in Legg-Perthes disease and in tuberculosis of the hip. In adolescents, chronic hip disease is usually associated with a slipped proximal epiphysis and is char-

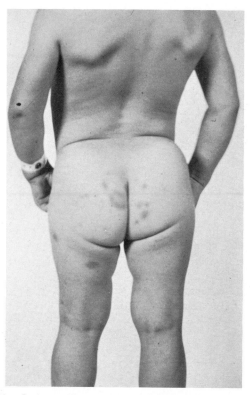

Figure 14–29. *Patient with congenital hip dislocation showing the asymmetry of skin wrinkles.*

acterized by external rotation deformity and complete loss of internal rotation of the hip.

Fractures of the hip occur most frequently in the aged. When the fracture is displaced, the leg lies in external rotation with slight shortening. Displaced and undisplaced fractures of the hip may also be diagnosed by auscultation. Place the stethoscope on the symphysis pubis and tap the patella lightly with a finger. On the intact side, the sound is carried up the femur, across the hip joint to the symphysis without interruption. If there is an intervening fracture or dislocation, however, the transmission of sound is less efficient, and the sound is diminished.

Posterior dislocations of the hip are common automotive injuries. There is usually evidence of direct injury to the knee, e.g., abrasion, lacerations, or even fractures of the patella, and the thigh lies in internal rotation, adduction, and some flexion. There is always measurable shortening. Since the sciatic nerve, particularly its peroneal portion, is often injured by the dis-

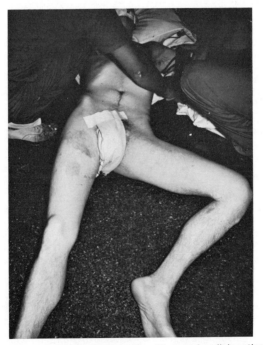

Figure 14–30. *Position of extremity with anterior dislocation of hip.*

placed head of the femur, sensory and motor function in the entire leg must be carefully evaluated. Anterior dislocations of the hip are rare and are distinguished by external rotation, abduction, and apparent lengthening of the extremity (Fig. 14–30).

Acute suppurative arthritis of the hip is an acute febrile disease accompanied by chills, inguinal adenopathy, and severe pain. Motion of the hip is quite limited and painful. Pain anterior to the hip in the groin may be associated with inguinal or femoral hernias. Pain behind the hip may be due to a bursitis over the ischial tuberosity (weaver's bottom). Bursitis, more frequent over the greater trochanter than in the shoulder,

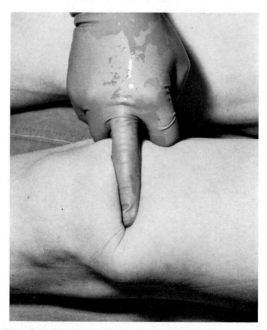

Figure 14–31. *Quadriceps tendon rupture. Note that the finger can easily be indented above the patella because of detachment of the tendon.*

causes pain that radiates down over the lateral aspect of the thigh to the knee. This pain is aggravated by internal rotation and adduction. Tenderness is easily localized by palpation at the top of the greater trochanter.

Tears of the large thigh muscles occur in athletes as a result of maximum effort or injury. The biceps femoris may be avulsed from the ischial tuberosity, the rectus femoris from the anterior superior spine. Contraction of the injured muscle is accompanied by a "balling up" of the free end of the muscle. Hard masses that develop in the muscle mass of the quadriceps after direct injuries are usually myositis ossificans. In the elderly, the quadriceps may occasionally be avulsed from its insertion into the top of the patella. In such a case the examining finger encounters no resistance to palpation immediately above the patella (Fig. 14–31) and the patient may be unable to actively extend his knee.

THE KNEE

The knee joint moves essentially as a simple hinge, the patella gliding over the femoral condyles as the joint is extended and flexed. It is the largest joint in the body, the suprapatellar pouch extending at least four fingerbreadths above the top of the patella. The joint is provided with medial and lateral collateral ligaments and cruciate ligaments to maintain stability. Since the patella is readily palpable, displaced fractures can be easily felt, and those that are undisplaced can be suspected because of local tenderness to palpation. Dislocations of the patella are readily diagnosed by the abnormal position of the bone, which is almost always displaced laterally. Recurrent dislocation is related to congenital maldevelopment wherein the patella is small and thickened and rides higher over the femoral condyles than is normal. The patella is very mobile, can sometimes be dislocated, and is usually associated with a knock-knee deformity.

The site of insertion of the patellar tendon into the tibial tuberosity is a frequent location of pain and swelling in adolescents. The pain is caused by mechanical stress at the insertion of

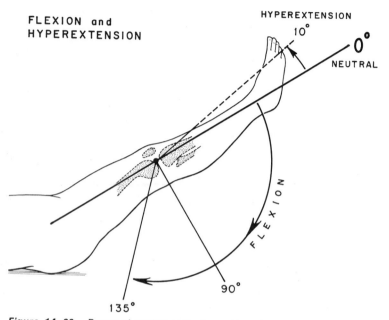

Figure 14–32. Range of motion of the knee. (American Academy of Orthopaedic Surgeons: Measuring and Recording of Joint Motion. Everett, Massachusetts, Glenwood Press, 1963.)

the powerful quadriceps muscle group, and the condition is termed Osgood-Schlatter disease. In adults, a bony prominence at the tibial tubercle may be residual evidence of this disease. One bursa lies behind the patellar tendon, and it may become swollen and painful. Another, the prepatellar bursa, lies between the skin and outer bony surface of the patella. A collection of fluid in this bursa can be differentiated from an effusion into the knee joint by its location and by its circumscribed extent.

Softening of the articular cartilage, chondromalacia, on the under surface of the patella or osteochondral fractures may result in a grinding or grating as the patella moves over the femoral condyles. This can be appreciated by holding the palm of the hand over the patella as the knee is moved. A lesser degree of chondromalacia can be detected by applying gentle pressure with the length of the examiner's index finger above the upper pole of the patella while the patient either actively

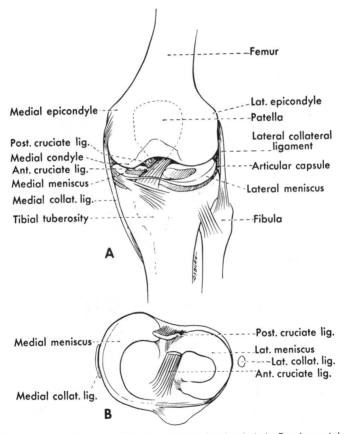

Figure 14–33. Anatomy of the knee joint. (Gartland, J. J.: Fundamentals of Orthopaedics. 2nd ed. Philadelphia, W. B. Saunders Co., 1975.)

contracts his quadriceps (if his knee is extended) or actively extends his flexed knee. A positive test is accompanied by accentuation of pain in the knee (Brittain's test). A clicking or grating just above the tip of the patella may be caused by a suprapatellar plica.

The amount of bowleg (genu varum) or knock-knee (genu valgum) (Figs. 14–34 and 14–35) is determined by inspecting both knees in full extension. Some degree of knock-knee is nor-

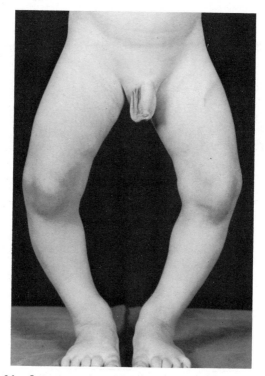

Figure 14–34. *Genu varum in a child of 1½ years. (Tachdjian, M. O.: Pediatric Orthopedics. Philadelphia, W. B. Saunders Co., 1972.)*

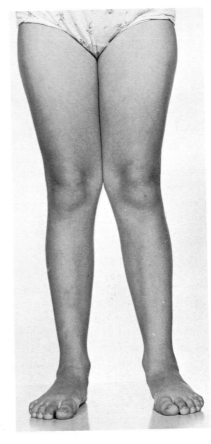

Figure 14–35. *Genu valgum in a young girl. (Tachdjian, M. O.: Pediatric Orthopedics. Philadelphia, W. B. Saunders Co., 1972.)*

mal in girls. Unilateral deformities may be due to injury or epiphyseal disease. In some patients the knee can be hyperextended; this "back knee" is usually the result of generalized hyperflexibility, but may be caused by a tight heel cord in association with an equinus deformity of the foot.

Pain in the knee is a common symptom and, as previously noted, it may be due to hip disease. Quadriceps atrophy constantly accompanies disease or injury to the knee. Locking or catching may result from a loose body, which either the patient or the examiner may be able to locate by palpation, or from tears of the menisci. An x-ray will usually indicate the source of the loose body.

The knee is frequently injured in sports. Since the semilunar cartilages, or menisci, are attached to the joint capsule along the joint line, tenderness to palpation along the joint margin suggests a tear of the menisci. The anterior horns of the menisci can be palpated on either side of the patellar tendon at the joint line in front. Local tenderness to palpation here may indicate a torn meniscus, especially if the prepatellar fat pad or the bursa behind the patellar tendon are not swollen and painful. An inability to completely extend and flex the knee, and pain on forced extension of the knee, may also indicate a torn and displaced meniscus.

Instability, or an abnormal increase in the range of motion of the knee, indicates a tear of one of the ligaments. Test the medial collateral ligament by forcibly abducting the knee (valgus strain) while the knee is in about 15 degrees flexion. Test the anterior cruciate ligament by a similar maneuver when the knee is in full extension. To evaluate the lateral collateral ligament, apply an adduction strain (varus strain) to the knee while the knee is in complete extension. To test the cruciate ligament, bend the knee to 90 degrees and first pull forward and then push backward on the upper end of the tibia. If the tibia can be pulled forward, the anterior cruciate is injured; if it can be pushed backward, the posterior ligament is damaged.

With the knee and ankle both at right angles, the foot should be in line with the thigh. With torsional, or twisting, deformities of the tibia, the foot may be turned in or out, and the patient will toe in or out as he walks. External tibial torsion is common in hyperflexible children with knock knees, everted ankles, and pronated feet. Internal tibial torsion occurs alone, resulting in bowlegs, or in association with clubfeet. The evaluation of tibial torsion should include examination of the hips for anteversion deformities.

THE LEG

Asymmetrical calf atrophy may be due to residuals of poliomyelitis, to the spastic hemiparesis of cerebral palsy, or to an old clubfoot deformity. Symmetrical calf atrophy, i.e., stork leg, especially if associated with a high arched foot, strongly suggests Charcot-Marie-Tooth progressive peroneal muscular dystrophy (Fig. 14–36). This diagnosis can be confirmed by finding atrophy of the first dorsal interosseous muscles of the hands. Observation of the patient or relatives may reveal a similar abnormality.

Symmetrical hypertrophy of the calf muscles in a child indicates progressive muscular dystrophy of the pseudohypertrophic type, the calf muscles possessing a characteristic doughy consistency on palpation. Such patients may be unable to stand from a seated position on the floor without help or without propping their arms on their legs and thighs as they stand (Gower's sign).

Rupture of the plantaris tendon in the back of the calf is caused by sudden forcible dorsiflexion of the foot against resistance. Pain is localized to the lateral side of the calf at the junction of the upper and middle thirds of the leg. Rupture of the Achilles tendon can be easily diagnosed by palpation of the defect in the tendon and by noting the lack of active plantar flexion. A large bursa that separates the Achilles tendon from the back of the ankle joint may become inflamed. Such Achilles tendinitis or bursitis is accompanied by pain, limitation of ankle motion, and local swelling along both sides of the tendon. There may be local crepitation on palpation or movement. Tendinitis of other tendons about the ankle also occurs and can usually be easily identified. No examination of the leg is complete without palpation of the pulse at the inguinal ligament (femoral artery), in the back of the knee (popliteal artery), behind the medial

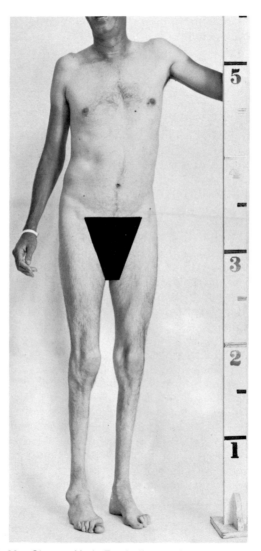

Figure 14–36. Charcot-Marie-Tooth disease showing muscle atrophy.

malleolus (posterior tibial artery), and on the dorsum of the foot (dorsalis pedis artery).

ANKLE AND FOOT

Although normal ankle movement is associated with a considerable degree of rotation, ankle motion is considered to take place in only one plane, as simple dorsiflexion-plantar flexion. Inversion and eversion of the foot takes place at the subastragalar joints. Limitation of dorsiflexion at the ankle joint is almost always caused by a tight heel cord or Achilles tendon. Loss of subastragalar joint motion regularly complicates fractures of the os calcis with destruction of the articular surfaces of this joint. Occasionally, as a result of failure of normal development, some of the tarsal bones remain bound together by bony bridges. This condition, called "tarsal coalition," ordinarily produces no difficulty until early adolescence, when the patient presents with a painful pronated foot associated with painful spasm of the peroneal muscles, i.e., peroneal spastic flatfoot.

Occasionally, anomalous bones of the foot are evident on x-ray examination. The only one of importance in physical examination of the foot is the accessory navicular, which presents as a mass on the medial side of the foot, below and distal to the ankle joint. It can be readily identified because the tibialis posterior tendon attaches to it. Small firm tumors about the dorsum of the foot and ankle are usually ganglia and are similar to those that occur around the wrist. Synoviomas are occasionally found about the foot and ankle. Hard calluses on the back of the heel are "pump bumps" and result from the irritation of ill-fitting shoes. Do not overlook "surfer's knots," hard granulomas that appear on the dorsum of the foot and in front of the ankle in surfing enthusiasts.

Ankle sprains are a common injury of daily activity. After such an injury there may be considerable local swelling and ecchymoses. The injured ligament can usually be located, first by careful palpation, and then by carefully applying stress to the

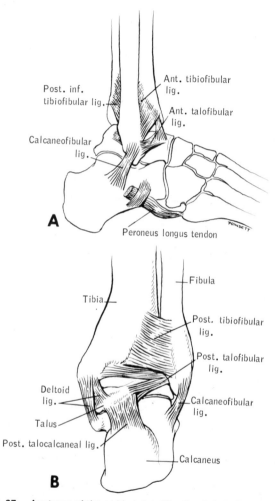

Figure 14–37. Anatomy of the ankle joint. (Gartland, J. J.: Fundamentals of Orthopaedics. 2nd ed. Philadelphia, W. B. Saunders Co., 1975.)

ankle at the extremes of its normal range of motion. As stress is applied to an injured ligament, pain is produced. If the ligament has been completely torn, the range of motion is greater than normal, and the ankle can be partially dislocated or subluxated. Such subluxations are most easily demonstrated in old injuries when the acute pain and swelling have subsided and protective muscle spasm is absent.

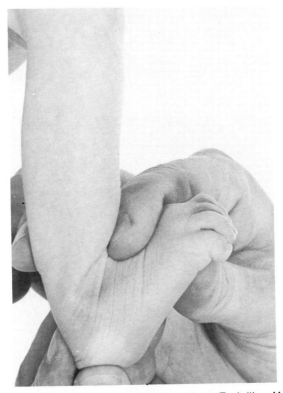

Figure 14–38. *Talipes calcaneovalgus in an infant. (Tachdjian, M. O.: Pediatric Orthopedics. Philadelphia, W. B. Saunders Co., 1972.)*

Dislocations and displaced fractures of the ankle and foot produce obvious deformities. Undisplaced fractures of the ankle should be suspected when there is local tenderness to palpation of bony structures. Since the distal ends of the tibia and fibula are subcutaneous, physical examination provides an accurate diagnosis in most cases. Fractures of the os calcis result in shortening and widening of the heel.

Talipes calcaneovalgus, a congenital deformity seen in infants, is marked by eversion and dorsiflexion of the foot, the dorsum of the foot touching the anterolateral aspect of the tibia (Fig. 14–38). The classic congenital clubfoot, talipes equinovarus (Figs. 14–39 and 14–40), is characterized by four components: metatarsus varus, i.e., adduction of the forefoot; inversion of the foot; a shortened Achilles tendon with an accompanying plantar

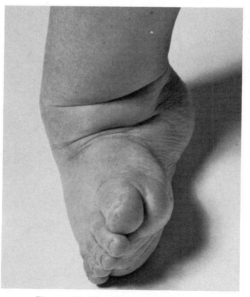

Figure 14–39. Clubfoot deformity.

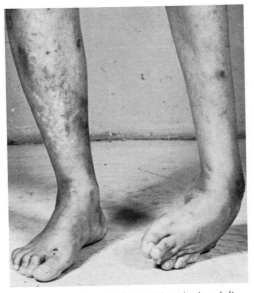

Figure 14-40. *Clubfoot deformity in adult.*

flexion contracture; and internal tibial torsion. Any patient with a congenital foot deformity must be carefully examined for congenital dislocation of the hips and for spina bifida, as well as other congenital anomalies. Internal tibial torsion and metatarsus varus may appear as single deformities. Occasionally only the first metatarsal is adducted, a condition called "metatarsus primus varus." This predisposes to foot difficulties in adults.

Pes cavus, or a high arched foot, occurring on one side is usually due to residual weakness of the calf muscle following poliomyelitis (Fig. 14–41). When such a condition occurs, the os calcis becomes almost vertical and the patient bears weight on the end rather than on the bottom of the heel. Bilateral pes cavus with atrophy of the calf suggests Charcot-Marie-Tooth disease. The characteristic foot deformity in Friedreich's ataxia is shown in Figure 14–42.

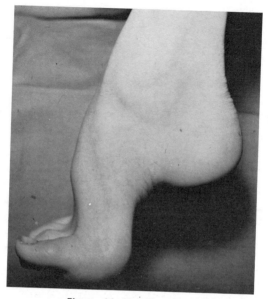

Figure 14–41. *Pes cavus.*

At birth the foot is fat and flat. As the child grows, the foot thins out and the muscles that support the arch develop. The normal arch appears in early childhood. In a hyperflexible child, the foot appears to be normal until the child stands and the foot bears weight. Then the flexible foot rolls out into pronation and eversion. By adulthood this may have become a flat or pronated foot (pes planus, Fig. 14–43). A rigid, painful foot that accompanies marked spasm of the leg muscles should make the examiner think of peroneal spastic flatfoot, an entirely different problem.

A bunion is a chronic bursitis over the medial aspect of the distal end of the first metatarsal. The cause of the bursitis is almost always an adduction deformity of the first metatarsal (metatarsus primus varus), an exostosis on the dorsum or medial

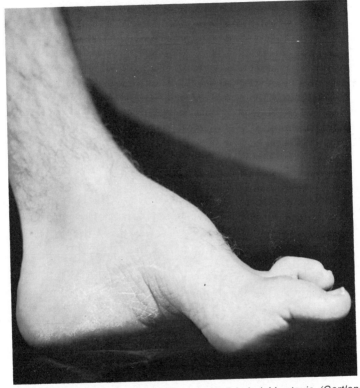

Figure 14–42. Foot deformity in patient with Friedreich's ataxia. (Gartland, J. J.: Fundamentals of Orthopaedics. 2nd ed. Philadelphia, W. B. Saunders Co., 1975.)

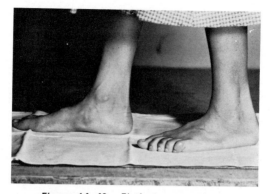

Figure 14–43. Flatfeet, or pes planus.

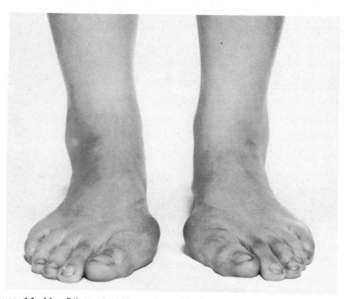

Figure 14–44. Bilateral hallux valgus (Tachdjian, M. O.: Pediatric Orthopedics. Philadelphia, W. B. Saunders Co., 1972.)

side of the head of the metatarsal, and a lateral deviation of the first toe—i.e., hallux valgus (Fig. 14–44). This is often accompanied by hammer toes, in which the metatarsal phalangeal joints are extended and the proximal interphalangeal joints are flexed. A callus or corn will form over the proximal interphalangeal joint. If the first metatarsal phalangeal joint becomes stiff as the result of arthrosis or injury, it is called hallux rigidus.

A bunionette is a small painful bursa over the lateral aspect of the head of the fifth metatarsal. It is called a "tailor's bunion" because it can be caused by irritation of the lateral side of the foot from sitting cross-legged. Podagra, an inflammation of the first metatarsal phalangeal joint, is due to acute gout. When such occurs, inspection of the ears may reveal the tophi of gout, confirming the diagnosis.

COMMON CLINICAL TERMS

Ankylosis—Abnormal immobility of a joint.

Contracture—Reduction in the range of motion of a joint, the result of scarring of soft tissue surrounding the joint.

Crepitation—A grinding sound and palpable sensation elicited when fragments of bone move against each other or when roughened joint surfaces move upon each other.

Kyphosis—Abnormal dorsal curvature of the vertebral column.

Lordosis—Abnormal anterior curvature of the vertebral column.

Subluxation—Displacement of articulating surfaces of a joint, short of complete dislocation.

Scoliosis—Abnormal lateral curvature of the vertebral column.

Valgus and varus—Terms used to describe the relationship of the distal portion of a limb to the proximal portion in reference to the midline. In *hallux valgus* the great toe is deviated *away* from the midline at the first metatarsal phalangeal joint. In *cubitus varus* the forearm is deviated *toward* the midline at the elbow joint. Bowleg (*genu varum*) and knock-knee (*genu valgum*) are self-explanatory.

COMMON CLINICAL SYNDROMES

Battered-child syndrome—These children are seen in the emergency room because of a history of a fresh injury. The patient is said to have fallen out of bed or the history may be conflicting and obscure. Examination reveals contusions in varying stages of resolution and x-rays may show fractures of ribs, clavicles, long bones, or the skull in various stages of healing. These injuries may have been inflicted by one or both parents, baby sitter, or other siblings.

Charcot-Marie-Tooth disease (progressive peroneal muscular dystrophy)—A hereditary neuromuscular disease transmitted as an autosomal dominant. The patient is first seen as a child because of a high arched foot and later because of difficulty in walking because of muscle weakness in the peronei and calf muscles. With progressive atrophy of the muscles below the knee the patient develops a "stork leg" deformity. This condition is associated with atrophy of the intrinsic muscles of the hands. The patient almost always has a family history of this condition.

Hemophiliac arthropathy—The bleeding tendency in hemophilia commonly manifests itself in repeated hemorrhages into the major joints, the knee, the hip, the elbow, and the shoulder. As a result of the pain, and the immobilization required for treatment, muscle atrophy and joint stiffness result. Almost every adult hemophiliac has physical impairment due to involvement of one or more of the joints.

Hysterical contractures—These are deformities caused by the continuous contraction of various muscle groups. Hysterical torticollis, hysterical clubfoot, and hysterical upper extremity contractures are the most frequent. They are manifestations of a conversion reaction. When long-standing, they may be accompanied by skin and muscle atrophy and disuse osteoporosis. In the lower extremities dependent edema may be severe.

Neuropathic joints of diabetics—The peripheral neuritis associated with severe diabetes may result in a neuropathic joint. There is gross destruction of the joint with collapse of bony and articular structures. In contrast to the neuropathic joints seen in *tabes dorsalis*—usually the knee, ankle, spine and hips—the joints most frequently involved with diabetic neuropathy are the first metatarsal phalangeal joint and the tarsal joints.

Sudeck's post-traumatic sympathetic dystrophy (Paul H. M. Sudeck, 1866–1938)—A painful condition which appears several weeks after a minor injury to the hand and forearm or to the foot and leg. The extremity is very painful, cool, and moist. The skin appears shiny and there is atrophy of the nails and hair. After the condition has been present for some time, x-rays may reveal extensive demineralization of the bone. This condition is related to causalgia and the shoulder-hand syndrome.

Volkmann's ischemic contracture (Richard von Volkmann, 1830–1889)—A claw hand deformity with partial or complete paralysis and fibrosis of muscles in the forearm and hand supplied by the median and ulnar nerves. There may be, also, partial sensory loss in areas supplied by these nerves. The condition almost always follows an episode of acute circulatory deprivation of the forearm associated with a supracondylar fracture of the humerus in childhood.

BIBLIOGRAPHY

Gartland, J. J.: Fundamentals of Orthopaedics. 2nd ed. Philadelphia, W. B. Saunders Co., 1975.

Howorth, M. B.: Textbook of Orthopedics. Philadelphia, W. B. Saunders Co., 1952.

Kelikian, H.: Hallux Valgus, Allied Deformities of the Forefoot and Metatarsalgia. Philadelphia, W. B. Saunders Co., 1965.

Litton, L. O., and Peltier, L. F.: Athletic Injuries. London, J. & A. Churchill, 1963.

15
EXAMINATION OF THE ENDOCRINE SYSTEM

The various manifestations of endocrine dysfunction may result from either deficiency or overproduction of a hormone. The methods of physical diagnosis are especially applicable to the diagnosis of endocrine dysfunctions, since physical changes induced by hormone abnormalities often precede the development of abnormal laboratory tests. Alteration in body contour, size, fat distribution, pigmentation, skin texture, circulation, and the general functional level of the nervous system may result from endocrine disease; however, these changes must be differentiated from those established by the individual's hereditary pattern, which may simulate classic endocrine syndromes.

THE THYROID GLAND

Question your patient regarding any change in weight, intolerance to temperature variation, or in bowel habits; also look for tremulousness, palpitation, torpidity, or insomnia.

Inspection, palpation, percussion, and auscultation are all applicable during examination. Generalized or local enlargements of the thyroid gland may be detected by inspection of the neck during swallowing, with the patient viewed from the side in

700

front of a light source. The term "goiter" is applied to any visible enlargement of the gland. Palpation of the thyroid is described in Chapter 5, Examination of the Head and Neck. Estimation of the size of the gland by palpation may vary by as much as 50 per cent. Enlargements of the gland are either uninodular, multinodular, or diffuse. Percussion is useful in detecting substernal goiter, since widened mediastinal dullness may be evident. Auscultation of the gland may reveal, in thyrotoxicosis, a bruit coincident with the arterial pulsation which persists when pressure is exerted on the stethoscope. This is in contrast to a venous hum in the neck which will usually disappear upon pressure. No attempt should be made to assess the status of thyroid function

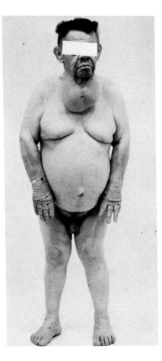

Figure 15–1. Cretin.

from the physical examination of the gland except for the presence of a bruit, which usually indicates the thyrotoxic state.

Hypofunction of the thyroid. Hypofunction may result from congenital absence of the gland, inborn errors in synthesis of thyroid hormone, Hashimoto's thyroiditis, malignancy, surgery, drugs, or unknown causes.

When thyroid function is deficient from birth, cretinism, which is characterized by mental deficiency and retardation in growth and development, ensues. The child retains infantile body proportions marked by a large head and short extremities, in addition to all of the features of adult hypothyroidism (Figs. 15–1 and 15–2).

Hypothyroidism appearing in the adult is characterized by the development of myxedema. Practically every system of the

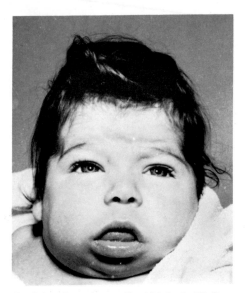

Figure 15–2. Cretinism in a six month old infant. (Di George, A. M.: Disorders of the thyroid gland. In Vaughan, V. C., III, and McKay, R. J.: Nelson Textbook of Pediatrics. 10th ed. Philadelphia, W. B. Saunders Co., 1975.)

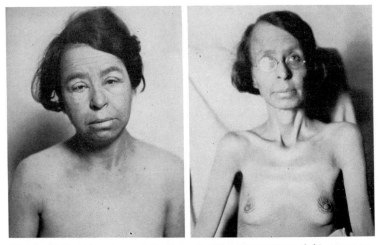

Figure 15–3. *Myxedema: left, characteristic appearance; right, same patient after three months of thyroid medication.*

body is affected by a generalized retardation in function. The subcutaneous structures become infiltrated with myxedematous material which, when present about the eyes, gives rise to the typical myxedematous facies. This is characterized by a look of extreme lethargy with accompanying periorbital edema, giving the eyes the appearance of having an epicanthal fold (Fig. 15–3). Loss of hair from the lateral portion of the eyebrows accentuates the facial appearance. The dulling of intellect is accompanied by a slowing and thickening of the speech which is further intensified by enlargement of the tongue. The lethargy may progress into a true coma that is characterized by a striking hypothermia. The hair becomes coarse and the skin dry and sallow, accentuated by a consistent anemia. The abdomen is protuberant and may show ascites. Some weight gain is noted, but extreme obesity is rarely seen in myxedema. The deep tendon reflexes, best examined at the biceps and ankle, are retarded both in contraction and recovery time. Characteristically, the patient develops an intolerance to cold. Both cretinism and myxedema may occur either with or without goiter.

Hyperfunction of the thyroid. The manifestations of hyperthyroidism are in many respects the opposite of those of myxedema. Increased heat production produces sweating, poor heat tolerance, and increased circulatory rate. The latter, manifested by tachycardia and widening of the pulse pressure, constitutes one of the prime features of hyperthyroidism and may be sufficient to produce peripheral capillary pulse, bruits over the large arteries, and hemodynamic cardiac murmurs, especially over the pulmonic area. Tachycardia during sleep is particularly characteristic of this state. Cardiac arrhythmias, especially atrial fibrillation, are common. The finding of a warm, moist palm constitutes one of the best points for differentiating hyperthyroidism from anxiety states, in which a cold, moist palm is found. Involvement of the nervous system is signaled by a fine tremor, a shortening of the contraction and relaxation phases of the deep tendon reflexes, and complaints of nervous irritability and inability to sleep. Muscular weakness is most evident in the quadriceps muscles and may progress to an actual thyrotoxic myopathy. Contraction of the levator palpebrae muscle produces retraction of the eyelid and widening of the palpebral fissure, giving the appearance of a "bright-eyed" state (Fig. 15–4). Other less common manifestations include generalized pruritus, retraction of the nail bed (onycholysis), generalized brown pigmentation, and lymphadenopathy.

Hyperthyroidism may occur as the result of a functioning adenoma, as a result of overmedication with thyroid preparations, or, most commonly, as a part of the constellation of Graves' disease, or exophthalmic goiter. In Graves' disease, in addition to hyperthyroidism, a diffuse goiter forms and infiltrative ophthalmopathy develops. Goiter formation is quite variable and in no way correlates with the degree of disturbed thyroid function. Multinodularity of the goiter appears in longstanding disease. The infiltrative ophthalmopathy does not correlate well with the degree of hyperthyroidism. A proptosis of 5 to 10 mm. above normal is measurable with the exophthalmo-

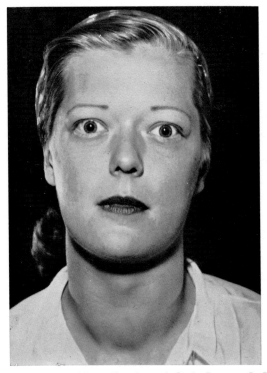

Figure 15–4. *Hyperthyroidism. (Stanbury, J. B., in Beeson, P. B., and Mc-Dermott, W. (eds.): Cecil-Loeb Textbook of Medicine. 11th ed. Philadelphia, W. B. Saunders Co., 1963.)*

meter and is often asymmetrical and frequently becomes more severe following treatment of the hyperthyroidism. In addition to protrusion of the eyes, there is often infiltration of the periorbital tissues, ulceration of the cornea, and the development of ophthalmoplegia. Failure of convergence (Moebius' sign), lid lag (von Graefe's sign), and failure to wrinkle the forehead on upward gaze (Joffroy's sign) bring out these weaknesses of the

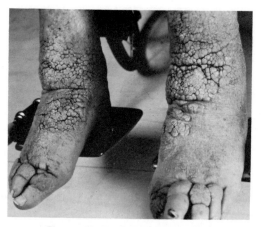

Figure 15–5. Pretibial myxedema.

ocular muscles. Pretibial myxedema, often seen in exophthalmic goiter, is characterized by subcutaneous thickening and the development of violaceous, raised, dry, nonpruritic lesions on the legs (Fig. 15–5). This syndrome is often associated with the presence in the serum of the long-acting thyroid stimulator. While hyperthyroidism and exophthalmic goiter frequently occur together, the spectrum of the disease is quite varied and either one may appear in the absence of the other.

THE PARATHYROID GLANDS

Patients with suspected parathyroid disease should be questioned with regard to muscle spasm or weakness, epigastric distress, excessive urination, and skeletal pain. Examination of the neck rarely reveals evidence of parathyroid enlargement. Hypoparathyroidism may be manifested by tetany, cataracts, and involvement of the central nervous system. Fully developed tetany is distinguished by a generalized increase in muscle tone and is particularly evidenced by carpopedal spasm with drawing of the fingers into the position of the obstetrician's hand, or main d'accoucheur (Fig. 15–6). Laryngospasm may give rise to stridor and embarrassment of respiration. Subclinical tetany may be detected by a twitching of the corner of the mouth on tapping the area over the mandibular joint (Chvostek's sign) or by the production of carpal spasm upon application of a tourniquet to the upper arm (Trousseau's sign). Papilledema may appear rarely. Involvement of the central nervous system may result in a coarse tremor that is referable to dysfunction of the basal ganglia.

Congenital hypoparathyroidism is characterized by short stature and rounding of the facies. A shortening of the fourth metacarpal is noted, giving rise to the "knuckle-knuckle-dimple-knuckle" sign. Moniliasis of the nail beds and Addison's disease may be found in association with the spontaneous forms of hypoparathyroidism.

Hyperparathyroidism is less likely to be accompanied by physical manifestations. When present, these physical manifestations include hypercalcemic encephalopathy, peptic ulcer, recurrent pancreatitis with abdominal pain, renal calculus forma-

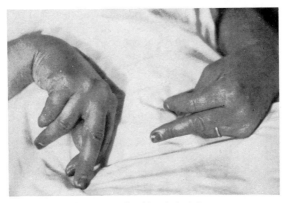

Figure 15–6. Hands in tetany.

tion, polyuria, bone pain, and deposition of calcium in the conjunctiva. Hypercalcemic encephalopathy is characterized by lethargy, disorientation, toxic psychosis, and a myriad of focal neurological deficiencies. The polyuria may give rise to a picture not unlike diabetes insipidus in that it is resistant to antidiuretic hormone. Band keratopathy, a cloudiness appearing about the margin of the cornea, occurs with prolonged hypercalcemia.

THE ADRENAL CORTEX

Weakness and abdominal pain are cardinal symptoms of adrenal disease. Physically, particular note should be made of pigmentation, texture of the skin and subcutaneous tissues, fat distribution, and postural changes in the blood pressure.

Abnormalities of adrenal cortical function are related to deficiencies or excesses of the principal hormones of the gland: cortisol as the glucocorticoid, aldosterone as the mineralocorticoid, and the adrenal androgens, which are largely by-products and of low physiological potency.

Destruction of the adrenal cortex gives rise to Addison's disease. The glucocorticoid deficiency thus evoked is manifested by weakness, hypoglycemic episodes, and pigmentation. Pigment distribution is generalized but differs from actinic pigmentation by involving the folds in the hands, old scars, and the areas inside the mouth, such as the buccal surfaces, the roof of the mouth, and the area under the tongue. The pigmentation is characteristically brown with a bluish tint and is reversible with glucocorticoid treatment (Fig. 15–7). Other causes of pigmentation which may simulate that of Addison's disease are lymphoma, gastrointestinal carcinoma, hemachromatosis, thyrotoxicosis, porphyria cutanea tarda, and chronic drug ingestion. Mineralocorticoid deficiency in Addison's disease causes a postural drop in blood pressure as an early manifestation and results from a decrease in the circulating blood volume. This is not specific for Addison's disease but may also be observed in states of dehydration, polyneuropathy, malnutrition, and exten-

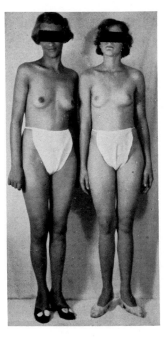

Figure 15–7. *Skin pigmentation of patient with Addison's disease (left) compared with normal.*

sive atherosclerosis of the large elastic arteries. Hyponatremia associated with this may give rise to a salt craving, abdominal cramping, and diarrhea.

Hyperfunction of the adrenal cortex presents as one or more of three classic syndromes: Cushing's disease, adrenal virilism, or primary aldosteronism.

Cushing's syndrome results from an excess of glucocorticoids. The resulting catabolic state brings about atrophy of the muscles in the extremities and retention of fat about the abdomen—the typical "Humpty Dumpty" appearance consisting of spindly legs, flattened buttocks, and a protuberant abdomen (Fig. 15–8). An accumulation of fat about the shoulders resem-

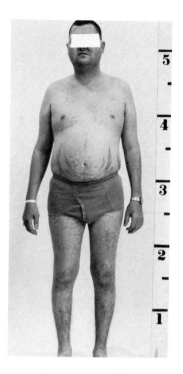

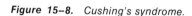

Figure 15–8. Cushing's syndrome.

bling a buffalo hump is not pathognomonic of Cushing's syndrome, since it is also seen with simple obesity. The patient with Cushing's disease rarely weighs over 200 pounds. Extreme obesity, while often presenting superficially some of the features of Cushing's syndrome, usually is manifested by large extremities with good muscle strength and development, whereas weakness of the extremities is a prominent feature of Cushing's syndrome. Degeneration of the subcutaneous structures gives rise to a thin skin, which breaks down with only slight trauma. Easy bruisability associated with subcutaneous atrophy is a feature (see Fig. 16–7). Pigmented striae may appear about the abdomen, but are not pathognomonic of Cushing's syndrome, since they may appear in obese adolescent males. Cushing's syndrome appearing in a child will cause stunting of growth and lead to a form of dwarfism. Hypertension is a common feature, as is a mild diabetic syndrome. Hirsutism with a fine lanugo-like hair is often noted.

Cushing's disease may result from overstimulation of the adrenal cortex by excess pituitary adrenocorticotropic hormone (ACTH) that arises in an adenoma of the pituitary, or from a regulatory abnormality in the pituitary hypothalamic mechanism. Cushing's syndrome may also appear as a result of a functioning neoplasm of the adrenal cortex, from bronchogenic carcinoma, and, most commonly, from overmedication with adrenocorticoid preparations.

Adrenal virilization in females is marked by breast atrophy, appearance of a masculine distribution of hair, amenorrhea, hypertrophy of the clitoris, and masculine development of muscles. (Fig. 15–9). When present in a child, an increase in the growth rate and premature closure of the epiphyses are noted, leading to an ultimate shortening of stature. When present in the male, it is striking only in the prepubertal boy with sexual precocity. Adrenal virilism may be caused by a functioning neoplasm of the adrenal cortex or by a metabolic block in the formation of cortisol. The resultant retardation in cortisol synthesis allows the pituitary to stimulate the adrenal cortex through excess formation of ACTH, thus increasing the production of adrenal androgens. This results in the production of congenital adrenal hyperplasia (adrenogenital syndrome). Enzymatic block in hydroxylation at C-21 of the steroid nucleus gives rise to the hypotensive type of adrenal virilism, whereas a block in C-11 hydroxylation results in the hypertensive variety of adrenal virilism (Bongiovanni's syndrome).

Overproduction of aldosterone gives rise to severe arterial hypertension and hypokalemic alkalosis, characteristically without edema formation. This may be due to adrenal hyperplasia or to a neoplasm of the adrenal cortex (Conn's syndrome).

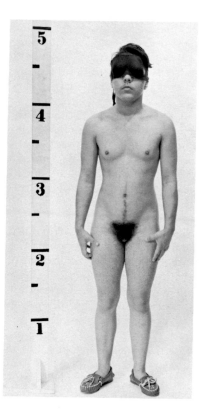

Figure 15–9. Adrenal virilization in a girl.

THE ADRENAL MEDULLA

A functioning neoplasm of the adrenal medulla (pheochromocytoma) gives rise to a hypertensive state, characteristically paroxysmal in nature but in some cases of a continuous type. The paroxysms are recognized by the appearance of pallor about the mouth, tremor, and a sudden rise in blood pressure. At times the attacks can be evoked by massage over the affected adrenal area. Glycosuria may also be present.

THE PANCREAS

Any patient suspected of having diabetes should be queried as to a family history of diabetes or of early family death from vascular disease, birth of large babies, episodes of weakness and sweating, weight changes, excessive urination, and foot infections. The disease may cause physical changes in all organ systems, but the examiner should especially note skin color, retinal changes, postural changes in blood pressure, abdominal and femoral bruits, peripheral pulses, and vibratory sensation.

Individuals with an insulin deficiency develop the syndrome of diabetes mellitus. Physical features are minimal initially but, when present, may include red cheeks, obesity, pallor and carotenemia, shortness of stature, xanthelasma, and staphylococcic pyoderma.

Classically, two types of diabetes mellitus are distinguishable: juvenile onset diabetes, characterized by polyuria, polyphagia, weight loss, and acidosis; and an adult type marked by obesity and the premature onset of vascular degenerative disease involving particularly the coronary and cerebral arteries and the arteries of the lower extremities. Most commonly arteriosclerosis obliterans develops at an early stage with accompanying intermittent claudication and dry gangrene. Look for attenuation of arterial pulsation in the dorsalis pedis and posterior tibial arteries, since gangrene of the foot may appear in some patients due to increased susceptibility to infection. Associated with diabetic neuropathy, these changes may give rise to punched-out, neurogenic ulcers at pressure points on the soles of the feet (Fig. 15–10).

Patients with juvenile onset diabetes are prone to develop microangiopathy. This is manifested by involvement of the arterioles of the retina and kidneys. Diabetic retinopathy is typically manifested by the formation of small microaneurysms, most commonly on the nasal side of the optic disc. Small yellowish exudates are also found which may coalesce, forming large lesions followed by scarring of the retina. Hemorrhage into the vitreous is followed by neovascularization and separation of the

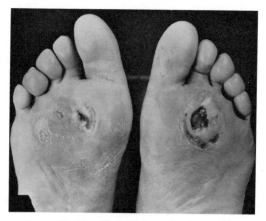

Figure 15–10. *Diabetic trophic ulcers of feet.*

retina. Microangiopathy in the kidneys leads to the appearance of Kimmelstiel-Wilson disease, which is marked by hypertension, generalized edema, and albuminuria.

Polyneuropathy is also a feature of diabetes and most commonly involves the sensory components. Femoral nerve involvement may be demonstrated by eliciting tenderness over the femoral triangle. Loss of vibratory sensation is a common early manifestation. Involvement of the visceral nerves may lead to postural hypotension, vertigo, and nocturnal diarrhea. Abdominal crises with vomiting and abdominal pain similar to that observed in tabes dorsalis are sometimes seen. Indeed, the manifestations of the polyneuropathy of diabetes may so closely mimic tabes dorsalis that the term "diabetic pseudotabes" has been applied.

Ketoacidosis is a frequent feature of diabetes mellitus and is characterized by rapid, deep respiratory movements (Kussmaul respiration) and the development of coma. The respiration, though increased in rate and amplitude, is quite regular and closely resembles that of someone sleeping soundly, although the patient may still be quite alert and anxious. The breath smells of acetone, and the patient shows evidence of dehydration. Softening of the eyeballs is a common feature, as is distention of the abdomen and absence of bowel sounds.

Hypoglycemia is marked by progressive cerebral dysfunction initially in higher cerebral functions and later involves the vital centers of the brain. Initially, hunger and sweating associated with weakness and tremor are prominent features. A decrease in body temperature is common, producing a cold and clammy skin. Hypoglycemia may result from an overdose of insulin, islet cell tumors, large fibrosarcomas, hypopituitarism, alcoholism, or from a regulatory disturbance known as functional, or reactive, hypoglycemia, which is marked by attacks after the ingestion of carbohydrates.

Tumors of the delta cells of the pancreas have been said to cause resistant peptic ulceration (Zollinger-Ellison syndrome).

THE GONADS

Gonadal dysfunction may cause alterations in puberal patterns, sexual function, menstruation, and general growth and strength. Particular note should be made of body proportions and measurements, as well as of the presence or absence of secondary sex characteristics.

Deficiency of testicular Leydig cell function results in eunuchoidism, the features varying according to the age of onset. When the deficiency appears before puberty, epiphyseal closure is retarded, resulting in a striking alteration in body proportions such that the individual has broad hips and disproportionately long extremities. As a result, the distance from the crown to the symphysis pubis may be shorter than from the symphysis to the floor. The span is greater than the height, the carrying angle of the elbow is increased, and the individual tends to be taller than normal. Muscular development is poor, and the pubic hair (escutcheon) does not extend up to the umbilicus as it should in the male. When the testicular deficiency appears after puberty,

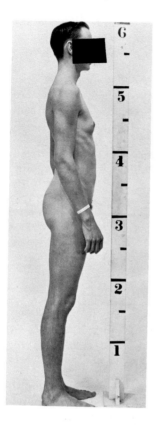

Figure 15-11. Klinefelter's syndrome.

changes are not so marked but include decreased hair growth, obesity, and the absence of baldness. The fine wrinkling of the skin is striking (see Fig. 5–12). A chromosomal abnormality characterized by the XXY pattern of sex chromosomes is associated with Klinefelter's syndrome. The findings are quite variable, and in some patients they may be minimal and include no more than a tendency to the eunuchoid body proportions previously described. Gynecomastia is a common feature, and secondary male sex characteristics may vary from normal to deficient (Fig. 15–11).

Ovarian deficiency occurring before puberty can produce a eunuchoid body build similar to that seen in the male eunuch. There will not, of course, be any development of the breasts and feminine body contours. Pubic and axillary hair will appear, however, if there is normal adrenal function.

Hypogonadism in either sex is often associated with anosmia (de Morsier's syndrome). In the male this is termed Kallmann's syndrome and is found in combination with hypertelorism and midline clefts.

Occasionally the ovary may produce an excess of androgen, with resulting masculine hair distribution, including the masculine extension of pubic hair toward the umbilicus and the development of clitoral hypertrophy. In many families, varying degrees of feminine hirsutism are common but do not indicate any disease state. In the Stein-Leventhal syndrome, there is a combination of hirsutism, obesity, and early onset of menstrual abnormalities. Actual virilism is rare in this syndrome.

THE PITUITARY GLAND

Anterior pituitary hypofunction may be evident by a deficiency in one or all of the target gland hormones, i.e., thyroid, adrenal cortex, or gonads, as well as by deficiencies of the other products of pituitary function not mediated through target glands, such as growth hormone and melanophore-stimulating hormone. When total absence of anterior pituitary function occurs, the term panhypopituitarism is applied. Each of the hormones of the anterior pituitary is controlled by releasing or inhibiting hormones elaborated in the hypothalamus. Thus, dissociated anterior pituitary dysfunctions commonly occur as a result of hypothalamic disease.

The patient with panhypopituitarism will show the typical picture of myxedema plus the signs of adrenal and gonadal insufficiency. Those symptoms of adrenal insufficiency due to lack of aldosterone, such as hypotension, will not be very evident, however. In addition, the hypopituitary patient will show a pallor or generalized depigmentation instead of the hyperpigmentation of Addison's disease.

Hypogonadism is marked in the male by a decrease in secondary sex characteristics and in the female by amenorrhea. In both sexes the loss of axillary hair is helpful in diagnosis. It should be remembered that loss of axillary hair is a normal occurrence in the older age group. In addition, in the immature person, the growth rate is checked or greatly retarded, leading to dwarfism. The hypopituitary dwarf characteristically has the appearance of a child of the age at which the disease had its onset (Fig. 15–12). Panhypopituitarism may appear in the postpartum state as described by Sheehan. In such patients there is often a history of severe blood loss and shock at the time of delivery and a failure to resume menses after delivery. Simmonds described a cachexia in panhypopituitarism, but this finding is quite rare and probably results from other causes (Fig. 15–13). This had lead to the frequent misapplication of the diagnosis of panhypopituitarism to individuals with anorexia nervosa who typically are young, psychoneurotic females who develop amenorrhea and severe weight loss. In contrast to persons suffering from hypopituitarism, these patients feel quite well and retain axillary and pubic hair. When disease involves the posterior pituitary or the hypothalamus, diabetes insipidus appears, in which large volumes of dilute urine are formed and polydipsia appears.

There is no syndrome of generalized hyperpituitarism. Acromegaly represents a syndrome of overproduction of growth hormone and is usually due to a neoplasm of the anterior pituitary. When it occurs in a prepuberal individual, it may lead only to abnormally rapid growth resulting in a form of gigantism. After the epiphyses close, growth can occur only in the membranous bone. This leads to characteristic changes in the skull and extremities. The face is changed by marked prominence of the frontal bone and enlargement of the nose. The lower jaw continues to grow, resulting in an overbite and the ap-

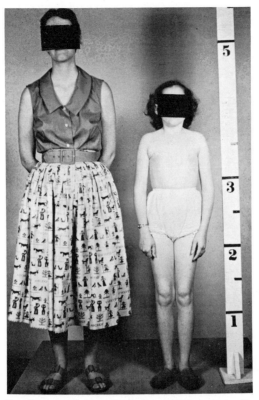

Figure 15–12. *Patient with hypopituitarism (right) compared to normal person of same age.*

pearance of prognathism (see Fig. 5–6). The hands and feet become thickened and take the form of a spade. The fingers lose their normal taper, and the hand develops a square appearance. Kyphosis is sometimes seen. The voice of the patient develops a resonant, ringing quality, resulting from enlargement of the nasal accessory sinuses.

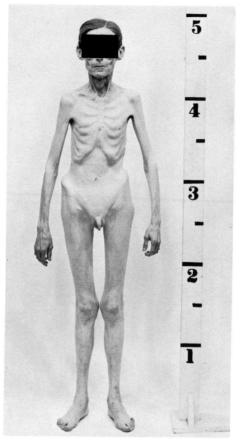

Figure 15–13. Simmonds' disease with cachexia.

Hyperpigmentation may result from chromophobe adenomas of the pituitary; however, this hyperpigmentation usually appears only in patients who have had ablation of the adrenals for Cushing's disease. The pigmentation is progressive and intense and is termed Nelson's syndrome.

MISCELLANEOUS SYNDROMES

Extreme obesity is not associated with any of the known classical endocrine diseases. Various combinations of obesity with other deviations in body characteristics have been described, and are often confused with endocrine disease. A combination of obesity, hirsutism, and diabetes has been described as the Achard-Thiers syndrome. The combination of obesity with hyperostosis of the inner table of the frontal bone is labeled

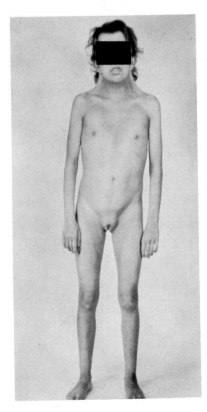

Figure 15–14. *Turner's syndrome.*

as the Stewart-Morel-Morgagni syndrome. Obesity, supernumerary digits, feeblemindedness, and retinitis pigmentosa occur in the Laurence-Moon-Biedl syndrome, and obesity with apparently small genitalia and delayed puberty in boys is called the Fröhlich syndrome. It is doubtful if any of these represent any primary endocrinopathy. Illustrated in Figure 15–14 is an example of Turner's syndrome, a form of primary hypogonadism associated with gonadal aplasia, infantile genitalia, lack of secondary sex characteristics, amenorrhea, webbing of the neck, short stature, and other congenital defects. The genetic constitution of individuals with this syndrome includes only a single X chromosome.

Multiple functioning endocrine adenomas (MEA syndrome) often occur as a familial characteristic. In the MEA I syndrome, endocrine tumors of the pituitary, pancreas, parathyroids, thyroid, and adrenal cortex occur together. In the MEA II syndrome, medullary carcinomas of the thyroid and pheochromocytomas occur together.

COMMON CLINICAL TERMS

Band keratopathy—Cloudiness about the margin of the cornea seen in hypercalcemia.

Escutcheon—The pubic hair outline. Androgens produce a diamond-shaped escutcheon, whereas the normal adult female configuration is that of an inverted triangle.

Myxedema coma—A state of obtunded consciousness, hypothermia, and hypoventilation resulting from severe myxedema.

Orthostatic hypotension—A drop in the blood pressure on standing seen in Addison's disease, dehydration, diabetic neuropathy, and atherosclerosis.

Thyroid bruit—Pulsating arterial vascular sound heard over the thyroid in thyrotoxicosis. Persists upon pressure with the stethoscope.

Virilism—A combination of hirsutism and clitoral hypertrophy seen in androgen excess states in females.

COMMON CLINICAL SYNDROMES

Bongiovanni's syndrome—Hypertensive type of adrenogenital syndrome due to 11-C hydroxylase deficiency in the adrenal cortex.

Conn's syndrome—Adenoma of the adrenal cortex producing aldosterone associated with hypertension and an absence of edema.

Eunuchoid habitus—The body conformation in hypogonadism characterized by a body segment which is shorter than the legs.

Gynecomastia—Hypertrophy of the male breast. The hypertrophy should include glandular tissue and not fat alone.

Hashimoto's thyroiditis—A progressive painless enlargement of the thyroid gland associated with atrophy of endocrine tissue, lymphocytic infiltration, and circulating antithyroid antibodies.

Kimmelstiel-Wilson disease—Nodular glomerulosclerosis associated with albuminuria, edema, hypertension, and retinopathy in diabetics.

Sheehan's syndrome—Panhypopituitarism following post partum pituitary necrosis due to hemorrhage and shock.

Stein-Leventhal syndrome—Obesity, hypomenorrhea, and relative sterility associated with sclerocystic ovaries.

Zollinger-Ellison syndrome—Gastrin-producing tumor of the delta cells of the pancreas associated with intractable peptic ulcer.

BIBLIOGRAPHY

Albright, F., and Reifenstein, E. C.: The Parathyroid Glands and Metabolic Bone Disease. Baltimore, Williams & Wilkins Co., 1948.

Fajans, S. S., and Sussman, K. E.: Diabetes Mellitus: Diagnosis and Treatment. Vol. III. New York, American Diabetes Association, 1971.

Means, J. H.: The Thyroid and Its Disease. 3rd ed. New York, McGraw-Hill Book Co., 1963.

Rimoin, D. L., and Schimke, R. N.: Genetic Disorders of the Endocrine Glands. St. Louis, C. V. Mosby Co., 1971.

Wilkins, L.: The Diagnosis and Treatment of Endocrine Disorders in Childhood and Adolescence. Springfield, Illinois, Charles C Thomas, 1966.

Williams, R. H.: Textbook of Endocrinology. 5th ed. Philadelphia, W. B. Saunders Co., 1974.

16
EXAMINATION OF THE HEMIC AND LYMPHATIC SYSTEMS

Physical signs associated with hematological disorders, when combined with a thorough history, may be diagnostic, subsequent laboratory and x-ray studies serving merely to confirm or modify the initial clinical impression. Though frequently sensitive and specific, these clues are quite varied in form and location, since they are related to involvement of the reticuloendothelial and lymphatic tissues present in most organs — notably the lymph nodes, spleen, liver, and bone marrow. The clues, on the other hand, may be secondary to changes in coagulation factors or to infiltration of abnormal cells into the tissues, particularly the skin.

GENERAL INSPECTION

Patients with severe sickle cell disease may show immature physical development with disproportionate lengthening of the extremities, consistent with associated hypogonadism. In this disease as well as in other congenital anemias, such as thalassemia major and congenital spherocytic anemia, the head may

724

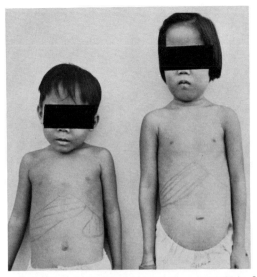

Figure 16–1. Prominent frontal basses and "tower skull" in Chinese children with thalassemia major. Note enlarged liver and spleen.

be disproportionately large, the forehead high, and prominent frontal and parietal bones evident, the result of rapid, excessive red cell production in the marrow of these bones. The bridge of the nose may be depressed (Fig. 16–1).

The gait may be abnormal as a result of joint changes, such as asceptic necrosis of the femoral head in sickle cell and hemoglobin S-C disease. The hemarthroses of congenital hemorrhagic disorders, e.g., hemophilia, may be crippling and may involve any joint. The gait may likewise be abnormal in patients with pernicious anemia when sufficient spinal cord or peripheral nerve injury exists. Numerous abnormalities may be observed in Fanconi's anemia (congenital panhypoplasia), such as dwarfism, microcephaly, patchy pigmentation of the skin, hypogenitalism, strabismus, and abnormalities of the digits (frequently of the thumbs), ears, forearms, and hips, in addition to the hematological abnormality.

The pallor of anemia may be less obvious, since it varies with degree and duration. If sudden loss of blood occurs, the skin is waxy white, the pulse rapid, and respirations shallow. If the loss is slow and prolonged, the skin becomes sallow; the nails lose their luster and become brittle and concave, and "spoon" nails (Fig. 16–2) may develop—the classic findings of iron deficiency anemia. Anemia caused by hemolysis results in an icteric tint, whereas lemon-colored skin, gray hair, and large ears are frequently present in pernicious anemia. Jaundice, cyanosis, or various degrees of pigmentation may mask a severe degree of anemia. The opposite of anemia, i.e., polycythemia of various types, produces a purple cyanosis with a ruddy, florid complexion and telangiectasia of the nose and cheeks (Fig. 16–3).

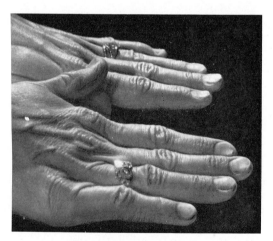

Figure 16–2. Spoon nails.

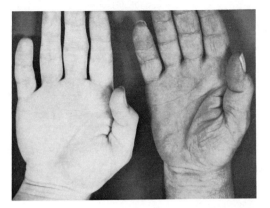

Figure 16–3. Polycythemia (right) compared with normal.

THE SKIN

Distinctive physical signs in the skin caused by hematological diseases are secondary to vascular changes, hemorrhage, or cellular infiltrates.

Vessel involvement in familial hemorrhagic telangiectasia (Osler-Weber-Rendu disease) results in a striking appearance, particularly in the elderly patient. The lesions are obvious on the face, lips, tongue, nasal mucosa, and tips of the fingers or toes (Figs. 5–21 and 16–4). In children, telangiectatic lesions are minute but grow larger with increasing age. The minute transient telangiectasia common in pregnancy should not be mistaken for generalized purpura. In children, a large disfiguring hemangioma may accompany thrombocytopenic purpura.

Purpuric lesions vary in appearance according, in part, to the causative mechanism. The lesions are small and generalized in thrombocytopenic purpura, although ecchymoses of varying size may appear. Anaphylactoid, or vascular, purpura differs

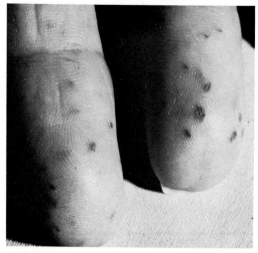

Figure 16–4. Lesions in familial hemorrhagic telangiectasia.

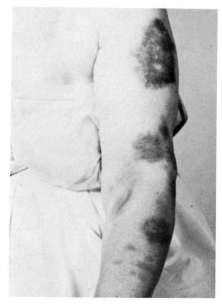

Figure 16–5. Ecchymoses of upper extremity in hypersensitivity state.

728

from thrombocytopenic purpura in both appearance and location. The former is usually seen on the buttocks, thighs, and legs, with the elbows being the next area of predilection. Careful inspection of the lesions reveals the small, reddened, swollen, tortuous vessels. If these vessels become occluded, edematous necrotic ulcers described as Henoch-Schönlein purpura may appear. The lesions in Waldenström's hyperglobulinemic purpura have a similar distribution but are orthostatic in nature and hence are limited to the legs and feet (Fig. 16–6). Remissions and exacerbations result in deep brown pigmentation over the affected areas. Ecchymoses secondary to a circulating anticoagulant, increased fibrinolysis, or congenital lack of a clotting factor

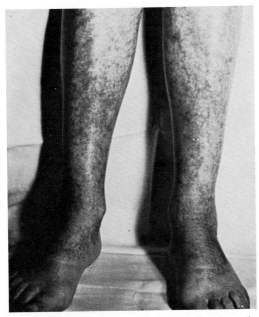

Figure 16–6. *Orthostatic changes and pigmentation in patient with Waldenström's hyperglobulinemic purpura.*

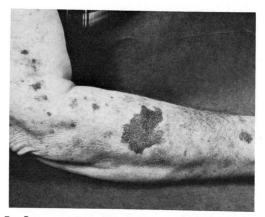

Figure 16–7. *Purpura of upper extremity in patient receiving cortico-steroids.*

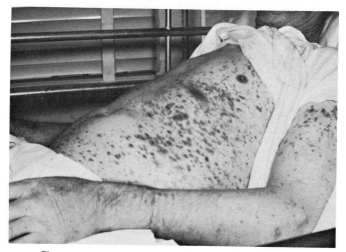

Figure 16–8. *Generalized purpura in acute leukemia.*

(as in classic hemophilia, or factor VIII deficiency), may extend throughout an entire fascial plane. This may be the presenting sign in carcinoma of the prostate with metastases. Purpura resulting from long-term corticosteroid therapy is usually limited to the arms (Fig. 16–7).

Purpuric lesions in leukemia and lymphoma differ from those of uncomplicated thrombocytopenia and usually result from cellular infiltration and hemorrhage (Fig. 16–8). The center of the lesion may be white, resembling that of subacute bacterial endocarditis.

Skin manifestations of leukemia and allied disorders may be generalized or discrete. They are usually red, purple, or gray and vary from slightly elevated to large discrete tumor masses.

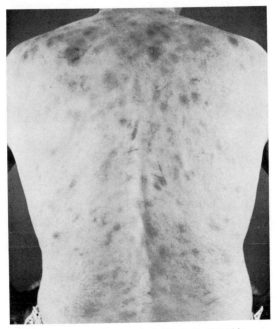

Figure 16–9. *Leukemic infiltrate in the skin.*

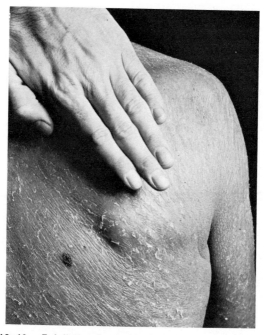

Figure 16-10. Exfoliative dermatitis in chronic lymphatic leukemia.

There may be pigmentation and vascularization of varying degrees (Fig. 16–9). At times a severe exfoliative dermatitis occurs, the skin becoming extremely red and thickened. The degree of desquamation may be quite startling (Fig. 16–10).

Previous sections describe the appearance of and methods of examining for enlarged lymph glands and tumor masses. It should be noted that masses may be continuous with bone in multiple myeloma and chloroma.

THE MOUTH

Hematological diseases frequently produce lesions in the oral cavity. The redness of the oral mucous membranes in polycythemia vera is indeed impressive. The tongue is enlarged and firm when it is the site of deposition of paramyloid in multiple myeloma. The papillae vary in appearance and may disappear so that the tongue becomes smooth, as in pernicious anemia and, rather strangely, also in chronic iron deficiency anemia. Purpura and telangiectasia may be seen in the mucosa of the nasopharynx and oral cavity. Small ulcers with a minimal amount of tissue reaction are typical of agranulocytic angina. Tonsillar tissue may be hypertrophic in lymphoid and reticular lymphomas. With modern antitumor chemotherapy there is a tendency for small, round, flat, white clusters of monilia to grow anterior to the tonsillar pillars and the base of the tongue in patients receiving these potent agents. In highly infiltrative leukemia, the gingiva hypertrophy to such an extent that the teeth appear sunken into the gums (see Fig. 5–27).

THE EYES

Examination of the eyes may reveal unilateral or bilateral exophthalmos caused by retrobulbar infiltration of abnormal cells. In polycythemia the conjunctival vessels are engorged and enlarged, producing the appearance of conjunctivitis. Scleral hemorrhages are brilliant red until entirely absorbed because the hemoglobin is continuously oxygenated. Fundus examination shows tortuosity of the vessels in sickle cell disease. Both hemorrhage and infiltration are observed in hemorrhagic and leukemic diseases. Hemorrhage into the aqueous humor is occasionally seen.

THE CHEST

Chest findings in hematological diseases vary with the type and degree of involvement by tumor tissue or bleeding. In severe anemia both right and left ventricular enlargement is common, and an apical systolic murmur is a usual finding. Mitral, aortic, and pulmonic diastolic murmurs have been occasionally described in sickle cell disease.

THE EXTREMITIES

Examination of the extremities may reveal, in addition to the skin lesions described, accentuation of peripheral vessels in multiple myeloma due to deposition of abnormal proteins in the vessel walls. Venipuncture in such patients frequently produces protracted oozing of blood. At times, the tips of the fingers, toes, ears, and nose may become discolored or gangrenous if cryoglobulins are present.

THE LYMPH NODES

Though many groups of lymph nodes are not readily accessible to examination, the cervicofacial, axillary, epitrochlear,

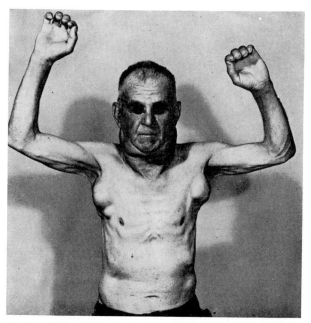

Figure 16–11.   *Enlarged cervical and axillary glands in lymphatic leukemia.*

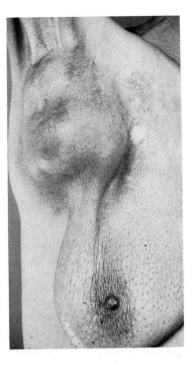

Figure 16-12. *Large axillary nodes in chronic lymphatic leukemia.*

femoral, and inguinal are easily palpated. The abdominal nodes can be felt only when they are quite large or unusually situated. We have had the discouraging experience of knowing the size and location of large periaortic lymph nodes, well visualized by lymphangiography, and not being able to locate them by examination, even though the patient was quite thin.

Lymph nodes should be palpated and measured, and note made as to whether they are discrete or matted together, fixed or movable, and whether hard, soft, or fluctuant. In some diseases they will be tender. There is rarely any difficulty in examining the cervicofacial, femoral, and inguinal nodes. Examination of the axilla must be done carefully or even large nodes will be missed. Have the patient either supine or sitting, with the

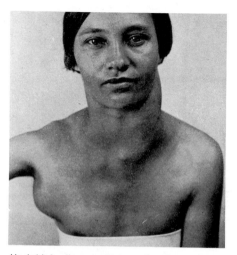

Figure 16–13. *Hodgkin's disease. Note collar-like enlargement of cervical glands and enlarged glands in the right axilla.*

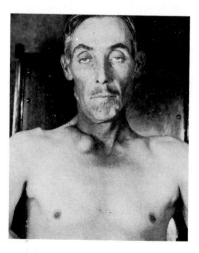

Figure 16–14. *Hodgkin's disease.*

arm supported and completely relaxed. Place your right hand high in the patient's left axilla while your left hand supports the shoulder. Be careful not to get too close to the chest wall until the fingers are in place, then gently palpate medially against the supporting thorax. Thorough examination of the entire superior, inferior, medial, and posterior areas, with attention to those lymph nodes along the pectoral border, is indicated. Reverse hands for the right axilla. To examine the epitrochlear nodes, shake hands with the patient, and with your other hand, palpate the distal medial area of the arm.

THE ABDOMEN, LIVER, AND SPLEEN

Techniques previously described in Chapter 11 apply here. When a mass is present in the upper left quadrant, identification may be difficult, since the spleen and kidney may feel quite similar and since retroperitoneal tumors or large pancreatic cysts may protrude into this region. Roentgenologic techniques can be helpful in defining the nature of a left upper quadrant mass. A horizontal spleen may not be palpable even when enlarged, whereas a lateral spleen may be palpable when normal in size.

Dameshek has published what he believes are short cuts in the diagnosis of splenomegaly (Fig. 16–15).

In addition to infantilism and hypogonadism, a painful continuous penile erection known as priapism may be seen in leukemia and sickle cell disease.

BONES AND JOINTS

Mention has been made of changes in the bones and joints that are obvious on general inspection. Extreme bone pain may be the chief complaint in the crises of sickle cell disease. Slight pressure over the sternum may cause pain in the patient with leukemia. Hemorrhage into a joint may cause a crippling decrease in the degree of motion and a permanent enlargement of

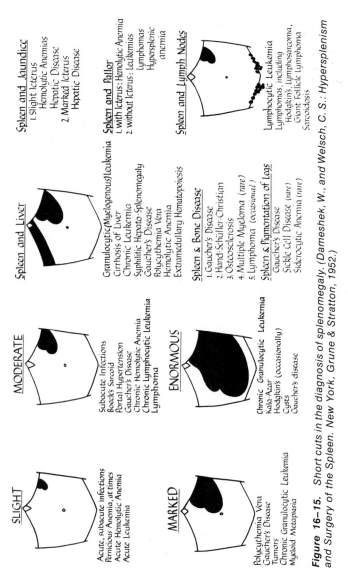

SLIGHT

Acute, subacute infections
Pernicious Anemia, at times
Acute Hemolytic Anemia
Acute Leukemia

MODERATE

Subacute Infections
Boeck's Sarcoid
Portal Hypertension
Gaucher's Disease
Chronic Hemolytic Anemia
Chronic Lymphocytic Leukemia
Lymphoma

MARKED

Polycythemia Vera
Gaucher's Disease
Tumors
Chronic Granulocytic Leukemia
Myeloid Metaplasia

ENORMOUS

Chronic Granulocytic Leukemia
Kala-Azar
Hodgkin's (occasionally)
Cysts
Gaucher's disease

Spleen and Liver

Granulocytic(Myelogenous)Leukemia
Cirrhosis of Liver
Chronic Leukemia
Syphilitic Hepato-Splenomegaly
Gaucher's Disease
Polycythemia Vera
Hemolytic Anemia
Extramedullary Hematopoiesis

Spleen & Bone Disease

1. Gaucher's Disease
2. Hand-Schüller-Christian
3. Osteosclerosis
4. Multiple Myeloma (rare)
5. Lymphoma (occasional)

Spleen & Pigmentation of Legs

Gaucher's Disease
Sickle Cell Disease (rare)
Siderocytic Anemia (rare)

Spleen and Jaundice

1. Slight Icterus
   Hemolytic Anemias
   Hepatic Disease
2. Marked Icterus
   Hepatic Disease

Spleen and Pallor

1. with Icterus: Hemolytic Anemia
2. without Icterus: Leukemias
   Lymphomas
   Hypersplenic
   anemia

Spleen and Lymph Nodes

Lymphocytic Leukemia
Lymphomas, including
Hodgkin's, Lymphosarcoma,
Giant Follicle Lymphoma
Sarcoidosis

Figure 16–15. Short cuts in the diagnosis of splenomegaly. (Dameshek, W., and Welsch, C. S.: Hypersplenism and Surgery of the Spleen. New York, Grune & Stratton, 1952.)

the joint. Hard tumors of bone may be found in multiple myeloma, and pathological fractures are frequent.

NEUROLOGICAL EXAMINATION

Hematological disease may involve all parts of the central and peripheral nervous systems through hemorrhage, cellular infiltration, or metabolic abnormalities. Thus neurological signs, if present, are quite varied and are related principally to the site or sites of involvement. This is especially true in pernicious anemia, in which both peripheral and central nervous system function may be disturbed. Peripheral neuropathy may be present in multiple myeloma.

COMMON CLINICAL TERMS

Ecchymosis—Subcutaneous hemorrhage, the color being dependent on the age of the lesion; it may vary from blue, purple, brown, and yellow. The area involved may be small or extend throughout an entire large fascial plane.

Glossitis—A soreness of the tongue, with visible and variable abnormalities, that may occur in various disorders such as pernicious anemia, iron deficiency anemia, sprue, and amyloid disease.

Hemarthrosis—A deformed joint due to hemorrhage that usually results in permanent changes. Prevalent in congenital hemorrhagic diseases where there may be repeated trauma to the same joint.

Hepatosplenomegaly—Enlargement of the liver and spleen to a degree that it is noticeable to the examiner.

Hypertrophic frontal bosses—Visible enlargement of the frontal bones, particularly observed in children having diseases with pronounced erythropoiesis, such as occurs in the congenital hemolytic syndromes.

Leukemia cutis—Visible and palpable raised cutaneous lesions varying in color (white, gray, brown) observed in leukemic diseases.

Lymphadenopathy—A visible and palpable enlargement of the lymph nodes.

Purpura—Visible small hemorrhagic spots in the skin and mucous membranes.

Splenomegaly—Enlargement of the spleen to a degree that it is determined by physical examination.

Telangiectasia—Small vascular lesions composed of enlarged vessels most frequently found on the skin of the face, the ears, the hands and feet, at the base of the fingernails, and the mucous membranes. There are congenital and acquired lesions.

COMMON CLINICAL SYNDROMES

Cooley's or Mediterranean anemia (thalassemia)—An anemia of varying severity and in the most severe cases there may be prominent frontal bosses and hepatosplenomegaly. Hemoglobin synthesis is abnormal; increased amounts of fetal hemoglobin are present.

Erythremia—A particular type of erythrocytosis of a chronic disease, with a marked increase in the red cells, and the clinical findings of a peculiar reddish purple skin color, usually splenic enlargement, and a variety of vasomotor and neurological changes.

Fanconi's syndrome—A congenital disease with pancytopenia and various and varied congenital abnormalities including brown pigmentation of the skin, dwarfism, microcephaly, hypogenitalism, and thumb abnormalities.

Gaucher's disease—A familial disorder with clinical findings of splenomegaly, skin pigmentation, bone lesions, and pingueculae of the sclera. A congenital defect in metabolism resulting in accumulations of glucocerebroside in various organs and tissues.

Hemophilia—A congenital lack of, or decrease in, antihemophilic globulin resulting in hemorrhage and deforming sequelae, particularly in the joints. The classic form is a sex-linked recessive disorder.

Henoch's purpura—A nonthrombocytopenic "allergic purpura" with abdominal symptoms including severe colic. The abdominal symptoms may occur before the purpura.

Pernicious anemia—A disease characterized by a waxy yellowish tint to the skin and a triad of changes including pallor, glossitis, and neurological changes.

Purpura hemorrhagica—Localized or generalized small, discrete, or confluent areas of hemorrhage in the skin and mucous membranes, due to various defects in the clotting substances and changes in the small vessels.

Schönlein's purpura—A nonthrombocytopenic purpura of the "allergic" type associated with rheumatoid pains and periarticular effusions. Abdominal pain may be present.

Sickle cell disease—Usually a term reserved for homozygous hemoglobin S-S disease with anemia, malnutrition, weakness, marked tortuosity of fundal vessels, and leg ulcers.

BIBLIOGRAPHY

Dameshek, W., and Welch, C. S.: Hypersplenism and Surgery of the Spleen. New York, Grune & Stratton, 1952.

Judge, R. D., and Zuidema, G. D.: Physical Diagnosis. 2nd ed. Boston, Little, Brown & Co., 1968.

Leavell, B. S., and Thorup, O. A., Jr.: Fundamentals of Clinical Hematology. 3rd ed. Philadelphia, W. B. Saunders Co., 1971.

Linman, J. W.: Principles of Hematology. New York, The Macmillan Co., 1966.

Stefanini, M., and Dameshek, W.: The Hemorrhagic Disorders. New York, Grune & Stratton, 1962.

Wintrobe, M. M.: Clinical Hematology. 6th ed. Philadelphia, Lea & Febiger, 1967.

Zelman, S.: Liver and spleen visualization by a simple roentgen contrast method. Ann. Intern. Med., 34:466, 1951.

17
PEDIATRIC EXAMINATION

The examination of a child requires a variety of techniques and methods that are, in general, different from those generally used with adults. First, familiarity with the rapid changes brought about by growth and development and, second, skill in dealing with individuals who are not always willing to be examined are essential. The first of these, knowledge of growth and development, is a lifelong pursuit and beyond the scope of this chapter. More properly this information contained in pediatric texts is the subject of extensive, ever-expanding study. Mastery of the literature on growth and development is not essential before undertaking the examination of children. However, you will require frequent assistance in interpreting observations, until such time as you become familiar with the normal changes accompanying growth and development. The purpose of this chapter is to describe the technique of examining children, to explain its significance, and to emphasize those aspects of the examination that differ from routines used with adults.

Children under five years of age often do not wish to be examined; they cry and struggle as soon as any effort is made to undress or uncover them. Examination of crying, struggling, negativistic children provides little information of value and may even lead to false conclusions. The observer skilled in

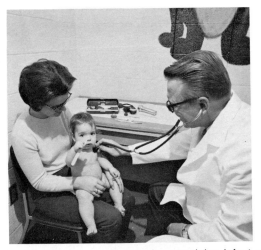

Figure 17–1. *Appropriate arrangement for examining infant on mother's lap.*

dealing with refractory children takes every opportunity to observe as much as possible before the child becomes stirred up. If the child is asleep in bed, relaxed on the mother's lap, or playing unconcernedly, observe color, form, movements, and vital signs as far as possible, for the information thus obtained may be the only valid results of an entire examination.

When you begin that part of the examination requiring physical contact with the child, commence by exploring those parts of the body that provoke the least anxiety, such as the parts of the body farthest away from the head, or if the child has pain, farthest from the area of pain. Observation and palpation of a child's hands and feet are the least disturbing to most young children and, at the same time, give some clue as to the amount of resistance likely to be encountered as you proceed to more difficult areas. Obviously, the more disturbing portions of the examination should be left to last, such as the examination of various body orifices and available cavities or funduscopic exam-

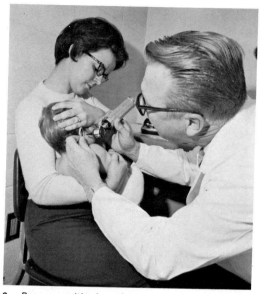

Figure 17–2. *Proper positioning of mother and child for otoscopic examination. Note particularly use of mother's hands in restraining infant's head and arms.*

inations. The better part of wisdom may be to defer the examination a few hours or to another day rather than complete it on a crying and struggling child merely for the sake of completion. The child three or four years old often tolerates a second attempt well, having apparently learned that the examiner intends no harm or pain. If it is essential to complete an examination and obtain valid information, sedation or, under some circumstances, even anesthesia is justified. Reference will subsequently be made to these exceptions to usual practice.

Children over five years old usually do not present difficulties in cooperation. Much can be learned from older children during the course of an examination by asking about their problems, complaints, and symptoms. Their responses to direct questions are often very revealing and amaze even parents, who never "dreamed" their child felt that way about his environment and the people in it. Neither refusal to answer nor the familiar "I don't know" should be construed as ignorance. These responses often reflect a situation too painful, in the psychological sense, for the child to discuss.

ANTHROPOMETRIC MEASUREMENTS

The routine measurement of height and weight beginning at birth and continuing with each subsequent examination during childhood is standard practice. Measurement of the greatest circumference of the head should also begin at birth and continue during the first three or four years. Results should be plotted on accepted growth charts so that you can compare the somatic growth and development of the individual to norms based on large numbers of children (Figs. 17–3 and 17–4). Scales used in weighing should be accurate and calibrated frequently.

THE NEWBORN

The common life-threatening conditions of this age period can be detected only by frequent, routine observation of vital functions and meticulous attention to the details of an infant's course. An examination carried out in isolated fashion without knowledge of vital functions and clinical course may contribute little, and may mislead the unsuspecting physician, who, observing no abnormal findings, concludes no problems exist. Significant anatomical malformations are present in about 5 per cent of the population at birth, but even experienced observers are able to identify only about one out of five anomalies by physical examination during the neonatal period. The remaining anomalies become manifest with the passage of months and even years.

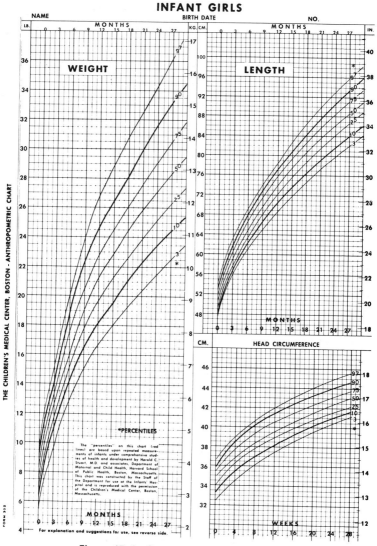

Figure 17-3 See opposite page for legend.

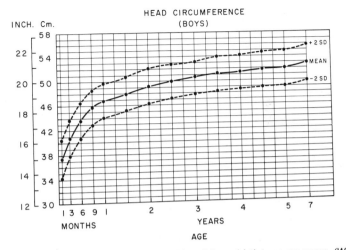

HEAD CIRCUMFERENCE
(BOYS)

Figure 17–4. Sample growth chart of head, from birth to seven years. (Westrop, C. K., and Barber, C. R.: Growth of the skull in young children — Part I: Standards of head circumference. J. Neurol. Neurosurg. Psychiatry, 19:52, 1956.)

At the moment of birth, direct your attention immediately to the competency of the cardiorespiratory system. Pay particular attention to the infant's color, cry, inspiratory effort, and muscle tone. Respiratory and cardiac rate and rhythm and air exchange in the lungs are checked by auscultation over the chest. A highly desirable routine for all premature infants or those expected to develop trouble by reason of complications during pregnancy, labor, or delivery is to initiate routine observations every hour or two on respiratory rate and rhythm, color, degree of sternal retraction, muscle tone, and state of activity (asleep, quiet, or restless). Such routine should begin at birth

Figure 17–3. Sample growth chart for infant girls. (The Longitudinal Studies of Child Health and Development, Harold C. Stuart, M.D., and associates, Harvard School of Public Health, Boston, Mass.)

and be continued for the next 24 or 36 hours or until all danger of respiratory insufficiency is thought to have passed. If signs of respiratory distress or insufficiency develop, a standard chest x-ray should be obtained, because auscultation and percussion are inadequate for detection of disease or anatomical malformation in the thorax of newborn infants.

Of particular importance in the newborn is recognition of jaundice, intestinal obstruction, and early evidence of infection. Since about one-third of all newborn infants become visibly icteric in the first three to five days, it is necessary to separate those who will develop very high levels of serum bilirubin (above 20 mg. per 100 ml.) from those with less involvement. Inspection of skin and sclerae to determine the degree of icterus can be misleading because of the nullifying effect of artificial light on yellow colors, the effect of different wall colors on yellow, and the fact that the degree of icterus in the skin does not correlate closely with the level of bilirubin in the blood. The only safe way to measure the degree of icterus is by chemical analysis of the amount of circulating bilirubin.

Most newborn infants do some spitting up, regurgitation, and even vomiting. The problem is to recognize anatomical obstruction. Abdominal distention may not be present. Palpation of the abdomen rarely helps. The presence of bile in the vomitus is considered evidence of anatomical obstruction until proven otherwise. The single, most helpful diagnostic examination is a simple x-ray examination of the abdomen, which may locate the source of trouble by demonstrating an unusual gas pattern in the gastrointestinal tract.

The first evidence of serious sepsis in the newborn infant may be a failure to gain weight, loss of weight, or a subnormal temperature. Physical examination may not reveal significant changes. Early diagnosis, the key to successful treatment, depends on willingness to obtain blood cultures and to examine spinal fluid on suspicion, rather than waiting for obvious physical signs of illness.

Head.   It is not always easy to palpate open suture lines in infants or to deduce from palpation whether they are open or whether premature synostosis has occurred. The surest and easiest way to determine their condition is by x-ray examination. Palpation of fontanelles is unsatisfactory if the infant is crying or struggling. Normally, in an infant at rest, the anterior fontanelle should be depressed slightly below the surface of the surrounding cranium. A "cracked-pot" sound obtained upon percussion of the infant's skull while the sutures remain open does not necessarily indicate a skull fracture. Bruits can frequently be heard over the orbital areas and do not necessarily indicate the presence of an aneurysm.

Unusual shapes of the head and its parts should be noted, since many of the recognized chromosomal aberrations are associated with abnormalities of the head and face. The size of the head and its rate of growth are the most important observations to be made and can be readily determined by measuring the greatest circumference with a tape measure. Palpation of the skull bones should be done in order to detect unusual depressions or swellings. Transillumination of the skull is one of the simplest and most informative of procedures. It requires a darkened room and a uniform source of light (usually a flashlight with a special collar to obtain a tight fit between light and scalp). An infant with hydrencephaly or subdural hematoma has an increased area of luminosity extending out from the perimeter of the light source.

Neck. The neck of small infants is usually short. The head can normally be passively rotated, so that the infant's chin points to the acromioclavicular joint without difficulty. Limitation of rotation of the head requires further examination, especially for hematomas of the sternocleidomastoid muscles. The presence of palpable lymph nodes in the necks of older infants and children is not uncommon in healthy children. The size of the lymph nodes, their discreteness, and any tenderness need to be taken into account in assessing their significance. The infant who lies day in and day out in the opisthotonic position without signs of other illness may be mentally retarded. A stiff neck along with pain on anterior flexion occurs in infants with dehydration, lobar pneumonia, pharyngeal and peritonsillar abscesses, or marked cervical adenitis. Conversely, infants and young children with meningitis may not have opisthotonos or a stiff neck.

Chest. Newborn infants at rest breathe mostly with the diaphragm; the chest may not expand at all during inspiration, but may actually contract as a result of strong diaphragmatic action. Respiratory rhythms during the first few weeks after birth are frequently periodic and even grossly irregular in normal infants. The main respiratory rate for the normal newborn infant is 40 per minute; rates of 65 per minute or higher are definitely abnormal. Auscultation of the lungs is helpful in determining the volume of air being exchanged in newborn infants; marked inspiratory efforts are not necessarily accompanied by increased tidal volumes. Breath sounds in infants normally have an amphoric quality and appear close to the ear. The diagnosis of pneumonia in both infants and children sometimes can be made only by x-ray examination. Partial suppression of breath sounds is the most frequent, and sometimes the only, physical sign of consolidation of underlying pulmonary tissue. Crying during examination of the chest grossly distorts all auscultatory signs. Auscultation of the nose and mouth with a stethoscope helps in evaluating the source of sounds transmitted to the lungs from the patient's nose and throat.

Heart and circulation. Crying interferes seriously with this part of the examination. Sedation may be necessary to obtain valid information. Usually a second effort at a later time will suffice and will preclude the necessity of resorting to sedation.

Findings vary considerably as the child undergoes normal growth and development. The thorax is barrel-shaped at birth, but becomes wider in its transverse plane during the first few months. The heart is relatively larger in infancy than in older individuals and it is located higher in the thorax during infancy because of the relatively higher elevation of the diaphragm. The heart is also more centrally placed and lies in a more horizontal position than in older children or adults. Cardiac and respiratory rates fluctuate widely in infants and children who are excited or under stress; these rates, as well as measurements of blood pressure, should be obtained while the individual is well relaxed or asleep.

The apex beat in infancy is maximal in the fourth interspace just outside the left nipple line. Locating the apex beat in young patients by inspection or palpation is usually more difficult than in older patients. By ten years of age the apex beat has moved down to the fifth interspace in the left midclavicular line. Infants and children with enlarged hearts frequently have significant precordial bulges. Overactive hearts sometimes cause heaving of the chest wall with each beat as well as an easily visible, diffuse apex beat. Color changes in the skin of infants are frequent because of labile vasomotor reflexes. Pallor and flushing can alternate in a period of minutes. Acrocyanosis, local cyanosis of the hands and feet, must be distinguished from cyanosis of central origin. The former is usually limited to the hands and feet and is related to local conditions in the skin capillaries.

Determination of heart size by percussion in infants and children is fraught with large errors except in cases of marked cardiac enlargement. Heart size can better be determined by attempting to locate the maximal apex beat, but even this method is not too satisfactory. Efforts to determine heart size by roentgen examination in infants who are a few months old are also subject to considerable errors because of superimposed thymic shadows and the variation in heart size with the phases of respiration.

Auscultation is particularly important in the diagnosis of specific cardiac conditions in the pediatric age group. The expert cardiologist relies heavily on auscultatory findings in the differential diagnosis of the many anatomical malformations encountered in children. Auscultation is also very helpful in distinguishing organic murmurs from the functional murmurs that frequently occur. The normal heart sounds of children have a greater intensity, higher pitch, and shorter duration than those of adults. The pulmonary component of the second heart sound is always greater than the aortic component of the second heart sound throughout infancy and childhood; these should be judged primarily over the area of the main pulmonary artery. Midsystolic clicks are not uncommon over the pulmonic area. A normal third heart sound can sometimes be heard at the cardiac apex after three years of age. Of the several innocent murmurs that can be heard in children, neonatal systolic murmurs heard intermittently prior to anatomical closure of the ductus arteriosus, systolic ejection murmurs over pulmonic area, venous hums, and cardiorespiratory murmurs that are extracardiac in origin are frequent.

Abdomen. Most infants do not object to gentle abdominal palpation. It is virtually impossible to evaluate the abdomen of a crying infant. Offering a bottle with water or milk in it or just a bare nipple will sometimes provide sufficient distraction to allow satisfactory palpation. Flexing the thighs on the abdomen is helpful in deep palpation (see Fig. 17–6). In examining the toddler or young child, it may be helpful to allow the child to remain sitting or lying on the parent's lap instead of supine on a table. Abdominal tenderness can be easily located when the child is in the sitting position. Palpation should begin with the thighs or the lower chest. If the child shows no objection to these maneuvers, palpation of the abdomen may begin, starting with the part least likely to be the focus of trouble and reserving the problem area for last. There are some ill children who will not respond favorably to patience and to due consideration on your part. Adequate examination of these patients may require sedation (Fig. 17–5). This should not be done with opiates or their derivatives, but with a drug that will induce sleep, such as Nembutal in the amount of 5 mg. per kg. of body weight, given per rectum in a saline solution. Sleep will be induced, but pain on palpation remains.

Inspection of the abdomen of the neonate presents some special problems. At birth the abdomen is flat or even scaphoid, but with the first breath a large amount of air enters the gastrointestinal tract and subsequently reaches the rectum within 18 hours. The entrance of air distends the abdomen and produces the normal, rounded belly of the newborn. This normal

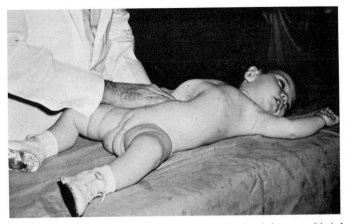

Figure 17–5. Method for deep palpation of infant's abdomen with infant sedated.

configuration continues for the first two years or so, largely because the colon during this period is relatively longer and because the intestine contains relatively more gas than in older individuals. The roundness of the infant's belly is considerably increased during the postprandial state as a result of ingested food and air. The gas pattern in the intestinal tract of newborn infants can be determined by simple x-ray examination. Knowledge of the pattern is most helpful in diagnosing the types and locations of obstruction. An abdomen that remains scaphoid after birth should arouse suspicions that viscera have been displaced upward into the chest through a Bochdalek diaphragmatic defect. Such hernias are usually on the left side, and produce a shift of the heart to the right. Heart sounds that are heard best on the right of the sternum should make one think, first, of a diaphragmatic hernia, and second, of a situs inversus. The newborn infant whose abdomen remains flat may have either a high (duodenal or pyloric) obstruction or a blind lower esophageal segment associated with a tracheoesophageal fistula.

An overdistended abdomen in the newborn is observed in obstruction of the distal small bowel or colon, in peritonitis, and in gastroenteritis. The umbilical stump of all newborns should be routinely examined to determine if there is a single umbilical artery or the usual two. The former condition is associated with a high incidence of congenital malformations of all types. In the first few days after birth, all umbilical stumps show the presence of some polymorphonuclear cells on histological examination, suggesting infection; clinically significant omphalitis, however, is manifested by erythema or induration of the surrounding skin or by purulent discharge. Visible peristalsis is not uncommon in infants with thin abdominal walls. Large waves the size of golf balls moving from left to right across the upper abdomen may indicate the presence of a pyloric tumor, but they are not pathognomonic.

The liver, and sometimes the kidneys, can be palpated in normal infants. Though the spleen is not normally palpable, its tip is frequently felt on first palpation, and can be readily displaced upward beyond reach. The liver edge remains palpable 1 to 2 cm. below the right costal margin during infancy and early childhood, but should not be felt below the costal margin after four to five years of age. Any mass in a baby's abdomen, other than the liver and kidneys and the usual fecal masses, is abnormal. Palpation of the liver and spleen in infants is best done by placing your hand lightly over the proper areas, rather than by using deep palpation.

Pyloric tumors are best palpated when the infant's stomach is empty and the infant is pacified by a nipple or bottle (Fig. 17–6). Repeated efforts to locate the olivelike pyloric mass just below the right costal margin and just to the right of the midline may be necessary. The experienced examiner usually is successful in palpating these tumors 90 per cent of the time.

Auscultation of the abdomen is not as helpful in the infant as it is in the older child or adult. Peritoneal irritation is usually accompanied by hypoactive bowel sounds; but, with a spreading peritonitis, bowel sounds may increase. Peritoneal irritation is best elicited by gentle percussion. A child who is three or four

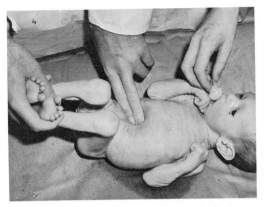

Figure 17–6. Method for palpating pyloric tumor.

years old can sometimes help in locating tenderness by responding to simple questions as to where it hurts.

Inguinal masses are always abnormal. Those that can be reduced are hernias; those that cannot be reduced may be incarcerated hernias, hydroceles, or lymph nodes. Abnormalities of the external genitalia of males or females indicate the need for careful and extensive evaluation of those parts of the genitourinary tract not available to external examination. Vaginal examination may at times require the administration of a general anesthetic.

Rectal examination, always uncomfortable, should be postponed until last. Rectal examination of the newborn infant affords an unusual opportunity to palpate the lower abdomen. The anus of the full-term infant will accept a small finger, even an index finger, unless you have unusually large hands. It is possible to palpate the internal inguinal rings in order to distinguish an incarcerated hernia from other inguinal masses, and to palpate the uterus and retrorectal masses. If the appendix is ruptured, a spongy, tender mass is frequently palpated in the cul-de-sac.

Neurological examination. This part of the examination varies more with age than any other. The usual, formal neurological examination of adults and children old enough to cooperate has no place in the newborn period and must be modified considerably for children under five or six years of age.

Neurological examination of the newborn infant is not a very productive procedure. The physical signs of cerebral lesions in this age period are usually of a general nature and are not pathognomonic; among the more common are general depression of physical activity, difficulty in being aroused, loss of vigor, irritability, jitteriness, whining, high-pitched cry, convulsions, and hypotonia. Focal signs, such as increased pressure over the anterior fontanelle, continued overlapping of cranial bones at suture lines, rapid increases in head circumferences, or a poor sucking reflex are infrequently observed, but when present are helpful evidence of underlying trouble. Focal convulsions almost always indicate generalized disease. Paralysis of an extremity is more likely the result of injury to a peripheral nerve than of injury to the central nervous system. A tonic neck reflex or a positive Babinski response may be present in normal newborn infants. Retinal hemorrhages are observed in up to 25 per cent of newborn infants and rarely have any alarming significance. Classic physical signs are lacking in meningitis in almost all cases among newborn infants; the diagnosis rests on lumbar puncture done on the basis of suspicion—which is often based on signs of infection elsewhere, together with tenuous evidence that the infant is "not doing well." The diagnosis of cerebral birth injury is the most difficult of all. Modern, skilled obstetrical practice has largely eliminated the danger of physical trauma, but it has done less well in circumventing the hazards of hypoxemia. Congenital malformations of the brain are readily diagnosed if gross evidence of hydrocephaly, microcephaly, anencephaly, or an encephalocele is present, but hydrencephaly—one of the most devastating of cerebral conditions—may go undiagnosed for weeks after birth for lack of either readily recognized general or focal signs.

In older infants, particular attention should be given to

motor, social, and mental development as part of the neurological evaluation. Delay in one area does not necessarily mean delay in the other two areas, but development in all three areas is usually parallel. The level of motor development is the easiest to assess, as there are striking landmarks that can be readily identified even by the beginner, such as good head control, sitting without support, crawling, standing, walking alone, and self-feeding. Social development is next easiest to evaluate, and mental development, or intelligence, is the most difficult. Tests for the latter have been developed for all age periods, beginning with infants about 16 weeks of age. At about eight months of age these tests have considerable reliability, i.e., if repeated, the results will be the same; however, their predictive value leaves a good deal to be desired in the case of individual children. A high degree of validity on psychological testing cannot be expected much before four or five years of age. It is important for the physician to gauge the level of mental development of infants and children he examines in order to make the correct interpretation of the neurological examination. Poor affect and impaired alertness may be related just as much to mental deficiency as to acute febrile illnesses or severe chronic disease. Neurological tests that require considerable cooperation from the patient, such as tests of hearing and vision, are much more difficult to interpret in mentally retarded children than in normal infants and children. In fact, the failure of young infants to respond to noise may be the result of either deafness or mental retardation.

Sensory examination of the child too young to cooperate is limited to tests for pain; correct interpretation requires consistent results on repeated testing. Those parts of the neurological examination that involve tests for ataxia, gait, and general motor ability frequently call for some modification of the routines used for adults. Watching a child manipulate toys or asking him to write and draw and perform tasks natural to him can be more revealing than putting him through a routine of testing that only confuses him. Correct interpretation of his behavior and performance will depend on knowledge of how children behave and perform at various age levels.

Vision. The presence or absence of vision in newborn infants can be tested by using a rotating striped drum and looking for nystagmus. Visual acuity can be measured with some precision after three years of age by using pictures of various sizes or the familiar E symbol. Ophthalmoscopical examination is as important in children as in adults. Sedation may be required, and dilation of the pupils is almost always necessary for funduscopic examinations of infants. Conjugate movement of the eyes in following objects is usually established after three months of age. Frequent or persistent deviation of the eyes after six months should be cause for concern.

Hearing. Parents are often aware that their child hears poorly, or not at all, before one year of age. Precise measurement of hearing loss depends on cooperation from the child being tested; children can rarely give this before five or six years of age. Lacking proper cooperation, it is most difficult to differentiate deafness from mental retardation, cerebral palsy, autism, and emotional disorders. Nevertheless, by the time children are three years old it is possible, in some instances, to carry out pure tone audiometric testing. Success at this early age depends frequently on the patience of the examiner and his willingness to repeat tests. Experienced audiologists, using less refined methods than pure tone audiometry, are often able to diagnose significant hearing losses in infants under one year old, but differentiating between deafness and mental retardation in the very young is not an easy task. The possibility of a partial loss of hearing in older children should be investigated by pure tone audiometry, since losses of 30 decibels are a serious handicap in a classroom setting.

COMMON CLINICAL TERMS

Acrocyanosis—Blue color of skin of hands and feet, usually seen in newborn infants, caused by sluggish capillary circulation.

Bililight—A lamp with a special wavelength placed over patient; used to break down unconjugated bilirubin in the circulation.

Croup—Hoarseness bordering on aphonia in the presence of partial laryngeal obstruction causing labored breathing.

Marasmus—Severe depletion of subcutaneous fat and soft tissue mass.

Poor skin turgor—On pinching, over abdomen usually, the skin returns slowly to its previous flat state; usually a sign of dehydration in infants and children.

Positive Kernig Sign—Sign of meningeal irritation in which the leg cannot be fully extended at knee when hip is flexed.

Projectile vomiting—Vomitus forcefully ejected 2 or 3 feet from the patient.

COMMON CLINICAL SYNDROMES

Battered-child syndrome—Applies to infants who are willfully traumatized or burned by another person, resulting in multiple ecchymoses, fractures or subdural hematomas, or burns of the skin.

Blue baby—Refers to a cyanotic infant who has congenital heart disease with a right to left intracardiac shunt.

Failure to thrive—A condition in which weight gain in infants and young children is significantly retarded for any reason.

Floppy baby—Infant with generalized hypotonia related to disease or injury of brain, spinal cord, or muscles, or to some chronic metabolic disturbance.

Hypernatremic dehydration—Seen in young infants with diarrhea or who have been given too much sodium chloride; infants are hypertonic and jittery, may convulse, and are not dehydrated in the usual sense, because dehydration is intracellular.

Intravascular coagulation defect—A bleeding tendency associated with a rapid fall in platelets, increased consumption of fibrinogen, deficiency of Factors VIII and V in blood, reduction of prothrombin, and increased production of split-end products of fibrinogen in blood and urine.

Respiratory distress syndrome (RDS)—Refers to newborn infants who are tachypneic, dyspneic, and cyanotic in the immediate postnatal period.

Reye's syndrome—Rapid onset of coma and convulsions in infants and young children during the course of some infection associated with hypoglycemia, fatty infiltration of liver and kidneys, and edema of the brain.

School phobia—Applies to school-aged children who refuse to go to school for a variety of reasons.

Shock (clinical)—A state in which the pulse is rapid and weak, hands and feet are cold to touch, the skin has a gray pallor, and there is generalized hypotonia accompanied by reduction in awareness of surroundings progressing to coma and death if not treated rapidly and appropriately.

Index

Note: Page references in *italics* indicate illustrations.

Abdomen
  auscultation of, 584–585
    in infants, 754
  examination of, 52, 548–589
    diagnostic probabilities and, 585
    in hematological diseases, 737
    in infants, 752–755
    position of patients for, 549
  inspection of, 550–566
    in newborn, 752
  palpation of, 566–582
    in infants, 752, *753*
    position of patient for, 567
  percussion of, 582–583
  rigidity in, causes of, 577
    palpation of, 580
  topographical anatomy of, *549*,
    550
Abdominal aorta, aneurysm of, 508
Abdominal distention, cardiac dullness and, 379, *380*
Abdominal muscles, testing of, 134
  weakness of, gait of patient in, 139
Abdominal reflex, clinical significance of, 580
  elicitation of, 145
*Abhandlung über Perkussion und
  Auskultation*, 16
Abortion, 635
Abruptio placentae, 636

Abscess
  lactation, *542*, 546
  lung, 353
    breath odor in, 210
  peritonsillar, 212
  retropharyngeal, 212
Abstraction ability, testing of, 130–
  131
Acalculia, as sign of cerebral dysfunc-
  tion, 129
Accommodation, of eye, loss of, 251
Achard-Thiers syndrome, 721
Achilles reflex, elicitation of, *145*
Acidosis, diabetic, coma in, 123
Acne, 102, 115
Acne rosacea, 237
Acne-seborrhea complex, 115
Acrocephaly, 228
Acrocyanosis, 751, 758
Acromegaly, 718
  facial features in, 180, *180*
Addison's disease, buccal membranes
  in, 210
  causes of, 708
  skin pigmentation in, 708, *709*
  tongue in, 205
Adductor muscle(s), of thigh, testing
  of, 134
Adductor reflex, elicitation of, 144
Adenocarcinoma, of cervix, 627

761

Adenoid(s), enlargement of, facial features with, 181
Adenomas, multiple functioning endocrine, 722
Adenosis, of breast, 545
Adiadokokinesis, 137
Adie's pupil, 159
Adie's syndrome, 298
Adrenal cortex, diseases of, 708–711
Adrenal gland, hypertension and, 388
Adrenal medulla, dysfunction of, 712
Adrenogenital syndrome, 603, 711
Agammaglobulinemia, tonsils in, 211
Agraphia, as sign of cerebral dysfunction, 129
Akinesia, 136
Akinetic mutism, 172
Allergy, dermatologic, 114–115
Alopecia, 114
Alopecia areata, 190
Alternate-cover screening test, 297
Amaurosis, 242, 245
Amblyopia, 275, 298
Amenorrhea, 635
Ametropia, 298
Amyloidosis, tongue in, 204
Anacrotic pulse, 400, *401*
Anemia, Cooley's, 740
  pernicious, 726, 740
    tongue in, 203, *203*
  physical findings in, 724–726
Aneurysm(s), 506–510
  aortic, Oliver sign in, 227
  arteriovenous, 508
  intracranial saccular, cranial bruits with, 179
  of carotid artery, 227, *227*
Angina, Ludwig's, tongue in, 203
  Vincent's, 211
Angina pectoris, 466–468, 510
Angioma(s), of lips, in Osler-Weber-Rendu disease, *194*, 195
  of scalp, cranial bruits with, 179

Ankle, anatomy of, *690*
  examination of, 689–697
Ankylosing spondylitis, 649, *649*
  iridocyclitis in, 249, 278
Ankylosis, 697
  temporomandibular, 183
Anisocoria, 256, *256*
Anomia, as sign of cerebral dysfunction, 130
Anosmia, 240
  hypogonadism and, 717
Anosognosia, as sign of cerebral dysfunction, 130
Anuria, 602
Aorta
  abdominal, aneurysm of, 508
  aneurysm of, Oliver sign in, 227
  coarctation of, 487, *487*
    blood pressure in, 389
    cranial bruits with, 179
  thoracic, aneurysm of, 506
Aortic insufficiency, 478
  jerking of head in, 175
  murmur of, 452, *453, 454*
  pulse in, 396, *396*
  throbbing of carotid arteries with, 219
Aortic stenosis, 479, 488
  pulse in, 397, *398, 401*
Aortic systolic murmur, 439, *440*
Apert's syndrome, 228
  exophthalmos in, 176
Apex beat, 510
Aphasia, 172
  global, 129
  motor, 125
  sensory (receptive), 126
  testing of, 127–130
Apnea, 351
Appendicitis, false diagnosis of, 578
  physical findings in, 579, *579*
Applanation tonometry, 283, 286
Apraxia, 172
  as sign of motor aphasia, 125

Apraxia *(Continued)*
  constriction, as sign of cerebral
    dysfunction, 130
  testing of, 127–130
Argyll Robertson pupils, 159, 299
Arrhythmias, of cardiac mechanism,
    411
Arteriosclerosis obliterans, 502
Arteriosclerotic heart disease, 466–
    470
Artery(ies), auscultation of, 459
  diseases of, 502–506
Arthritis, of hip, 680
  rheumatoid, hands and, 669, *671*
Arthropathy, hemophiliac, 698
Asbestosis, 308
Ascites, 586
  abdominal inspection for, 554
  cirrhosis of liver and, 554, *555*
  with cardiac failure, *554*
Asterixis, 141
Asthma, 352
Astigmatism, appearance of optic
    disc in, 254
  pinhole test and, 245
Ataxia, 172
Ataxia-telangiectasia, tonsils in, 211
Atelectasis, 319, 351
  mediastinal displacement and, 322
Athetosis, 142
  speech disturbance and, 127
Atrial fibrillation, 370, 407
  pulsus irregularis perpetuus in,
    405, *406*
Atrium, septal defect in, 485
Atrophy, in peripheral vascular dis-
    ease, 496
  of calf muscle, 687
  optic, 162
Auditory nerve, evaluation of func-
    tion of, 168
Auenbrugger, Leopold, 9, *9*
Auenbrugger's sign, 371
Auscultation, 49

Auscultation *(Continued)*
  of abdomen, 584–585
    in infant, 754
  of arteries, 459
    carotid, 220
  of blood pressure, 384–387, *385*
  of blood vessels, 459
  of chest, 334–351
    errors in, 339
  of head, 181, 179
  of heart, 413–460, *418, 419*
    in infants, 751
  of lungs, *311*, 334–351
  of neck, 220
  of thyroid gland, 215
Auscultatory percussion, 377
Auscultatory sounds, 335
Austin Flint murmur, 450, *451*
Ayerza's disease, 471

Babinski reflex, elicitation of, 145,
    146
Back, examination of, 53, 637, 649–
    657
  inspection of, 638–639
  palpation of, 655
Bacteria, dermatologic infection and,
    116
Bacteriuria, 602
Bagassosis, 308
Balanitis, 594
Band keratopathy, 248
  in hypercalcemia, 708, 722
Barrel chest, 312, *312*
Bartholin's gland, palpation of, *616*,
    617
Basal ganglia, disease of, Hunting-
    ton's chorea as, 142
    motor function in, 132
    speech disturbance and, 127
Baseball finger deformity, 666
Battered-child syndrome, 639, 697,
    759

Battle's sign, 190
Bauxite pneumoconiosis, 308
Behavior, of patient, during neuro-
        logic examination, 119–123
    factors influencing, 23, 25, 26
    with cerebral hemisphere dys-
        function, 130
Bell's palsy, 186, *187*, 228
    decreased blink reflex in, 258, 260
Bell's phenomenon, *187*, 260
Benign familial tremor, 140
Beryllium pneumoconiosis, 308
Biceps reflex, elicitation of, *143*, 144
Bichat, Xavier, 8
Bililight, 758
Biot's respiration, 318, *319*
Bismuth line, of gums, *198*, 199
Blepharochalasis, 263
Blink reflex, examination of, 257–
        260
Blocker's node, 647, 661
Blood pressure, 384–390
Blood vessels, auscultation of, 459
Blue baby, 759
Blumer's shelf, 586
Boerhaave syndrome, 587
Bone(s), facial, examination of, 189–
        190
    in hematological diseases 737, 738
    maxillary, sarcoma of, 238, *239*
Bongiovanni's syndrome, 711, 723
Borborygmus(i), 586
    auscultation of, 584
Boss(es), frontal, hypertrophic, *725*,
        739
Boutonnière deformity, 666
Bowel(s), auscultation of, 584
    obstruction of, *550*, 557
Bowleg deformity, 684, *684*
Bradycardia, 395
Brain, diffuse disease of, behavior of
        patient with, 130
    speech disturbance and, 127
    ectopic, 178

Brain *(Continued)*
    lesions of, homonymous quad-
        rant defect and, 161
    tumors of, cranial bruits with, 179
Brain stem, lesions of, sensory loss
        and, 158
Branham's sign, 509
Breast
    accessory, 544
    carcinoma of, 519, *522–526*, 532–
        535
        inflammatory, 545
    cystic disease of, 538, 545
    examination of, 52, 517–547
        history of patient in, 518–519
    fibroadenoma of, 537
    hypertrophy of, 538–541, *539*, *540*,
        545
    infections of, 541–542
    inspection of, 519–521, *520*, *521*
    intraductal papilloma of, 535, *536*
    Paget's disease of, 521, *526*, 535–
        536, 546
    palpation of, 521, 524, 526–528,
        527–531
    traumatic fat necrosis of, 543, *543*,
        546
    tumor of, fixation of, 526, *528–
        529*
        papillary, 546
Breath, as diagnostic aid, 209–210
Breath sounds, classification of, 49
    normal, 340–345
    transmission of, *342*, *343*
Brittain's test, 684
Broadbent's sign, 368, 465
Bronchial breathing, 341, 343–345,
        344
Bronchiectasis, 352
Bronchitis, acute, 351
    chronic, 352
Bronchophony, 349
Bronchus(i), obstruction of, 319
    vesicular breathing and, *342*

Brudzinski's neck phenomenon, 171
Brudzinski's sign, 170
  elicitation of, 171
Bruit(s), cranial, auscultation of, 179
  of thyroid gland, 701, 722
    Graves' disease and, 217
Buccal cavity, examination of, 210–212
Budd-Chiari syndrome, 587
Buerger's disease, 504, 510
Buerger's test, 495
Bulla(e), 102, *106, 107*
Buphthalmos, 266
Burrow(s), skin, 113
Byssinosis, 308

Calf muscle, atrophy of, 687
  hypertrophy of, 687
    congenital, 645, *646*
Camptocormia, 133, *133*
Capillary pulse, 412
Carcinoid syndrome, 587
Carcinoma. See name of body part.
Carcinoma en cuirasse, 544
Cardiac cycle, phases of, *360*
Cardiac dullness, 379–381
  absolute, 379
  decrease in area of, 381
  in abdominal distention, 379, *380*
  increase in area of, 381
  pericardial effusion and, 381, *382,
    463, 463*
  pleural effusion and, 322, *322,* 380
  position of heart and, 380
  relative, 379
Cardiac failure, ascites with, *554*
Cardiac irregularities, 387
Cardiac murmur(s), 434–439. See
  also *Heart murmur(s).*
Cardiac outlines, 379
  percussion of, 377, *377, 378*
Cardiovascular disease, 460–493. See
  also name of disease.

Cardiovascular system, examination
  of, 39, 358–516. See also *Heart*
  and names of specific diseases.
Carotid artery(ies), aneurysm of, 227,
  227
  auscultation of, 220
  inspection of, 219
  throbbing, aortic valve insufficiency
    and, 219
Carotid body, tumors of, 224, *225*
Carotid sinus syndrome, 228
Cassidy syndrome, 587
Castleman-Bland syndrome, 471
Cataract, 249
  onset of, 250
Caviar tongue, 207, *208*
Cazenave's disease, 237
Cerebellar disease
  abnormal movements with, 139–142
  gait of patient in, 139
  motor function in, 131–133
  muscle coordination in, 136
  muscle tone in, 135
  pendulous reflex in, 147
  speech disturbance and, 126
Cerebral cortex disease, Huntington's chorea as, 142
  muscle coordination in, 137
Cerebral hemisphere dysfunction
  abnormal position of eye with, 165
  behavior of patient with, 130
  sensory loss and, 158
  speech disturbance and, 125–127
  testing of, 127–131
Cerebral hemorrhage, coma in, 123
Cervicitis, types of, *625,* 626
Cervix, carcinoma of, classification
  of, 627
  squamous cell, 626
  examination of, 623–628
  lesions of, 623, 626–627
Chadwick's sign, 630
Chalazion, 265, *265*

Chancre, of lips, 192, *193*
  of male genitalia, 596, *597*
Chancroid, in female, *612*, 613
  in male, 595
Charcot joints, 642, *642*
Charcot-Marie-Tooth disease, 687,
  688, 698
Chemodectoma, 224
Chemosis, 265, 270
Chest
  asymmetric expansion of, 319
  auscultation of, 334–351
    errors in, 339
  evaluation of, 305–311
  examination of, 52, 311–351
    in newborn, 750
  in hematological diseases, 733
  inspection of, 312–319
  palpation of, 320–325
  percussion of, 325–334
  topographical anatomy of, 301–
    304, *303*
Chest sounds, classification of, 49
Cheyne-Stokes respiration, 317, *318*,
  351
Chiari-Frommel syndrome, 636
Chicken breast, 313, *314*
Chloasma, of forehead, *96*
Cholangitis syndrome, 587
Cholecystitis, Murphy's sign in, 572
Chondromalacia, 643, 682
Chordee, 602
Chorea, 172
  jerking of head with, 176
  motor dysfunction in, 142
Choriocarcinoma, 623
Choroiditis, 277
Chvostek's sign, 707
  elicitation of, 184
Ciliary flush, 269
Clavicle, fractures of, 659
Cleft lip, 191, *191*
Clinical process, 20–54
  approach to patient in, 24–26

Clinical process *(Continued)*
  physical examination in, 46–47
    outline for, 48–54
  physician-patient relationship in,
    20–24
  study of patient in, 26–46
    interview in, conducting of, 31–
      44
      outline for, 44–46
      structuring of, 30–31
Clonus, 146
Clubbing, of fingers, 351, *667*
Clubfoot deformity, 692, *692*, *693*
Coarctation, of aorta, 487, *487*
  blood pressure in, 389
  cranial bruits with, 179
Cold, exposure to, 505
Collapsing pulse, 397
Colles' fracture, 664
Coma, causes of, 122
  myxedema, 722
Comedones, 112
Compulsions, as indicator of psycho-
  neurosis, 42
Concretio cordis, 465
Condylomata acuminata, in female,
  614, *614*
  in male, 595
Condylomata lata, *613*, 614
Congenital heart disease, 484–491
  acyanotic, 485–489
  cyanotic, 489–491
Conjunctiva, ocular, examination of,
  269
  palpebral, examination of, 267,
    268, 269
  hemorrhage in, in endocarditis,
    482, *483*
Conjunctivitis, 270–272
Conn's syndrome, 711, 723
Contractions, premature, of pulse
  rhythm, 403, *403*, *404*
  pulsus bigeminus and, 407
Contracture, 697

Contracture *(Continued)*
  Dupuytren's, 669, *670*
  hysterical, 698
  Volkmann's ischemic, 699
Contralateral reflex, 171
Convergence, of eyes, 164
Cooper's ligament, 544
Cornea, disorders of, 272–276
  examination of, 248
Coronary insufficiency, acute, 468
Cor pulmonale, 471, 511
Corrigan pulse, 397
Cortex, adrenal, diseases of, 708–711
Corticospinal tract disease, muscle
    coordination in, 137
  muscle reflex in, 147
Corvisart, Jean Nicolas, 11
Costen's syndrome, 201
Cough, evaluation of, in examination
    of chest, 309
Coup de sabre, 183, *184*
Courvoisier's sign, 586
Cranial nerve(s), dysfunction of,
    auscultation of head in, 171
  evaluation of function of, 159–170
  ocular muscles and, *165*
Cremasteric reflex, elicitation of, 145
Crepitation, 643, 697
Cretinism, *701*, 702, *702*
  lens opacity with, 250
  tongue in, 204
Cri du canard, 212
Cri du chat syndrome, 241
Cross-bun skull, 178
Croup, 758
Crust(s), skin, *106, 107*, 109
Cruveilhier-Baumgarten murmur,
    460
Cryptorchidism, 601
Cubitus valgus, 662, 663
Cubitus varus, 662, 663, 697
Cushing's syndrome, 389, 709–711,
    710
Cyanosis, 310, 351, 510

Cyst
  Bartholin duct, 617
  branchial cleft, 218, *219*
  dermoid, 178
  mesonephric duct, 622
  ovarian, 632
  sebaceous, of scalp, 178, *178*
  synovial, 644
  thyroglossal duct, 217, *218*
Cystic disease, of breast, 538, 545
Cystitis, 602
Cystocele, 617, *618*
Cystosarcoma phyllodes, 519, 537,
    537, 545

Dacryoadenitis, tear deficiency in,
    248
Dalrymple's sign, 266
Dandruff, 108, 115
Decerebration, 122, 136
Deep tendon reflex (DTR), abnor-
    malities of, 146
  elicitation of, 142–145
  localization of patterns of, 147, 149
  sensory supply of, *148*
*De Humani Corporis Fabrica Libri
  Septem,* 7
Dehydration, hypernatremic, 759
de Kleyn syndrome, blue sclera in,
    276
De l'Auscultation Médiate, 14
Delusions, as indicator of psycho-
    neurosis, 42
de Morsier's syndrome, 717
de Musset's sign, 175, 478
Depression, emotional, behavior of
    patient with, 121
de Quervain's disease, 665
Dermatitis
  contact, 102, 114
  exfoliative, 117
    cataract with, 250
    in lymphatic leukemia, 732, *732*

Dermatitis *(Continued)*
  infected, crusts in, 109
  poison ivy, 114
  seborrheic, 115
Dermatitis venenata, 114
Dermatosis(es), bullous, 117
  localized pruritic, 115
  papulosquamous, 115–116
  pigmentary, 117
Dextrocardia, 488
Diabetes, cataract with, 250
  hair in, 190
  late onset, vitreous opacities with,
    251
Diabetes mellitus, breath odor in, 209
  characteristics of, 713–715
  lips in, 192
Diagnosis, 54–72
  accuracy and precision of, 69
  by hypotheses, 55–57
  certainty of, 58
  conditional probabilities in, 64–66
  credibility of, 61
  definition of, 57–59
  differential. See *Differential diagnosis.*
  evaluation of observations in, 59–
    61, 66–69
  formal logic of, 57–72
  laboratory, history of, 16–19
  operational, 71
  physical, history of, 1–19
  possibilities in, partition of, 62,
    64, 67
  role of physician in, 57
  sensitivity and specificity of, 70
  steps in, 59, *60*
Diastole, 510
Diastolic murmurs, 50, 444–455
Dicrotic pulse, 399, *399*
Differential diagnosis, definition of,
    27, 63
  hypothesis and, 55
  of gastrointestinal distention, 558–
    565

Differential diagnosis *(Continued)*
  of jaundice, 570–573
Dilantin, gums and, 199
Diphtheria, ocular muscle paralysis
    with, 251
  tonsils in, 211
Diplacusis, 240
Diplopia, 172, 189, 293
Direct tenderness, abdominal, 580
Discomfort, defined, vs. pain, 35
Discrimination, sensory, testing of,
    152–154
  two-point, 153
Disease. See also name of disease and
    body part.
  cutaneous signs of, 88
  defined, vs. illness, 1–3, 32
  diagnosis of, 54
  factors describing, 35–37
Dissecting aneurysm, 508
Distention, abdominal, cardiac dull-
    ness and, 379, *380*
  gastrointestinal, 557
    differential diagnosis of, 558–
      565
Divergence, of eyes, 164
Doctrine of the Four Humours, 5
  Galen and, 6
Double simultaneous stimulation
    test, 154
  of visual field, 160
Down's syndrome, tongue in, 204
Drug eruption, 115
  fixed, 115
  generalized, 116
Dullness
  cardiac. See *Cardiac dullness.*
  of percussion note, 327, *327,* 332
    shifting, 334
    zones of, patient position and,
      331, *331*
  retrosternal, increased, 382, *383,*
    384
  shifting, abdominal, 586

Dupuytren's contracture, 669, *670*
Dysarthria, 172
Dysgraphia, as sign of cerebral dysfunction, 129
Dysmenorrhea, 635
Dyspareunia, 635
Dysphagia, 240
  with peritonsillar abscess, 212
Dysphonia, 240
Dyspnea, 351
  evaluation of, in examination of chest, 305
Dystonia musculorum deformans, 142
Dysuria, 602

Ear
  anatomy of, 230–232
  carcinoma of, *232*, 233
  deformities of, 233, *233*
  examination of, 51, 230, 232–236
Ecchymosis(es), *728*, 729, 739
Ectasia, 298
Ectropion, 626
Eczema, atopic, *91*, 114
  nummular, 115
Edema, 510
  angioneurotic, of eye, *260–261*, 261, 262
  conjunctival, 265
  corneal, 248, 273
  facial, in nephritis, *259*, 261
  of legs, in hepatic cirrhosis, *556*
  of penis and scrotum, 594
  of vulva, 609, *612*
  pulmonary, 354
Effusion
  of eyelids, *258*, 261
  pericardial, cardiac dullness and, 381, *382*, 463, *463*
  pleural, 353
    cardiac dullness and, 322, *322*, 380

Effusion *(Continued)*
  pleural, point of maximal impulse and, 365
    tactile fremitus and, phonogram of, *324*
Egophony, 350
Ehlers-Danlos syndrome, 299
  skin in, 183, *185*
Eighth cranial nerve, disease of, nystagmus and, 166
  evaluation of function of, 168
Eisenmenger's syndrome, 490, 511
Ejection click, 430, *431*
Elastodystrophy, systemic, 299
Elbow, examination of, 662–664
Electrocardiogram, 491
Elephantiasis, of male genitalia, 594
Eleventh cranial nerve, evaluation of function of, 169
Embolus, pulmonary, 355
Emphysema, interstitial, 348
  pulmonary, 352
    decrease in cardiac dullness with, 381
Empyema necessitatis, 319, *320*
Encephalitis, coma in, 122
  motor tics and, 142
Encephalocele, 178
Endocarditis, 482–484
Endocervicitis, 626
Endocrine system, examination of, 700–723. See also name of specific gland.
Endolymphatic hydrops, 228, 241
Endometriosis, 623, 636
Endophthalmitis, ciliary flush with, 269
  hypopyon with, 249
Enroth's sign, 266
Enterocele, 617
Enuresis, 603
Epicondylitis, 663
Epididymis, enlargement of, 601
Epigastrium, palpation of, 575

Epiphoria, 259
Episcleritis, 277
Epistaxis, 240
Epithelioma, 96
  basal cell, *105*
Epulis, 199, *200*
Erb's palsy, 661
Erysipelas, of vulva, 609
Erythema, 114
Erythema multiforme, *106*
  conjunctiva in, 271
Erythremia, 740
Escutcheon, 722
Essential hypertension, 389
  physical findings in, 470
Eunuchoidism, 715, 723
  skin in, 184, *186*
Examination. See also name of body
    part or system.
  pediatric, 742–759
  pelvic, 607–617
    patient position for, 607, *608*
  physical, 46–47
    basic maneuvers in, 47, 48–50
    equipment for, 47, 48
    order of procedure in, 50–54
    outline for, 48–54, *81–84*
    preparing for, 48
  rectal, 590, 601–602
    in newborn, 755
    with low back pain, 657
  rectovaginal, 632, *633, 634*
Excoriation(s), skin, 109, *110*
Exophthalmos, in Apert's syndrome,
    176
  in cavernous sinus thrombosis, 262,
    262
  in hyperthyroidism, 266, *266*
  in oxycephaly, 176
Expiration, of air, forced, 317
Extinction, sensory test for, 154
Extracardiac functional murmurs,
    457

Extremities. See also name of specific
    extremity.
  examination of, 53, 637–699
  in hematological diseases, 734
  inspection of, 638–639
Eye(s)
  diseases of, 272–297
  examination of, 51, 242–300
    external, 257–270
    of fundus, 252–255
    of ocular media, 245–252
    of pupillary reflex, 255–257
    of visual acuity, 159, 242–245
    tests for, 159
  in hematological diseases, 733
Eyelid(s), effusion of, *258*, 261
  eversion of, 267, *268*
  examination of, 260–267

Face, examination of, 179–189
Facies, Hippocratic, 181
  leonine, 181, *181*
  myxedematous, 703, *703*
Fallot's tetralogy, 489, *490*, 511
Fanconi's syndrome, 725, 740
Farmer's lung, 308
Fasciculation(s), of muscles, facial,
    168
  flaccidity and, 135
Fetor hepaticus, 209
Fibrillation, atrial, 370, 407
  pulsus irregularis perpetuus in,
    405, *406*
Fibroadenoma, of breast, 537
Fibrocystic disease, of breast, 538,
    545
Fibrodysplasia elastica, 299
Fibroma, of gums, 199
Fibrosis, of palmar fascia, 669, *670*
  pulmonary, 355
Fifth cranial nerve, evaluation of
  function of, 166

Finklestein's test, 665
First heart sound, 49, 421–423
Fissure(s), skin, 109
Fistula(s), arteriovenous, cranial
        bruits with, 179
    bronchopleural, 352
    carotid cavernous, auscultation of,
            179
        orbital congestion in, 265
        palpation of eyeball in, 179
Flaccidity, 172
    of muscles, 135
Flatfoot deformity, 694, *696*
Flipper deformity, of hand, 669, *671*
Floppy baby, 759
Floppy valve syndrome, 511
Fluid, detection of, in abdominal
        cavity, 580, 581
    within joint, 643
Fluid wave, 580
    examination for, *581*
Fluorosis, 197, *197*
Folliculitis, multiple, *108*
Folliculosis, 271
Foot, examination of, 689–697
Foot-drop gait, 138
Fourth heart sound, 50, 428–430
Fourth sound gallop, 50
Fremitus, tactile, evaluation of, 323–
        325
        palpation for, *323*
        pleural effusion and, phonogram
            of, *324*
Frey's syndrome, 187
Friction rub(s), 49, 351
    pericardial, 373, 433, 434
    pleural, 49, 347
Friction sound(s), over heart, 433
Friedreich's ataxia, foot deformity
        in, *695*
Friedreich's sign, 462
Fröhlich syndrome, 722
Functional murmur(s), 456–458

Fundus, optic, abnormalities of, 162
    examination of, 252–255
    normal, *161*
Fungi, dermatologic infection and,
    116
Funnel chest, 313, *313*
Furunculosis, 234
Fusion, of retinal images, 293
Fusion reflex, 291

Gait, disturbances of, 138–139
    evaluation of, 138, 639–640
    in hematological disorders, 725
Galactocele, 545
Galen, 6
Gallbladder, palpation of, 568
Gallop rhythm(s), 432
Gangrene, in peripheral vascular
    disease, 496
Gardner's syndrome, 178
Gargoylism, corneal clouding in, 248
Gastrocnemius muscle, testing of,
    133
Gastrointestinal distention, 557
    differential diagnosis of, 558–565
Gaucher's disease, 740
Gaze, deviations of, 293–297
    positions of, 293, *294*
Genitalia
    female, examination of, 605–636
        external, 608, *609*
        patient's history and, 605–607
        pelvic, 607–617
            patient position for, 607,
                608
            preventive medicine and, 635
        speculum, 617–622
    male, examination of, 590–601
Genu valgum, 684, *685*
Genu varum, 684, *684*
Geographic tongue, 205, *206*

Gerhardt's dullness, 381
Gibbus, of spine, 649, *650, 651*
Gland(s). See name of gland.
Glaucoma, 286–291
  angle closure, 287
    clinical signs of, 282
  ciliary flush with, 270
  congenital, blue sclera in, 276
    buphthalmos from, 266
    disorders of cornea and, 273
  corneal edema with, 248, 249
  hypersecretion, 288
  infantile, 289
  open angle, 287, 288
    secondary, 290
    treatment of, 289
Glomerulonephritis, facial edema
  with, *259,* 261
Glossitis, 739
Gluteus maximus muscle, testing of,
  134
Goiter, colloid, myxedema and, *217*
  of thyroid gland, 701
  toxic, cranial bruits with, 179
Gonads, dysfunction of, 715–717
Goniometer, 643, *641*
Goniotomy, 290
Goodell's sign, 630
Gout, ear and, *231,* 233
  of hands, *667*
Gower's sign, 687
Gradenigo's syndrome, 241, 299
Graham Steell murmur, 454
Granuloma inguinale, in female, 613
  in male, 597
Graphite pneumoconiosis, 308
Graves' disease, 228
  hyperthyroidism and, 704
  pulse in, 394
  thyroid bruit in, 217
  thyroid gland in, 215
Grönblad-Strandberg syndrome, 299
Gums, Dilantin and, 199
  examination of, 196–202
Gunstock deformity, 663

Gynecomastia, 540, *541,* 545, 723
  in Klinefelter's syndrome, 716
  with hepatic cirrhosis, *555*

Hair, as diagnostic aid, 190–191
Hallucinations, as indicator of
  psychoneurosis, 41
Hallux rigidus, 697
Hallux valgus, *696,* 697
Hamartoma, of eye, 265, 279
Hamman's sign, 348
Hand, examination of, 666–673
Harada's syndrome, 241
Hashimoto's thyroiditis, 702, 723
Head
  auscultation of, 171, 179
  examination of, 45, 51, 175–212
    in newborn, 748
    of face, 179–189
      bones of, 189–190
    injury to, coma in, 123
    palpation of, 171
    percussion of, 171, 179
Hearing, evaluation of, in newborn,
  758
  sound and, 415
  tests for, 168, 234
Heart. See also *Cardiac.*
  auscultation of, 413–460, *418, 419*
    in infants, 751
  diastolic beat of, 368, *369*
  examination of, 52
    in newborn, 750–752
  inspection of, 361–371, *362*
  palpation of, 371–375, *371, 372*
  percussion of, 375–384, *378*
  rate of, 368
  rhythm of, 368
  topographical anatomy of, 359,
    361
Heart block, 407, 408
Heart disease
  arteriosclerotic, 466–470

Heart disease *(Continued)*
  chronic valvular, 475–482
  congenital, 484–491
    acyanotic, 485–489
    cyanotic, 489–491
  hypertensive, 470
Heart failure, 474
Heart murmur(s). See also *Heart sound(s), Murmur(s),* and type of murmur or valve involved.
  character of, 437
  definition of, 510
  functional, 456
  loudness of, 438
  production of, mechanism of, 435, *436*
  transmission of, 438
Heart sound(s), 420–431. See also *Heart murmurs* and *Murmur(s).*
  classification of, 49
  ejection clicks as, 430, *431*
  first, 49, 421–423
  fourth, 50, 428–430
  in infants, 751, 752
  midsystolic click as, 430, *431*
  opening snap, as, 50, 427
  second, 50, 423–427
  third, 50, 427
Heart valve(s), diseases of, 475–482. See also name of disease.
  function of, 435
  location of, areas of sound and, 417, *417*
    during systole and diastole, 435, *436*
Heberden's nodes, 669, *672*
Hegar's sign, 630
Hemangioma, of eye, 265, 279
  of lips, 195
  of neck, 224
  unilateral hypertrophy of face and, 183
Hemarthrosis, 739
Hematemesis, 240, 586
Hematocele, 601

Hematoma, with temporal bone fracture, 190
Hemiatrophy, facial, 182, *183, 184*
Hemic system, disorders of, 724–741
Hemiplegia, 135
  capsular, 172
Hemophilia, 740
  arthropathy with, 698
Hemoptysis, 241, 309, 351
Hemorrhage, cerebral, coma in, 123
  of eye, anterior chamber of, 249
    conjunctival, in endocarditis, 482, *483*
    subconjunctival, *269,* 270
    vitreous body of, 251
  splinter, in endocarditis, 482, *483*
  subarachnoid, coma in, 123
Hemp worker's disease, 308
Henoch's purpura, 729, 740
Hepatosplenomegaly, 739
Hermaphrodism, 594
Hernia(s), inguinal, 591
  in female, 608
  palpation of, *592*
  umbilical, *553*
Herpes, of penis, 595
  of vulva, 609
Herpes labialis, 192, *192*
Herpes simplex, decreased blink reflex in, 258
  dendritic ulcer of, 273
Herpes zoster, 102, *106*
  decreased blink reflex in, 258
  involvement of eye in, 273, *274*
Herpes zoster oticus, 241
Hip
  disease of, 677
  dislocation of, congenital, 677, *678*
    posterior, 679, *679*
  examination of, 673–681
  fractures of, 678
  range of motion of, 673, *674–675, 676*
Hippocratic facies, 181
Hippocratic method, 5

Hirschsprung's disease, 557, *566*, 587
History, of patient, examination of
    breast and, 518–519
  examination of female genitalia
    and, 605–607
  family, 38–39
    outline for, 44, *78*
  medical past, outline for, 45, *78*
  neuropsychiatric, 40–44
    outline for, 46
  personal, 37–38
  social, 37
    outline for, 45
  medical. See also *Medical record.*
    conducting interview for, 31–44
    outline for, 44–46
    structuring interview for, 30–31
Hoarseness, lesions of tenth cranial
    nerve and, 169
Hodgkin's disease, *736*
  cervical lymph nodes in, 221, *222*
Homans' sign, 501
Homonymous hemianopsia, 161, 173
Hordeolum, 261, *264*, 265
Horner's syndrome, 163, 299
Humoral pathology, 5
  Galen and, 6
Huntington's chorea, 142
Hurler's disease, corneal clouding in,
    248
Hutchinson's teeth, 196, *196*, 197
Hutchinson's triad, 197
Hydrocele, of canal of Nuck, 609,
    611
  of testis, 600, *600*
Hydrocephalus, 176, *177*
Hygroma(s), cystic, 224
Hypalgesia, 172
Hyperactivity, of patient, during
    neurological examination, 120
Hyperacusis, 241
Hyperopia, appearance of optic
    disc in, 254
  pinhole test and, 245
  size of pupil in, 256

Hyperparathyroidism, 707
Hyperplasia, of gums, 199
Hyperresonance, of percussion note,
    332
Hypertension, 388
  physical findings in, 470
Hypertensive heart disease, 470
Hyperthyroidism, 704–706, *705*
  exophthalmos in, 266, *266*
Hypertonicity, of muscles, 135
Hypertrophy, of breast, 538–541,
    539, 540, 545
  of calf muscle, 687
    congenital, 645, *646*
Hyphema, of eye, anterior chamber
    of, 249
Hypoactivity, of patient, during
    neurological examination, 120–123
Hypoacusis, 241
Hypoglycemia, 715
  coma in, 123
Hypogonadism, 718
Hypoparathyroidism, 707
  cataract with, 250
Hypopituitarism, 718, *719*
Hypopyon, of eye, anterior
    chamber of, 249
Hypotension, 390
  orthostatic, 722
Hypothalamus, pituitary dysfunc-
    tion and, 717
Hypothyroidism, 702–704
  muscle reflex in, 146
Hypotonicity, of muscles, 134
Hypotony, 283
  corneal edema with, 249
Hysteria, blindness and, 242
  conversion, sensory loss in, 156
  gait of patient in, 139
  stance of patient in, 133, *133*

Ileus, 586
Iliopsoas muscles, testing of, 134

Illness, clinical manifestations of, 54
  defined, vs. disease, 1–3, 32
  diagnosis of, 54
  factors describing, 35–37
  patient insight to, 43
  recording of, 34
  somatic aspects of, 34
Illusions, as indicator of psychoneurosis, 41
Impetigo, crusts in, 109
  pustules in, 102
Indentation tonometry, 283, 286
Infantilism, male genitalia and, 591,
  593
Infarction, of lung, 353
Infection(s), dermatologic, 116
  of breast, 541–542
Inguinal area, examination of, 590–
  591
Injury, facial, 189
  of neck, muscle spasms with, 225
Inspection, 48
  of abdomen, 550–566
    in newborn, 752
  of back and extremities, 638–639
  of breast, 519–521, 520, 521
  of carotid artery, 219
  of chest, 312–319
  of heart, 361–371, 362
  of muscle body, 134
  of neck, 213
  of shoulder, 657, 659
Inspiration, of air, forced, 317
    percussion note in, phonogram
      of, 329
Insufficiency, acute coronary, 468
Intercostal muscles, testing of, 134
Intercourse, patient's history and,
  606
Interventricular septal defect, 442
Intestine, auscultation of, 584
  obstruction of, 550, 557
Intoxication, coma in, 122
  hyperactivity of patient in, 120
  tremors with, 140

Intracranial pressure, coma in, 123
Intravascular coagulation defect, 759
Inventum Novum, 9
Iridectomy, 287
Iridencleisis, 289
Iridocyclitis, 277
  chronic, keratic precipitates in,
    248, 279
  ciliary flush with, 269
  clinical signs of, 278
  hypopyon with, 249
  pupil size in, 257
  systemic disorders and, 249
Iridodialysis, 257

Jaundice, differential diagnosis of,
  570–573
  in newborn, 748
Jaw(s), locked, 212
  lumpy, 228
  tumors of, 201
Joffroy's sign, 705
Joint(s), in hematological diseases,
  737, 738
  motion of, evaluation of, 640–645.
    See also Range of motion and
    name of specific joint.
  neuropathic, of diabetics, 698
  testing of sensation in, 152
Judgment, of patient, testing of,
  130–131
Jugular veins, pulse in, 219

Kallmann's syndrome, 717
Kartagener's syndrome, 241, 488
Keloid(s), 111, 113
Keratitis, interstitial, 275, 275
Keratitis profunda, 275
Keratoconjunctivitis, 270
  epidemic, 272
Keratoconus, 276

Keratopathy, band, 248
    in hypercalcemia, 708, 722
Keratosis(es), 116
    multiple seborrheic, *104*
    senile, *101*
Kernig's sign, 170, 759
Ketoacidosis, 714
Kidney(s), hypernephroma of, *576*
    palpation of, 574
    tumor of, *576*
Kimmelstiel-Wilson disease, 714, 723
Klinefelter's syndrome, 603, 716, *716*
Klippel-Feil syndrome, neck in, 213
    position of head in, 175, *176*
Klumpke's palsy, 661
Knee, anatomy of, *683*
    examination of, 681–687
    range of motion of, 681, *682*
        abnormal, 686
Knock-knee deformity, 684, *685*
Koplik's spots, 210
Kussmaul, Adolph, 16
Kussmaul respiration, 316
    in diabetes, 714
Kyphosis, 649, *650*, 697

Laennec, René Théophile Hyacinthe,
    12, *12*
Lagophthalmos, 186
Laryngoscopy, 240
Larynx, examination of, 240
Lateral medullary syndrome, 173
Laurence-Moon-Biedl syndrome, 722
Lead poisoning, gums in, 197, *198*
Leg, examination of, 687–689
Leiomyoma, of uterus, 630
Lens, of eye, examination of, 249–
    251
Leonine facies, 181, *181*
Leprosy, facial features in, 180, *181*
    facial muscle paralysis in, 186
Leriche syndrome, 503, 511, 603
Leukemia, acute monocytic, hyper-
    plasia of gums in, 199, *199*

Leukemia *(Continued)*
    lymphatic, 221, *734*, *735*
    skin in, *730*, 731, *731*, 732
    spleen in, *575*
Leukemia cutis, 739
Leukoplakia, of cervix, 626
    of lips, 195
    of tongue, 203, *204*
Lichen planus, 96, 116
    papulosquamous lesions of, *101*
Lichen simplex chronicus, 115
Lichenification, 111
Lip(s), carcinoma of, *105*, *194*, 195
    examination of, 191–196
Lipoma, of labia majora, 609
    of neck, 223, *223*
Lipschütz ulcers, 613
List, of spine, *651*, 652, *652*
Little League elbow, 663
Liver
    cirrhosis of, ascites and, 554, *555*
        edema of legs in, *556*
        gynecomastia with, *555*
    disease of, parenchymal, breath
        odor in, 209
        tremor with, 141
    palpation of, 568, *569*
        in hematological diseases, 737
        in infants, 754
Lordosis, 649, *650*, 651, 697
Ludwig's angina, tongue in, 203
Lung(s)
    abnormal sounds of, 345–351
    abscess of, 353
        breath odor in, 210
    anatomy of, 302, *303*, 304, *306–
        307*
    auscultation of, *311*, 334–351
    carcinoma of, 354
    disease of, chronic obstructive, 352
    expansion of, percussion limits of,
        330, *330*
        posterior, testing of, 320, *321*
    infarction of, 353
    volume of air in, 315

Lupus erythematosus, butterfly lesion of, 237, *238*
  chronic discoid, papulosquamous lesions of, *100*
Lupus vulgaris, of ears, 233
Lymph nodes
  cervical, enlargement of, *734, 736*
    malignant disease of, 220–223, *222*
    pathological changes in, indications of, 220
    tuberculosis of, 220, *221*
  disorders of, 734–737
  preauricular, enlargement of, 272
Lymphadenopathy, 739
Lymphangioma(s), of lips, 195
  of neck, 224, *224*
  of tongue, 204, *205*
  unilateral hypertrophy of face and, 183
Lymphatic system, disorders of, 724–741
  diseases of, 498–500
Lymphogranuloma venereum, 613
Lymphosarcoma, 221

Macule(s), 95, *96*
Mallory-Weiss syndrome, 587
Mammography, 544
Maple bark stripper's disease, 308
Marasmus, 759
Marfan's syndrome, 511
  palate in, 211
Marie-Strümpell disease, 649, *649*
Masseter muscle, hypertrophy of, 188
Mastitis, lactation, 546
Mastodynia, 518
Maximal impulse, point of, 361, 362–367
  palpation of, *371*, 372
MEA syndrome, 722
Measles, 210

Medical history. See *History, medical,* and *Medical record.*
Medical record, 72–87, *75–85*
  data base in, 72, *76–84*
  function of, 72
  initial plan in, 74
  problem list in, 73, *75*
  progress notes in, 74
  usage of, 72
Meigs' syndrome, 636
Melanin, 114
Melanoma(s), malignant, 116
  of eye, 280
    hemorrhage and, 249
  of vulva, 609
Melanosis oculi, 276
Melena, 586
Meniere's syndrome, 228, 241
Meningitis, cerebrospinal, Kernig's sign in, 170
  coma in, 122
  rigidity of neck with, 225, *226*
Menopause, 635
Menorrhagia, 635
Menstruation, patient's history of, 605
Midsystolic click, 430, *431*
Mikulicz's syndrome, 228
  enlargement of parotid glands in, 187, *188*
Milia, 113
Milroy's disease, 498, *499*
Miner's elbow, 664
Miosis, 255, 279
Miscarriage, 635
Mitral insufficiency (regurgitation), 441, *442*, 477
  murmur of, *449,* 450
Mitral stenosis, 476, *477*
  murmur of, 447–450, *448*
  pulse in, 398
Moebius' sign, 705
Moles, 116
Mondor's disease, 532, *534,* 546
Morgagni, Giovanni Battista, 8

Motor system, examination of, 131–142
Motor tics, 141
Mouth, as diagnostic aid, 210–212
in hematological diseases, 732–733
Multipara, 636
Munchausen's syndrome, 603
Murmur(s). See also name of murmur.
cardiac, 434–439. See also *Heart murmur(s).*
classification of, 50
continuous, 444, *445*
diastolic, 50, 444–455
functional, 456–458
systolic, 50, 439–444
Murphy's sign, 572, 586
Muscle(s)
coordination of, evaluation of, 136–138
examination of, 645–647
extraocular, paralysis of, 296
inspection of, 134
masseter, hypertrophy of, 188
ocular, nerve supply of, *165*
paralysis of, 251
in leprosy, 186
of face, tonic spasm of, 184
spasm of, with neck injury, 225
strength of, evaluation of, 131–134, 645
tone of, testing of, 134–136
Myasthenia gravis, ophthalmoplegia with, 165
ptosis with, 163, *164*
Mycosis fungoides, 96, *103*
Mydriasis, 255
Myocardial disease, 473
Myocardial infarction, acute, 468–470
Myocarditis, 473
Myopia, pinhole test and, 245
size of pupil in, 256, 266
Myositis ossificans, 647, 661

Myotonia, 132
muscle reflex in, 147
Myotonic dystrophy, lens opacity with, 250
Myxedema
colloid goiter with, *217*
hair in, 191
hypothyroidism and, 702–703, *703*
muscle reflex in, 146
pretibial, 706, *706*
tongue in, 204

Nasal fossae, inspection of, 238, *239*
Neck, anatomic structures of, *213*
examination of, 51–52, 175, 212–227
in newborn, 749
Necrobiosis lipoidica diabeticorum, *90*
Nelson's syndrome, 720
Nephritis, chronic, urea frost in, *89*
edema of lips with, 192
facial edema in, *259*, 261
Nerve(s). See also specific nerve.
cranial, dysfunction of, auscultation of head in, 171
ocular muscles and, *165*
testing of, 159–170
facial, paralysis of, 186, 228
peripheral, disease of, muscle tone in, 135
sensory loss of, 154–156
Nervous system
examination of, 53–54, 118–174
in hematological diseases, 739
in newborn, 756–758
of cranial nerves, 159–170
of higher functions, 123–131
of motor function, 131–142
of reflexes, 142–146
sensory, 149–159
testing of, 150–152

Neurodermatitis, disseminated, 114
  localized, 96, 115
Neurofibroma, unilateral hypertrophy of face and, 183
Neurological system. See *Nervous
  system.*
Neuromas, 223
  plexiform, 224
Neuropsychiatric history of, patient,
  40–44
  outline for, 46
Nevoxanthoendothelioma, hyphema
  of eye and, 249
Nevus(i), 114, 116
  elevated, 96
  flat, 95
  port-wine, 179
Newborn, examination of, 745–758
Ninth cranial nerve, evaluation of
  function of, 169
Node(s)
  blocker's, 647, 661
  Heberden's, 669, *672*
  lymph. See *Lymph nodes.*
  Osler's, 484, 672
  Parrot's, 178
  Virchow's, 223, 586
Nodule(s), skin, 96, *104*
Nose, examination of, 45, 51, 230,
  236–240
Nosebleed, 240
*Nouvelle Méthode pour reconnaître les
  Maladies internes*, 11
Nullipara, 636
Nystagmus, 165
  eighth cranial nerve disease and,
    168
  optokinetic, 291
    test for, 292
  testing for, 169

Obsessions, as indicator of psychoneurosis, 42

Obstruction, of bowels, *550*, 557
Occlusion, of teeth, 200, *201*
Occupation, patient history of, in
  examination of chest, 305, 308
Ochronosis, 276
Ocular conjunctiva, examination of,
  269
Ocular media, examination of, 245–
  252
Ocular motility, abnormalities of,
  291–297
Olfactory nerve, testing of, 159
Oliguria, 603
Oliver sign, 227
On the Seats and Causes of Disease, 8
Opacity, corneal, 273
  focal, location of, 247, *247*
  of lens, 250
  vitreous, 251
Opening snap, 50, 427
Ophthalmodynamometer, 282, *283*
Ophthalmoplegia, internuclear, 173
  with myasthenia gravis, 165
Ophthalmoscope, use of, 246, *246*,
  252
Opisthotonos, 228
Optic chiasm, lesions of, visual field
  defects and, *160*, 161
Optic nerve, evaluation of function
  of, 159
Orbicularis oculi muscles, paralysis
  of, in leprosy, 186
Orthopnea, 351
Ortolani's sign, 677
Osgood-Schlatter disease, 682
Osler's nodes, 484, 672
Osler-Weber-Rendu disease, angioma
  of lip in, *194*, 195
  skin in, 727, *728*
Osteochondritis dissecans, 643, *644*
Osteogenesis imperfecta, blue sclera
  in, 276
Osteoma, 178
Osteomyelitis, of jaw, 201

Physical examination. See *Examination, physical.*
Pierre Robin syndrome, 200
Pigeon breeder's disease, 308
Pinguecula, 272
Pinhole test, 245
Pinprick, perception of, testing for, 150
Pituitary gland, dysfunction of, 717–720
Pityriasis rosea, *98*, 116
Placenta previa, 636
Plaque(s), skin, 96, *103*
    xanthelasmic, 263, *263*
Pleural effusion, 353
    cardiac dullness and, 322, *322*, 380
    point of maximal impulse and, 365
    tactile fremitus and, phonogram of, *324*
Pleural friction rub, 49, 347
Pleurisy, 353
Plexus, brachial, injury to, 661
Plica polonica, 191
Pneumoconiosis, 308
Pneumonia, 353
Pneumonitis, hypersensitivity, 308
Pneumothorax, 322, 354
Podagra, 697
Poliomyelitis, muscle atrophy with, 225
Poliosis, 264, 279
Polycythemia 726, *727*
Polyneuropathy, 155
    diabetes and, 714
Polyps, cervical, 626
Polythelia, 544
Porphyria cutanea tarda, skin pigmentation in, *89*
Posterolateral column syndrome, 173
Posterior urethral syndrome, 604
Precordium, examination of, 370
Preeclampsia, 636
Pregnancy, patient's history of, 605
    pelvic signs of, 630

Pregnancy *(Continued)*
    striae of, 553
Presbyopia, 250
Pressure, intracranial, coma in, 123
    intraocular, disorders of, 248, 281–291
        measurement of, 283–286
    intrathoracic, respiration and, 314–316, *316*
        tension pneumothorax and, 322
Presystolic thrill, 374
Priapism, 603
Primigravida, 636
Procidentia, of uterus, 617, *619*
Proptosis, 265, *266*
Proteinuria, 603
Pruritus, 114
Pruritus vulvae, 609
Pseudoathetosis, 153
Pseudoxanthoma elasticum, 183
Psoas sign, in appendicitis, 579
Psoriasis, 94, 116
    lesions of, 108, *109*
Pterygium, 272
Ptosis, 172, 262
    third cranial nerve palsy and, 159, 163
Puddle sign, 582, *583*
Pulmonary disease, occupational causes of, 308
Pulmonary insufficiency, 480
    murmur of, 452
Pulmonary stenosis, 480, 488
Pulmonary systolic murmur, 441
Pulse, 390–413. See also type of pulse.
    characteristics of, 392–413
    inequality of, 390
    in peripheral vascular disease, 497
    palpation of, 391, *392*
    rate of, 393–395
    rhythm of, 402–410
    size of, 395
    tension of, 410
    venous, 413, *414*

Pulse (*Continued*)
  vessel wall and, 411
  wave type of, 396–401
Pulse deficit, 407
Pulsus alternans, 387, 398, *398*
Pulsus bigeminus, 407, *408, 409*
Pulsus bisferiens, 400, *401*
Pulsus celer, 393, 396
Pulsus durus, 393, 410
Pulsus frequens, 393
Pulsus irregularis, 393
Pulsus irregularis perpetuus, 405,
  406, 407
Pulsus magnus, 393, 396
Pulsus mollis, 393, 410
Pulsus paradoxus, 400
Pulsus parvus, 393, 396
Pulsus rarus, 393, 395
Pulsus regularis, 393, 402
Pulsus tardus, 393
Pulsus trigeminus, 410
Pupil(s), abnormal reactions of, 159
  Argyll Robertson, 159, 299
  size of, muscle control of, 255–257
  tonic, 298
Pupillary reflex, examination of,
  255–257
Purpura, 739
  lesions of, 727, 729, *729, 730*, 731
Purpura hemorrhagica, 740
Pustule(s), 102, *108*
Pyorrhea alveolaris, 196

Quadriceps reflex, elicitation of, 144,
  144
Quinsy, 212

Radiodermatitis, skin in, 182
Râle, 49, 345, 346
Ramsay Hunt syndrome, 241
Range of motion
  of angle, 689

Range of motion (*Continued*)
  of cervical spine, 647, *648*
  of elbow, 662, *662*
  of hip, 673, *674–675, 676*
  of knee, 681, *682*
    abnormal, 686
  of shoulder, 657, *658*
  of spine, 654, *656*
  of wrist, 664
Ranula, 207, *208*
Rapid filling wave, 365, *366*
Raynaud's disease, 505, 511
Rebound sign, 137
Rebound tenderness, abdominal, 580
Rectal examination, 590, 601–602
  in newborn, 755
  with low back pain, 657
Rectal shelf, 586
Rectocele, 617, *619*
Rectovaginal examination, 632, *633,
  634*
Rectus muscle, weakness of, abnormal position of eye in, 164
Reflex(es). See also name of reflex.
  abdominal, clinical significance of,
    580
    elicitation of, 145
  blink, 257–260
  contralateral, 171
  deep tendon. See *Deep tendon re-
    flex.*
  depressed tendon, muscle flaccidity
    and, 135
  examination of, 142–146
  lesions affecting, *147*
  pathological, 145–147
  pupillary, examination of, 255–257
  superficial, 145
Reiter's disease, 604
  hypopyon of eye in, 249
Renal hypertension, 389
Resonance, of percussion note, 326,
  327
  vocal, 349–351
Respiration, patterns of, 314–319

Respiratory distress syndrome (RDS), 759
Respiratory tract infection, tongue in, 204
Reticular activating system (RAS), lesions of, 121
Retina, detachment of, 251
  nerve fiber distribution of, 253, *253*, 254
Retinocerebral angiomatosis, 300
Retinochoroiditis, 277, 278
Retraction sign(s), from breast lesions, 519, *523*, *524*, 532, *533*, *534*, 544
Retrosternal dullness, increased, 382, *383*, *384*
Reye's syndrome, 759
Rhabdomyosarcoma, 224
Rhagades, 192, *193*
Rheumatic fever, odor in, 210
Rhinolalia, 228
Rhinophyma, 237, *237*
Rhinorrhea, 228
Rhonchus, 49, 347
Rigg's disease, 196
Rigidity
  abdominal, causes of, 577
    palpation of, 580
  decerebrate, 136
  of muscles, 135
  of neck, with meningitis, 225, *226*
Ringworm infestation, loss of hair with, 190
Rinne's test, 168
Risus sardonicus, 184
Roger's disease, 442
Romberg's disease, skin in, 182, *183*, *184*
Romberg's sign, 133
Rotch's sign, 382
Rubeosis, hemorrhage of eye and, 249

Saddle nose, *236*, 237
Sarcoidosis, of cervix, 626

Sarcoma, of maxillary bone, 238, *239*
  of vagina, 623
Sarcoma botryoides, 623, *624*
Scabies, of penis, 595
  of vulva, 611
Scale(s), skin, 108, *109*
Scalp, angioma of, cranial bruits with, 179
  sebaceous cysts of, 178, *178*
Scapula(e), congenital deformity of, 654
  winging of, 659
Scarlet fever, tongue in, 203
Scars, 111
Schirmer test, 274
Schizophrenia, behavior of patient with, 120
  catatonic, 121
Schönlein's purpura, 729, 740
Sclera, disorders of, 276
Scleritis, 277
Scleroderma, of face, 182, *182*
  of hands, *668*
Scleromalacia perforans, 277
Sclerosis, 114
Scoliosis, *653*, 654, 697
Scotoma, 298
Scotopic vision, 298
Screwdriver tooth, 197
Scrofula, 228
Scrotal tongue, 205, *207*
Scrotum, edema of, 594
  elephantiasis of, 594
  examination of, 599–601
Second heart sound, 50, 423–427
Semi-stupor, 122
Sensory discrimination, testing of, 152–154
Sensory dysfunction, patterns of, 154–159
Sensory loss, gait in, 139
  muscle incoordination with, 138
  nerve compression and, 669
  peripheral nerve, 154–156
  testing of, 150–152
Sequoiosis, 308

Seventh cranial nerve, evaluation of function of, 167
Sheehan's syndrome, 636, 718, 723
Shifting dullness, abdominal, 586
Shock, clinical, 759
Shoulder, dislocation of, 661
  examination of, 657–661
  motion of, 657, *658*
Sickle cell disease, 740
  physical findings in, 724–726
Siderosis, 308
  of iris, 250
Sign. See also name of sign.
  diagnostic probability of, 64–66
  factors describing, 33
  in diagnosis of illness, 54
Silicosis, 308
Silo filler's disease, 308
Silver fork deformity, 664
Simmonds' disease, 718, *720*
  hair in, 190
Sinus, cavernous, thrombosis of, 262, *262*
  infected preauricular, 188, *189*
Sinus irregularity, of pulse rhythm, 403
Sinusitis, frontal, 178
Sixth cranial nerve, dysfunction of, abnormal position of eye in, 164
Sjögren's syndrome, 187, 299
  enlargement of parotid glands in, 187
  tear deficiency in, 274
  xerostomia in, 209
Skin
  examination of, 48, 50, 88–117
  hyperpigmentation of, 720
  in Ehlers-Danlos syndrome, 183, *185*
  in hematological diseases, 727–732
  in scleroderma, 182, *182*
  in radiodermatitis, 182
  lesions of, 95–113
    combined primary and secondary, 111

Skin *(Continued)*
  lesions of, primary, 95–108
    secondary, 95, 108–112
    special, 112–113
  of eunuch, 184, *186*
  pigmentation of, in Addison's disease, 708, *709*
    in porphyria cutanea tarda, *89*
  sensory nerve supply of, *148*
  temperature of, in peripheral vascular disease, 496
  tumors of, 96, *105*, 116
  turgor of, poor, 759
Skoda, Josef, 15, *15*
Skodaic resonance, of percussion note, 333, *333*
Skull, auscultation of, 179
  cross-bun, 178
  percussion of, 179
  tower, 176, *177*
Smallpox, odor in, 210
Smith's fracture, 665
Smoking, history of, in examination of chest, 305
Snellen chart, 243, *244*
  test letter of, *245*
Sound(s). See also type of sound.
  classification of, 49, 50
Spastic gait, 138
Spasticity, 122, 135, 172
Speculum, ear, 233, *234*
  vaginal, examination with, 617–622
    introduction of, 618, *620–621*
Speech, disturbances of, 124–127
  testing for, 127–129
  twelfth cranial nerve disease and, 170
  nasal, 169
  scanning, 126
  stammering, 127
  stuttering, 127
  telegraphic, 125
Spermatocele, 601
Spider nevus, *556*

Spina bifida cystica, 654, *655*
Spinal cord, lesions of, sensory loss
    and, 156–158
  posterolateral column syndrome
    of, 173
Spine
  cervical, examination of, 647–648
  mobility of, evaluation of, 170
  motion of, *656*
    evaluation of, 654
  palpation of, 171
  percussion of, 171, 655
Spleen, in leukemia, *575*
  palpation of, 573, *574*
    in hematological diseases, 737
    in infants, 754
Splenomegaly, 739
  diagnosis of, *738*
Splinter hemorrhage, in endocarditis,
  482, *483*
Spondylitis, ankylosing, 649, *649*
  iridocyclitis in, 249, 278
Spoon nails, 726, *726*
Sprengel's deformity, 654
Sprue, tongue in, 203
Sputum, evaluation of, in examina-
  tion of chest, 309
Stammering, 127
Stance, evaluation of, 639–640
Staphyloma, 267, 276, 298
Static reflex, 292
Steeple head, 176, *177*
Stein-Leventhal syndrome, 717, 723
Stenosis, aortic, 479, 488
    pulse in, 397, *398, 401*
  mitral, 476, *477*
    murmur of, 447–450, *448, 449*
    pulse in, 398
  pulmonary, 480, 488
  subaortic, 488
  tricuspid, 451, 481
Steppage gait, 138
Stereognosis, 153
Stereopsis, 293
Stethoscope, Laennec's, 12, *13*
  types of, 336–339, *337, 338*

Stewart-Morel-Morgagni syndrome,
  722
Still's disease, iridocyclitis in, 249
Stimulus(i), auditory, impaired per-
    perception of, 126
  testing of, 168
Stokes-Adams syndrome, 511
Stress incontinence, 603, 606, 617
Striae, of abdominal skin, 553
Stridor, 351
Sturge-Weber syndrome, 300
  cranial bruits in, 179
  hemangioma of eye in, 280
Stuttering, 127
Sty, 261, *264, 265*
Subaortic stenosis, 488
Subarachnoid hemorrhage, coma in,
  123
Subluxation, 697
Sudeck's post-traumatic sympathetic
  dystrophy, 698
Superficial reflexes, elicitation of, 145
Sydenham's chorea, 142
Symblepharon, 271
Symptoms, diagnostic probability of,
  64–66
  factors describing, 33, 35–37
  in diagnosis of illness, 54
Synchysis scintillans, 251
Syndrome. See name of syndrome.
Synechia(e), 257, 279, 290
Syphilis
  Argyll Robertson pupils in, 159
  congenital, shape of head in, 178
    rhagades from, 192, *193*
    teeth in, 196, *196*, 197
    uveal inflammation of, 275, *275*
  hair in, 190
  in female, lesions of, 613, *613*, 614,
    614
  nose in, *236*, 237
  secondary, 116
    nodules in, 96
    papulosquamous eruption in,
      100
  tertiary, lesions of, 96, *104*

Syringomyelia, sensory loss with, 157
System review, 39–44
  outline for, 45–46, *79–84*
Systole, 510
  movement of heart during, 362, *363*
Systolic ejection murmur, *426*, 439
Systolic retraction, 367
Systolic thrill, 375

Tachycardia, 393, 510
  paroxysmal, 394
Tachypnea, 316, 351
Talc pneumoconiosis, 308
Talipes calcaneovalgus, *691*, 692
Talipes equinovarus, 692, *692*, *693*
Taste, loss of, with facial nerve paralysis, 187
  testing of, 167
Tears, vision disturbances and, 247, 273
Teeth, examination of, 196–202
  fluorosis of, 197, *197*
  Hutchinson's, 196, *196*, 197
  screwdriver, 197
Telangiectasia(s), 113
  hereditary, *194*, 195
  familial hemorrhagic, lesions of, 727, *728*, 740
Telangiectasis, 114
Temperature, of skin, in peripheral vascular disease, 496
  perception of, testing for, 151
Temporal bone, petrous portion of, abscess of apex of, 241
Tenderness, abdominal, 580
Tendinitis, in shoulder, 659
Tendon, rupture of, Achilles, 687
  biceps, 660, *660*
  quadriceps, *680*, 681
Tennis elbow, 663
Tenosynovitis, stenosing, 665, 669
  tuberculous, *666*

Tenth cranial nerve, evaluation of function of, 169
Test(s). See also name of test.
  of hearing, 168, 234
  of visual acuity, 243–245, *244*, *245*
Testis(es), enlargement of, 601
  examination of, 599–601
  torsion of, 601
  undescended, 601
Tetanus, facial features with, 184
Tetany, Chvostek's sign in, 184
  detection of, 707
  hands in, *707*
Tetralogy of Fallot, 489, *490*, 511
Texture, perception of, testing for, 153
Thalamus, lesions of, sensory loss and, 158
Thalassemia, 740
Third cranial nerve, dysfunction of, ptosis and, 159, 163
  palsy of, unilateral dilated fixed pupil in, 159, 163
Third heart sound, 50, 427
Third sound gallop, 50
Thomas test, 673, *676*
Thoracic aorta, aneurysm of, 506
Thoracic outlet syndrome, 506
Thrills, palpation of, 373–375
Throat, examination of, 230, 240
Thromboangiitis obliterans, 504
Thrombophlebitis, 501
  of thoracoepigastric vein of breast, *534*, 546
Thyroid gland, auscultation of, 215
  dysfunction of, 700–706
  palpation of, 215, *216*
Tibial muscle, anterior, testing of, 134
Tietze's syndrome, 659
Tinea capitis, *94*
Tinea infection, of nails, *95*
Tinea versicolor, *99*, 116
Titubation, 133, 139
Tone(s), of auscultatory sounds, characteristics of, 335

Tones *(Continued)*
of muscles, evaluation of, 134
Tongue, as diagnostic aid, 202–209
atrophy of, 170
carcinoma of, 202, *202*, 204
in hematological disease, 733
strawberry, 203
Tongue muscles, lesions of, speech
disturbance and, 124
Tonometer, application of, 284–286,
285
identification of glaucoma with, 288
Tonometry, 283–286
Tonsils, appearance of, as diagnostic
aid, 211
Tophi, of ear, *231*, 233
Torticollis, 142, 225, *226*
Torus mandibularis, 199
Torus palatinus, 211
Touch, perception of, testing for, 151
Tower skull, 176, *177*
Tracheal tug, 227
Trachoma, conjunctiva and, 269
tear deficiency in, 248
Transverse myelitis, 173
Traumatic fat necrosis, of breast,
543, *543*, 546
Tremor, benign familial, 140
intention, 136
of head, in parkinsonism, 175
types of, 140, 141
Triceps reflex, elicitation of, *143*
Trichinosis, systemic, edema of eye-
lids in, 261
Tricuspid atresia, 491
Tricuspid insufficiency (regurgita-
tion), 442, *443*, 481
Tricuspid stenosis, 451, 481
Trigeminal nerve, branches of, *167*
evaluation of function of, 166
Trigger thumb, 669
Trismus, 228
Trousseau's sign, 707
Truncus arteriosus, 491
Tuberculosis
cutaneous, of ears, 233

Tuberculosis *(Continued)*
genital, 603
of cervical lymph glands, 221, *221*
of cervical lymph nodes, 220, *221*
of cervix, 626
of hip, lordosis in, *650*
of spine, gibbus and, *650*, 651
of tongue, 204
pulmonary, 355
Tularemia, oculoglandular, conjunctiva in, 272
Tumor(s)
buccal, 210
metastatic, of eye, 280
of brain, cranial bruits with, 179
of breast, fixation of, 526, *528–
529*
papillary, 546
of carotid body, 224, *225*
of frontal bone, 178
of kidney, *576*
of neck, 223
differentiation of, 220
of nose, 238
of ovary, 631
of parotid glands, 188
of skin, 96, *105*, 116
of testis, 601
of uterus, 630
pyloric, palpation of, in infant,
754, 755
Turner's syndrome, 229, *721*, 722
neck in, 213
palate in, 211
Twelfth cranial nerve, evaluation of
function of, 170
Two-point discrimination, 153
Tympanitic percussion note, 327
Typhoid fever, loss of hair in, 190
tongue in, 203

Ulcer(s)
aphthous, 206
diabetic, of foot, 713, *714*

Ulcer(s) *(Continued)*
  gangrenous, *503*
  in peripheral vascular disease, 495
  Lipschütz, 613
  of tongue, 205
  skin, 109
    of sporotrichosis, *112*
    tuberculous, *111*
    varicose, 501, *502*
Urea frost, in chronic nephritis, *89*
Uremia, breath odor in, 209
Uremic syndrome, 604
Urethra, carcinoma of, 616
  detached, 617
Urethritis, 595
Urethrocele, 617
Urticaria, *102*
Uterus, bimanual examination of,
    628–635, *629*
  masses in, palpation of, 577
  procidentia of, 617, *619*
Uvea; 298
  disorders of, 277–280

Vagina, carcinoma of, 623
  examination of, 622–623
  lesions of, 622
Vaginitis, types of, 609, 610
Valves, of heart. See *Heart valve(s).*
Valvular heart disease, chronic, 475–
    482
van der Hoeve syndrome, blue sclera
    in, 276
Varicocele, 599
Varicose vein(s), 500, *500, 502*
  of lips, 195
  of tongue, 207
Vascular disease, peripheral, 493–
    510
  aneurysm as, 506–510
  history of patient in, 493–495
  of arteries, 502–506
  of lymphatic system, 498–500
  of veins, 500–501

Vascular disease *(Continued)*
  peripheral, physical examination in,
    495–497
Vascular encephalotrigeminal angio-
    matosis, 300
Vein(s)
  auscultation of, 460
  diseases of, 500–501
  jugular, pulse in, 219
  varicose, 500, *500, 502*
    of lips, 195
    of tongue, 207
Venous pulse, 413, *414*
Ventricle(s), failure of, 475, 476
  septal defect in, 485
Ventricular filling murmurs, 444–451
Vergence, 298
Verrucae, 595
Version, 298
Vertigo, 241
  eighth cranial nerve disease and,
    168
Vesalius, Andreas, 6
Vesicle(s), skin, 102, *106*
Vesicular breath sounds, 340, *341*
Vessel(s), blood, auscultation of, 459
  great, transposition of, 489
  peripheral, examination of, 53
Vibration, perception of, testing for,
    151
Vincent's angina, 211
Virchow, Rudolph, 8
Virchow's node, 223, 586
Virilism, adrenal, 711, 722
  male genitalia and, 591, *593*
Virilization, adrenal, 711, *712*
Virus(es), dermatologic infection
    and, 116
Vision, evaluation of, in newborn,
    758
  photopic, 298
  scotopic, 298
Visual acuity, evaluation of, 159,
    242–245
Visual field, defects of, 161
  evaluation of, 159–161

Visual fixation reflex, 291
Vital signs, recording of, 50
Vitiligo, 96, *97*, 264, 279
Vitreous body, examination of, 251
Vocal resonance, 349–351
Vogt-Koyanagi syndrome, uveitis in,
    279
  vitiligo in, 264
Voice sounds, classification of, 49
  transmission of, *325*
Volkmann's ischemic contracture,
    699
Vomiting, projectile, 759
von Graefe's sign, 266, 705
von Hippel-Lindau syndrome, 300
von Recklinghausen's disease, neuro-
    fibroma of gums in, 200
    neurofibromatosis as, 224
Vulva, carcinoma of, 614
  diseases of, 609–614
  edema of, 609, *612*

Waardenburg's syndrome, 191, 241
  poliosis in, 264
Wart(s), penile, 595
  venereal, 595, *596*
Water-hammer pulse, 397
Wave, fluid, 580
    examination for, *581*

Weaver's bottom, 680
Weber's test, 168
Weight, perception of, testing for,
    153
Wheal, 96, *102*
Wheeze(s), 49, 347
Whipple's triad, 588
Whooping cough, ulcers of tongue
    in, 205
Wrist, examination of, 664–665
Wryneck, 225, *226*

Xanthogranuloma, hyphema of eye
    and, 249
Xanthoma, tuberous, 264
Xerostomia, 209, 228
Xiphisternal crunch, 345
X-ray, diagnostic use of, in cardiac
    disease, 492

Yo-Yo testis syndrome, 604

Zeis, gland of, obstruction of, 261,
    264
Zollinger-Ellison syndrome, 588, 715,
    723